FOUNDATIONS OF EDUCATION

AN EMS APPROACH

FOUNDATIONS OF EDUCATION

AN EMS APPROACH

NATIONAL ASSOCIATION OF EMS EDUCATORS

SECOND EDITION

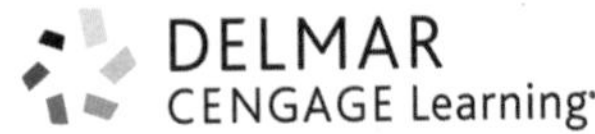

Australia • Brazil • Japan • Korea • Mexico • Singapore • Spain • United Kingdom • United States

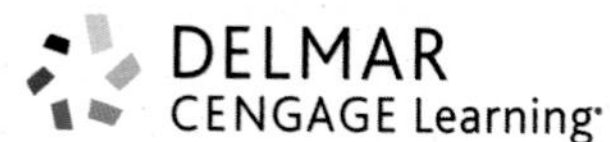

Foundations of Education: An EMS Approach
National Association of EMS Educators (NAEMSE), Second Edition

Vice President, Careers & Computing: Dave Garza

Director of Learning Solutions: Sandy Clark

Senior Acquisitions Editor: Janet E. Maker

Managing Editor: Larry Main

Senior Product Manager: Jennifer Starr

Editorial Assistant: Leah Costakis

Vice President, Marketing: Jennifer Baker

Marketing Director: Deborah Yarnell

Associate Marketing Manager: Erica Glisson

Senior Production Director: Wendy Troeger

Production Manager: Mark Bernard

Senior Content Project Manager: Jennifer Hanley

Senior Art Director: Casey Kirchmayer

Library of Congress Control Number: 2012933743

ISBN-13: 978-1-111-13488-4

ISBN-10: 1-111-13488-X

Delmar
5 Maxwell Drive
Clifton Park, NY 12065-2919
USA

Cengage Learning is a leading provider of customized learning solutions with office locations around the globe, including Singapore, the United Kingdom, Australia, Mexico, Brazil, and Japan. Locate your local office at: **international.cengage.com/region**

Cengage Learning products are represented in Canada by Nelson Education, Ltd.

To learn more about Delmar, visit **www.cengage.com/delmar**

Purchase any of our products at your local college store or at our preferred online store **www.cengagebrain.com**

Printed in the United States of America
1 2 3 4 5 6 7 16 15 14 13 12

Dedication

To our EMS instructor colleagues, who give so much of themselves to so many students—simply because that is who they are.

Dedication

To the memory of my father, Joseph H. Cason, one of my first and best teachers, who taught life and love and service to his country, family, community and God by an example I can only hope to follow.

— *DC*

For my parents, Anne and John Tubman, whose life lessons were my most valuable.

—*KDM*

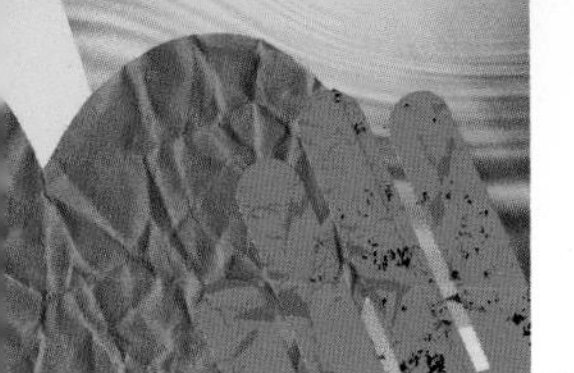

CONTENTS

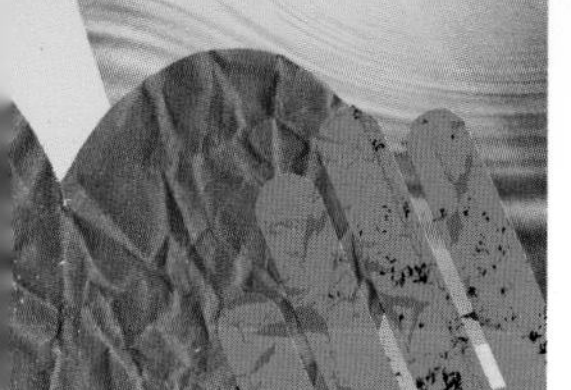

FOREWORD

Fasten your seatbelt . . .

Over the past 40 years, Emergency Medical Services has evolved from a vaguely recognized network of disconnected response organizations to become an integral part of a highly complex health care system. A significant portion of the more than 15 million patients who access EMS services each year do so as their primary point of entry for all health services, whether they have an actual "emergency" or not. We are truly gatekeepers for a broad array of inpatient, outpatient, and social services for a public that is often bewildered by the complexities of the system, but unified in its trust of EMS and its practitioners. As health care evolution has emphasized care in the outpatient setting, a growing percentage of hospitalized patients enter through the "doors" of the EMS system.

These forces have significantly "raised the bar" for the EMS profession at all levels. Our clinical sophistication has increased, both in breadth across a multitude of medical specialties, and in depth within emergency and critical care. The recent recognition by the American Board of Medical Specialties of Emergency Medical Services as a medical subspecialty offers testimony to the importance and credibility of this evolving practice of out-of-hospital medicine. In line with this practice, integrated relationships between EMS clinicians and other health care professionals will require increased foundational knowledge and enhanced communication at all levels. The health care system's strong emphasis on patient safety increases EMS clinicians' responsibilities to provide accountable, accurate, and reliable care. These responsibilities begin with the education of our providers and the skillfulness of their teachers.

Simply stated, this new environment has created a need for a better-educated and more masterful clinician who can effectively practice both the art and science of out-of-hospital medicine and integrate them with other disciplines. Today's EMS personnel provide an array of clinical services unimaginable at the dawn of EMS: traditional 911 response; interfacility transport; transfer of critical patients dependent upon life-sustaining technology; utilization of highly selective criteria to identify patients who require care in ST segment Elevation Myocardial Infarction (STEMI), stroke, trauma, or pediatric specialty facilities; public health screening and immunization; collaborative clinical practices that utilize technology to enable physicians to "see" patients in remote locations. And these services are provided in a remarkable variety of physical settings including ambulances, fire/rescue vehicles, hospitals, fixed wing aircraft, helicopters, factories, mines, offshore drilling platforms, battlefields, community health settings, military installations, and people's homes. There have even been EMTs in space.

What does this all mean for us?

As EMS educators at all levels, we have the privilege and responsibility to prepare these clinicians during a period of unprecedented emphasis on educational quality. In the six years since the first edition of this textbook was published, the *National EMS Education Standards* have been released, providing educators with the opportunity and responsibility to adapt curricula to better match both local community needs and the educational attributes of both educators and students. State requirements for paramedic programs to be accredited by the Committee on Accreditation of Education Programs for the EMS Professions set the stage for well-prepared EMS educators to partner with our colleagues from other health care professions to create meaningful programs that employ exciting new tools, like high-fidelity simulation, online synchronous and asynchronous platforms, and competency-based evaluation tools.

This book will be a valuable partner for you through this time of change and professional growth. It has updated the most popular features of the first edition, including the Case in Point and Teaching Tips, to help you to polish and refine your classroom strategies. The role of classroom research continues to be emphasized throughout the text to instill and maintain a focus on evidence-based practice, both in the field and in the classroom. The Legal and Administration chapters have been updated to provide guidance to new instructors, while remaining a valuable resource to those with more experience. And a new chapter has been added on Simulation, with information that will be invaluable to novice and experienced educators alike.

As experienced EMS educators, we believe the profession is entering the most exciting period in EMS education since our inception in the early 1970s. We thank you for your service, and encourage you to use this book as but one tool to expand your educational practice to meet the needs of the health care community. But hang on; it will be a fast ride.

Scott Bourn, PhD, RN, EMT-P
President-elect NAEMSE 2011-2013

D. Randy Kuykendall, MA, NREMT-P
President, NASEMSO 2010–2012

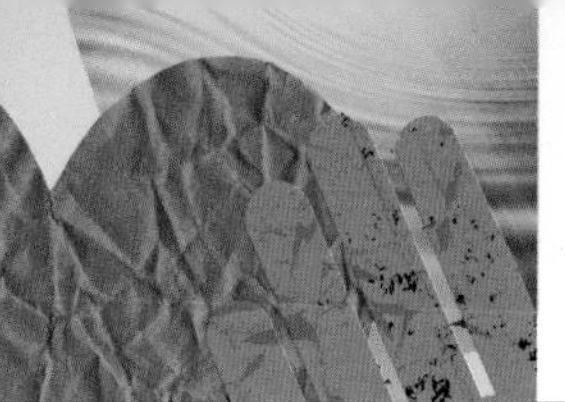

PREFACE

Foundations of Education: An EMS Approach, second edition, is designed to provide Emergency Medical Services (EMS) educators with an overview of teaching philosophy, strategy, and techniques to promote effective student learning and evaluation. This will enable EMS faculty to maximize their effectiveness in the classroom, to transition to teaching the *National EMS Education Standards*, and to provide tools to assist them to meet practice guidelines that comply with state and national program-accreditation guidelines.

Organization of This Book

Part I: Instructor Roles and Responsibilities

The introductory chapters outline attributes of instructors and detail the various roles of EMS educators.

Part II: The Student

Factors that influence student needs and student learning such as how adults learn, learning styles, and classroom diversity are described in the second part of the book.

Part III: Foundations

This section introduces instructors to elements in the learning environment that influence effective teaching and learning, including how EMS faculty can use technology to enhance the students' learning. It outlines core elements needed to design instruction in a legal and ethical manner. This section takes instructors through a lesson-planning process based on understanding the need to meet each learning domain and to construct learning objectives that clearly describe the desired outcomes in students in all domains.

Part IV: Delivering the Message

Delivering the message elaborates on the many strategies instructors use to promote student learning when they are alone or in groups, or while in the classroom, skills laboratory, or at a distance, or in field and clinical settings.

Part V: Evaluation

Significant attention is devoted to elaborating on the methods for sound, reliable, and valid assessment and student evaluation using a variety of tools needed to assess learning in all domains. This section also assists instructors to determine the need for and process to implement remediation plans.

Part VI: Administration

The Administrative Issues chapter addresses the complexity of planning, delivering, and evaluating educational programs within academic and nonacademic settings. This knowledge will help program directors to ensure programs are managed legally, ethically, and within sound business principles.

Features of This Book

This book is written from an EMS perspective with features incorporated to assist instructors to see how educational principles can be applied within EMS, and specifically how they might be used within their own classrooms. Although EMS instruction varies from region to region and from institution to institution, some fundamental issues and problems remain the same across the industry. The authors have framed these issues within an EMS context to help readers see how to transition the information directly to their program.

- *By EMS Instructors, for EMS Instructors:* Written specifically for educators teaching EMS and focused on specific challenges and needs of those teaching EMS, this book presents ideas that can be used in a variety of EMS educational settings that include emergency service-based organizations and college and university settings.
- *Practical Approach:* "How to" examples blend essential educational theory with practical information applicable to a variety of EMS educational settings, and provide a framework for an introductory EMS education curriculum.
- *Case in Point:* These scenarios illustrate how principles or problems are specifically addressed within an EMS setting.
- *Teaching Tips:* These specific examples enable instructors to envision how to apply the concepts directly within their own classrooms.
- *Articles:* These engaging topics offer sidebar discussions on important points that are presented in the chapters.

New to This Edition

- A recognition and application of the National EMS Education Standards provides the tools for meeting state requirements as well as national paramedic program-accreditation requirements.
- An extensively revised Instructional Technology chapter highlights cutting-edge teaching techniques and new technologies that help enhance classroom instruction and engage students in the learning process.
- A new chapter on Simulation offers a look at the lab setting and how to implement this teaching tool into the curriculum.
- Extensively revised Legal and Administration chapters offer guidance on managing these responsibilities within and beyond the classroom.

Supplement to This Book

The publisher, in partnership with the National Association of EMS Educators, is pleased to offer additional tools and resources for instructors to support the information presented in this book. FREE access to a companion website offers examples of student-centered activities, articles on relevant topics, helpful links, additional references, and more!

The learning materials described in this section are designed as further reference for the book, and are offered in addition to the EMS Educator course Part I & Part II conducted by the National Association of EMS Educators. The NAEMSE EMS Educator course Part I represents the didactic component and practical application of the beginning education process to become an EMS Instructor. The NAEMSE Part II Instructor Course is geared toward the experienced instructor and is representative of the 2002 National Guidelines for EMS Educators. It provides educators and program directors with the tools and information needed to further build their leadership skills and better evaluate programs, students, and faculty. For more information on these courses, please visit http://www.naemse.org.

About the Editors

Deb Cason

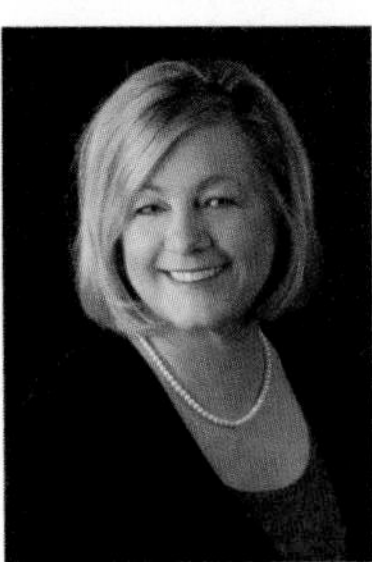

Debra Cason RN, MS, EMT-P is associate professor and program director for Emergency Medicine Education at University of Texas Southwestern Medical Center at Dallas, overseeing initial EMT and Paramedic programs and continuing-education activities for various local fire departments. She serves on the Committee on Accreditation for EMS Professions (CoAEMSP) and NREMT Boards, and is past president of NAEMSE. She was project director for the National EMS Education Standards development.

Kim McKenna

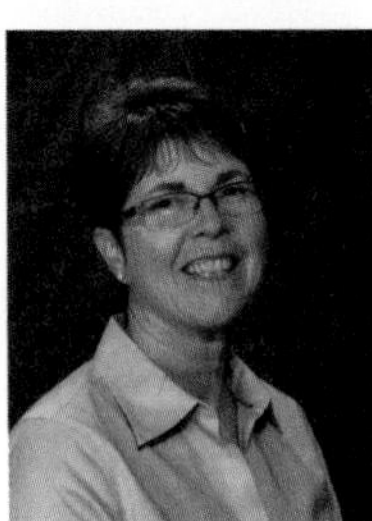

Kim D. McKenna MEd, RN, EMT-P is the director of education for the St. Charles County Ambulance District and an adjunct professor at Lindenwood University in St. Charles, Missouri. Kim is a paramedic, registered nurse, educator, EMS author and editor who has been involved in emergency care, fire service, and EMS education for more than 25 years. She served as the Emergency Medical Responder Project Level Leader on the National EMS Education Standards Task Force, and is presently a member of the board of directors of the National Association of EMS Educators.

About the Authors

Bill Raynovich

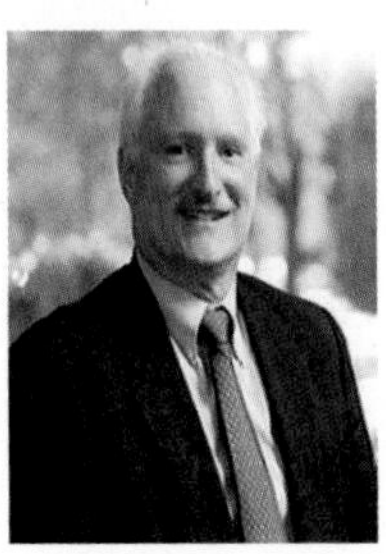

Contributing Coauthor: Chapters 1, 2, and 3

Bill Raynovich EdD has been active in EMS for more than 45 years. He had a faculty appointment at the University of Pittsburgh from 1978 through 1988. He developed and directed the Reading Hospital and Medical Center Paramedic Training Institute from 1987 through 1996. He started the University of New Mexico–Albuquerque BS EMS degree program in 1996, and was the senior program manager of the EMS Academy through 2004. In 2004, he accepted the position of EMS education director at Creighton University in Omaha, Nebraska, where he currently serves as an associate professor and director of EMS Education. Bill has served on the board of directors of NAEMSE and the CoAEMSP.

Together with:

Cy T. Stockhoff, MS, NREMT-P
Professor, Outreach Coordinator
Central New Mexico
Community College

Michael G. Miller, MS, BSEMS, RN, NRP
Assistant Professor and Paramedic
Program Director
School of Pharmacy and Health Professions
Creighton University–EMS Education

Bruce Walz

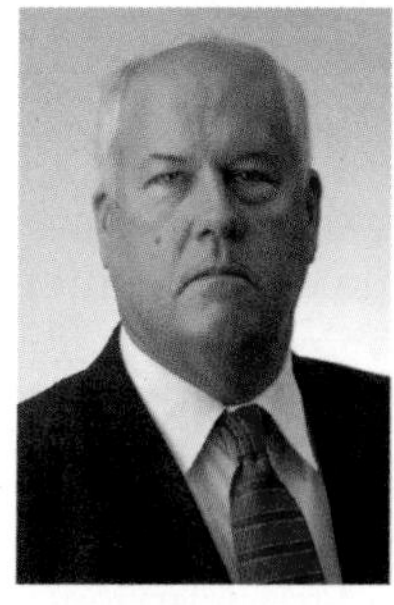

Contributing Author: Chapters 4, 9
Contributing Coauthor: 24

Bruce J. Walz, PhD is professor and chair of the Department of Emergency Health Services at the University of Maryland, Baltimore County (UMBC). He has been in the university system of Maryland since 1979, having served with the Maryland Fire and Rescue Institute until 1987 when he joined the faculty of UMBC. He served as a group leader for the development of the 1998 National Standard Paramedic Curriculum and the 1999 National Standard Intermediate Curriculum as well as the National EMS Education Standards. He is a charter member of the National Association of EMS Educators and served as president in 1998. He has been on the board of Advocates for EMS and is a past president. Additionally, he serves as a site visitor for the Committee on Accreditation of Educational Programs for the EMS Professions (CoAEMSP). Bruce Walz has also been active in the volunteer fire service since 1970, serving in many administrative and line positions including president and chief officer. He is nationally certified as a Fire Officer IV and Fire Instructor IV.

Art Hsieh

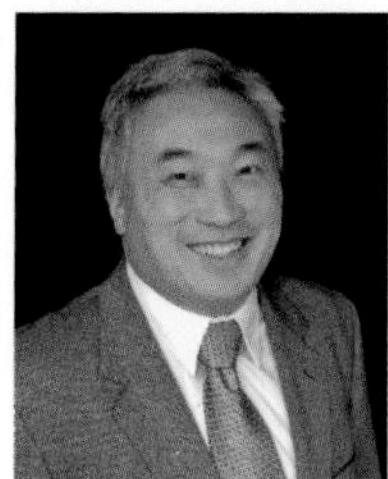

Contributing Author: Chapter 5

Art Hsieh, MA, NREMT-P has been in the EMS profession since 1982, earning his master's degree in adult education in 2000. He has worked as a volunteer, line medic, educator, and chief officer in private, third service, and fire-based EMS. He has directed both primary and EMS continuing-education programs, and currently is on the faculty at Santa Rosa Junior College, Public Safety Training Center in California. A past president of the National Association of EMS Educators, and a scholarship recipient of the American Society of Association Executives, Art is a published textbook author, editorial columnist, and has presented at conferences nationwide.

LeAnne Hutson

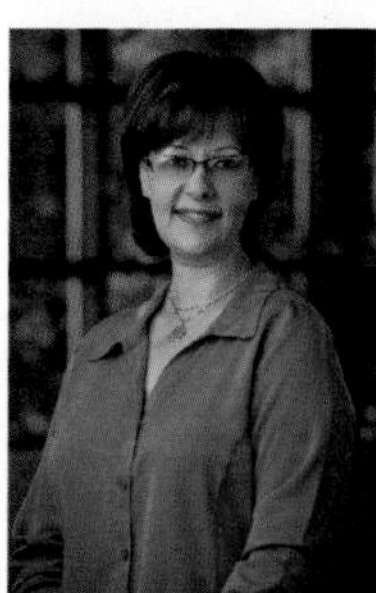

Contributing Author: Chapter 6

LeAnne M. Hutson is an assistant professor and program director of the Medical Laboratory Sciences Program at the University of Texas Southwestern Medical Center. She is also a doctoral student in educational leadership and policy studies.

Walt Stoy

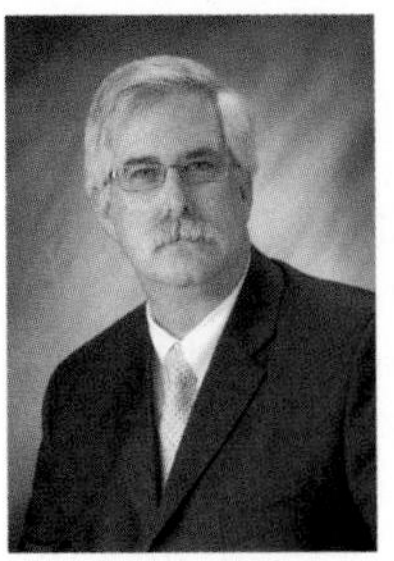

Contributing Author: Chapters 7, 8, and 23

Walt Alan Stoy, PhD, EMT-P is professor and director of emergency medicine at the School of Health and Rehabilitation Sciences at the University of Pittsburgh, and the director of Educational and International Emergency Medicine at the Center for Emergency Medicine. He is internationally renowned for his efforts in EMS and is recognized by his peers and colleagues as a groundbreaker and national leader in the field of EMS education. Dr. Stoy has served as the project director of the 1998 EMT-Intermediate & Paramedic: National Standard Curricula Revision Project. He has served as principal investigator to the 1994 EMT-Basic: National Standard Curriculum and project director to the 1995 First Responder: National Standard Curriculum.

He has over 35 years of experience in EMS and served as the founding president of the National Association of EMS Educators. Additionally, Dr. Stoy has written more than 60 instructional guides and published his educational work, using both print and visual media including Instructional Guides for the Street Medicine Series, the Hands On Series, and the Advanced Cardiac Life Support Series.

Donna Hammaker

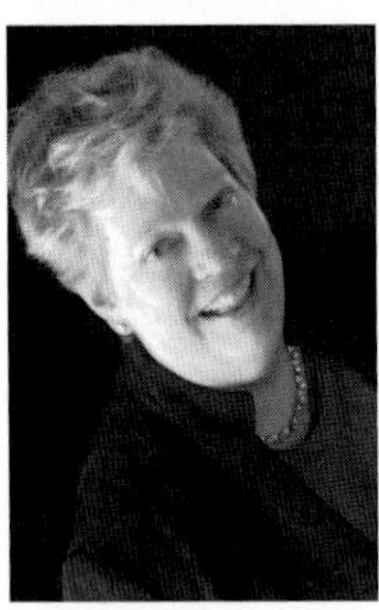

Contributing Coauthor: Chapter 10

Donna K. Hammaker, a health-law attorney, holds a faculty appointment at Immaculata University in Pennsylvania where she teaches health law and serves as director of the National Institute on Health Care Management and Law. Before entering academia, Donna was a member of the Pennsylvania Bar, admitted to practice before the U.S. District Court, Eastern District of Pennsylvania, and the U.S. Court of Appeals for the Third Circuit. She was also president and chief executive officer of Collegiate Health Care, the nation's first interuniversity managed-care organization. She has served on the adjunct faculty and taught graduate management and health law at Pennsylvania State University, Rutgers University, Saint Joseph University, and Widener University. Donna recently authored *Health Care Management and the Law* and coauthored *Health Care Ethics and the Law*, also published by Delmar Cengage Learning.

Together with:

Sarah J. Tomlinson, JD, MBA
Fox Rothschild, a national law firm;
Health Law Scholar, NIH-CML.

Gleb Epelbaum, MBA
Student at Temple University
Beasley School of Law;
Adjunct Law Scholar, NIH-CML.

Curt Varone

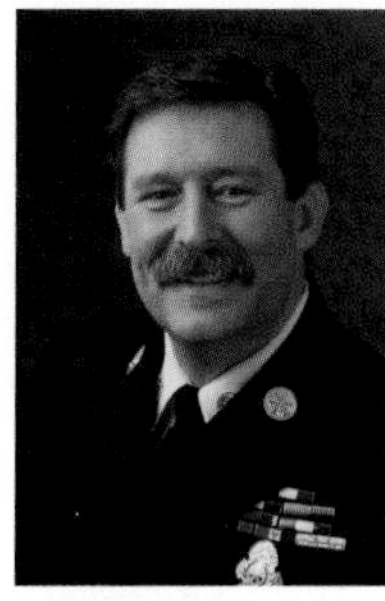

Contributing Coauthor: Chapter 10

Curt Varone has over 39 years of experience in the fire service, retiring in 2008 as a deputy assistant chief with the Providence, Rhode Island, Fire Department. He is a practicing attorney licensed in both Rhode Island and Maine, and served as the director of the Public Fire Protection Division at the National Fire Protection Association. Curt has written two books, *Legal Considerations for Fire and Emergency Services*, and *Fire Officer's Legal Handbook*, also published by Delmar Cengage Learning. He writes the Fire Law column for *Firehouse Magazine* and is a deputy chief with the Exeter (RI) Fire Department.

Heather Davis

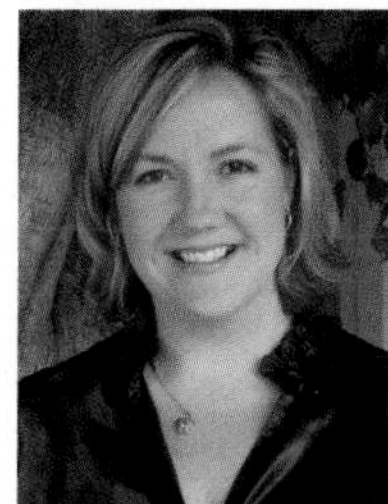

Contributing Author: Chapters 11 and 12

Heather Davis is the program director for the University of California–Los Angeles Paramedic Education Program in the David Geffen School of Medicine. Her previous position was the education program director for Los Angeles County Fire where she managed education programs for over 3,000 EMTs and paramedics. She holds a master's of science degree from New York Medical College, and is earning her doctorate in education from the University of Southern California. She is a published author and national speaker.

Julie Coffman

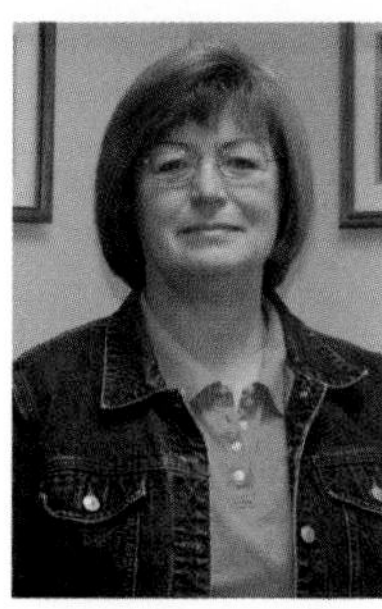

Contributing Author: Chapter 13

Julie Coffman graduated in 1981 from Mississippi University for Women with a bachelor's of science degree in microbiology and attended Baptist Medical Center School of Medical Technology in Birmingham, Alabama, where she received her national registry in Medical Technology. She has an associate degree in Fire Science from Jefferson State Community College and a master's degree in public and private management from Birmingham Southern College.

Julie started her fire/EMS career in 1983 as a volunteer firefighter in Hamilton, Alabama. She completed EMT Paramedic training at the University of Alabama in Huntsville in 1985 and became a career firefighter in 1987. In 2003, she accepted a position at the Alabama Fire College as curriculum coordinator. She has served as the program director for the EMS program, deputy director of administration, and is currently the director of certification. She has served on the Committee on Accreditation for the ProBoard Fire Service Professional Qualifications System for six years.

Madeline O'Donnell

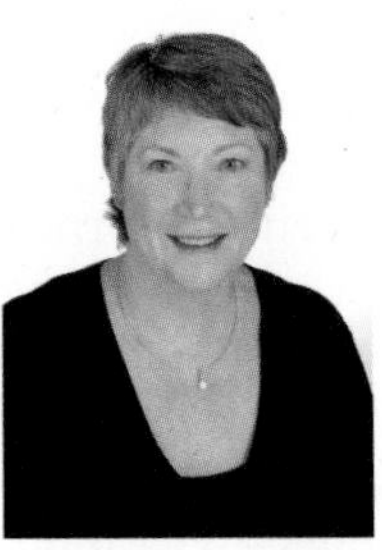

Contributing Author: Chapters 14, 15, and 17

Madeleine O'Donnell, BNg, BEd, MEdS, EdD, now retired, continues to teach health sciences at Flinders University, Adelaide, South Australia. She previously served as the principal educator for SA Ambulance Service, South Australia, where she was responsible for state-wide coordination and administration of all aspects of education, policies and procedures, including teaching, writing curriculum and syllabus for the paramedic program, and staff development and education. Her career has included that of clinical associate of intensive care and anaesthesiology at Flinders University, South Australia. She is an international speaker, a respected consultant, and a member and active participant in many professional and community-related organizations.

Greg Friese

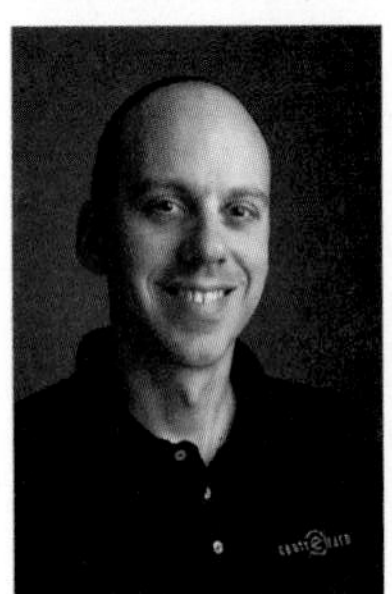

Contributing Author: Chapter 16

Greg Friese, MS, NREMT-P is the director of education for CentreLearn Solutions, LLC. He specializes in the development, production, and distribution of e-learning content for emergency responders in formats like Flash movies, online videos, podcasts, and blog posts. He believes that EMS education should honor student's knowledge, experience, and time. Greg is committed to making EMS education engaging, experiential, and exciting. Greg is also a leading advocate for the use of social media and social networks for EMS agencies and training organizations. Greg is an EMS World editorial advisory board member, and regularly contributes to EMS publications and websites. Greg is a regular conference presenter, the cohost of the EMSEduCast—the podcast by and for EMS educators—the founder of the EverydayEMSTips.com blog, a paramedic, Wilderness Medical Associates lead instructor, marathon runner, and participant in many online EMS communities.

Together with:

Mickey Moore
Deputy Director
Georgia Department of Public Health
State Office of EMS and Trauma
Atlanta, GA

David Page

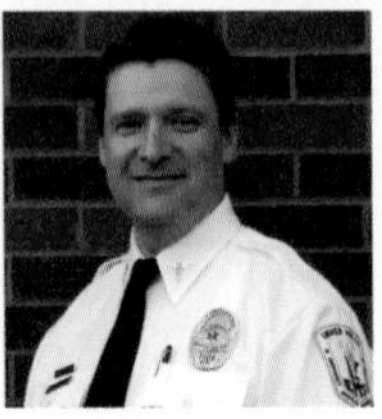

Contributing Coauthor: Chapters 18 and 19

David Page, MS, NREMT-P is a full-time paramedic instructor at Inver Hills Community College and a field paramedic with Allina EMS in Minneapolis/St. Paul, Minnesota. He has over 25 years of active EMS street experience and is an award-winning speaker and contributor to many national EMS organizations. He authors a monthly research review column in the *Journal of Emergency Medical Services (JEMS)* and serves on the advisory board for the journal. He is a charter member of the National Association of EMS Educators (NAEMSE) and a current board member of the University of California–Los Angeles Prehospital Care Research forum. Dave is also co-creator of FISDAP, a national Web-based EMS tracking, research, and testing project. He was awarded the prestigious Minnesota State Colleges and Universities "Educator of the Year" award in 2011, and the National Association of EMS Educators "Legends That Walk Among Us" award in 2009.

Together with:

Marshall J. Washick, BAS, NREMT-P
Peer Review and Research Coordinator
HealthEast Medical Transportation

Michael McLaughlin

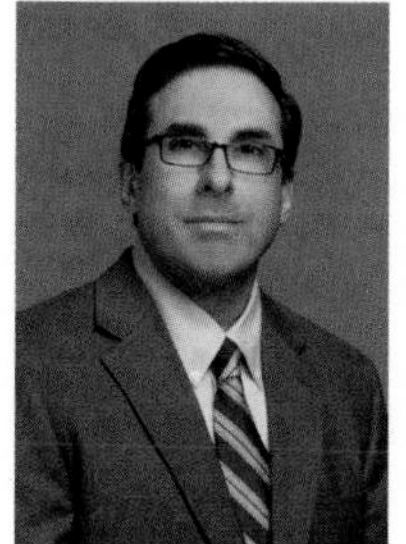

Contributing Coauthor: Chapter 18

Michael McLaughlin is the dean of Health Occupations and director of the Healthcare Simulation Center at Kirkwood Community College in Cedar Rapids, Iowa. He has been active in EMS for over 10 years, working as both a paramedic and flight paramedic. In addition to his duties at Kirkwood College, he currently works part time as a paramedic for Keokuk County Ambulance Service in Sigourney, Iowa.

Mark Terry

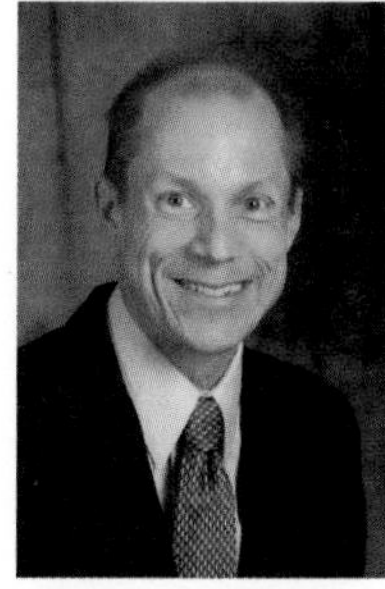

Contributing Author: Chapters 20, 21, and 22

Mark Terry, MPA, NREMT-P is the deputy chief of operations for Johnson County Med-Act. He has been a nationally registered paramedic since 1987, serving in Kansas City area EMS systems. Mark has been active in the EMS community in local, regional, and national venues. He has worked with the American Heart Association, National Association of EMS Educators, National Association of EMTs, National Registry of EMTs, and the states of Missouri and Kansas.

Connie J. Mattera

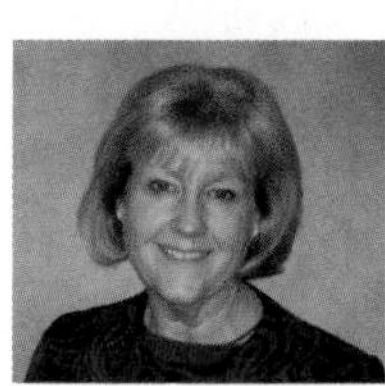

Contributing Coauthor: Chapter 24

Connie J. Mattera, MS, RN, TNS, EMT-P is the EMS administrative director for the Northwest Community EMS System in Arlington Heights, Illinois. She is the senior editor for the State of Illinois Trauma Nurse Specialist Course, is a member of the State of Illinois Governor's EMS Advisory Council, chairs the State EMS Education Committee and serves on the EMS Planning and Legislative Committee. She is a frequent faculty member at local, state, and national conferences and has published multiple articles in nursing and EMS journals. She is honored to serve on the editorial board of *JEMS* magazine, the board of directors of the National Association of EMS Educators and the executive board of Advocates for EMS. Connie serves as one of the national faculty for the NAEMSE Instructor 1 and 2 courses.

Together with:

Douglas K. York, PS, NRP
Director, EMSLRC
University of Iowa Hospitals and Clinics

About Our Founding Authors

We would like to recognize the original authors of the first edition, who laid the foundation through their research and writings, contributing greatly to the framework of the second edition.

Angel Clark Burba, MS, NCEE, EMT-P, EMT-B
Associate Professor and EMS Program Director
Howard Community College
Columbia, Maryland

Alice "Twink" Dalton, RN, NREMT-P, MS, CNS
Director, EMS Division
Mountain View Fire Protection District
Longmont, Colorado

Bill Garcia
Field Engineer II
Closed Circuit/Hyperbaric Systems
Army 7th Special Forces Dive Locker
Eglin Air Force Base, Florida

George W. Hatch, Jr., EdD, LP, EMT-P
Executive Director
Committee on Accreditation of Educational Programs for the EMS Professions
Rowlett, Texas

Sandy Hunter, PhD, NREMT-P
Professor
Eastern Kentucky University
Richmond, Kentucky

Gary L. Ireland, MA
Iowa EMS Bureau Chief (Retired)
Iowa Department of Public Health
Des Moines, Iowa

Christopher J. Le Baudour, MS Ed, NREMT
Director of Education and Outreach
Verihealth Ambulance Service, Inc.
Petaluma, California

Ranaye J. Marsh, PhD
Independent Education Management Professional
Springfield, Missouri Area

Christopher Nollette, Ed.D., NREMTP, LP
Director, Emergency Medical Services
Ben Clark Training Center
Moreno Valley College
Riverside, California

Judith A. Ruple, PhD, RN
The Ruple Group/Education Consultants
The Villages, Florida

Jane Smith, MA, NREMT-P
CEO
San Francisco Paramedic Association
San Francisco, California

Acknowledgements

Along with the editors and authors, we would like to recognize the individuals who contributed the engaging articles that appear in this edition:

Tia Radant, MS, NREMT-P
Interim Director of Emergency Services
Inver Hills Community College, MN

—Chapter 3, Learning Disabilities in the EMS Classroom

Maj. Z. Heather Yazdanipour, CCEMT-P
Clinical Services Coordinator I
Emergency Medical Services Authority Western-Division

—Chapter 16, Turn on the Tech: Pedogogical Perspective on the Tech-Savvy Student

Todd M. Cage, MEd, NREMT-P
Instructor/Paramedic
Mayo Clinic, MN

— Chapter 19, A Model for Teaching Team Leadership

Dean Vokey, BEd, MAdEd, ACP
Quality and Learning Department
Emergency Health Services, Nova Scotia

—Chapter 19, Cultivating Preceptors: Developing a Culture of Preceptorship

A special thank you to our reviewers, whose meticulous review of the technical content offered valuable insight for the development of the second edition:

Amy Aggelou
Instructor/Clinical Coordinator
School of Health and Rehabilitation Sciences
Pittsburgh, PA

Brenda M. Beasley, RN, MS, EMT-P
Department Chair, Allied Health (retired)
Calhoun Community College
Wedowee, AL

Richard Beebe, MS, RN
Associate Director of Training and Education
Mohawk Ambulance Service
Albany, NY

Terry DeVito, EdD, RN, EMT-P
Paramedic Program Coordinator
Capital Community College
Hartford, CT

Joseph W. Ferrell, MS, NREMT-P
Regulation Manager
Iowa Department of Public Health
Des Moines, IA

Steve Kanarian
Lead Paramedic Instructor
City University of New York, LaGuardia Community College
Long Island City, NY

Mary Murray
Instructor
University of Pittsburgh
Department of Sports Medicine and Nutrition
Pittsburgh, PA

Meredith Hansen
Chief, Academic Support Division
U.S. Army Department of Combat Medicine
Fort Sam Houston, TX

Michael Price, AS, NREMT-P
Program Developer for EMS Education
Central Piedmont Community College
Charlotte, NC

Bill Raynovich, EdD
Associate Professor and Director of EMS Education
Creighton University
Omaha, NE

Gina Riggs
EMS Director
Kiamichi Technology Centers
Poteau, OK

Gabriel Romero, MBA, NREMT-P
Director of Testing
FISDAP
St. Paul, MN

Sherm Syverson, BS, NREMT-P
Director of Education
F-M Ambulance/Bismarck State College
Fargo, ND

John Todaro, BA, NREMT-P, RN, TNS, NCEE
Executive Director
Lowcountry Regional EMS Council
North Charleston, SC

Patricia Tritt, RN, MA
Director of EMS and Trauma
HealthONE Swedish Medical Center
Englewood, CO

Lance Villers, PhD, EMT-P
Associate Professor and Chair
University of Texas Health Science Center
San Antonio, TX

Dean Vokey, BEd, MAdEd, ACP
Quality and Learning Department
Emergency Health Services, Nova Scotia

Bruce Walz, PhD
Professor and Chair
Department of Emergency Health Services at the University of Maryland
Baltimore, MD

Michael Ward, BS, MGA, NREMT-B
Assistant Professor of Emergency Medicine/EHS Director
George Washington University
Washington, DC

John Young
Program Director
Poquoson Fire
EMS Training Center
Portsmouth, VA

Thank you to the following individuals and institutions who contributed to the photography:

Mike Gallitelli, photographer, Metroland Photo, Inc.

Anthony Caliguire, paramedic instructor, and Hudson Valley Community College, Cardio respiratory and Emergency Medical Services Program

LifeNet of New York, an Air Methods Company

Albany Medical Center

Albany Medical College–Patient Safety & Clinical Competency Center

Deb Cason, editor, and University of Texas Southwestern Medical Center at Dallas

Kim McKenna, editor, and St. Charles County Ambulance District

Of course, we owe a debt of gratitude to the team of professionals at NAEMSE and at Delmar Cengage Learning without whom this book would not have been possible. We sincerely appreciate the professionalism of our partners at Delmar Cengage Learning; especially Janet Maker for having the vision to take on this project, Jennifer Starr whose organization, attention to detail and leadership saw the project through to completion. And to Joann Freel, NAEMSE Executive Director, and her staff, thanks for continuing in your quest to realize the vision of NAEMSE.

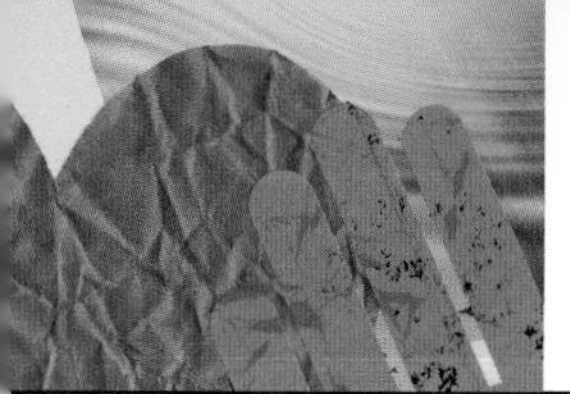

INTRODUCTION

Since its grassroots "pass the hat" inception in 1995, the National Association of EMS Educators (NAEMSE) has been committed to providing resources to develop the practice of EMS education as reflected in its mission statement which reads,

> to Inspire and Promote Excellence in EMS Education and Lifelong Learning within the Global Community.

As the association has grown in numbers and maturity, so has our collective knowledge and experience in education. Most of the authors of *Foundations of Education: An EMS Approach* came into EMS education the same way we did—from clinical practice. Fortunately we had wise educators who willingly shared educational principles at conference sessions and whetted our appetite to learn more, even to inspire some of us to go back for more formal education in issues related to teaching. NAEMSE has provided programs and educational resources and inspired over 5,000 EMS instructors to become better educators through EMS instructor courses taught nationally. Although this has not been a required text for the course, both new and seasoned instructors from a variety of educational venues have utilized this textbook and consequently enhanced their teaching role. Many have been reenergized with updated ideas, techniques, and methodologies.

This textbook's first edition was written in service to NAEMSE's mission and has provided a foundational resource for novice and expert educators since its publication in 2005. This edition continues to deliver a framework for excellence to all EMS educators, regardless of whether they teach in an ambulance service, fire district, military branch, hospital, private entity, or within a college or university system.

Much has transpired in the world of EMS education since the publication of the first edition of *Foundations of Education: An EMS Approach.* Most of these changes reflect implementation of the key elements of the industry vision document, the 2000 *EMS Education Agenda for the Future: A Systems Approach.* In 2005, *National EMS Core Content* that defined the domain of EMS knowledge was released. The Institute of Medicine nudged the agenda forward in their 2006 report, EMS at the Crossroads, with recommendations for a uniform national EMS Scope of Practice, which subsequently was published in 2007, and national paramedic program accreditation tied to national certification, which is slated for implementation in 2013. The *National EMS Education Standards* followed in 2009. The Standards represent a large shift in how EMS educators approach the design of education. The bedrock for a solid EMS program design based on the Education Standards is competent educators.

This seven-year evolution in EMS policy profoundly influences whom we teach, how we teach, what we teach, and the accountability to our students, to our schools, and to our community for quality of the instructional programs. All of these changes further the need for us to practice as professional educators who are knowledgeable about teaching and learning strategies, classroom management, assessment and evaluation, technology in learning, legal implications in education, program infrastructure design, and administering programs of excellence to meet state and national accreditation guidelines.

This edition was written with those specific challenges in mind. Each author's content builds on the contributions of the first edition to reflect how current educational knowledge and theory uniquely apply to EMS students, educators, and programs. Specific examples highlight how to apply solid educational principles to meet the challenges of today's EMS classroom. *Foundations of EMS Education: An EMS Approach,* second edition, was written by experienced EMS educators from diverse regions and backgrounds, acknowledging that, although our practice may vary, we all have common needs and face similar challenges in our attempt to promote excellence in Emergency Medical Services delivery.

Debra Cason, RN, MS, EMT-P
Editor

Kim D. McKenna, MEd, RN, EMT-P
Editor

Resources

Institute of Medicine (2006). Emergency Medical Services: At the crossroads. In Committee on the Future of Emergency Care in the United States Health System (Ed.), *Future of Emergency Care*. Washington, DC.

National Highway Traffic Safety Administration (2009). *National EMS education standards*. (DOT HS 811 077A). Washington, DC: U.S. Department of Transportation.

National Highway Traffic Safety Administration (2007). *National EMS scope of practice model.* Washington, DC: U.S. Department of Transportation.

National Highway Traffic Safety Administration (2005). *Emergency Medical Services core content*. Washington, DC: U.S. Department of Transportation.

National Highway Traffic Safety Administration (2000). *Emergency Medical Services education agenda for the future*. Washington, DC: U.S. Department of Transportation.

PART I

Instructor Roles and Responsibilities

A career as an educator is one of the most noble and challenging callings. Few individuals possess all of the qualities that are required to become a great educator, including the knowledge, aptitude, ethics, self-motivation, leadership skills, and empathy that are necessary to make a meaningful contribution to the profession. Educators play vital roles in the advancement of their professions and many Emergency Medical Service (EMS) educators also face the onerous challenge of teaching critical content with limited time and resources. EMS students not only must acquire considerable knowledge and skill, they must also master the concepts so they can apply them quickly and accurately, often in uncontrolled and unpredictable environments. The instructor's goal, therefore, is to teach students the knowledge, skills, and professional behaviors required of a competent practitioner.

The EMS educator is the essential facilitator of this complex learning process. As with any long and challenging journey, the path to becoming an excellent educator begins with the first step. This first part of the text outlines the attributes of effective EMS educators, and explains their roles and responsibilities. As experience and knowledge are acquired and teaching becomes more refined, it may be of value to return to these early chapters in Part 1 to reflect on how these concepts contribute to professional growth and formation of mastery in education.

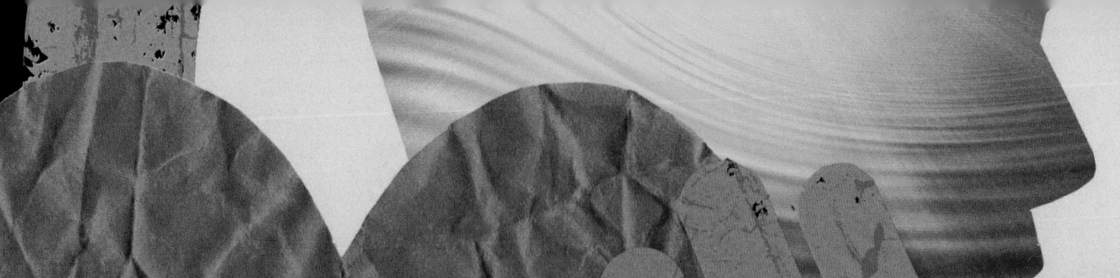

1 Attributes of Effective Educators

In a completely rational society, the best of us would be teachers and the rest of us would have to settle for something less! – Lee Iacocca

An educator begins his or her career with a clean slate, but rarely gives much thought to how he or she wishes to be remembered at the end of a teaching career. Because the first weeks and months are critical in forming the type of instructor one will become, every new educator should carefully reflect on the kind of instructor he or she wants to be. Periodic self-reflection is important to examine the steps and progress he or she is making toward reaching that ultimate goal. Every new educator should consider the attributes that can make not just effective instructors, but extraordinary instructors, and strive to emulate those attributes.

With a clear vision of the type of educator one wants to become, new educators can face the many external pressures from students, administrators, and regulators that come with the job. In the absence of a clear vision of who one wants to be, educators risk growing complacent and stale, or even bitter and jaded. Emergency Medical Services (EMS) educators, similar to EMS practitioners, can choose to lead a career defined by high standards of diligence, caring, compassion, and integrity. This chapter can help educators to identify their teaching philosophy, as well as attributes that contribute to becoming an effective educator. Furthermore, in this chapter, the educator will gain a clear understanding of what it means to be professional and ethical. Finally, this chapter also explores creativity and strategies to develop a successful career as an EMS educator.

Any discussion of the attributes of effective EMS educators should begin with a review of the qualities of effective practitioners within that specific field. The National Emergency Medical Services Education Standards describes 11 professional clinical behaviors and judgments of emergency responders.[1] The EMS educator should strive to embody these same characteristics, which include the following:

- Integrity
- Empathy
- Self-motivation
- Neat appearance and personal hygiene
- Effective communication
- Self-confidence
- Effective time management
- Teamwork and diplomacy
- Respect
- Patient advocacy
- Careful delivery of services

CHAPTER GOAL: This chapter will help educators identify their teaching philosophy as well as attributes that contribute to becoming an effective educator. It will also provide guidance on professional and ethical behaviors and strategies to develop a successful career as an EMS educator.

Attributes

In this chapter, instructor attributes are broken down into three major categories: professionalism, ethical behavior, and creativity. An *attribute* is an abstraction of a characteristic of an entity or substance. Instructors should be professional, ethical, and creative.

Professionalism

Professionalism is the first major attribute of a good instructor. In this chapter, *professionalism* is defined and then its elements are explored. These are outlined in Dr. Herbert M. Swick's elements of

Swick's Elements of Professionalism[2]

1. Professionals subordinate their own interest to the interest of others.
2. Professionals adhere to the highest ethical and moral standards.
3. Professionals respond to social needs, and their behaviors reflect a social contract with the communities served.
4. Professionals demonstrate core humanistic values, including honesty, integrity, caring, compassion, altruism, empathy, respect for others, and trustworthiness.
5. Professionals exercise accountability for themselves and for their colleagues.
6. Professionals demonstrate a continuing commitment to excellence.
7. Professionals exhibit a commitment to scholarship and to advancing their field of study.
8. Professionals deal with high levels of complexity and uncertainty.
9. Professionals reflect upon their actions and decisions.

THREE ADDITIONAL CHARACTERISTICS OF PROFESSIONALISM

10. Professionals create a nonpolitical classroom environment.
11. Professionals respect confidentiality.
12. Professional educators strive to have their students surpass them in both mastery of the content material and actualization of being a professional.

professionalism.[2] In addition, three other attributes of professionalism that are specific to education are described.

Professionalism Defined

In recent years, much attention has been devoted to the issue of professionalism in medical education and practice.[3–10] Certain professional associations, such as the American Medical Association (AMA), have become concerned about how both the body of knowledge and the delivery of medical care have affected the physician's time-honored responsibilities toward patients. Medical educators have also been concerned about the impact a physician's behavior can have on the professional development of medical students and residents; hence, the recent call for a renewed focus on professionalism.

Swick proposed a list of nine characteristics that define professionalism.[10] Although Swick's work focused on professionalism as it relates to physicians, many of his thoughts and concepts are applicable to educators in every field. The definition and understanding of professionalism must be grounded both in the nature of the profession (education) and in the nature of the professional field (in this case, EMS). Furthermore, professionalism must be considered on two levels: the individual and the collective.

In addition to those listed in Swick's work, medical professionals must exhibit three additional characteristics if they are to meet their obligations to their patients (students), their communities, and their profession.[10] These are (1) assuring a nonpolitical classroom environment, (2) respecting confidentiality, and (3) striving to have their students surpass them in both mastery of the content material and actualization of being a professional.

Elements of Professionalism

1. Professionals subordinate their own interest to the interest of others.

Because most educators have numerous responsibilities, they sometimes confront conflicts of interest in their work. These conflicts may arise, for instance, between the policies and demands of the educational institution and those of the health systems that employ the students. For example, employers who send students to complete their EMS education may pressure the school to modify the students' hours to accommodate their needs, causing the students to miss important content. When such conflicts arise, educators must ensure that the students' interests and needs remain paramount. Instructors must constantly advocate for their students. Professionalism in the field of education reflects the educator's willingness to put students' needs before his or her own.

2. Professionals adhere to the highest ethical and moral standards.

Because it is believed that professional work has a moral value, educators are compelled to behave ethically in both their personal and their professional lives. Educators must realize early in their teaching profession that they are never "off duty," just as some EMS professionals are never truly "off duty" in their communities. An educator's behaviors will be judged against the highest ethical standards, whether he or she is in the classroom, providing patient care, or taking a day off at the beach. The ethics of educators is an important and complex topic that warrants separate discussion. (See Ethics for the Educator later in this chapter.)

3. Professionals respond to social needs, and their behaviors reflect a social contract with the communities served.
Any profession best meets its obligations when its members attend actively to community and social needs. Sullivan's concept of civic professionalism stresses the importance of social leadership.[11] One way in which EMS educators can begin to fulfill their social contract is to form advisory groups from within the community to help guide educational services. It is not enough that educators think they know what is best for the community they serve; they must actively seek out the opinions of those within the community. This involves gathering information on the scheduling of courses, the number and type of courses offered, and suggested additions and deletions to the curriculum.

4. Professionals demonstrate core humanistic values, including honesty, integrity, caring, compassion, altruism, empathy, respect for others, and trustworthiness.
Although most experienced educators agree that it is difficult to write learning objectives for social values, no argument has been put forth about their importance as part of the foundation of any health professional's education. Values such as compassion, altruism, integrity, and trustworthiness are so central to the nature of the educator's work that no educator can be truly effective without holding deeply to such values. Unfortunately, it is possible to turn out students who excel in their skills and knowledge, but who lack social values. The care delivered by these students, once they become practitioners, may be insensitive, overly aggressive, and laden with risk for the provider, the patient, and the employing agency.

Teaching Tip >> *The most effective way to impart to students the values of honesty, integrity, caring, compassion, altruism, empathy, respect for others, and trustworthiness is to be a good role model for these values by living them every day and in every interaction.*

5. Professionals exercise accountability for themselves and for their colleagues.
Educators enjoy relative academic freedom and autonomy in the classroom as one of the most highly valued principles of education. However, academic freedom and autonomy do not mean that standards

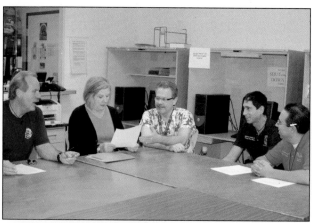

Figure 1.1

An advisory group can provide important input for the educational program, thus enhancing the value of the program to the community.

of practice and accountability for performance can be ignored or altered. Educators must adhere to educational and clinical practice standards at the institutional, state, and national levels. The best way to ensure that educators are upholding standards of practice is to have a well-developed peer-review process in place **(Figure 1.1)**.

Several methods are commonly used to develop a peer-review process. The key is to have as many different perspectives as possible from which feedback is obtained. Peer review is different from student evaluation. Although student evaluations are an important feedback tool, they come from a relatively unsophisticated audience. Having the head of the department or program sit in on a classroom session and provide feedback is the most common form of peer review. Equally valuable, and sometimes less intimidating, is having a peer instructor provide this service. Note that the instructor doing the peer evaluation does not have to be a subject matter expert, but he or she should be an experienced educator. Another means of procuring peer review is to obtain feedback from state or national testing organizations. Still another type of peer review is feedback that can be obtained from agencies that employ graduates from the course. Lastly, do not forget to talk with clinical instructors. They are invaluable sources of information regarding student strengths and weaknesses. The ideal would be that all these peer-review feedback processes would become formal and routine aspects of every school's evaluation process. At the paramedic level, programs are required to evaluate each of these elements to meet the Committee of Accreditation of EMS Programs (CoAEMSP) accreditation requirements.

6. Professionals demonstrate a continuing commitment to excellence.
All professions are based on intellectual work, a specialized body of knowledge, and expertise; thus, the commitment to maintain one's competency within the field is an important professional quality. Demands to stay current with the body of knowledge require educators to maintain the highest standards of excellence through the continuing acquisition of knowledge and development of new skills. This can be challenging in that the amount of new material in every field of science is growing at an exponential rate. In many professions, required periodic refreshers and testing of instructors have been considered means of ensuring that educators remain current in both their discipline as well as teaching methodology.

Subject Knowledge

To fulfill the sixth element of professionalism—*Professionals demonstrate a continuing commitment to excellence*—instructors must stay current with any and all sources of valid information and must maintain an updated and accurate knowledge base. Several common, appropriate resources for staying up-to-date include fellow instructors, students, other health care professionals, patients, periodicals, and conferences and continuing-education opportunities. One of the most challenging areas for instructors to address is staying up-to-date in both the academic arena as well as the clinical arena. Two strategies are commonly used to address this challenge. One method of keeping the instructor current is to take the summer off from teaching and work clinically in a hospital or on an ambulance. This is an excellent way to sharpen clinical skills and remain current in the field. If this is not possible, there must be a concerted effort to balance academic and clinical expertise. It is also critically important that educators keep current with the professional literature. New research and clinical procedures and practices are constantly being introduced, while well-established practices and therapies sometimes fall out of use or are discovered to be harmful.

Fellow Instructors

An instructor should maintain a list of colleagues who have special knowledge in a particular area of the curriculum, as well as a list of instructors who have a special gift for presenting information, running labs, or conducting meaningful classroom experiences. These instructors may constitute a personal advisory group, which can help an educator to focus on his or her commitment to personal excellence. All educators should strive to build a strong network of collegial contacts with other educators regionally and nationally. This network will be invaluable in serving as teaching resources and for leads and ideas about ways to educate in the most effective ways possible.

Students

If an instructor has a student with particular expertise in a given area, the instructor might consider using that student as a resource. This should be considered carefully, in some cases it may be perceived negatively by other classmates. Of course, it is wise to first **mentor** the student in the development of the presentation, or to gently ease the student into the presentation by informally asking the student to comment on his or her experience in the given area—with advance permission, of course.

Student advisory groups can play a very important role. The program should include a student representative on the advisory board as a minimum. Many programs have found it effective to designate student teams and student task responsibilities. For instance, students can be assigned a day of the week for set-up or take-down duties, and they may be responsible for stocking labs or cleaning equipment, such as manikins. These assignments have validity when they match the actual responsibilities of the professional work environment.

Other Health Care Professionals

Instructors should maintain a list of other health care professionals who have expertise in a given area of the curriculum. These people can be contacted as content experts, guest lecturers, lab assistants, or curriculum and exam reviewers. An example of this would be the use of a respiratory therapist in a high-fidelity manikin simulation involving a respiratory failure case. Nurses, physicians, and preceptors may also provide valuable input in the classroom when given specific learning objectives. Additionally, EMS instructors and students should interact with multidisciplinary teams, if possible, to see how various aspects of patient evaluation and care are met with different health care providers.

Patients

Clinicians and educators can learn tremendously from each patient encounter. Often, at their first meeting, patients know more about the pathophysiology and treatment of their diseases than the clinicians do. They certainly know infinitely more about how it *feels* to have a particular disease than any health care provider who has not had that disease can possibly know. One can learn a great deal from patients by listening carefully with an open mind **(Figure 1.2)**. Finally,

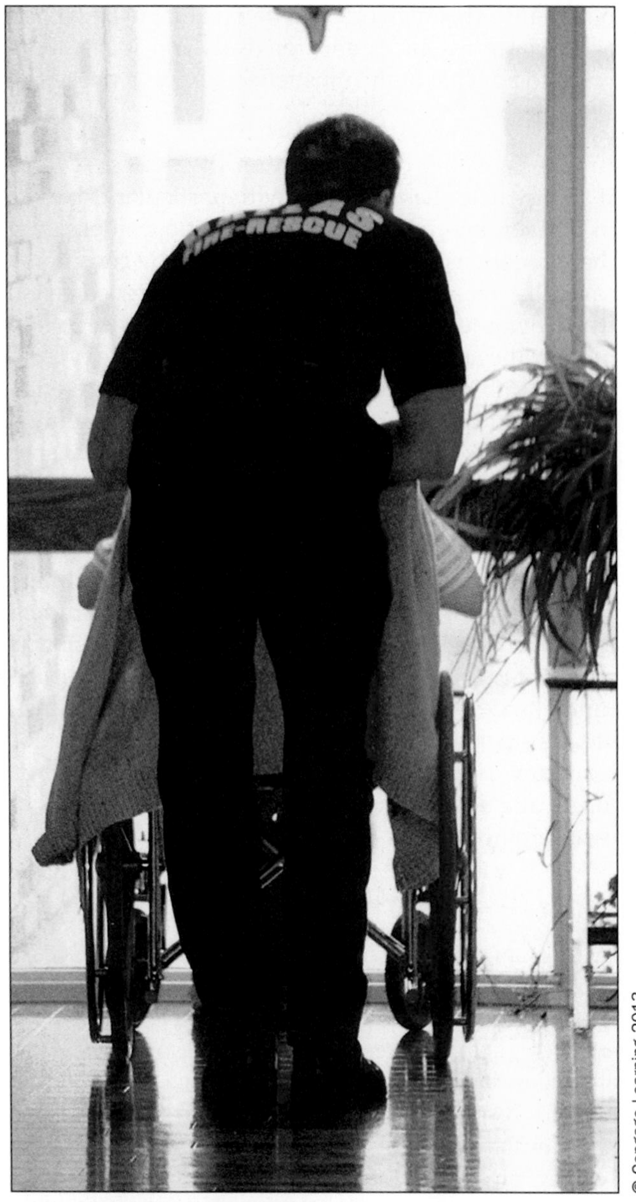

© Cengage Learning 2013

Figure 1.2

Instructors should encourage students to learn from their patients.

some patients with chronic or unusual illnesses, as well as family members, may be open to teaching health care professionals about their disease experiences. They may even view the opportunity to come into the classroom or clinic to teach as a welcome sign of respect and a chance to contribute meaningfully. Examples could be: having a diabetic patient present a session on an insulin pump; a patient with chronic renal failure presenting on continuous ambulatory peritoneal dialysis (CAPD); or a family member describing their experience with a hospice patient. The instructor should establish learning objectives for the session and facilitate it to ensure they are met.

Periodicals

The EMS educator should subscribe to at least one professional peer-reviewed journal and one professional educational journal. Membership in professional organizations is essential to keeping up with the developments of the profession and networking with peers who share problems and solutions. Educators must be strong advocates with their administrators and librarians to assure that funds for the appropriate professional journals for their professions are included in their institutional budget.

Educational Resources

There are many educational resources readily available to both the new and the seasoned instructor to improve teaching skills. These resources include other educators' materials, government agencies or professional associations, and periodicals. A list of examples of each is provided in this section, but it is only a start. It would be impossible in the scope of one chapter to list all the resources available to instructors.

Numerous educators post their materials on the Web. The instructor can find PowerPoint presentations, test questions, classroom exercises, screencasts, videos, and other classroom-management tools readily available. Two effective ways to search for these materials are to search for the medical topic you are interested in with either the suffix "PowerPoint" or "lecture" or "video" added to the topic. Another approach is to search the specific educational tool you need; "medical math problems," "teaching medical math," "drug calculations," and so on.

Professional association, manufacturer, and government websites often have position statements, PowerPoint® presentations, videos, and screencasts, or other current, accurate information that can be used to develop lessons. The Trading Post of the National Association of EMS Educators (NAEMSE) contains EMS-specific educator resources. The National Highway Traffic Safety Administration office of EMS publishes many vision and position documents, educational resources, research, National EMS Education Standards, and educator guidelines. The website and publications of the Centers for Disease Control and Prevention have up-to-date, accurate information related to diseases, EMS trauma triage guidelines, other trauma issues, disaster, and terrorism. Many other agencies and associations have valuable information that can be used as references for lesson preparations, as foundations for discussion assignments, and as resources for student projects.

Finally, there are a number of periodicals that instructors can subscribe to. They include

EMS Association and Government Resources

Emergency Medical Services for Children (EMSC)
American Heart Association (AHA)
Federal Emergency Management Association (FEMA)
National Registry of EMTs (NREMT)
Committee on Accreditation of Emergency Medical Services Professions (CoAEMSP)
National Institutes of Health (NIH)
National Association of State EMS Officials (NASEMSO)
National Association of EMTs (NAEMT)
National Association of EMS Physicians (NAEMSP)
American College of Emergency Physicians (ACEP)
International Association of Fire Chiefs (IAFC)
International Association of Fire Fighters (IAFF)
Society for Academic Emergency Medicine (SAEM)
Individual state EMS Office websites

educational journals such as *Domain3*, *Journal of Simulation*, *Adult Education Journal*, and *Adult Education Quarterly*. These journals present the latest research on instructional techniques. EMS and medical journals also include policy statements, articles, or research on education or instructional techniques relevant to EMS education. Referring to these journals informs evidence-based practice for both instructors and students. They include: *Prehospital Emergency Care (PEC)*, *Journal of Emergency Medical Services (JEMS)*, *Annals of Emergency Medicine*, *Pediatric Emergency Care*, *Academic Emergency Medicine*, *Journal of Emergency Primary Health Care*, *Circulation*, and many others.

Teaching Tip >> *Require every student in every course to turn in two articles from clinical or educational peer-reviewed journals. The purpose of this exercise is for students to learn about the professional journals and to get to know where they are located. Also, require students to provide the address of one website resource. In addition to the learning opportunity that this activity provides to students, instructors generally receive numerous interesting articles to read, along with 10 to 15 new Web addresses per class.*

Conferences

Educators have a responsibility to learn current patient care methods and teaching strategies, and conferences provide the perfect learning opportunity. EMS educators should not limit themselves to local, regional, or even state conferences, but should attend national conferences as often as possible. Furthermore, the educator should not limit himself or herself to discipline-specific conferences. There are wonderful national conferences on distance education, how to give presentations, technologies in education, testing and measurement, and student counseling **(Figure 1.3)**. There are many benefits to attending national conferences that go beyond learning new instructional methodologies or learning about new treatment modalities and clinical practices. These include opportunities for career networking and the "cross pollination" of programs. The networking opportunities provide avenues for contacts to find available instructors for future recruitment, and for contacts for future possible positions in other locations and institutions. Being tied into a national network is invaluable for assisting educators, students, and colleagues with job searches and, often, when the time comes to relocate for career advancement, contacts to find the best possible position in the best location.

7. Professionals exhibit a commitment to scholarship and to advancing their field of study.

In all professions, one of the most basic defining elements of members is the commitment to advance the body of knowledge of that discipline. This commitment to **scholarship** can be manifested as a desire

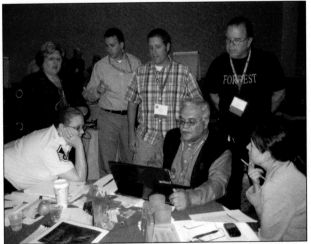

Figure 1.3

Instructors can keep abreast of new clinical topics, as well as educational techniques, by networking at conferences.

to share one's knowledge for the benefit of others—whether students, other instructors, or members of the community. All professionals should be strongly committed to supporting research within their area of study. This requires the following:

- A functional knowledge of research methods
- The ability to conduct literature searches or reviews
- Evaluation of research for use in the classroom
- Presentation of research to students to instill a commitment among the next generation of professionals

Without formal and informal forums at which instructors can routinely gather and share knowledge, any profession is severely limited in its ability to advance. Introducing students to research early in your program provides a foundation upon which you can build a learning environment where evidence-based practice is emphasized and valued.

8. Professionals deal with high levels of complexity and uncertainty.
Uncertainty and ambiguity have long characterized the practices of medicine and education. Instructors, similar to health care providers, must be able to exercise independent judgment to make appropriate decisions in the face of complex and often unstable circumstances, and usually with incomplete information. Instruction that is simple and repetitive, or that does not involve a great deal of judgment, does not require the independent decision making that is a hallmark of these professions.[12] Furthermore, while commercially prepared lessons can be invaluable for the novice, instructors who rely strictly on canned curricula and do no more than repeat the work of others without adjusting the material for a given audience, adding personal insights, or developing creative approaches of delivery, fall far short of the term "professional educator."

9. Professionals reflect upon their actions and decisions.
Professional educators must be able to reflect objectively on the decisions they have made, as well as on their actions, to learn from their experiences. These self-reflective activities not only improve their knowledge and skills, they also bring balance to their professional and personal lives.

NOTE: Although the nine Elements of Professionalism discussed here are based largely on definitions developed by Dr. Swick, the following three additional characteristics are proposed for the educator's consideration.

10. Professionals create a nonpolitical classroom environment.
Instructors must create a safe, nonpolitical environment for their students. Local, state, and national politics have no place in the classroom environment. In fact, all students should be treated with respect regardless of their socioeconomic or political background. Moreover, some health professions inherently have political controversies such as which national certification to obtain, or, in the EMS field, issues related to paid providers versus volunteer providers. All points of view should be respected; however, some are not appropriate or relevant to include in classroom discussions. Certain topics, however, are appropriate for critical, professional discussion such as different perspectives on rural and urban medical care. When questions arise about sensitive or controversial issues, the professional educator must present all sides of the argument in an unbiased and balanced manner.

11. Professionals respect confidentiality.
All health care professionals are acutely aware of the issues associated with patient confidentiality. Educators must be equally sensitive to these issues when they discuss their students with colleagues. Information on individual student performance, personality, and strengths and weaknesses should be considered strictly confidential. The professional educator has a legal responsibility to refrain from sharing this information inappropriately. (See Chapter 10: Legal Issues.)

12. Professional educators strive to have their students surpass them in both mastery of the content material and actualization of being a professional.
A key requirement of being a professional is the understanding that it is a dynamic process. Being a professional is not an end point or a destination. Being a professional means that one is on a lifelong journey as a learner and practitioner, and it is the educator's mission to impart this understanding to students.

Developing A Philosophy of Education

For any educator, knowing oneself and one's core beliefs about instruction lays the foundation for planning and delivering effective education. In *The Skillful Teacher*, Stephen Brookfield suggests that instructors "adopt a critically reflective stance towards their practice."[13] This stance, developed as a teaching philosophy, gives direction and purpose to actions and decisions made while designing learning, or when teaching in the classroom. Lindeman supports this when he says, "The person who is vividly aware of his activity, as well as the goal toward which the activity is directed, becomes conscious of his powers and limitations."[14] A philosophical statement can guide an instructor in the same way the mission, vision, and values of an organization drive its key actions, decisions, and strategies. A well-thought-out philosophy provides a framework for reflection on action when teaching. It is important to recognize that a teaching philosophy is not a static document. As instructors grow and gain experiences, their teaching philosophy will change to reflect their changing views about themselves and their relationships to students, to learning, and to teaching.

Lorraine Zinn suggests that, while defining a working **philosophy of education**, the first step is to examine what the educator believes about the adult learners in the areas of the learner, the overall purpose of education, the content or subject, and the learning process. Examining one's beliefs about the role of the adult educator is another important step.[15] There is no "perfect" teaching philosophy; the differences in instructional philosophy mirror the rich diversity seen in great EMS educators. See an example of David Royse's approach in the text box "Developing a Teaching Philosophy".

Developing A Teaching Philosophy[16]

David Royse, in his text *Teaching Tips for College and University Instructors*, proposes that all educators should construct a teaching philosophy that represents what is most important to them as educators. In identifying his own philosophy, Royse considered the instructors who had influenced him positively, both personally and professionally, as well as those who had affected him with their poor teaching and interpersonal skills. His philosophy of important issues includes the following:

- Create a sense of community in the classroom. Students learn more and enjoy learning when they feel connected to one another and to the instructor.
- Ensure that education is a two-way, interactive process. The instructor is neither infallible nor an authority on all matters.
- Give respect to each individual person in the classroom.
- Be accountable to the students. Make sure to prepare appropriately and be on time for class, as well as to offer timely, high-quality feedback to students.
- Make sure that learning is fun. Include humor as part of all classes.
- Apply learning to issues and problems in the world today.
- Hold lifelong learning as a goal.

Ethics for the EMS Educator

EMS educators are members of two professions: teaching and health care practice. To fulfill the second element of professionalism—*Professionals adhere to the highest ethical and moral standards*—they must comply with the requirements and standards of each. EMS educators who are EMS practitioners are subject to the laws of professional ethics that are in force within the jurisdictions and services in which they work. In addition, as members of the teaching profession, all educators are subject to the regulations and ethical guidelines of the institutions or facilities at which they teach.

EMS educators undoubtedly serve as important role models for students in that the classroom experience is frequently the student's first exposure to the EMS profession. Therefore, EMS educators must understand the importance of ethical standards of behavior. They should have a strong sense of the special obligations that come with serving as an educator, especially since their responsibilities frequently extend beyond the classroom to out-of-class activities with students, both in the community and in other professional activities. They should also recognize their responsibility to serve students and to help students achieve their goals. This responsibility for moral integrity and dedication to the welfare of students must originate within the educator.

The following good practices concerning ethical and professional responsibility can assist new instructors and remind experienced ones of the basic ethical and professional code of their profession. This is by no means to be considered a disciplinary code, although the norms of conduct are relevant when questions concerning propriety arise in an institutional context. The primary purpose of these practices is to provide general guidance to EMS educators concerning their ethical and professional responsibilities to students, to colleagues, and to the profession and the general public.

Responsibilities to Students

Because of their inevitable function as role models, educators should be guided by and adhere to ethical and professional standards. As educators, scholars,

RIGHTS OF LEARNERS[17]

Learners have a right to the following:

- A clear indication of expectations for a course or program
- Reasonable access to the instructor and resources
- Due process when challenging the judgments and actions of the teacher
- Treatment with dignity and respect at all times
- A learning environment that is fair, safe, and productive

RESPONSIBILITIES OF TEACHERS[17]

Teachers have a responsibility for the following:

- Accurately represent the work of others (avoiding plagiarism)
- Maintain professional, vocational, or academic competence
- Maintain confidentiality in matters related to evaluation and assessment
- Ensure that what is taught matches what was promised
- Ensure that what is tested or evaluated matches what was taught

counselors, mentors, and friends, EMS educators can profoundly influence students' attitudes concerning professional competence and responsibility. Educators must help students recognize the responsibility they have to their profession and to the community at large.

Educators should aspire to excellence in teaching and to mastery of the theories and practices of the subjects they teach. Furthermore, they should prepare conscientiously for class and employ teaching methods appropriate for the subject matter and objectives of their courses. Similarly, classes should always be convened as scheduled or, when impossible, rescheduled at a time that is reasonably convenient for students; if needed, an alternative means of instruction should be provided.

Educators should provide a class syllabus or handbook that clearly outlines the objectives and requirements of a course, including applicable attendance and grading rules. Further, the educator should review these with the class, ensuring that each student fully understands them. It is advisable to have students sign a statement acknowledging receipt of the handbook and syllabus and acceptance of its contents.

A primary obligation of the educator is to treat students with politeness and respect. Educators can do this by creating a learning environment that fosters a stimulating and productive debate in which the pros and cons of important issues are fairly acknowledged and discussed. Allowing students to explore new ideas without fear of censure or criticism within the learning environment is essential to the free exchange of ideas. Educators should nurture and protect intellectual freedom for their students and colleagues.

The Ethics of Student Evaluation

Educators have a fundamental obligation to fairly, accurately, honestly, and constructively evaluate student work. This is a crucial aspect of respecting and nurturing students.

Exams and assignments should be conscientiously designed to meet the expectations of student performance, and evaluation materials should match learning objectives and stated goals. Moreover, student work should be evaluated with impartiality. The instructor may enhance impartiality by blinding the review of student material, that is, the student is not identified until after the review has been completed. Another way to achieve impartiality with essay-type exams is by using a **rubric**, or *grading template*, that outlines all of the important points that must appear in the student's written work. (See Chapter 22: Other Evaluation Tools.)

The standards for assigning grades should be consistent with standards recognized within the facility or institution. Students should be informed about evaluation methods in the syllabus and a clearly defined basis on which grades are assigned. Instructors should offer an explanation if students ask why they received a certain grade. In addition, instructors should grade and provide feedback to students in a timely fashion. When evaluation criterion are clearly defined and followed by the instructor, students will typically not win an appeal for a failing grade.

The Ethics of Counseling

Educators should make themselves reasonably available to counsel students about academic matters, career choices, and professional interests. Furthermore, they should offer timely and accurate information.

When counseling students, educators must make every effort to hold student information confidential. They should not disclose any information unless required to do so by institutional rule or applicable law. In most cases, instructors have an obligation to inform administrators if they believe a student intends to harm self or others. Before providing counseling, educators should inform students of the possibility of such disclosure.

Educators should strive to be as fair and complete as possible when communicating evaluative recommendations for students. If information disclosed in confidence by the student to the educator makes it impossible for the educator to write a fair and complete evaluation/recommendation without revealing the information, the educator should inform the student and refuse to provide the evaluation/recommendation unless the student consents to full disclosure.

Educators must be aware that counseling is a profession with levels of graduate degrees of education, professional licensing, and extensive experiential learning. Thus, educators cannot venture into the counseling arenas of mental health, marriage, and other significant life issues without incurring the liabilities and practice risks involved in that profession's boundaries and scopes of practice. EMS educators should limit their student-counseling activities to the performance of students, how well they are learning, their attitudes about their learning, and ways to improve their learning through supportive tutoring, remediation, or other appropriate means. When a student expresses any psychological or mental health issues, or possibly concerns about learning disabilities, the educator should refer the student to appropriate counselors and psychological services for further assessment and interventions. Educators must report student statements or behaviors that indicate the intent to harm self or others to the appropriate authorities immediately.

The Ethics of Diversity

Educators must make the learning environment a hospitable community and comfortable setting for all students. Discriminatory conduct based on such factors as race, color, religion, national origin, sex, sexual orientation, disability or handicap, age, or political beliefs is unacceptable in the education community. It is important for educators to be sensitive to the harmful consequences of instructor or student conduct, or comments in classroom discussions or elsewhere that perpetuate stereotypes or prejudices.

The Ethics of Personal Relationships with Students

Educators must be careful to avoid comingling personal and professional roles in interactions with students, even with seemingly harmless situations such as having a student babysit or wash a car for fair payment. It is especially important that the educator not engage in a sexual relationship with a student or subject a student to a hostile academic environment based on any form of sexual influence. Sexual harassment of a student would guarantee an end to the educator's career. *Sexual harassment* is defined as conduct that involves unwelcome advances, requests for sexual favors, and other verbal or physical conduct of a sexual nature. Whenever an educator has professional responsibility for a student, such as in teaching, evaluating, supervising, or advising the student as part of a course, this conduct is inappropriate.

Even when an educator has no professional responsibility for a student but maintains a relationship with that student, the educator should be sensitive to the perceptions of other students. Students may perceive that a student who has a sexual relationship with an instructor may receive preferential treatment from other instructors within the institution.

An educator who is closely related to a student by blood or marriage, or who has a preexisting close relationship with a student, generally should avoid any role involving professional responsibility for that student.

Ethical Responsibilities as Professional Educators

The community of EMS educators has a basic responsibility to refine, extend, and transmit knowledge regarding the teaching and practice within their specific discipline. Educational institutions and programs also have a responsibility to maintain an atmosphere of freedom and tolerance in which knowledge can be sought and shared. Educators are obligated, in turn, to make the best and fullest use of that academic freedom to fulfill their responsibilities to enrich the profession and practice of EMS education.

As previously discussed, educators have a responsibility to be current in the knowledge of the subjects that they teach. In teaching, as well as in research, writing, and publication, the scholarship of others is indispensable to one's knowledge and growth. To stay current in any health care field requires continuous study and lifelong learning. To this extent, the educator must remain a student. Moreover, in some institutions, educators have a responsibility to engage in their own research and publish their conclusions. In this way, educators participate in an intellectual exchange that tests and improves their knowledge of the field to the ultimate benefit of their students, the profession, and society.

The educator's commitment to truth requires intellectual honesty and open-mindedness. Although an educator should feel free to criticize another's work, distortion or misrepresentation of a colleague's work is always unacceptable. When using any intellectual work of another author—whether another educator or a student—the original author must be acknowledged every time the ideas are used or transmitted. Appropriate ways to acknowledge contributions of others is through shared authorship, attribution by a footnote or endnote, or discussion of the original author's contributions within the main text or within a presentation.

An educator has a responsibility to preserve the integrity and independence of research and to promote the development of new knowledge. Sponsored or compensated research activities or presentations should always be acknowledged with full disclosure of the personal interests. Conflicts of interest should be acknowledged and brought forward for discussion among educators and students. It is best to err on the side of conservatism when one is addressing conflict-of-interest situations. If an instructor believes there might be a conflict, there probably is; so it is wise to disclose the possibility to others with whom or for whom he or she is working. For example, it is important to self disclose when speaking about a specific device, drug, or procedure at a conference if the speaker is being paid an honorarium by the manufacturer of the device or drug. If the speaker had any grant money provided by the sponsor of the device, the audience has the right to know that the presentation was being funded by the product manufacturer and could then evaluate the validity of the research.

Ethical Responsibilities to Colleagues

Educators should treat colleagues and staff members with politeness and respect. Additionally, they should comply with institutional rules or policies requiring confidentiality concerning oral or written communications. Such rules and policies typically exist with respect to personnel matters and evaluations of student performance.

As is the case with students, sexual harassment or discriminatory conduct involving colleagues or staff members on the basis of race, color, religion, national origin, sex, sexual orientation, disability or handicap, age, or political beliefs is unacceptable.

Ethical Responsibilities to the EMS Community and the General Public

An EMS educator occupies a unique role as a bridge between the EMS community and students who are preparing to become members of that community. Educators must accept the responsibilities of their professional status. At a minimum, they should adhere to the Code of Rules of Conduct of state-licensing or certification divisions. Conduct by an EMS educator or provider that warrants discipline should be a matter of serious concern to the educator's school and to the general public.

One of the traditional but less frequently performed obligations of EMS educators is to engage in uncompensated public service. As role models for students and as members of the professions, educators should strive to fulfill this responsibility. They can meet this obligation in a variety of ways, including direct patient contact through public aid programs, lecturing in continuing-education programs, educating public school pupils or other public groups concerning the profession and other health issues, and by teaching community health and safety programs.

Conclusions Regarding Ethics

This chapter serves to assist new educators and to remind experienced ones about the basic ethical and professional code of their profession. The educator must understand what constitutes good practice in terms of ethical and professional responsibility. Additionally, educators must recognize their responsibility to serve students and to help students achieve their goals. This responsibility to serve students requires moral integrity and a dedication to providing what is in the best interest of the students.

Every educator has the responsibility to adhere to the code of the profession and to be aware of the ethical and professional conduct requirements of the system in which he or she is teaching. It is important for EMS educators to remember that they have an ethical responsibility to students, colleagues, their profession, and the general public. Because it is paramount that the professional educator should uphold high standards within the profession, breeches of ethical conduct should not be taken lightly.

Creativity

Creativity is an attribute essential to achieving excellence in education. A dedicated and highly skilled clinical provider who provides excellent compassionate patient care will still not rise to greatness in the classroom without creativity. Reaching the hearts and minds of students requires the EMS educator to be able to place oneself in the place of the student who does not have a depth of experience and knowledge and who requires a rich context for meaningful learning to take place. It is through originality, adaptability, and meaningful exchanges between the instructor and the student that effective learning takes place.

Creativity in Teaching

According to Thomas L. Schwenk and Neal Whitman, all effective instructors have one attribute in common—they present creative lessons that stimulate their students and make learning easier.[18] An educator can achieve this kind of creativity by starting with the lesson plan and asking if there is something he or she can do to make the learning more creative.

Creativity is defined as any activity that is novel and useful and results in contributions to human experience. Novel approaches in the classroom may involve the use of interesting modalities of communication, the application of inventive or unorthodox teaching techniques, and the provision of memorable and meaningful educational experiences through graphic demonstrations or imagery. Useful approaches may include providing correct, up-to-date, and relevant information, along with opportunities to develop good problem-solving skills and good patient care attitudes. If these qualities are combined into a grid, four possible types of instructor are revealed **(Figure 1.4)**.

Creative educators are both novel and useful. They reveal the "inner relevance" of what they teach.[19] Creative instructors exhibit three characteristics:

1. They are selective in choosing their teaching methodologies.
2. They pay attention to delivery.
3. They teach beyond the printed material, beyond the textbook.

On the opposite side of the spectrum of creative and excellent educators, there are ineffective educators, such as charlatans and pedantic bores.

Charlatan

Instructors can be **charlatans**—persons who claim knowledge or skill that they do not possess—when they focus more on being novel, entertaining, and well liked than on transmitting essential information and designing a meaningful learning experience. Students generally love charlatans. As a result, all will appear to be going well until students have to sit for the state or national exam. That is when students discover that their instructor has not adequately prepared them for the exam.

One sign that an instructor is a charlatan is that he or she excessively uses "war stories." Additionally, charlatans rarely have prepared teaching materials and rely more on personal interaction than on content. Moreover, charlatans can be spotted by the fact that they rarely take responsibility for their students' failures—failure is always someone else's fault. Charlatans focus on themselves rather than on meeting the students' learning needs.

	USEFUL	NOT USEFUL
NOVEL	Creative teacher	Charlatan
NOT NOVEL	Pedantic bore	Old goat

Figure 1.4

Types of instructors.

CASE IN POINT

Two months in advance, an instructor recruited one of the best physicians from the local hospital to present a talk. She sent him a copy of the course schedule and learning objectives for the lecture, so that the physician would know exactly where the students were in their learning process when he arrived. She also invited him to review the test questions that she had on the topical material, as well as to write any questions that he felt were important to include. She then sent a reminder 30 days in advance, offering to print any handouts and to make sure that any ancillary audiovisual presentation materials were "loaded and ready to go." His office confirmed his appointment, saying that he would bring anything he needed with him.

The surgeon arrived on time and in good spirits. His lecture was entertaining and filled with valuable clinical tips and anomalies. He spoke of fascinating complications and tragic deaths due to occult anomalies. He brought alive the imagery of the heroic clinical team working feverishly to save the lives of those *in extremis.* The class gave him a warm applause and stood in line to speak with him after the lecture.

The instructor sat and listened in dismay. The guest physician ignored the content objectives. She would have to squeeze another 1-hour lecture into the already full course. The physician had been entertaining and charming, but if the students took their national board examinations based on the lecture, they were certain to fail. However, the students loved the lecture and his evaluations were excellent.

Pedantic Bore

It is certainly better to be a pedantic bore than a charlatan—at least students receive useful information from a pedantic bore. Rarely is anyone who is interested in teaching in health care a born and unredeemable pedantic bore. Pedantic bores are made, not born. The primary reason that educators may be boring is that they truly find the content material boring, or they may be so overbooked that they are simply trying to survive **(Figure 1.5)**.

> **Teaching Tip** >> *Instructors should not attempt to lecture on something they do not really own. If the instructor has enough time to really prepare to present a topic, he or she will tend to get pretty excited and will really start to employ the creative process.*

Becoming More Creative

By acting more creatively, an instructor can actually become more creative.[20] Instructors should not be afraid to try new methods in the classroom, or even to fail. Creativity may be viewed more as a process than as a product.[21] In fact, the four stages of this process have been identified as preparation, incubation, illumination, and verification.

Stages of Creativity

In the *preparation stage*, the instructor investigates the subject, deciding on what he or she wants students to value or know. It is often very helpful for instructors to brainstorm with other instructors at this point. The more possibilities one explores, the more likely one is to discover effective and creative approaches to presentation.

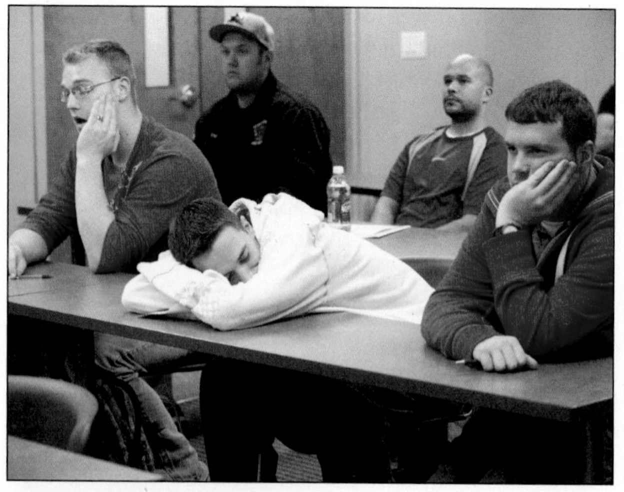

Figure 1.5

A sleeping student is a sure clue that the class is boring.

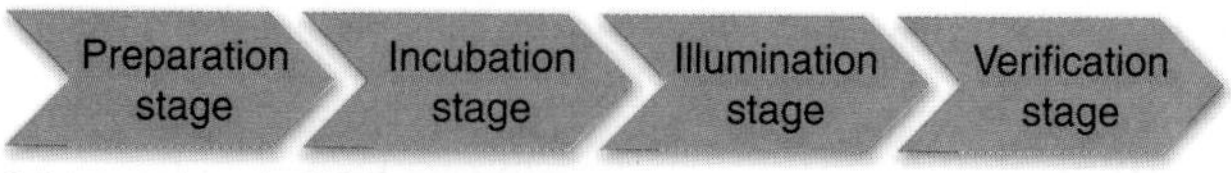

Preparation stage → Incubation stage → Illumination stage → Verification stage

Figure 1.6

The four stages of creativity: preparation, incubation, illumination, and verification.

During the *incubation stage*, the instructor does not devote conscious thought to teaching the assignment, but continues to work at the subconscious level. Not allowing oneself time for the incubation stage of the process defeats the whole process of creativity. The educator must allow time for doing the subconscious and deliberative creative work, and this process cannot be rushed. Instructors who chronically overbook themselves can expect to do less than their best work.

In the *illumination stage*, the creative instructor becomes aware of how the topic can be presented. It is at this point that the organization of the content is combined with a plan on how to present it.

In the *verification stage*, the instructor teaches, and the validity of the instruction is tested. At this point, the reflective educator should contemplate whether or not he or she had the desired impact on the students **(Figure 1.6)**.

> **Teaching Tip** >> *The number-one way educators sabotage themselves is by not allowing themselves sufficient time to prepare. When they do not schedule adequate time to be creative, update their material, or simply review their lesson plans before presenting, they give students less than their best.*

Positive Attributes

Along with being creative, other basic positive qualities contribute to one's becoming an effective instructor. Chickering and Gamson reviewed 50 years of research on effective teaching. They identified seven common principles of good teaching practice, which were later validated by additional research findings. They concluded that effective teaching involves the following:[22]

- Frequent contact between students and faculty
- Encouragement and cooperation among students

- Use of active-learning techniques
- Prompt feedback
- Emphasis on time on task
- Communication of high expectations
- Respect for diverse talents and ways of learning

Negative Attributes

The positive attributes of effective instructors have been described throughout most of this chapter; however, it is equally important here to point out certain negative attributes that can define an instructor. Provided in the following paragraphs is a brief list of characteristics that generally are considered to be negative characteristics within the classroom environment. The educator who becomes familiar with these styles of teaching will likely have greater success in avoiding them.

Dominating instructors have difficulty organizing and running discussions. They demonstrate low levels of participation in student activities, especially if they do not learn to control this negative characteristic.

Noncurrent (out-of-touch) instructors have difficulty clarifying issues, beliefs, and problems. They also tend to have problems explaining, informing, and demonstrating.

Egocentric (the world revolves around them) instructors have difficulty referring students to other people and offices. They try to be their students' only source of information. In addition, these instructors find it almost impossible to defend other faculty, course directors, or agencies. They lay blame for any problem in the course to some external source, rather than taking responsibility.

Burned-out instructors find it nearly impossible to motivate or encourage students.

Curriculum-based versus student-based (those who place more importance on the curriculum than on the student) instructors find it very difficult to clarify questions and to construct tests. They have trouble getting into a student's head and seeing the class from the student's perception.

Charting A Successful Career Path As An Educator

Every individual goes through life and career cycles. Educators experience exhilarating triumphs and thrills during the first day of a new class, or at a graduation ceremony when an at-risk student graduates and gets a job with a premier employer. At other times, the administrative burdens of lesson planning, preparing routine reports, getting ready for an accreditation inspection, or teaching a class of seemingly disinterested students and hearing endless excuses and appeals, can take a toll and wear down a dedicated and well-balanced instructor. Educators can help chart a path to career success that avoids a downward cycle of apathy and burn out.

It is important for educators to establish a clear set of career goals and produce quality work. Every educator should constantly cultivate a professional image. This begins with learning the structure, mission, and goals of the organization. Educators need to identify available resources and stay visible, while avoiding petty political spats and gossip. It is also advisable to realize that it is not healthy or productive to stay in a job that is not meeting the needs the educator has for career growth and satisfaction.

It should be no surprise that, for most educators, job satisfaction is linked to salary, benefits, and long-term job security.[23] Other extrinsic rewards that promote job satisfaction include publications, presentations, and grant funding.

There are, however, intrinsic motivators equally important to job satisfaction in education. Satisfying one's personal ideals, such as a passion for high-quality teaching, is linked to job satisfaction. New instructors experience stress related to a heavy workload, isolation, scholarly inactivity, perceived lack of support and collegiality, and uncertainty about institutional requirements.[24,25] These stressors can be lessened through mentorship by experienced faculty.

Enhancing one's knowledge through continuing professional development is another strategy to lessen stress and promote excellence and career advancement. Professional development, even in the middle of an educator's career, has been shown to improve faculty knowledge, behaviors, and satisfaction.[24]

Mentors in Education

If the school does not assign a mentor, new instructors should seek one or more to assist integration into their new teaching setting. Mentor roles vary, and in some cases new educators may have more than one mentor with expertise in a variety of areas. The role of the mentor is to guide, advise, and coach the new instructor.[24] Effective mentors can provide assistance with lesson-plan development, syllabi, or other learning activities. The experienced instructor can direct the novice faculty to resources within the facility and familiarize them with the culture of the institution.

Most importantly, the mentor serves as a sounding board as the new instructors reflect on successes and failures in their new role.

Even experienced instructors seek career mentors to develop interests or to broaden professional knowledge. An external mentor is someone who is experienced, influential, and well respected in the field. Educators should find someone in the profession who has somewhat more experience, who has succeeded in gaining respect and advancement, and who can provide guidance and support. Mentors are important for providing contacts and opportunities in the field. Educators should look beyond the organization toward the full professional network for career mentors.

Developing a Network of Colleagues

Having a network of contacts has many benefits. Often, the best jobs are those that are learned about by word of mouth. Having a variety of contacts in the local EMS and educational communities makes the educator valuable to the employer. It also makes the educator a person who can get things done. The more professional contacts an educator has in the field, the more opportunities for collaboration and involvement in meaningful projects.

Continuing Professional Development

Through lifelong learning, the educator can assure that he or she is always employable by constantly developing and maintaining expertise demanded by the marketplace. As the base of general knowledge continues to expand, it becomes harder and harder to be a generalist, either as a clinician or an educator.

The term *continuing professional development* encompasses a wide range of activities that can improve an EMS instructor's knowledge, enhance the chance for advancement, and promote job satisfaction. It incorporates three broad areas: (1) self-directed learning; (2) formal professional development; and (3) organizational development.[26]

Most of an educator's continuing professional development is self-directed and occurs on a day-to-day basis. This self-directed learning occurs as an instructor prepares a lesson, participates in curriculum planning, teaches, conducts research, participates on committees, and reads professional materials.

The availability of professional-development programs is generally broad. It includes web-based, local, national and international continuing-education seminars and conferences. Topics available through this format vary widely. Instructors' ability to attend this type of education may depend on financial support from their employers if travel is involved. Professional development may also include furthering one's own formal education by obtaining a specialty certification, degree, or advanced degree.

Organizational (or staff) development is targeted education designed to improve or change performance within an institution. The amount and quality of organizational development varies widely by institution.

Factors That Influence Professional Development

According to Zinn, throughout an educator's career there are four main influences that can either support or serve as barriers to an educator's success and satisfaction. They are interpersonal relationships, institutional structure, personal considerations and commitments, and intellectual and psychosocial characteristics.[26] If absent, the supporting factors within each of these areas can become barriers. In some cases the instructor can influence them to promote success, while in others they will be out of the instructor's control and the only solution may be a job change.

Positive interpersonal relationships are essential for job satisfaction and success. They include demonstrating positive relationships with coworkers and administrative staff in a manner that models respect, recognizes achievement, and provides encouragement. They promote a supportive work environment. The educator should model these behaviors.

Institutional structures can influence the educator's success and development. Institutional factors that promote success in education include providing resources and time for the educator to attend professional development. An important institutional attribute is a climate that promotes collaboration and collegiality rather than competition among faculty.

Personal factors play a substantial role in an educator's professional development and can determine progress to a successful career. Having a strong network of family and friends to provide support for long and irregular work hours, travel, or interruptions for student crises can help performance. Major life crises such as deaths, divorce, or significant illness can have short- or long-term career implications.

The educator's individual, intellectual, and personal characteristics powerfully impact development.

A strong work ethic with a commitment to excellence is essential. Instructors must believe in themselves and that their actions make a difference. The educator's ability to see where their role fits within the success of their students, their school, and their field is critical. And just as important is the enjoyment of challenge and change, because both are inevitable to learn and grow as educators.

Changing Jobs

For some EMS educators, remaining in the same satisfying job for a prolonged period can be rewarding and there is no desire or need to change. Other educators enjoy the challenge of job change to learn new skills or to take on new opportunities. In other cases, job dissatisfaction related to conflict or misalignment with institutional goals may lead to a desire for change. Staying in an unsatisfactory position for a prolonged period of time can lead to poor performance. Regardless of the reason for job change, it should be planned in a thoughtful manner.

Vertical promotions are not the only way to advance careers. There are a limited number of higher positions available in EMS. This can create a "bottleneck" effect. Lateral moves, even within an organization, such as from one department to another, or from a proprietary company or a municipal agency to a college or university, can enrich the educator's experience portfolio. It may be possible to find a niche in a different type of organization, or find a preference for doing continuing education over doing primary education. Advancing up the career administrative ladder can also distance an educator from students and teaching as administrative duties increase. It is not for everyone.

The best career-advancement opportunities may occur in other organizations. This makes sense because career opportunities and progressive changes are occurring all the time, all over the world. The number of especially prestigious or exciting positions available at any given time in any profession is generally very small. Thus, being mobile and willing to relocate to where an opportunity presents itself makes it more likely that an educator will find an appealing position. The EMS educator should be careful about seeking another similar position in the same community with a competing agency. First, it is quite likely that the exploration, and even considering the position, may quickly or eventually get back to the educator's employer. Second, once the move to the competing agency has been made, it better be the right decision and a good fit, as a return to the original employer is not likely to be possible, at least for many years and changes of administration, if ever.

There is more to being successful than just "doing a good job." Career advancement does not happen by luck or chance for most people, but through opportunities they as individuals have created through the careful artistry of career development.

Teaching Tip >> *The best ways to avoid developing negative teaching characteristics are the following:*

- *Equally balance decisions between what is good for the course and what is good for the students.*
- *Be a student. This, more than anything else, helps instructors to see things from the students' perspective.*
- *Remember that students need different levels of support at different times in the class.*
- *Be constantly alert to pressures in one's outside life that may creep into the classroom.*
- *Do not overcommit. It is better to say "no" to teaching a class than to teach it poorly.*

Summary

To teach effectively, educators must decide what kind of instructor they want to become; they must possess a teaching philosophy; and they need to be able to identify attributes of effective teachers. A clear understanding of the definition and characteristics of *professionalism* can help to clarify one's long-term career goals of becoming an effective, and maybe even an extraordinary, educator. Having a good grasp of (1) how being professional also means being ethical, and (2) how striving for excellence is essential, helps to guide educators along their journey. Moreover, an understanding of the concepts of *novel* and *useful* teaching strategies can help instructors to focus on what they need to be doing along the way. Finally, periodic review and contemplation of the attributes of an effective instructor—and the negative characteristics—help one to develop into the best instructor that one can become.

Glossary

charlatan Persons who claim knowledge or skill that they do not possess.

mentor An experienced person guiding a less experienced person toward a goal.

philosophy of education A personal statement that reflects the educator's beliefs and attitudes about their approach to education.

rubric A structured grading tool that outlines specific assignment criteria and the value assigned if each is completed.

scholarship High standards and/or quality of academic achievement.

References

1. National Highway Transportation Safety Administration, National Emergency Medical Services Education Standards (2009, January). Department of Transportation, HS 811 077A, (p. 53).
2. Swick, H. M. (2000). Toward a normative definition of medical professionalism. *Academic Medicine, 75*, 612–616.
3. Blumenthal, D. (1994). The vital role of professionalism in health care reform. *Health Affairs, 13*(Part I), 252–256.
4. Cruess, R. L., & S. R. (1997). Professionalism must be taught. *British Medical Journal, 315*, 1674–1677.
5. Hensel, W. A., & Dicky, N. W. (1998). Teaching professionalism: Passing the torch. *Academic Medicine, 73*, 865–870. Abstract.
6. Relman, A. S. (1998). Education to defend professional values in the new corporate age. *Academic Medicine, 73*, 1229–1233. Abstract.
7. Reynolds, P. P., (1994). Reaffirming professionalism through the education community. *Annals of Internal Medicine, 120*, 609–614.
8. Swick, H. M. (1998). Academic medicine must deal with the clash of business and professional values. *Academic Medicine, 73*, 751. Abstract.
9. Swick, H. M., & Simpson, D. E. (1995). Fostering the professional development of medical students. *Teaching and Learning in Medicine, 7*, 55–60.
10. Wynia, M. K., Latham, S. R., Kao, A. C., Berg, J. W., & Emanuel, L. L. (1999). Medical professionalism in society. *New England Journal of Medicine, 341*, 1612–1616.
11. Sullivan, W. M. (1995). *Work and integrity: The crisis and promise of professionalism in America*. New York, NY: Harper Collins.
12. Southon, G., & Braithwaite, J. (1998). The end of professionalism? *Social Science and Medicine, 46*, 23–28.
13. Brookfield, S. D. (2006). *The skillful teacher: On technique, trust, and responsiveness in the classroom* (2nd ed.). San Francisco, CA: Jossey–Bass (p. 24).
14. Lindeman, E. C. (1926). *The meaning of adult education* (1961 ed.). New York, NY: New Republic (p. 33).
15. Zinn, L. M. (2004). Exploring your philosophical orientation. In: M. W. Galbraith (Ed.), *Adult learning methods* (pp. 39–74). Malabar, FL: Krieger Publishing.
16. Royse, D. (2001). *Teaching tips for college and university instructors*. Boston, MA: Allyn & Bacon.
17. Pratt, D. D. (2004). Ethical reasoning in teaching adults. In: M. W. Galbraith (Ed.), *Adult learning methods: A guide for effective instruction* (3rd ed.). Malabar, FL: Krieger (p. 173).
18. Schwenk, T. L., & Whitman, N. (1987). *The physician as teacher*. Baltimore, MD: Williams & Wilkins.
19. Kestin, J. (1970). Creativity in teaching and learning. *American Science, 58*, 250–257.
20. Stein, M. I. (1974). *Stimulating creativity*. Vol 1: *Individual procedures*. New York, NY: Academic Press.
21. Whiting, C. S. (1958). *Creative thinking*. New York, NY: Reinhold Press.
22. Chickering, A. W., & Gamson, Z. F. (1987). Seven principles for good practice in undergraduate education. *American Association of Higher Education (AAHE) Bulletin. 39*, 3–7.
23. American Society for Healthcare Engineering (ASHE) Higher Education Report (2007). Community college faculty: Overlooked and undervalued. *ASHE Higher Education Report* (Vol. 32, pp. 1–161).
24. Lumpkin, A. (2009). Follow the yellow brick road to a successful professional career in higher education. *The Educational Forum, 73*, 200–214.
25. Reybold, L. E. (2005). Surrendering the dream: Early career conflict and faculty dissatisfaction thresholds. *Journal of Career Development, 32*(2), 107–121.
26. Caffarella, R., & Zinn, L. F. (1999). Professional development for faculty: A conceptual framework for barriers and supports. *Innovative Higher Education, 23*(4), 241–254.

2

EMS Educator Roles

We teach to change the world. The hope that undergirds our efforts to help students learn is that doing this will help them act toward each other and their environment with compassion, understanding, and fairness. — Brookfield, 1995

The roles of EMS educators encompass far more than simply teaching students in classrooms and practical laboratories. EMS educators must have a thorough understanding of the broader scope of educator responsibilities, one of which is teaching with a team mentality. Although an educator may spend considerable time as the only instructor in the classroom, a team approach to EMS education is essential in EMS education programs as hospital and field personnel play important roles in paramedic education. The team approach also enriches the quality and breadth of EMS learning experiences. To facilitate a team approach to teaching, it is important to identify the common titles and roles of the other team members and assure that they are fully committed and involved in the educational process.

CHAPTER GOAL: This chapter explores EMS educator roles and responsibilities.

EMS EDUCATOR SPECIFIC ROLES

Nearly every higher level institution and almost all larger EMS education programs have EMS educators filling all or most of the positions listed below; however, in many moderately sized or smaller programs, several positions may be combined. All of the EMS educator specific roles fall into four broad general categories:

Program Director: The EMS educator with overall responsibility for the program. The program director is accountable to the institutional administrators, state agencies, accreditation bodies, and students. The program director is ultimately responsible for getting the program approved (authorized) by the institution, the state or local regulatory agencies, and the accreditation body, when necessary. The program director is responsible for securing the facility, equipment, supplies, instructors, clinical and field training sites, and funding. The program director is also responsible for selecting and evaluating faculty, assuring the quality of the instruction, and complying with all regulatory and accreditation standards.

Program Medical Director: The physician responsible for medical oversight of the program, thus reviewing and approving the curriculum, monitoring, either directly or indirectly, the quality of instruction, and assuring terminal competency through monitoring testing and program evaluation.

Primary Instructor: A person who possesses the appropriate academic or allied health credentials, an understanding of the principles and theories of education, and the required teaching experience necessary to provide quality instruction to students.

Secondary Instructor: A person who possesses the appropriate academic or allied health credentials and an understanding of the principles and theories of education, and who may have *limited* teaching experience. Secondary instructors are responsible for assisting primary instructors and providing instruction to students. In some situations, they may be responsible for lab exercises in which students practice psychomotor skills. The secondary instructor may even conduct classes on specific topics within his or her realm of expertise. The teaching skills that the secondary instructor possesses determine his or her specific responsibilities within the classroom. In some programs the faculty member in this role is defined as adjunct or contract instructor.

Other instructor roles that may be found in an EMS education program depend on the size, nature, and resources of the institution that offers the training. These roles are often combined in smaller programs. They may include:

Program or Course Coordinator: The educator responsible for all program logistics, such as scheduling facilities, assuring ready and properly staged equipment, assuring adequate available supplies, scheduling secondary instructors, as well as seeing that all other routine functions of the program operate smoothly. In many programs, these responsibilities fall within the responsibility of the program director.

Lecturer: A content expert who presents didactic instruction in traditional instructional settings.

Practical Lab Instructors: Expert field and hospital practitioners, for example, experienced paramedics, nurses, or other health professionals who teach in laboratory settings, most often in psychomotor-skills labs, and practical scenarios.

Clinical Coordinator: The person who schedules and tracks hospital and other clinical-training rotations, communicates with clinical programs, and monitors student clinical progress.

Field Coordinator: The person who schedules and tracks field EMS rotations, communicates with field clinical programs, and monitors student field clinical progress.

Preceptor *(or Field Training Officer)*: Practicing paramedics or other health professionals who teach EMS students in the hospital or field clinical setting by (1) demonstrating clinical procedures, (2) coaching the performance of clinical procedures through increasing stages of competency, (3) evaluating clinical performance, and (4) determining or recommending terminal competency. (See Chapter 19: Tools for Field and Clinical Learning for additional information.)

The National Association of State EMS Officials (NASEMSO) provides slightly modified definitions of EMS instructor roles and qualifications in a National EMS Education Standards transition document **(Table 2.1)**.[1]

Responsibilities of the Program Director

The program director represents a specific category of instructor. The Committee on Accreditation of Educational Programs for the Emergency Medical Services Professions (CoAEMSP) has set the following responsibilities and qualifications for EMS program directors.

Responsibilities: The program director must be responsible for all aspects of the program, including, but not limited to the following:

- The administration, organization, and supervision of the educational program
- The continuous quality review and improvement of the educational program
- Long-range planning and ongoing development of the program

Table 2.1 NASEMSO EMS Instructor Roles

Role	Expectations	Experience	Education/Licensure
Program Director	Administrate, plan, coordinate, develop curricula, supervise	Director/Manager 2 years of field experience EMS instructional experience	Degree from post-secondary school Education degree
Lead Faculty	Deliver content, skills instruction, remediation	2 years of field experience Experience in other instructional role	Postsecondary degree Instructional methods education
Adjunct Faculty (Subject-matter expert/content expert)	Deliver targeted content, skills instruction	1 year of experience at level taught or in specific discipline	High school diploma
Assistant Instructor	Skills instruction	1 year of experience at level taught	High school diploma

Adapted from NASEMSO, 2011

- The effectiveness of the program and the systems that are in place to demonstrate the effectiveness of the program
- Cooperative involvement with the medical director
- Adequate controls to assure the quality of the delegated responsibilities

Qualifications: CoAEMSP requires that program directors meet specific education and experience qualifications. They suggest that the program director:

- Possess a minimum of an associate's degree for advanced emergency medical technician instruction and a minimum of a bachelor's degree when teaching a paramedic program from a regionally accredited institution of higher education;
- Have appropriate medical or allied health education, training, and experience;
- Be knowledgeable about methods of instruction, testing, and evaluation of students;
- Have field experience in the delivery of out-of-hospital emergency care;
- Have academic training and preparation related to Emergency Medical Services at least equivalent to that of program graduates;
- Be currently certified in the United States to practice out-of-hospital care, and currently certified by a nationally recognized certifying organization at an equal or higher level of professional training than that for which training is being offered;
- Be knowledgeable concerning current national curricula, national accreditation, national registration, and the requirements for state certification or licensure.[2]

The program director and primary instructor may be the same person in a small program. Typically the program director has a reduced teaching load to address the many demands of running the program that are not associated with the direct duties of teaching.

Responsibilities of the Primary (Lead) Instructor

The primary EMS instructor may be called upon to provide leadership or supervision over a series of courses, or even over an entire EMS education program. Additionally, he or she may be called upon to provide the coordination of individual courses within a program.

Frequently, primary instructors are responsible for documenting student progress and course work progression. They have a responsibility to provide timely feedback to students concerning their progress toward successful completion of the courses. In some circumstances, student progress and feedback (with the student's written permission) may be shared with others, such as the student's employer, parents, or sponsors. This information may not be shared with anyone without a student's specific written permission. (See Chapter 10: Legal Issues for EMS Educators.)

Course coordination, an important role of primary instructors, may include coordinating guest instructors, or special-topics instructors, and scheduling and supervising all secondary instructors. Moreover, the primary instructor is most often responsible for guiding the development, maintenance, and assignment of clinical rotations and field internship rotations.

The primary instructor, when serving in the capacity of a program or course director, may also be chiefly responsible for the development of policies and procedures for courses or for the program. Course and program policies may govern activities such as the selection and screening of students, student discipline, course or program evaluation, and responses to data regarding outcomes such as pass rates, employer feedback, and feedback from graduates.

Additionally, the primary instructor is often asked to identify sources of disciplinary problems and to suggest solutions. In such situations, he or she must be able to work closely with the medical director, institutional administrator, other faculty, and students to resolve problems in the classroom or clinical setting.

Finally, primary instructors are frequently involved in determining the need or type of remedial instruction students will receive or be required to undergo, and they may also be involved in providing the remedial instruction themselves. Thus, they must be able to assess both the students and their situations to identify the root causes of problems, and then be able to develop workable strategies to help the students succeed.

Responsibilities of the Secondary Instructor

The roles of secondary instructors are defined by the primary instructor. Their scope of assigned responsibilities usually involves direct teaching in the classroom and labs, and may extend to clinicial instruction in the hospital and the field. The two main responsibilities of secondary instructors are to provide instruction to students and to support primary instructors as needed and assigned. Secondary instructors may be required to possess only entry-level teaching competencies and are often not expected to perform with the same proficiency as the program's more "experienced" instructors. Because the primary instructor often sets the tone for the class, the secondary instructor must be aware of course expectations, acceptable presentation styles, and both formal and informal "rules and regulations" that have been established by the primary instructor for the class. The optimal relationship between the primary and the secondary instructor is one in which mentoring and professional growth take place for both individuals **(Figure 2.1)**.

In summary, the primary instructor has overall responsibility for the learning experience. Together, primary and secondary instructors are expected to work as a team to deliver the curriculum, mentor and support each other, and assure the program and the students continually strive to meet high standards. The breadth of responsibility assigned to both levels of instructors reinforces the need for participation in a program of teaching instruction before one enters the field of education.

Continuing Education and Service-Based Educators

Another category of instructor is the continuing education (CE) (also referred to as "in-house" or "service-based") instructor. While the responsibilities of a CE instructor versus an instructor teaching entry-level EMS programs are very similar, the focus of content and the stressors of the classroom are very different. Entry-level program instructors must teach according to national education standards. Typically, they are preparing students for an independent third-party examination. These examinations reference questions and skills to nationally accepted standards and are not focused on local protocols. Entry-level instructors must be very familiar with the National EMS Education Standards[3] as well as the content of the major certification courses: Advanced Cardiac Life Support, Pediatric Advanced Life Support, Basic Life Support, and Prehospital Trauma Life Support, or International Trauma Life Support as examples. CE and service-based instructors focus on local protocols, identified system-quality problems, and state recertification or relicensure requirements as well as new equipment, drugs, and evidence-based changes in practice. Monitoring peer-reviewed publications to identify current research relevant to prehospital emergency care helps the CE instructor teach according to current scientific evidence.

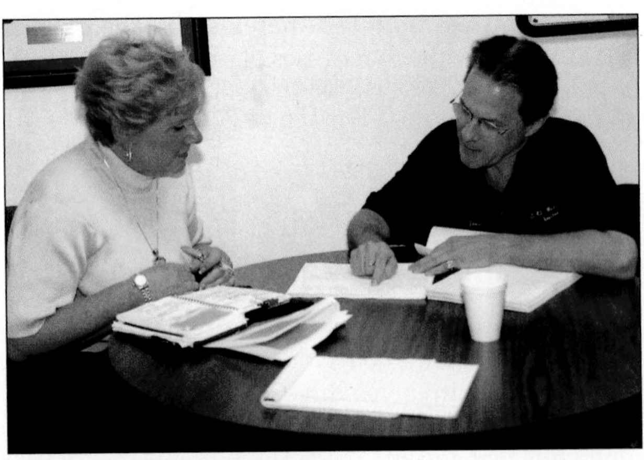

Figure 2.1
Mentoring a new instructor is a rewarding experience for both primary and secondary instructors.

CE instructors are often tasked with assuring continued competence of employees. They must ensure that employees, or other EMS professionals for whom they are accountable, maintain minimum education requirements for relicensure and for other critical competencies identified within their system. Additionally, in-house and some CE instructors are responsible for introducing information related to new standards of care, new policies, and new equipment within their system, and to verify that each person has mastered the knowledge and skill associated with them. Often the in-house instructor is also assigned to remediate employees when the internal quality-improvement process identifies deficiencies in their knowledge or skill.

Institutional instructors typically do not have the added pressure of having to instruct as well as test their fellow employees. This can be an unexpected source of stress if not addressed well before the beginning of the course. It is important that management, instructional staff, and students have clearly defined expectations addressing successful completion prior to the start of the in-house courses and education activities.

Student Expectations of Educators

Erving Goffman wrote extensively about student expectations of educators and the ways that educators can sabotage themselves by failing to meet these expectations. The following information about role expectations is adapted from his work.[4]

All EMS students have certain reasonable expectations of their instructors. Since every new and seasoned educator was once a student and is likely to return to that role time and again, it would seem that he or she would have a solid understanding of student expectations. However, when one is taking on the role of educator, it is always helpful to reflect on those basic expectations that students have and keep them in mind when preparing to enter the classroom (**Table 2.2**).

The educator's level of experience, training, and position give the educator a different worldview than that of his or her students. In accordance with this, educators are generally expected to suppress their feelings and to convey a professional demeanor that is stoic, pleasant, and welcoming. This is similar to the expectation that the caregiver will comfort a dying patient by touching the patient's hand and saying something such as, "We are going to do everything that we can to take good care of you."

Educators have many modalities for expressing themselves and conveying their role in addition to the words that they speak. Facial expressions, posture, and tone of voice and inflection are just as powerful, or even more powerful, in communicating the educator's attitude and in setting the tone for the course as the instructor's words. The expressive repertoire also includes the insignias of office or rank, uniforms or clothing, age, and grooming. Just as the EMT dresses in uniform for quick identification and acceptance by patients, so should the EMS educator dress for respect and professionalism.

Students expect educators to have the ability to communicate the course content. Educators can spoil the impression they want to make by forgetting content, appearing nervous or self-conscious, or giving way to inappropriate outbursts of laughter or anger. Additionally, students expect their instructors to provide them up front with an uncomplicated and straightforward view of the course and all essential materials.

Table 2.2	Student Expectations
Professionalism	A calm, pleasant, and stoic demeanor A positive and welcoming attitude Appropriate appearance and conduct, even in settings other than the formal classroom or learning laboratory
Competence	Ability to clearly communicate content and ideas, expressing complex and difficult concepts in ways that make them understandable and memorable Ability to demonstrate skills
Investment in student success	Positive, encouraging attitude that shows that learning can be achieved

Educators can sabotage themselves in a number of ways in trying to establish their role and authority within the classroom. Most notably, students easily sense when an educator is not personally invested in their success; they may react negatively to the educator's perceived indifference. Moreover, students neither expect nor need their educators to be on the same social plane that they are on. Thus, an educator's appearance and manner should set him or her apart from students. Confusion is likely to occur if instructors *appear* to have greater professional status than their students but *act* in an equalitarian, intimate, or even apologetic manner.

Students expect educators to behave as educators at all times. Educators are never "offstage" or "off-the-record" when students are present. Educators must be aware of the environments, or regions, in which they perform their roles. Front regions, such as classrooms and offices, are areas where educators perform formal roles for the observation of their students. But even in back regions, such as hallways, faculty lounges, and out-of-class community settings, where educators may wish to relax and express their "true feelings," they must remember that they are always subject to student expectations and are never truly offstage. The *Case in Point* on page 24 demonstrates how a primary instructor and a teaching assistant violated the boundary expectations between students and instructors.

Educator Responsibilities

Many new educators assume that the bulk of their time will be spent in preparing and delivering lectures. The reality is that educators have many additional duties and must have the skills and characteristics to adapt to these other responsibilities. Although it is true that whenever an instructor teaches a new class, he or she can expect to dedicate considerable time and effort toward the preparation and delivery of course materials, this "advance" work will decrease each time the class is taught. Additional administrative duties and responsibilities will generally increase and expand and will increasingly consume a large part of the educator's time.

Preparing for the Class

Good teaching appears effortless. This is true in performances in sports, the arts, and clinical care. Professional competence is smooth and seamless. Amateurish performances appear jerky and look extremely difficult.

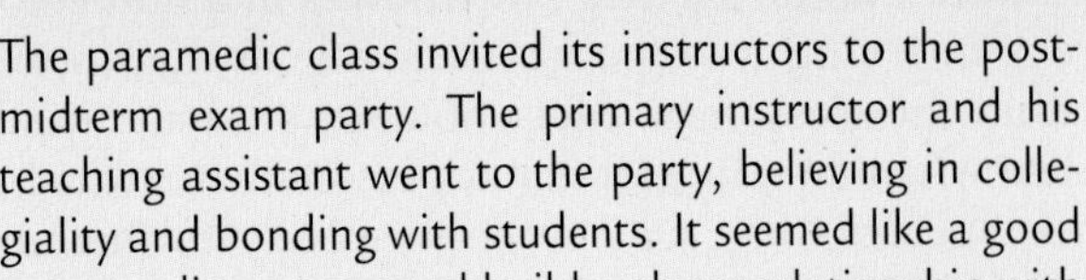

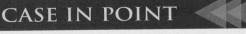

The paramedic class invited its instructors to the post-midterm exam party. The primary instructor and his teaching assistant went to the party, believing in collegiality and bonding with students. It seemed like a good way to relieve stress and build a closer relationship with the class.

However, one student at a distant table and out of sight of the instructors, began drinking straight shots of whiskey between beers and started to become intoxicated. Two other students, sitting near the instructors, were becoming argumentative over a personal matter. The lead instructor maintained his composure and suggested that they hold off on any arguments while the party was going on. The two students looked at him and resented what they perceived as a look of disapproval. A third student, an attractive young woman, began openly flirting with the teaching assistant, who was flattered and enjoyed the attention but kept his professional bearing and dismissed the attention with just an innocent smile. After all, it was just a harmless party. It was time to relax.

Everyone left an hour later and drove home. None of the students should have been behind the wheel of an automobile. Fortunately, there were no accidents, and no traffic violations were received.

Three days later, the lead instructor was called into the dean's office and was confronted about the party. "I understand that you went out and socialized with the class after the midterm exam. Is that correct?"

"Yes, it is," the lead instructor responded, growing nervous. "Is something wrong? Did something happen?"

The dean leaned forward with hands on his desk and spoke in a very deliberate and controlled voice. "Yes. Something happened. You drank socially with some underage students. You were involved in an argument between two students. You have a complaint filed against you and your teaching assistant for inappropriate conduct. You have very likely compromised your ability to lead this class any further. At minimum, you have compromised your ability to keep this class on a professional plane. You will need to write a letter of explanation to be considered by the faculty review committee. I do not know what the outcome will be."

No formal action was ever taken. The verbal warning was sufficient. It was a hard lesson. The educator is always on stage and is never on the same social plane as the students.

Dr. Harry Wong's Tips for the First Days of School[5]

1. Greet students "honestly" and with energy
2. Begin with an activity to facilitate name learning
3. Have info (policies, outlines, etc.) posted or ready to hand out
4. Give class the idea that you are a person
5. Give them your expectations, rules, and class policies
6. Have an activity planned to give them a feel for what is ahead
7. Establish good control
8. Know (a) What you are doing; (b) Your classroom procedures; and (c) Your professional responsibilities
9. Know positive and high expectations come from ATTITUDE
10. Create a classroom climate both for your students and yourself
11. Celebrate the first day of school
12. Dress appropriately and professionally to model success
13. Use your students' names and correct pronunciations
14. Practice effective classroom management—FROM THE BEGINNING
15. Initiate a task-oriented and predictable environment
16. Have your classroom ready
17. Stress large-group organization and student procedures
18. Make first assignment on first day interesting, short, easy, and successful
19. Two things important to state: your name and your expectations
20. Teach student behaviors: (a) discipline; (b) procedures; (c) routines
21. Have a hard copy of your plan and follow it (discipline plan)
22. Introduce discipline plan on the first day of school; post it and give a copy to each student
23. Spend more time discussing consequences than rules
24. Consequences should be reasonable and logical
25. Communicate your discipline plan effectively (tell students why the rules are needed)
26. Establish your procedures

How do those professional athletes, musicians, and clinicians make their performances look so easy? They prepare in advance with countless hours of practice and preparation. To achieve the appearance of effortless and smooth instruction, the educator needs to prepare a game plan and build a resource collection well in advance of the first class session.

CASE IN POINT

It was just another day of the week. The ECG rhythm class was from 8:00 AM to 10:00 AM. The materials and handouts were ready. The lab was scheduled from 10:00 AM to noon, so equipment had to be set up early that morning, a task that the teaching assistant handled. A curriculum committee meeting was planned to take place over lunch. The state conference was in three months; the objectives, description, and handouts were due next week. Cardiac case scenarios were scheduled for this afternoon; they needed to be pulled from last year. The cardiac module exam was Friday, and it still had to be finalized and printed. The exam needed to be reviewed and weak questions that scored low point biserial item discriminators and homogenous distractors had to be "switched out" or improved. Student evaluations from the respiratory module had just been reviewed and summarized. Two students failed the respiratory exam and needed counseling and remediation. The county EMS Council is to meet from 7:00 to 9:00 this evening to discuss the latest legislative initiative to cut funding. It is a critical meeting that cannot be missed. The local EMS chief had just called to say that one of the internship students did not know the local protocols and was rude about it when confronted. The student was sent home and was not welcome back. A vendor stopped in to demonstrate the latest in spinal immobilization equipment.

It was 7:00 AM, and the alarm had just gone off. It was just another day in the life of an EMS educator.

Developing Adjunct Materials to Stimulate Class Discussion and Learning

It is helpful for the instructor to have preplanned scenarios, discussion topics, activities, and quizzes that have been developed and made available well before the first class meets. These adjunct materials should support and coordinate lessons that are being taught. Audiovisual materials, for example, can be used to support lectures and presentations, but they may take a surprising amount of time to develop. The Internet is an excellent source for images, but use of these images requires that the educator must have the resources to scan existing photographs or download and edit videos. Creating a file of supporting classroom activities for each block of course material is time intensive but worthwhile. Each year it should be revisited to ensure that the content is keeping pace with current evidence-based practice.

Ordering and Operating Equipment

A surprising amount of time and effort can go into ordering, maintaining, and cleaning equipment. Anything that can be done to help minimize this work, time, and energy spent will be helpful. For instance, an instructor may set up a routine for periodic ordering of new supplies and equipment; assign students to help clean, repair, and move equipment and supplies on a schedule; and acquire adequate room to store, organize, and maintain the equipment (**Figure 2.2**).

Developing Class Materials and Handouts

Nearly every accredited higher education institution formally credits full-time educators with three hours of work, or activities, for each hour of instruction. The two extra hours are for preparatory and follow-up times. Preparation includes reviewing the material to be taught in advance and keeping up with current practices and literature, as well as a period of time for mental preparation, as it is educationally unsound to "just walk in cold" to present as an instructor. Follow-up time includes returning equipment and supplies, meeting with students to answer questions, and grading assignments. Adjunct instructors, those not working as full time educators with the institution, are often paid a flat rate for each hour they teach. For the adjuncts, the 3:1 hourly rate is included in the

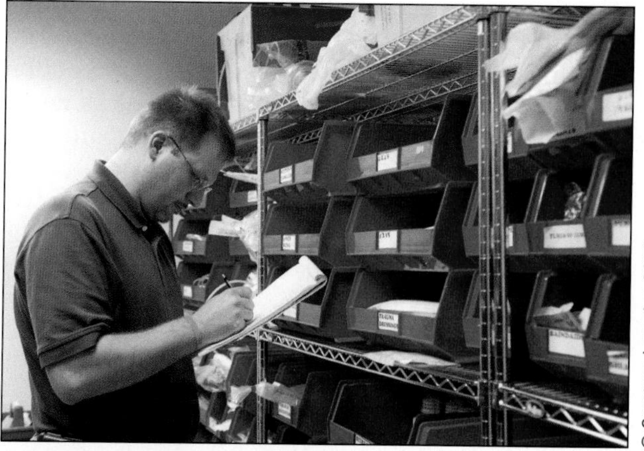

Figure 2.2

The instructor may need to assume responsibility for ordering equipment and supplies.

flat hourly rate for teaching. Tasks associated with developing and maintaining class instructional materials and handouts should take much more time than it takes to deliver the material. It is essential that the educator schedule sufficient time for this work every semester. For the first time that one is teaching a class, a good rule of thumb is to schedule at least three times as much time for preparation as for instruction. After the first time, it may be sufficient to schedule one hour of preparation for each hour of instruction. However, instructors who teach the same lecture with the same materials year after year eventually find themselves the object of student scorn. Updates and revisions are essential, particularly in the health care field.

Participating in Professional Activities

It is critically important that educators participate in professional activities outside the educational organization. Professional associations and conferences provide an excellent way for educators to stay current both in content-related areas and in new teaching methods and strategies. In addition, professional networking can contribute significantly to a program's success through the sharing of resources and ideas. Every EMS educator should consider joining local, state, and national EMS educator associations.

Teaching the Class

The role of today's teacher involves much more than showing up and delivering a "canned" lesson. Teaching to promote maximal student learning is a planned, purposeful event that includes consideration of advanced assignments, appropriate content delivery methods, student-centered learning activities, and evaluation methods. Once the plan is determined, the instructor must coordinate assembly of appropriate resources to execute the lab, lecture, discussion, evaluation, or other activity that is planned. The first time an instructor prepares a new lesson often takes hours of planning. And the planning is never finished. The instructor must diligently prepare each time the lesson is repeated and make revisions based on (1) effectiveness of prior strategies; (2) new knowledge, equipment, or evidence that alters content; or (3) the learning needs of the specific students within the current classroom.

Organizing and Leading Discussion Sessions

It is important that a portion of each class be devoted to discussion of the curriculum. Two of the most valuable and effective ways of achieving this are (1) to start each lecture or session with a brief overview of the learning objectives, and (2) to follow each session with a brief summary of the key learning points. (See Part IV: Delivering the Message, Chapters 11-19, for a more in-depth look at teaching methods.) As has been mentioned previously, developing an engaging discussion that prompts students to share their ideas and views is a time-consuming but worthy investment of time.

Preparing for Lab Procedures and Assignments

In EMS clinical education, practical sessions, or "labs," tend to account for approximately half of the total amount of time spent in the course. These should include practical skills workshops, patient assessment exercises, and patient care scenarios. Developing labs is just as time intensive as developing lectures. Preparing for invasive labs, such as intravenous and medication administration workshops, generally takes much more time than inexperienced educators may imagine. Instructors should allow enough time to obtain and set up the necessary equipment and supplies, and to schedule and brief any secondary instructors. If secondary instructors are paid employees, then additional recruitment and hiring time may be needed. The hiring and orientation process can take months in some cases.

When simulation is used in the lab setting, additional advanced planning is needed to assure that the appropriate cases are developed to meet the objectives. If live patients are used for simulation, models will need to be coached prior to the education setting to accurately portray the desired patient situation. In addition, simulated physical injuries or conditions may need to be moulaged prior to the lab session. If a high-fidelity manikin is used, selected vital signs and patient findings may be preprogrammed. Lab simulations are developed to meet specific higher-level learning objectives. Clear direction should be provided regarding the setting, patient presentation, treatment expectations, and patient outcomes based on either optimal or poor treatment. The lab session should be linked to the content so students recognize that specific higher objectives are being practiced or assessed. (See Chapter 18: Tools for Simulation.)

Developing and Grading Tests

The development of valid tests is a highly specialized skill. A great deal of time, energy, and expense goes into ensuring that a test is valid. (See Part V: Student Evaluation, for more information on evaluation.) The test should be based on the desired learning outcomes and on the content that has been presented to meet those objectives. There should be a clear link between the standards, the objectives, the content, and the assessment. The educator should ensure that the right number of questions, at the right level of Bloom's taxonomy, are assessed for any given topic. Asking only recall questions that depend on rote memory will not serve an EMS student well when the outcomes require higher levels of performance. Most EMS educators develop their own bank of test questions from which to generate their tests. Although this saves considerable time, the high stakes examinations must be validated and updated.

Reviewing for Tests

It is common in EMS education for educators to conduct review sessions before tests are given. However, students rarely come to these review sessions prepared with questions. To avoid teaching directly to the test, the instructor might require that only student questions will be answered during the review. Another alternative would be to consider preparing a number of challenging applied-patient problems for students to discuss. In this way, the instructor will be able to give the students a thorough review without giving away the specific material included on the test.

Evaluating Student Performance

It is time consuming for the educator to develop fair and effective criteria for grading student performance. Developing grading criteria is more of a process than a single event, and the educator should never stop trying to improve the evaluation process. Good educators have multiple performance references to use in evaluating their students' performance—participation, test scores, practical skills scores, projects, and scenario testing, for example. Developing, reevaluating, refining, recording, and providing feedback on these different reference points takes time and effort. The State of EMS Education Research Project (SEERP)[6] found it troubling that attendance was used as a factor in measuring student performance by over half of the educators who were surveyed. Attendance alone does not indicate competency. Grading should be structured to measure student achievement of specific, measurable, learning outcomes. The instructor should communicate results of student evaluation to students confidentially and in a timely manner to allow them the opportunity to adjust their performance if necessary.

Improving Performance through Evaluation (Feedback)

The EMS educator has the responsibility and capacity to assure a positive and constructive learning environment. While students and educators may complain about aspects of the program, spending time listening to their criticisms with an open mind and communicating to them the importance placed on their complaints, the educators are able to channel the energy in the program toward an open dialogue and ultimate program improvement. Students are typically focused on their goal of passing the course.

Teaching Psychomotor Skills

When a competent instructor demonstrates and explains procedures, most students readily comprehend them and feel comfortable with what they have seen. However, that does not mean that most students will be able to perform the procedure themselves. Teaching students a procedure requires that each step be broken down, demonstrated, explained, and followed as soon as possible by student performance of each step with careful monitoring and coaching. Once students master the steps, they should be coached through several complete sequences. Finally, they should be given the chance to perform the skill in the context of patient care scenarios.

Administrative Tasks and Duties

Although the primary role of an instructor is to be in the classroom or clinical or field setting, administrative tasks comprise an essential secondary function. The number of administrative tasks assigned to instructors depends on their position and the type of teaching setting. The program director is often tasked with the greatest number of administrative duties; however, each instructor has essential duties in this area.

Holding Instructor Meetings

Departmental meetings, whether formal or informal, are a necessary part of staying connected with the broader picture **(Figure 2.3)**. The educator should eagerly participate in faculty meetings, as curriculum development and educational design are best accomplished collaboratively. Sharing information about student progress and performance is also important, so that problems can be identified and a plan of action initiated. Collaboration with fellow instructors can ensure that key content areas are being reinforced throughout the curriculum. Additionally, clinical issues or procedures may need to be reviewed together to promote instructor consistency.

Developing a Budget

Education is a business. Facilities, instructional materials, and instructors cost money. Sources of revenue are required to fund an educational program. Thus, developing and maintaining a budget is a significant

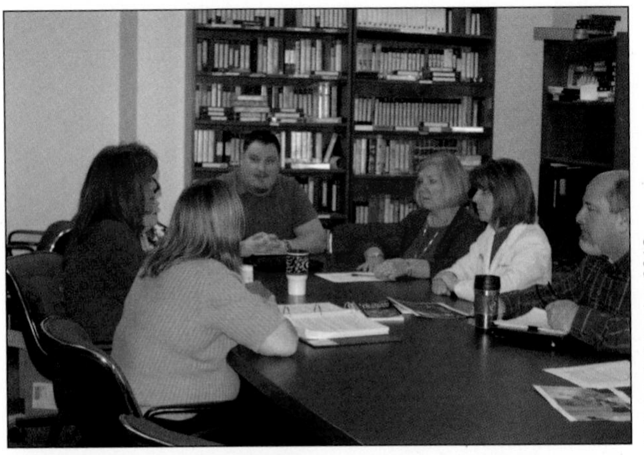

Figure 2.3

It is important to hold faculty meetings to discuss important topics, such as student progress, curriculum development, and exam item development.

part of the education administrator's responsibilities. This often means seeking out external sources of funding, such as grants and donations. Each instructor has a role in budget accountability by using resources carefully, monitoring student class size to ensure that an excess number of faculty have not been scheduled, and documenting expenses accurately.

Evaluating Personnel

Scheduling times for evaluating and providing frequent feedback for educators and any educational support personnel is a vital and necessary part of the EMS education administrator's job. The administrator's role includes working with primary and secondary instructors to ensure that they are developing appropriate skills as educators. It may also be helpful for the administrator to periodically clarify job responsibilities.

Maintaining Departmental Records and Reports

Records of enrollment, curricula, counseling, schedules, attendance, grades, attrition, and successful completion are all critical to the educational institution. These constitute fundamental legal documentation. Reports to various agencies are also required and may seem endless. The Committee on Accreditation of EMS Professions (CoAEMSP) requires documentation of student progress and evaluation in all areas of the program. Additionally CoAEMSP requires an annual report from accredited programs to document their outcome evaluation of the program's success toward achievement of program goals and objectives. These documents are also significant in helping with and supporting future decisions, such as justifying the hiring of additional staff or the purchase of more equipment.

Attending Committee Meetings

In addition to the vital role of teaching, most educators in academic institutions are expected to improve the overall environment of the organization and the community. This includes serving on a variety of educational committees whose work can range from long-term curriculum development to admissions, to academic affairs of the college, and to handling student grievances.

Attending Advisory Committee Meetings

All EMS programs, especially paramedic programs, should have an advisory committee that meets at least annually. The advisory committee should have representatives from all segments of the community in which the EMS program operates. Individuals involved on an advisory committee should include representatives of employers of graduates, hospital personnel, regulatory agency representatives, graduates, members of the local medical community, current student representatives, and consumers. Program personnel, such as program director or course coordinator and medical director, as well as program faculty, are also included but are usually *ex officio* members. Specifically, the goal of the advisory committee is to make recommendations for improvement and to provide feedback on the program and on how it is meeting the community's EMS educational needs. Difficult program challenges, such as requesting major funding for capital investments and recommendations for changes in admission requirements, are more likely to succeed and are often less contentious when put forward with advisory-committee involvement.

Programs seeking CoAEMSP accreditation will be required to show input from their advisory committees as part of their accreditation reporting. All programs should have at least annual advisory-board, or committee, meetings. Program directors should strive to make the membership of the advisory committee representative of all stakeholders as defined in CoAEMSP standards. Two groups often overlooked are students in the program and the lay public.

Participating In State and Local Rule-making Committees

Educators who do not participate in their EMS regulatory committees at the local, state, or national level lose their ability to effectively voice their concerns and opinions on many vital issues. Also, most, if not all, accredited higher-education institutions place great value on involvement with national, state, and regional leadership, regulatory and accreditation agencies and activities. Further, regulators, who do not have the involvement of the educators, when they are developing regulations, may adopt rules that are inappropriate or that present great problems to the educational programs that otherwise might have been avoided.

Maintaining Clinical Expertise

A difficult task, particularly for full-time educators, is maintaining clinical competency. Although educators can attend classes or read journals to keep abreast of new technology and cutting-edge content, clinical skills may be more time consuming to maintain. Often, the educator must work or volunteer part time for an EMS service to maintain patient care skills. Some academic institutions encourage instructors to work clinically by having a 35-hour work week or a 9-month contract. When possible, some educators participate actively with students in hospital and field settings, thus maintaining a level of clinical interaction.

Student Issues

Instructors must prepare to spend considerable time outside of the regular classroom time to perform other student-related duties. Time devoted to student-related issues can include meeting with students to review progress or discuss performance issues, providing referrals for life crises, motivating them toward success, or writing letters of recommendation.

Student Conferences

Some students, particularly those who are not progressing satisfactorily, need one-on-one time for feedback, tutorial help, and counseling (**Figure 2.4**). Each student should, at minimum, have the opportunity to talk with the primary instructor privately at the course midpoint to discuss his or her progress. If the student is progressing satisfactorily, this meeting can be brief. On the other hand, if the student is failing to meet minimum class standards, the educator must be prepared to give the student specific information pertaining to his or her performance deficits, along with concrete examples of how to improve this performance. Records of these meetings must be placed in students' files.

Clear guidelines regarding how to reach the instructor outside of class should be established. Students should know how and when it is appropriate to contact faculty, and how quickly a response should be expected. A back-up contact should be made available for emergency contact, particularly when students are in clinical rotations.

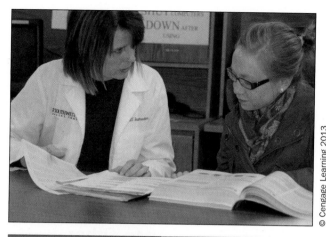

Figure 2.4

Student-teacher conferences provide students with valuable feedback about their performance.

Student Advisement

Students need routine advisement in all three domains of learning: cognitive, psychomotor, and affective. Frequent assessment of and advisement in these three domains is the gold standard programs strive for but rarely reach. While this may seem an impossible goal, there are several proven techniques that greatly increase individual and programmatic ability to advise students.

The use of grading *rubrics* is a very powerful tool. A rubric is a table that clearly defines the grading criteria for a given task. Rubrics can be used for providing feedback in all three domains. Providing feedback in the affective domain can be challenging. Using a rubric can assist the instructor and student to identify key behavioral characteristics to measure to provide feedback in the affective domain. A rubric can also be used to measure and provide feedback for scenario testing in a lab setting. The advantages of using a rubric for grading are the following:

- It clearly defines the grading criterion.
- It forces the instructor to look at all students exactly the same way.
- It makes grading much more objective.
- It allows students to select their grades and make informed decisions on where their focus should be.

- It helps eliminate the emotional aspect of grading.
- It can be done almost instantaneously.

If rubrics are developed for grading and providing feedback on all appropriate aspects of the class and program and used to review students' daily progress, advisement becomes a continuous process rather than a spot check.

There are many websites with many premade rubrics or templates to construct your own rubric. Simply typing in the search term "rubric" yields many free websites with sample grading templates.

Referring Students to Other People and Offices

Another role of the educator is to refer students to appropriate counseling resources or potential employers. The educator might refer a student to a career opportunity, to remedial classes, or for diagnostic testing, as might be the case with a student with a suspected learning disability.

Counseling Students on Personal Issues

Because the educator instills respect and trust, some students will approach their instructor for personal advice and guidance. Sometimes, even when not seeking advice and guidance, a student may bring personal issues to the instructor. Most educators spend a small part of their week dealing with student personal issues. It is paramount that the educator respect the student's feelings and confidentiality in these matters. It is also critically important that privacy is provided for these discussions. Developing a list of internal and community resources and having them readily available for making referrals is also essential. Common issues that can be expected include pregnancies, work terminations, evictions, physical abuse, personal illness, illness of a loved one, loss of financial aid, substance abuse, harassment from other students, learning disabilities, and conflicts in schedules. Knowing the institution's policies and resources on these issues goes a long way in helping the educator to determine what role to have in these issues. It is also critically important that the educator know the responsible professional limits and liabilities of acting in the role of counselor. The profession of counseling is now licensed in most states, and several levels of professional counseling licenses are available, including Licensed Mental Health Counselor and Licensed Professional Clinical Counselor. An educator who means well might offer counseling and comfort to a student who later attempts suicide or commits some violent act; the educator could be liable for practicing as a counselor without a license. The instructor must also notify the student of the limits of confidentiality. In instances where the student discloses information that represents a threat of harm to themselves or to others, the educator has an obligation to take appropriate action according to institutional policies.

Motivating Students to Complete Class Assignments

Some students do not require motivation to complete class assignments on time, but many do. The educator must take time and energy from his or her already busy schedule to devise strategies that encourage students to meet performance requirements, rather than simply nagging them to do so. Enforcing deadlines, and dealing with students who do not meet deadlines, requires time and energy initially, but pays off in the long run. Educators can include two items in the curriculum to assist this effort. First, every assignment and due date should be printed on the course syllabus that is distributed and reviewed on the first day of class. Second, the consequences of missing the deadlines must be spelled out. Many educators are very clear about the assignments in their syllabus, but do not explain the consequences of failing to complete assignments, making a faulty leap in logic that suggests that students will intuitively understand the ramifications. Finally, every student must be treated in the same way. If one student receives extra time to complete an assignment, then all other students in the class must receive the same.

Writing Letters of Reference

It is appropriate for students to request letters of reference or recommendation from their educators. An instructor may wish to set guidelines that determine what type of recommendation will be provided. Recommendation procedures should follow policies established by the school. A good place to publish these criteria is in the course syllabus. Some common requirements for letters of reference include a student's taking more than one course with the educator, earning above-average grades (generally a B or better), exhibiting positive, professional learning attitudes, not having disciplinary problems, and doing something to contribute positively to the class or program (e.g., helping with a research project or guest lecturing).

When writing a recommendation, include the following elements:

- The name of the person to whom the application is being sent. Encourage the student requesting the letter of recommendation to supply this name. Avoid addressing letters of recommendation: To whom it may concern. If the student indicates that he or she just wants a generic letter for possible future use, offer to write the letter at a later date when the student has all the appropriate information.
- When writing an academic or employment letter of recommendation, writers should first state the relationship they have to the student, including how long they knew the student and in what capacity, for example, director, advisor, instructor, or friend. Next the instructor should describe the moral character, dedication, maturity, and types of skills of the student. In an academic context, focus on ambition or desire to learn, a passion or drive for the field of teaching or clinical care, leadership skills and experiences, dedication to coursework, and so on. If the letter is for employment, focus on those attributes that indicate the student will make a good employee. Include comments on attendance, being a team member, coping with change, and self-motivation.
- The letter writer should back comments up with concrete examples, via anecdotes of how a student performed in class, on tests, in the lab, and so on. Honors and awards could be mentioned in the context of overall academic performance. Admissions committees want to see candidates who stand out from the crowd, so do not hesitate to use superlatives to describe the student. Was she the most organized in the class? Most willing to work as part of a team? Most curious? The writer should quantify such statements: "Mary was in the top 5 percent of the class when it came to lab work." Some selection committees request a ranking of the student.

A good letter of recommendation typically has several characteristics. Someone who knows the person fairly well and who is familiar with the student's academic history, personal traits, and goals should write the letter. For example, it could be a professor or other faculty member, an advisor, a college administrator, a teacher, and sometimes an employer—especially if the job or internship is related to the person's academic and career pursuits.

Academic letters of recommendation illustrate a student candidate's leadership skills, character, integrity, intellect, initiative, drive, and readiness to excel amid myriad pressures. The best reference letters present a picture of a student who is not one-dimensional, but instead, well rounded.

Advising Students on a Career

In most cases, students take EMS courses in hopes of obtaining a job. A vital part of the EMS educator's job is developing contacts within the local EMS community to help place students. Hosting career days is another way some schools meet this need. Educators must stay current on various job requirements, salaries, and employment practices. Students also seek information on further education and options for advancement and the instructor should be ready to provide information at the institution or elsewhere.

Tutoring Students

A few general approaches can be taken to providing remedial tutoring. One is to set aside time on a regular basis each week. A second ideal approach is to seek available tutorial resources within the institution or larger community. A third approach is to assign tutorial responsibilities to a secondary instructor, if one exists.

Some precautionary notes apply to providing tutoring, however. The first is to be careful to set limits on the time that services will be provided, as some students have a need that is impossible to fill. If unlimited tutoring is offered, some students will take up that offer. Not only will the educator's time be drained, but the student may still fail, and the failure becomes the responsibility of the educator. A second cautionary note is that it is best to tutor only in open groups, never by private or exclusive appointment. If in-class tutoring is not sufficient, students may be referred to fee-for-service tutoring. The program faculty should not provide this paid service as it could represent a conflict of interest.

Encouraging the Class

Nearly every class hits a slump at some point. This usually occurs about three-quarters of the way through the class. Remember that a major role of the educator is that of coach. Many educators find that they give motivational talks to nearly every class at some point, if not several points, during the class duration. If time permits, introduce a motivational or team-building activity at this point in the program. Consider inviting former graduates to return and discuss their careers. Plan graduation activities if you are nearing the end of the program. Keeping their eye on the end goal is often a strong motivator for students whose motivation is waning.

Clarifying Issues, Beliefs, and Problems

No matter how brilliant the lectures, no matter how well crafted the syllabus, key points and policies must be reiterated multiple times. This is a matter of human nature. There is no point in being despondent over the need to do this. Use diverse strategies to reinforce key material. Supplement reading and lecture with other activities such as discussion groups, games, scenarios, or case studies that allow students to integrate the knowledge in higher-level contexts. This not only increases retention, it promotes transfer of learning to the real world of EMS.

Teaching Tip >> *Anything worth saying is worth repeating three times—especially to tired, overloaded, overwhelmed students.*

Common Role Adjustments

Overall, the educator is expected to handle the teaching load and to continue on the path toward growth and scholarly excellence. Perhaps the most challenging aspect is balancing one's professional and personal lives. The second most challenging aspect is keeping one's clinical skills sharp.

The roles and expectations of the beginning EMS educator are new and very different from those of the EMS care provider. These new roles and expectations are more than just an extension of those clinical roles. They require a new set of assertive behaviors, for the power structure and length of relationships with students are completely different from those between care provider and patient. These new roles and expectations challenge and test the educator's teaching abilities.

One of the first and most important challenges facing the new educator is that of establishing authority and credibility in the classroom. After establishing authority, the educator must be able to exercise that authority prudently. This textbook and other education literature offer effective guidelines for establishing and exercising authority as an educator; however, there are no foolproof guidelines that apply in every situation. Each class, as a group, and each educator, individually, are unique.

Four characteristics of the educator help establish authority in the classroom: experience, expectations, knowledge, and goals.

Experience versus Authority

In general, an older educator relies more on teaching experience than on the authority of a title or position. Often, new educators learn the hard way that the title of "instructor" does not automatically impart esteem or credibility in a class. New instructors often learn that humility and deferential behaviors are typically more powerful with students than is authoritarian bluster. The educator's ability to deal with the thousand and one challenges of teaching far outweighs any badge of authority that goes with the title "instructor." This same phenomenon can be seen in the streets, where respect for EMS caregivers is earned through competent performance.

CASE IN POINT

The new EMS educator recently hired by the local community college had 10 years of experience in EMS and had been a practicing paramedic for seven of those last years. She was highly respected for her clinical skills, and she had a great personality to go with it. She was perfect for the instructor position at the local community college. Today was her first day in class.

She was a little nervous as she walked into class as lead instructor for the first time to face 23 students. She was more nervous than she had ever imagined she could be, realizing that she was now responsible for maintaining course continuity, covering the entire curriculum, covering for guest lecturers who did not show up, resolving disputes, counseling, providing discipline, developing and administering exams, and assigning grades. It hit her for the first time–what it meant to be the lead instructor–just as she introduced herself in her new role.

With genuine humility, a professional demeanor, and a little humor, she won over the class. She began, "Hello, this is my first day of class. You have a lot to teach me. I hope that we enjoy our journey of learning together. We're going to begin by introducing ourselves to one another. I'll start by telling you a little bit about my background, and why these folks asked me to come here to be your lead instructor."

Expectations versus Discipline

Seasoned educators inspire students to follow and obey them simply by their professional demeanor—the way that they impart their knowledge and understanding. It is this expectation of leadership and performance more than any badge of authority that will maintain order and discipline in the classroom. The seasoned instructor rarely needs to resort to disciplinary action for misconduct in the classroom. Setting high professional and academic expectations early in the course will prove to be a valuable strategy in avoiding the use of unnecessary discipline. Most caregivers have witnessed similar scenarios in the field. Crews may naturally follow a senior paramedic or EMT whom they respect, regardless of rank or title; other supervisors or chiefs become frustrated when they are unable to lead their subordinates.

Teaching Tip >> *Remember that it is always better to set high expectations at the beginning of a class, then be willing to back down a little, than to try to raise expectations later. Students will continually surprise their instructors, if given the chance to strive for high goals.*

Knowledge versus Insignia

No title, rank, or uniform will make up for a lack of content knowledge. It is hopeless for an educator to hide behind a title or position when faced with a question to which he or she does not have an answer. Seasoned educators know that students will ask questions they cannot answer. They expect these questions and honor them. Indeed, no EMS educator or any educator in any profession is expected to know every answer to every possible question. Educators who feel confident are not intimidated or threatened by questions that they cannot answer. When a question arises that they cannot immediately answer, they feel confident in telling students that they will get back to the class with the answer as soon as possible. It is also acceptable to inquire whether another student has the answer, or to assign a student to research the answer and report back to the class. Immature educators—those not yet confident in their authority or abilities—will often make up an answer or try to deflect the question. Both of these strategies leave students frustrated, and the educator's authority is undermined as a result.

Teaching Tip >> *An effective strategy in dealing with difficult questions is to address them on the first day of class. The instructor might say that occasionally students will ask a question that he or she will not be able to immediately answer. When that happens, the instructor will write the question in the corner of the blackboard, and it will stay there until, together, they find the answer to the question.*

This approach does three things. First, it validates the students' right to ask questions. Second, it keeps the instructor off the pedestal of "infallible." Lastly, it keeps the educator honest and reliable in the promise to find answers to student questions.

Goals: Firm Grasp versus Cookbook

Experienced EMS providers know what they want to accomplish for each patient, and they generally know several ways to go about it. The same is true for experienced educators. What worked in one class may not work in another. It is more important that educators have their own teaching philosophy and a clear understanding of what students need to learn than merely a series of lesson plans in cookbook fashion. The instructor should keep the educational goals in mind, and should constantly ask whether what he or she is teaching today brings him or her closer to those goals.

Summary

It is paramount that educators be well grounded and comfortable in the content that they are expected to teach. Many other issues will place demands on their time and energy, but they cannot be weak in content areas. Educators also must realize that teaching is a team sport; new instructors should actively seek out resources outside the classroom to help them address some of the issues that may otherwise overwhelm them. Secondary instructors can be a valuable addition to any class, but they may not know intuitively what to do. When an educator works with secondary instructors, the time taken to mentor them will be returned many times. Finally, new educators must seek a balance between teaching obligations and personal commitments, as well as the need to maintain current clinical skills. Attention to this balance must be a high priority and should begin on the first of day of class.

Glossary

clinical coordinator Schedules and tracks hospital and other clinical training rotations.

field coordinator Schedules and tracks field EMS rotations.

lecturer Content expert who presents selected didactic material.

practical lab instructors Persons who teach in laboratory settings.

preceptor Practicing paramedics or health professionals who instruct EMS students in hospital or field clinical setting.

primary (lead) instructor A person who is qualified to provide leadership or supervision over a series of courses or entire EMS program.

program coordinator Educator responsible for program logistics.

program director Assumes overall program responsibility.

program medical director The physician responsible for medical oversight of the program and assuring terminal competency through monitoring testing and program evaluation.

References

1. National Association of State EMS Officials (2010, December). EMS instructor qualifications. *Implementation of the National EMS Education Agenda Website.* Retrieved 08/19/2011, from http://www.nasemso.org/EMSEducationImplementationPlanning/Toolkit.asp
2. Committee on Accreditation of Education for the Emergency Medical Services Professions (2011, July). Standards and guidelines. Retrieved 08/19/2011.
3. National Highway Traffic Safety Administration (2009). *National EMS education standards.* (DOT HS 811 077A). Washington, DC: Department of Transportation.
4. Goffman, E. (1959). *Presentation of self in everyday life.* New York, NY: Anchor Books.
5. Wong, H. K., and R. T. (2009). *The first days of school: How to be an effective teacher*. Mountain View, CA: Harry K. Wong Publications
6. Ruple, J. A., Frazer, G., Hsieh, A., Bake, W., & Freel, J. (2005). The state of EMS education research project: Characteristics of EMS educators. *Prehospital Emergency Care, 9*(2), 203–212.

PART II

The Student

Emergency Medical Services (EMS) students are as different from one another as are the patients they will eventually treat. They span a spectrum from working adults looking for a second career to high school students who are still discovering themselves. They come from diverse backgrounds with varying levels of knowledge and life experience. Yet, each must grasp concepts and apply information that is often expected of physicians, anesthesiologists, social workers, and even psychiatrists.

This part of the text provides valuable information about the general attributes of today's EMS learners. Educators find that an understanding of the basic principles of education, including information about their students' various learning styles and factors of a supportive learning environment, help them meet their teaching goals and ultimately, produce effective, well-rounded EMS personnel.

Remember that EMS students are all unique individuals, each with their own strengths and weaknesses, and each deserving of respect. By respecting the individuality of each student and the strengths and weaknesses of each, we can earn and expect their respect in return.

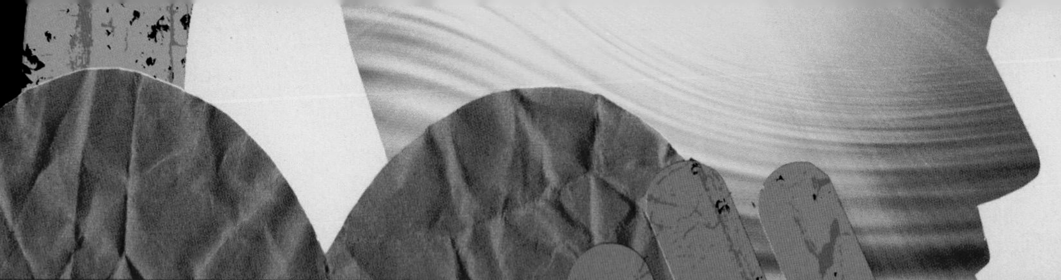

3 Principles of Adult Learning

Theories and goals of education don't matter a whit if you do not consider your students to be human beings. — Lou Ann Walker

The Emergency Medical Services (EMS) educator needs to become familiar with the principles of adult learning, since the typical EMS student is an adult. The learning styles, needs, responses, and expectations of adults differ from those of younger learners. Even when educators teach Emergency Medical Responder (EMR) or Emergency Medical Technician (EMT) courses to adolescents in high school, the instruction and learning follow more adult principles than those involved in teaching children.

An educator can develop techniques that enhance student comprehension and retention by striving to understand and incorporate basic principles regarding adult learning into his or her teaching strategies. Even in the environment of ever-evolving educational theory, several concepts regarding adult learning are commonly accepted and useful in application.

This chapter is an overview of what is known about how adults learn and retain information, which will help educators to clarify the educational needs of adult learners. The most logical place to start such a discussion is with the basic concept of adult learning, or *andragogy.*

CHAPTER GOAL: This chapter is an overview of what is known about how adults learn and retain information, which will help educators to clarify the educational needs of adult learners.

Pedagogy Versus Andragogy

In 1968, Malcolm Knowles introduced the concept of **andragogy**—the art and science of teaching adults. He used the term "andragogy" to separate adult learning principles from those centered on children, or **pedagogy**.[1] Andragogy is based on certain basic assumptions, which are examined here.

Autonomy and Self-Direction

Adults expect and enjoy independence, or a certain amount of **autonomy**, in what they learn and how they learn it. They like to have control, and they feel comfortable taking control of their learning. Moreover, for adults, learning is a process of sharing with the instructor, as well as with other students. The instructor, however, is responsible for facilitating and encouraging the student's self-direction, as opposed to simply supplying students with facts. Brookfield suggests that direction and guidance from the educator are essential because many adults actually need help in determining their learning needs.[2]

Adults approach education with the expectation of learning new skills and knowledge, and they focus on the final goal. Ultimately, they want to be well-prepared to practice competently and to pass the state or national exam. In light of this, the adult is less tolerant of wasted time and tasks that have no apparent value. In fact, educators should expect more criticism from the adult learner than from the younger learner, especially when the student feels that his or her expectations are not being met.

Problem-Centered Orientation

Adults are "relevancy oriented," which means they have a need to know *why* they are being told to learn something before they are receptive to learning it. Therefore, educators must ensure that instruction is **problem centered**, rather than subject centered. For example, paramedic students may not value the instruction in the fundamentals of human anatomy and physiology until that depth of knowledge becomes relevant to specific medical conditions and how they are encountered and treated in the field.

Life Experience

By the time a person reaches adulthood, he or she has naturally accumulated many enriching life experiences. This gives the adult learner the advantage of being able to relate new facts and concepts to real-life experiences—a fact that enhances and reinforces the adult learning experience. Because adult EMS classes typically include students with wide-ranging levels of expertise and educational backgrounds, the instructor can draw upon the experiences of those adult learners and incorporate them into the instruction. In this adult learning model, all members of the class share information and experiences with one another. In fact, in some areas of the curriculum, students may have more information and experience than the instructor does. With this in mind, the educator should strive to ensure that class communication is multidirectional and is more a dialogue than it is a lecture.

Goal Orientation

Adults are pragmatic by nature. In other words, they want to be able to apply the information they learn immediately, or at least have some understanding of how their learning will be of direct benefit to them. Adults generally do not tolerate studying anything that they cannot apply to tasks they expect to perform. Moreover, adults appreciate an educational program that is organized with clearly defined course components that can help them to achieve their goals.

Although Knowles himself, along with others,[2–5] have recently questioned the validity of the differences between andragogy and pedagogy, the previously mentioned attributes of adult learners can at least aid the educator in developing teaching techniques that will motivate adults to learn. Currently, learning is viewed as a continuum from childhood into adulthood; this is why the validity of different adult and child learning processes has been questioned. Indeed, there seems to be a continual transition from a pedagogical, or childlike, perspective (teacher-centered) to an adult, or andragogical, perspective (student-centered and self-directed). The transition varies from individual-to-individual, and there are no discrete points that appear to occur—that is, no magical change suddenly takes place between high school graduation and higher education.

Other Characteristics of Adult Learners

Adult learners typically display characteristics that can be divided into two broad categories: physiologic and psychosocial. Although adults are much more diverse than children are physiologically, sociologically, and psychologically, general characteristics and central tendencies are presented here; the educator must keep in mind that individuals vary broadly.

Physiologic Variables

Physiologic variables in adult learners specifically relate to how changes in vision, hearing, energy levels, and overall health affect learning. These variables involve the natural process of aging and maturing.

Lighting

Instructors must provide adequate lighting to ensure that older students can view presentations and take notes. Long courses that rely heavily on audiovisual projections for most presentations can tax the eyes of the mature learner. This is particularly true when there are students with visual impairment in the class. (See Chapter 5, Diversity.)

Task Performance

Although the adult's capacity to learn can remain essentially unchanged with age, the older learner has slower reaction times and, in some cases, less efficient senses on which to depend for learning, such as sight and hearing.[6] In addition, the older learner may have reduced ability to quickly process visual information or interpret rapid speech.

Adjustment to External Temperature Changes

For an adult to learn successfully over an extended sitting period, a comfortable temperature and environmental setting is required. This is important to note because sometimes it is necessary to teach in less than ideal environments. Making a room comfortable with adequate temperature control will add significantly to the adult's ability to learn.

Distractions

For nearly all younger generation students, smartphones, laptop computers, and wireless pad devices have become a way of life. What may be completely ordinary behavior to younger students, who routinely check on social media updates and the latest "news" announcements on their mobiles, may be intolerable distractions to adult instructors and learners. The

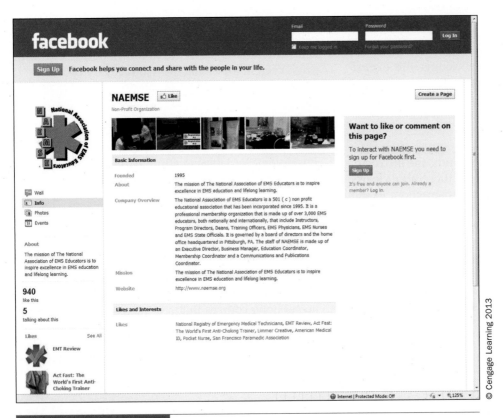

Figure 3.1

Social media can be used to enhance class activities.

educator can help to create a productive environment for adult learning by banning electronic devices in the classroom, but this may be a losing battle in the long run. A better alternative is currently evolving in which instructors are coopting the social media **(Figure 3.1)** to incorporate their use into the instruction in the form of "backchannel" communications. Other learning distractions include televisions, background office and emergency radio chatter, and emergency apparatus coming into and out of a station. The educator must be aware of these environmental distractions and must work to minimize them as much as possible.

Psychosocial Variables

The psychosocial differences between adult learners include the differences between adults' and children's learning behaviors. For instance, adult learners may vary in their established attitudes, beliefs, and values and they may be even more rigid in their thinking than younger learners. Through years of living, adults have acquired set patterns of behaviors, along with set ideas and beliefs about right and wrong, and fact and fiction. These patterns may have to be "unset" or challenged for learning to take place. New ideas and ways of doing things cannot be forced on adult learners; they must be soundly demonstrated through logic and good evidence. Adult learners must understand and believe the new knowledge or technique before they will be willing to abandon their beliefs.

Success

The educator must strive to create learning situations that afford the greatest potential for learning success; this includes taking special care not to embarrass the adult learner. When adult learners are placed on the defensive, they are less likely to be open to learning and are more likely to be protective of their thoughts and feelings; they may perceive the classroom as an unsafe learning environment. The saying "praise in public and criticize in private" clearly applies to the adult learner. This does not mean that the educator should structure all learning and assessment activities so all learners can succeed on their first attempt. "Failure" in a safe learning environment can be a healthy, meaningful experience when effective coaching and feedback are provided. Students must accept that not every clinical call will go well. They must learn to objectively reflect on their performance to determine how it can be improved in the future.

Respect

Returning to school is often a momentous decision for the adult learner, and attendance often represents a considerable investment. Having made this important and commendable decision, the adult learner expects—and deserves—to be treated with respect. The resourceful educator draws upon the wealth of knowledge and experiences that these learners bring with them to enrich the class for all students. It is the instructor's responsibility to demonstrate respect toward each student and to ensure an environment of mutual respect among all class members.

Critical Thinking Skills

The adult learns best by adding new information to an already existing framework, and has greater difficulty remembering isolated facts. The educator must seek the most effective approach to developing and presenting course material. Knowing the educational and professional backgrounds of students is important in making these determinations. With this knowledge, the educator can add new information to the students' existing frameworks—or expertise.

Teaching Tip >> *The educator should get to know his or her students' backgrounds, so he or she can better integrate new ideas with those ideas students already know. Linking new information to old is a particularly effective way to aid information retention in the adult learner.*

Practical Limitations and Considerations

The adult learner has competing responsibilities, and the EMS instructor who does not consider these factors risks losing very good students. These limitations and considerations may involve scheduling challenges, scarce time, financial stresses, conflicts between job and family responsibilities, and transportation problems. It is important that the educator respect the challenges that each student faces **(Figure 3.2)**.

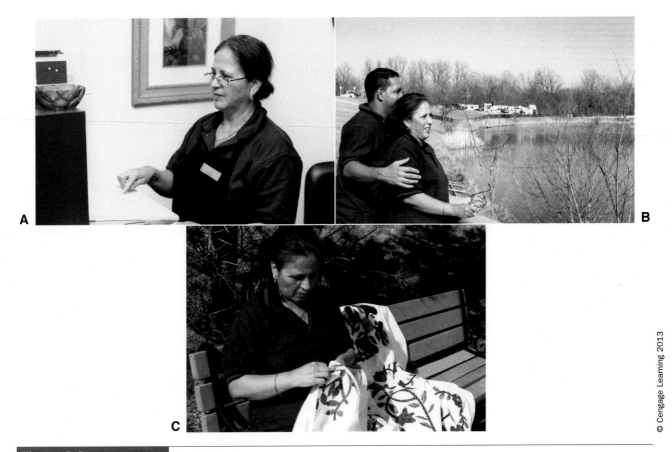

Figure 3.2

Teaching adults means teaching people with varied life experiences and responsiblities.

Principles for Teaching Adult Learners

With adult learners, instructors should:

- Involve students in the planning process
- Actively engage students in the learning process
- Incorporate a variety of teaching methods to meet the needs of students with a variety of learning styles
- Focus on "real world" problems
- Emphasize how the learning can be applied
- Practice information quickly after it is presented
- Relate the material to the learner's past experience
- Allow debate and challenge of ideas
- Listen to and respect the opinions of learners
- Encourage learners to be resources to the instructor and to one another
- Use students to evaluate learning
- Give learners control
- Reinforce positive behavior whenever possible

Motivation

Adults typically have different motivators for learning than do younger students. The instructor can apply an important classroom-management and performance-enhancement tool by understanding what motivates students, because motivation creates the desire to learn. By knowing what motivates students, the instructor can understand student behavior and choose relevant motivational tools. For example, if a student who is trying to support his family on his EMT wages is reminded that the top five students in a paramedic class will be guaranteed interviews for openings at one of the most highly respected regional ambulance services, he may be strongly motivated to excel in the program. Research by Fernandez, Studnek, and Margolis found that paramedic licensure required for employment was one of the independent variables that predicted passing the National Registry of EMTs written examination.[7] Furthermore, understanding one's own motivation for personal excellence in teaching is vital to maintaining high-level activity and instruction in one's classroom.

Teaching Tip >> *Active listening is one of the most effective ways to receive information and is a skill that few instructors master. During class, it is tempting to divide attention between several students at once, but that is not always effective. The instructor should self-monitor how actively and attentively he or she listens to students. Active listening may help the instructor identify what motivates his or her students.*

Intrinsic and Extrinsic Motivators

Motivators are divided into two groups: intrinsic (internal) and extrinsic (external).[8] *Intrinsic motivators* are internal drives for behavior, such as a desire to help others or to serve the community, a need for personal or professional growth and development, a need to boost one's self-esteem, a desire to achieve, and a need to be competent and to succeed in one's life. Another intrinsic motivator is to make or maintain social relationships, or to relieve boredom. Adults are usually more highly motivated by these intrinsic factors than by extrinsic factors.

In contrast, *extrinsic motivators* come from outside of the individual person. Examples of extrinsic motivators include the possibility of a promotion, a bonus, additional vacation time, or the need to find or maintain a job.

Once an instructor knows and understands his or her students' motivators, he or she can use language, examples, and incentives relevant to each student's motivators.

Maslow's Hierarchy

A discussion of motivation would be incomplete without including Abraham Maslow, one of the most respected seminal pioneers in the field of human motivation. **Maslow** worked on his **hierarchy of needs** theory over a period of years (1943, 1954, 1971), making alterations as he sought to understand the subject. In fact, the hierarchy has evolved over the decades. His theory has influenced many fields, including education, and can be helpful to the instructor as he or she seeks to identify and understand student needs and motivation.

Maslow, a humanist, believed that a person strives for a higher potential and desires to reach higher levels of his or her calling to become a fully functioning person—or, as he describes it, to achieve "self-actualization." Moreover, individual persons can grow and actualize their potential in the right

CASE IN POINT

A construction company foreman is confident and competent at his job. The other workers look up to him, and he prides himself on being an excellent contractor and manager. His group is enrolled in a mandatory first aid class as part of their company's safety program. The instructor is dreading teaching this group because she is concerned that they will not be interested in the material. However, she learns before the class that the foreman has a strong will to succeed, in addition to a healthy ego and a desire not to "look bad" in front of his subordinates.

The instructor knows that she has a useful tool by which to motivate this group by identifying the foreman as the team leader and encouraging and supporting his learning. By helping *him* to succeed, she will ensure that he will stay motivated to master the material, while simultaneously motivating the others who respect him to perform well also and learn the information.

Additionally, the instructor uses examples that are relevant to the students' experiences. She describes accidents and injuries that could occur on a construction job site. When teaching spinal immobilization, she uses the example of a roofer who falls while laying shingles. When teaching hemorrhage control, she uses the example of a framer who cuts himself while using a power saw. The students are able to see the relevance of the class to them personally, and they are more motivated to pay attention and practice the skills presented in class. In fact, several students pursue supplemental learning beyond the classroom by attending additional classes in construction site safety.

environment; but in a less-than-healthy environment, individuals do not grow to meet their potential.

Maslow's theory consists of a hierarchy of levels of *basic* human needs, then *higher* needs, or "growth" needs, which can be attained only when the more basic needs have been met. At the lowest level of the hierarchy, basic needs are physiologic, such as oxygen, food, water, and a reasonably constant body temperature. An individual who is deprived of any of these basic physiologic needs would be controlled by them and would desperately seek to attain them. Until these needs are satisfied, an individual cannot move to the next level. Students who are distracted by a classroom environment that is too hot or too cold. or who fail to have sufficient breaks to meet personal needs, may be distracted from learning.

Safety and security needs, the next level in the hierarchy, describes the ability to be free from fear of physical danger and also free from fear of deprivation of the basic physiologic needs. These needs include feeling secure about maintaining property and having a job to ensure food and shelter. Safety is most often presumed by most adults until a serious emergency or a major disruption in some social structure occurs. Examples of events that have raised safety concerns and questions of needs in recent decades include the 9-11-2001 attacks and the Oklahoma City bombing. Young children, on the other hand, almost constantly feel the effects of insecurity and have need to feel safe when they are in new places and around strangers. Likewise, the student must feel safe in the classroom to fully participate in learning. A classroom environment that allows bullying or sarcasm may inhibit students from speaking out or engaging in the learning experience for fear of being mocked or belittled by anyone.

The next level in the hierarchy is the need for love, affection, and "belonging." Maslow explains that individuals strive to overcome loneliness and separation from family, friends, and society. This level of need includes not just receiving love and affection, but also giving love and affection. If there is difficulty attaining a sense of belonging, individuals may substitute achievement. Student teams or groups can promote a sense of belonging. Likewise, a classroom of inclusion where all students are shown that their opinions and contributions are valued contributes to an atmosphere where students feel that sense of belonging.

The next and final level of Maslow's hierarchy of basic needs includes esteem. An individual has the strength and motivation to strive to fulfill this need only when the more basic needs have been met. Humans must have a stable, high level of respect for themselves and respect from others. Becoming competent and gaining recognition (validity from others) produces feelings of self-confidence, power, and usefulness to society. As with the other levels of need, individuals may not always seek to fill these needs through constructive behavior, but sometimes through disruptive or immature actions. In the classroom, everyone must be offered and encouraged the opportunity to participate in all activities. Allowing one person in a group or class to lead in every exercise or activity does little to improve the self-esteem of others. It is the instructor's responsibility to ensure all are given equal opportunities to demonstrate their ability to excel.

Once all these basic needs have been met, an individual, according to Maslow, is ready to pursue the higher level, or "growth," needs. Although Maslow initially identified only self-actualization needs, after more study he identified four specific levels: cognitive needs, aesthetic needs, self-actualization needs, and self-transcendence needs. Again, each of these levels of need is attempted only after lesser needs have been met. Cognitive needs include knowing, understanding, and exploring. Aesthetic needs include order and beauty. Self-actualization is reaching one's potential, or, as described by Maslow, "What a man can be, he must be." This is an intrinsic motivation; it is not related to what others think is important. Self-transcendence is a connection to something beyond the ego; it involves helping others to find self-fulfillment and to reach their potential. Offering nontraditional learning opportunities or activities within the curriculum allows students to experiment and to demonstrate their creative talents. This enriches the student experience and the classroom environment, allowing some students the chance to reach toward those higher needs.

Instructors must be able to talk to students and must attempt to understand life events that may impact their motivation. An instructor may be assisted in understanding and addressing the specific needs of students by considering Maslow's hierarchy and determining where students stand within this hierarchy **(Figure 3.3)**.

Honors

Presenting Honors or awards can be a two-edged sword. There is no doubt that recognition is a strong motivator for some students.

However, there are some programs where every student is recognized for something to avoid any individual student being left out. In reality, presenting any form of recognition or award is the act of singling out a student.

Awards must be thoughtfully chosen and reflect achievements or qualities that are worthy of special recognition. Time and effort must be invested to make the selection fair and objective. Criteria for granting awards must be disseminated to students in advance of the selection process.

If done appropriately and professionally, awards can acknowledge exceptional performance or behaviors demonstrated by the students who are selected.

Many programs use rubrics to calculate the awarding of honors. This has the advantage of making the process as transparent and objective as possible.

Careful consideration should be given to presenting awards or end-of-class certificates. Certainly, accomplishments should be celebrated. Completing

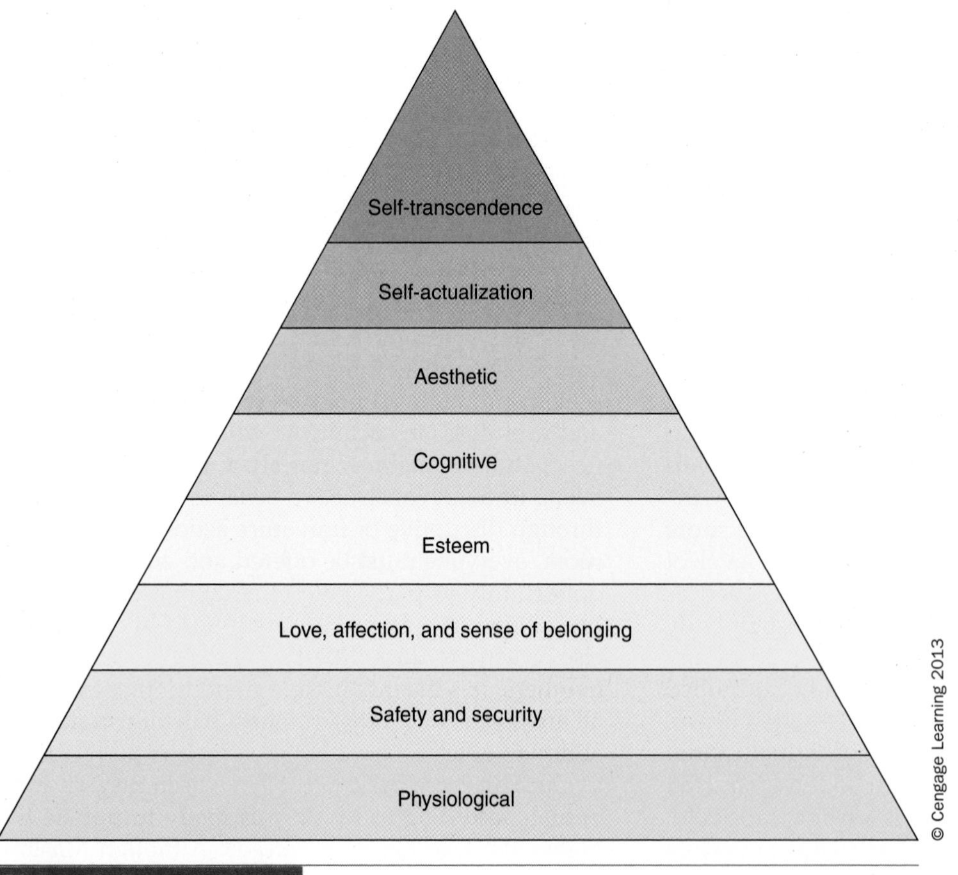

Figure 3.3
Maslow's hierarchy of needs.

any one of the four levels of EMS education can be a significant achievement for an individual student. These moments should be celebrated, but not at the expense of those students who failed to progress. If there is no formal graduation ceremony, some programs reserve the last day of class to present course completion certificates. They also use this time to register students who have successfully completed their coursework for either their state or national examinations. Students who have not successfully completed the course do not need to attend the last day. This practice avoids embarrassment for students who have not met the requirements for certification. It is common for schools to allow students who have made satisfactory progress, but lack some clinical hours or final course requirements to graduate, to "walk" and participate in the graduation ceremony. Their official graduation certificate is awarded when the entire program is complete.

CASE IN POINT

A student (Bob) is enrolled in an advanced EMT class. He has taken several other EMS courses and is well known by the instructional staff. He is gifted with natural academic talent and has not had to truly apply himself in any class he has taken so far. During the academic portion of the class, he has routinely announced his top standing academically to the great annoyance of his fellow classmates.

During the live intravenous (IV)-start lab, each student is given 10 attempts to start five successful IVs. Failure to accomplish this task results in a failing grade and prevents the students from progressing to the clinical portion of the class. Bob missed his first four IV attempts. He was able to start two successful IVs on his fifth and sixth attempts, but required significant coaching. On his seventh attempt he was unsuccessful. He now has three attempts left and needs three successful IV starts. To add more pressure, he is the only student in the class who will need to use all 10 attempts to complete this portion of the lab.

Bob received significant extra training after his missed fourth attempt. While he did not like the idea of remediation, his skills improved dramatically and he was able to successfully start his next two IVs. However, when he missed his seventh attempt, he became very negative and could be heard saying "I can't do this" under his breath.

The lead instructor knows Bob's problem is not psychomotor skills. Bob's problem is confidence. She instructs Bob to focus on other skills for the rest of the day. At the end of the class she asks Bob for a few minutes and discusses what she believes his problem to be. She asks Bob to take the five days before the next class meeting to visualize in his mind successfully completing the steps. She instructs him to clearly see himself successfully completing the remaining IVs. Bob returns the following week and successfully starts all three of the remaining IVs.

Positive Affirmations

Developing a positive mindset is one of the most powerful instructional strategies for giving feedback on performance. Using positive-thinking techniques, visualization, and positive affirmations are highly effective methods to increase levels of performance in stressful situations. They are, however, the most generally underutilized motivational techniques used in EMS education. Most experienced master educators know that a student's attitude is the most important factor in training.

Barriers to Learning

Not all learners come to the classroom adequately motivated. The phrase "barriers to learning" can be used to describe conditions or situations in which motivation is lacking, but can also include many other factors. Common barriers include family and career responsibilities that result in lack of time, money, or confidence. Learning disabilities can present a major impediment to student learning. Additionally, scheduling problems **(Figure 3.4)**, bureaucracy ("red tape"), and problems with childcare and transportation are often difficult barriers to overcome. Lack of confidence or self-efficacy can also be a significant barrier

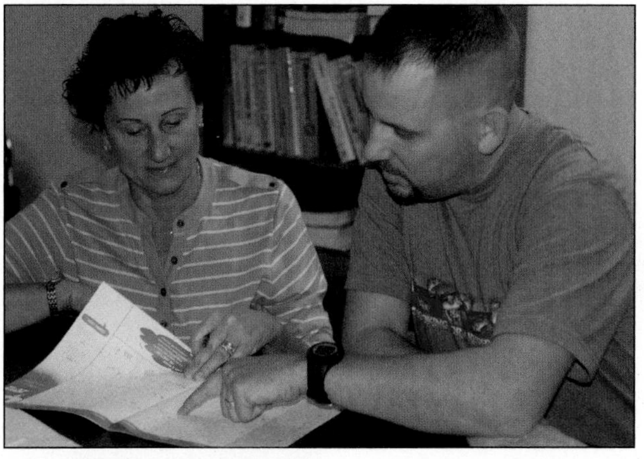

Figure 3.4

Scheduling problems and bureaucracy can be significant barriers to learning.

Learning Disabilities in the EMS Classroom

by Tia Radant

Learning disabilities (LDs) can be a confusing and intimidating topic for educators. Knowing what a learning disability is and what it is *not* can help the EMS student succeed. *Learning disability* is defined by the National Center for Learning Disabilities as "a neurobiological disorder that affects the brain's ability to receive, process, store, and respond to information."[a] According to Dr. Sheldon H. Horowitz, the definition of learning disability includes the following criteria:

- At least average intellectual capacity
- A significant (and unexplained) discrepancy between achievement and expected potential
- The exclusion of mental retardation, emotional disturbance, sensory impairment, cultural differences, or lack of opportunity to learn
- Central nervous system dysfunction as the basis of the presenting problem(s)[b]

Learning disabilities are not only for children; they are not a choice, nor are they a condition that comes and goes at different times in a person's life. Interestingly, Attention Deficit Hyperactivity Disorder (ADHD) is not categorized as a learning disability, though many of the steps an instructor can take to help a student with LD can benefit a student with ADHD. Information on ADHD can be found at http://www.add.org.

So how will the instructor know if a student has a learning disability? The average EMS instructor will not be able to diagnose a learning disability but rather identify clues that would suggest the student may benefit from further testing with a qualified professional. A student can visit their primary health care provider to begin the process of diagnosis.

The most common warning sign in a classroom is a *contrast between the perceived ability of a student and that student's achievement.* The student may excel in one portion of the class while struggling in others. Or maybe a student is very bright, engaged, and curious; however, struggles to complete assignments and tests successfully. The National Center for Learning Disabilities identifies the following as potential signs of a learning disability:

- Often spelling the same word differently in a single document
- Reluctance to take on reading or writing tasks
- Trouble with open-ended questions on tests
- Weak memory skills
- Difficulty in adapting skills from one setting to another
- Slow work pace
- Poor grasp of abstract concepts
- Inattention to details or excessive focus on them
- Frequent misreading of information
- Trouble filling out applications or forms
- Easily confused by instructions
- Poor organizational skills[c]

When one or more of these signs appear frequently and cause a disruption in everyday life or learning, the EMS instructor should discuss the warning signs with the student and recommend testing by a qualified professional.

When a student excels in one area of learning, for example, on psychomotor skills, and struggles in another area, such as written exams, it may be time to refer the student for further evaluation. This discrepancy in achievement should cause the instructor to ask, "What can I do to help this student achieve his or her full potential?" A variety of accommodations may be available to students. These may include:

- Extended time on exams
- Private space for written tests
- Tutoring
- A note taker
- Audio recording of lectures
- Alternative assignments

Early identification, assessment, diagnosis, and/or intervention and ongoing monitoring can help a student succeed who otherwise may have been discouraged or even have failed the course.

Adult students may disclose a previously diagnosed learning disability and ask for accommodation. A student's declaration of learning disability must be supported by documentation from an appropriate professional before accommodation is made. The EMS instructor must become familiar with state and local laws and institutional regulations surrounding accommodations for adult students. Section 504 of the Rehabilitation Act and the

continues

continued

Americans with Disabilities Act Amendments Act are federal laws which provide some protection for college students. A student's individualized learning plan (IEP) from high school is not valid for accommodation in college. It is also a good idea to learn what accommodations are allowed by your state EMS agency and the National Registry of EMTs. Once a student has a documented disability, the instructor may need to provide the accommodations requested if it is reasonable. Knowing what accommodations are allowed will help ensure a smooth process for the instructor and the student.

An instructor can support students with learning disabilities by designing learning in systematic and strategic ways. Offering a structured course with clearly identified course schedule and expectations will help students succeed. Here are a few ways to incorporate structure into the EMS classroom:

- Outline tasks a student must complete during skills practice
- Provide clear oral and written directions for homework assignments
- Develop grading which incorporates high stakes for late work or missed clinical shifts
- Allow opportunities for students to review exams with instructor feedback

After talking with a student who is struggling in class, concern for the student and efforts to advocate for his or her success may be the most important factor in their success. Adults with learning disabilities have often struggled to overcome the challenges of school for many years.

Despite classroom accommodation, EMS providers must be capable of performing all essential functions of the job regardless of any accommodation that was provided during school. Students who are concerned they will not be able to safely and effectively meet the requirements of a job in EMS should consult with EMS instructors, employers, and industry experts.

For more information visit the National Center for Learning Disabilities at http://www.ld.org

[a] http://www.ncld.org/ld-basics
[b] http://www.ncld.org/es/ld-basics/ld-explained/basic-facts/the-neurobiology-of-learning-disabilities
[c] http://www.ncld.org/es/ld-basics/ld-explained/early-warning-signs/problem-signs-is-it-ld

to learning, as can resentment or disinterest due to required, or involuntary, education.

Educators should understand that such barriers exist, and that they may be able to effect positive change in students through their role as mentor, guide, and advocate. The educator must strive to decrease barriers whenever possible and must encourage learners to explore ways to overcome their personal barriers. Encouraging attention to intrinsic motivators (e.g., success, helping others) may also be helpful. These barriers might otherwise limit students' ability to grow as prehospital EMS providers and to become lifelong learners.

Selected Learning Theories

This section examines several selected theories of learning and offers practical lessons that educators can gain from these theories. Although dozens of theories, preferences, and concepts are associated with learning in educational psychology, five of the more common types have been selected for discussion here. These include self-directed learning, the theory of margins, transformational learning, experiential learning, and context-based learning.

Self-Directed Learning

The theory of **self-directed learning** involves many related concepts, such as self-planned learning, self-teaching, autonomous learning, and independent study. Distributed learning and distance education are also frequently used modalities for self-directed learning.

Self-education has been described as nothing more than the manner in which information is acquired—that of learning without an instructor present.[9] However, the absence of an instructor, although an important characteristic of self-directed learning, is only *one* of several characteristics of self-directed learning. At least three additional characteristics are particular to self-directed learning, namely:

- A longer learning time period
- A wider range of studies
- A higher level of subject mastery and critical thinking

Self-direction in learning comes from a lifelong learning perspective. Kidd supports this view in the following passage: "It has often been said that the purpose of adult education, or of any kind of education, is to make the subject [student] a continuing, 'inner-directed,' self-operating learner."[10]

Self-direction in adulthood is a process in which the learner assumes primary control of what he or she desires to learn. Moore describes a self-directed learner as an individual who can

> identify his learning need when he finds a problem to be solved, a skill to be acquired, or information to be obtained. He is able to articulate his need in the form of a general goal, differentiate that goal into several specific objectives, and define fairly explicitly his criteria for successful achievement. In implementing his need, he gathers the information he desires, collects ideas, practices skills, works to resolve his problems, and achieves his goals. In evaluating, the learner judges the appropriateness of newly acquired skills, the adequacy of his solutions, and the quality of his new ideas and knowledge.[11]

A related view of self-directed learning that stresses the phases of a leaning process has been offered by Knowles:

> In its broadest meaning, "self-directed learning" describes a process in which individuals take the initiative, with or without the help of others, in diagnosing their learning needs, formulating learning goals, identifying human and material resources for learning, choosing and implementing appropriate learning strategies, and evaluating the learning outcomes.[12]

The EMS instructor can apply this theory by creating a classroom environment that includes two elements. First, implement an *institutional* process in which students are made responsible for identifying their learning needs and deciding on the strategies they plan to use to reach them. Then, promote self-directed learning from the point of view of an *internal* process. In other words, the student is encouraged to set his or her own goals in terms of learning outcome. By doing so, students take responsibility for their own learning.

For example, the instructor might plan an activity on the first day of class that requires students to immediately assume responsibility for their own learning. The instructor can assign students to define their career choice (EMT, AEMT, or paramedic) by investigating a variety of resources, and to write a paper with their definitions, observations, and findings. Instructors who ensure that students have initial success with their self-directed assignments can help motivate them in their studies and, in the process, can help them become lifelong learners.

Entry-level EMS education is, by its nature, driven by specific competencies and deadlines that somewhat restrict self-directed learning because of its limitations. By definition, self-directed learning allows students to decide what to learn—an entire program based on this concept would not be practical in EMS. In addition, this type of learning may take longer to achieve as students define their objectives and develop their plans for learning.

Self-directed learning does, however, offer many advantages. Knowles felt it increases learning because it is based on individual learner initiative; it is an essential element needed to move toward maturity; it makes the learner take responsibility for his or her own learning; and it develops essential independent learning skills needed to stay current as knowledge evolves.[13] The ability to independently continue learning is an important skill for EMS professionals. EMS instructors should provide tools for learners to pursue self-directed learning. Guiding students to find

CASE IN POINT

The EMT instructor looked at the requirements of the National EMS Education Standards for the EMT course and tried to imagine how to possibly cover all of the material adequately. He thought there was no possible way to have the students learn to be proficient in their skills, understand what they were doing, and still cover every topic during class. Yet he realized that they were all very motivated adults. He concluded that surely they could learn much of this on their own. With that in mind, he devised a self-learning plan that would help to improve his class in several ways.

First, he took the required bloodborne pathogens and Health Insurance Portability and Accountability Act (HIPAA) of 1996 materials that had been added to the curriculum and placed them into a self-directed learning module that had to be completed and passed (by a written test) before students could even register for the courses. This would be his first "commitment filter" because competition to get into the class was so strong.

Second, he took the medical terminology, hazardous materials, and weapons of mass destruction (WMD) modules and, from these, created self-directed learning modules that had to be completed by students during class at specific points in the schedule. The medical terminology module was required within one week of the start of class. The hazardous material module was required to be completed by the fourth class. Completion of the WMD module was required by the end of the program, but it had to be submitted before students could take the certification exam.

By shifting this content to self-learning modules, the instructor increased contact hours for content related to patient care skills and materials that the students would use on most of their EMS calls. He ended up with a better-prepared, less frustrated, better-performing class.

appropriate resources and seeking opportunities to encourage independent learning within the classroom empowers them to become self-directed learners after graduation.

Theory of Margins

The theory of Power-Load-Margins, commonly called the **Theory of Margins**, provides a model for looking at how much ability (*power*) a student has compared with how much learning the student needs to accomplish (*load*). *Margin* is the difference between "power" and "load." This theory is one way of describing the pressures placed on an individual during the learning process. In general, the less "margin" an individual has, the more likely he or she is to succeed.

Research Behind the Theory

Howard Y. McClusky, an experimental psychologist, examined adult learning and introduced the Theory of Margins in the early 1960s.[14] He believed that the theory was essential for understanding adult lives, especially as adults age and the various demands of family and career pressures increase.

According to McClusky, the key factors of adult life are the "load" that the adult carries in living and the "power" that is available to that person to carry the load.[15] He described *load* as the demands, both self and social, that are required by a person to maintain a minimal level of autonomy. He described *power* as the individual's resources, abilities, possessions, and position on which he or she can draw to cope with the load; and *margin* as the difference between the "power" and the "load." The greater the margin a person has, the more likely it is that he or she can deal with the load, because he or she has greater reserve capacity. A student with an overwhelming load, caused by the need to work a full-time job and take care of children and possibly an ill parent, may have no margin for handling any additional duties or stressors, including even the most minimal educational load.

McClusky further divided "load" into two groups of interacting elements: external and internal. The *external load* consists of tasks involved in normal life requirements (e.g., family, work, and community responsibilities). *Internal load* consists of life expectancies developed by the people themselves, such as aspirations, desires, and future expectations. Power consists of a combination of external resources and capacities such as family support, social abilities, and economic abilities. It also includes various internally acquired or accumulated skills and experiences that contribute to effective performance, such as resiliency, coping skills, and personality.

Practical Application of the Theory

Instructors can affect their students' margins in both positive and negative ways. McClusky's Power-Load-Margin theory can be applied to the degree that instructors contribute to the increase or depletion of "margin" in the lives and capacities of adult students.[16] Day and James at the University of Wyoming,[17] in a series of interviews with adult students, found numerous examples of instructor-generated "load" that they categorized into four areas: attitude, behavior, task, and environment.

One of the most surprising findings of this research was that the attitudinal and behavioral dimensions of the instructor-generated "load" were identified more than three times as often as the task dimension.

Examples of Instructor-Generated Load[8]

Instructors attributed greater "margin" to students.

ATTITUDE

- Instructor treats learner as an inferior person
- Instructor ignores learner's opinion
- Instructor is too impatient
- Instructor is too rigid

BEHAVIOR

- Instructor has distracting mannerisms
- Instructor mumbles or is difficult to understand
- Instructor is disorganized
- Instructor avoids eye contact

TASK

- Instructor gives inappropriate assignments
- Instructor's guidelines for evaluation/grades are unclear
- Instructor gives busywork
- Instructor allows too little time to complete assignments

ENVIRONMENT

- Learning environment is too hot or too cold
- Lighting is poor
- Desks and chairs are uncomfortable
- Noise or other distractions can be heard from neighboring classrooms

In other words, adults adjust their "margins" to deal with the expected task demands assigned to them by the instructor better than they do with interpersonal issues. Unexpected demands, such as an instructor's attitude and behaviors, create barriers to a student's ability to satisfactorily complete a learning objective.

Day and James identified several ways in which instructors can minimize the effects of instructor-generated "load."[17] These techniques include the following:

1. Recognize and understand that "margin" exists in adult students.
2. Understand that the concerns of students do not center merely on the content of the course.
3. Recognize that an instructor can contribute both positively and negatively to the "load" in learners, and that he or she does so through behaviors, the learning environment, attitudes, and the structure and content of classes.
4. Address issues of "margin" during the first class and occasionally revisit the topic at appropriate times, such as a week or two before a major examination.

The Theory of Margins provides a framework for discussion of how much work a given EMS course typically requires, and of how much time a student has to devote to the course. In addition, it gives both the instructor and the student a conceptual model by which to discuss how illness, personal problems, and work and family problems can add up to an unmanageable situation. Perhaps the most powerful component of this model is the way that an educator's attitude, lack of organization, or use of busywork can dramatically narrow a student's "margin," thus reducing his or her performance and chance of success in a class.

CASE IN POINT

An EMS instructor taught EMR as a contract course to a group of government workers. The course was conducted onsite, and students were detailed from their offices to the class. The class met for seven hours each day over a seven-week period. By the fourth week of class, the instructor noticed that several students frequently returned late from lunch, or not at all, for the second half of the day. He knew that none of those students would be eligible to take the state certification exam because of their absences. On questioning the students, the instructor discovered that most participants were supervisors or upper management personnel who could not afford to take the entire workday away from their offices, even though the highest administrative level required the training course. Students agreed that they could come for half-day sessions and were willing to do so, as they really enjoyed the course and valued what they were learning. The instructor proposed that the program should meet for half-day sessions for the remainder of the time. He was also able to convince the administration to allow him to offer two mornings of makeup sessions, so all the absent students could make up the classes they had missed. In this manner, he was able to have all students complete the training program. He and the administrators agreed that future contract courses would be offered as only half-day sessions.

This instructor applied the Theory of Margins by increasing the "power" the students had (by responding to their need and allowing them to help devise a solution) and decreasing their "load," thus increasing their "margin."

Transformational Learning

The theory of **transformational learning** emerged with the work of Jack Mezirow,[18,19] and it is defined as "learning that initiates and creates deep and lasting personal changes," sometimes known as a "paradigm shift."[20] In transformational learning, acquisition of specific knowledge and skills is often secondary to the deeper and lasting change in perception and thought. Although EMS educators generally are not oriented toward intentionally seeking out transformational-learning opportunities for their students, such experiences often appear unexpectedly for the students simply due to the nature of EMS and exposure to dramatic and unexpected life and death events. Many instructors can recall times when a student approached them at some point during or after the class and said, "EMS has changed my life. Now I know what I want to do." EMS educators should be on the lookout for those seminal moments that can transform the lives of students and influence their entire careers.

Research Behind the Theory

Transformational learning is based on the concepts of *meaning perspectives*, or one's overall worldview, and *meaning schemes*, or smaller components that contain specific knowledge, values, and beliefs about one's experiences.[18] A number of meaning schemes work together to generate one's meaning perspective. Meaning perspectives are shaped during childhood and youth, and they form the basis for a person's view of the world from his or her perspective. They operate as perceptual filters that determine how an individual will organize and interpret the meaning of his or her life experiences.

CASE IN POINT

A student came into her instructor's office frustrated and ready to quit. She told the instructor that she could not do the drug calculations no matter how hard she tried. The instructor, similar to every paramedic program instructor who has taught drug calculations, sat and listened attentively. Yes, drug calculations are one of the most challenging tasks for some students to learn, and some students *never* master the calculation skills that are essential to be a paramedic. However, this was a very bright student who had a block for some reason; she *believed* that she simply could not learn these calculation tasks.

The instructor thought about the student's background and about why she might not be learning the skill. He realized that she was a licensed cosmetologist, a beautician who ran her own business. He looked at her and said, "Don't you have to calculate your business expenses every month? Project the supplies you need and order them? Calculate how much they will cost? Calculate the costs of your utilities, lease, taxes, and other business expenses? Don't you have to anticipate how many customers you will have, how long it will take you to serve each one, and schedule them?" He continued, "How is all of that any more complicated than drug calculations? Isn't it all the same, except for changing dollars to milligrams, and ounces to bottles, instead of milligrams to kilograms?"

Suddenly, the student's face changed. She smiled. Her eyes lit up. She said, "I got it!" She left the office, passed her pharmacology tests with high scores, and became a practicing paramedic. Today, she is also a critical-care nurse. She had a *transformational learning experience* that occurred unexpectedly in one brief moment—just by being asked the right questions at the right time.

Meaning perspectives naturally change and evolve as the number and depth of life experiences increase. However, there are occasions when significant events occur that may induce powerful emotional responses within the individual. These life-changing events may include intensely personal issues such as divorce, death of a loved one, health crises, financial upheavals, or unexpected job changes, or they may involve large-scale incidents such as disasters and accidents. When these events occur, the individual must assess the information and decide whether it fits within his or her current meaning perspective. No transformative learning occurs as long as the information fits comfortably. However, if the event is so significant as to create upheaval and conflict in what one believes, a transformative learning experience may occur, as the new information shifts the meaning perspective to a new position.[19]

Practical Application of the Theory

Although transformational learning has powerful potential for enhancing and accelerating a student's self-actualization processes, an EMS instructor must consider some important points in attempting to understand these processes. Baumgartner advises instructors to consider ethical questions that may arise in the planning and delivery of transformational learning.[21] Baumgartner also discusses the dynamics and the balance of power in the classroom, emphasizing the necessity of a trusting and caring relationship between students and instructors. Students who see the instructor as an authority figure may be reluctant to challenge conventional values, beliefs, and interpretation of facts. Thus, Baumgartner recommends that educators must have a formal code of ethics and a forum for adult educators in which mutual support and exploration of the dynamics of transformational learning are encouraged.

Transformational learning can frequently elicit strong emotional responses from both the student and the instructor, often unexpectedly. Because of their powerful potential, the instructor should take the time to deal with transformational learning moments when they occur. For example, a class discussion about medical maladies among the homeless leads to a larger discussion of the exact nature of homelessness itself. The instructor gives a research assignment to a group of interested students, instructing them to find relevant information about the topic. As the students research the topic, several of them find the information to be very powerful and alter their preexisting thoughts regarding the homeless. As a result, they feel better prepared and more empathetic to the homeless patients they contact in the field.

Experiential Learning

Experiential learning can be explained simply as learning by doing. Kolb developed an early experiential learning model (based on work by Dewey, Piaget, and Lewin), but many new experiential models have developed over time. At first glance, this principle appears simple, but to learn rather than just do, the learner must move through a cycle that involves an experience, followed by meaningful reflection to see the experience from several perspectives. Abstract thought then follows to derive concepts and key ideas from the experience. Finally, there is critical thinking and problem solving to try out these new

CASE IN POINT

The EMT course covered the topic of child abuse and neglect. During the lesson, the instructor noticed that one student was withdrawn and very quiet. This was out of character for the student. The instructor approached the student during the break to see if he was ill, or if something was bothering him. The student related a story from his own childhood. He explained how his best friend had been the victim of child abuse. He told how he had watched his friend endure several years of abuse, and that he had been sworn to secrecy. Because they were both young children at the time, he thought that he was doing the right thing by not telling. He spoke of the feelings of loss when his friend moved away suddenly and he never heard from him again. He told the instructor how this experience had caused him to want to become an EMT, so he could help other children in similar situations. The instructor urged the student to share his story with the rest of the class, and when the break was over, he did. All students were riveted during his story, and one other student shared a similar experience with the class. This led to a much deeper discussion of the topic than could have been possible from the instructor's lecture alone. The whole class could clearly see how this experience had transformed the life of the student involved.

ideas by actively testing them in another situation **(Figure 3.5)**.[22,23]

Later theorists felt that the Kolb model neglected the individual learners and the important role their characteristics and past experiences play in learning. In addition, the critical relationship of emotion in situational learning was emphasized. A positive experience that enhances self-esteem, peer trust, and confidence is more likely to contribute to meaningful learning.[23] Negative emotions, such as fear, must be acknowledged for the student to move forward.

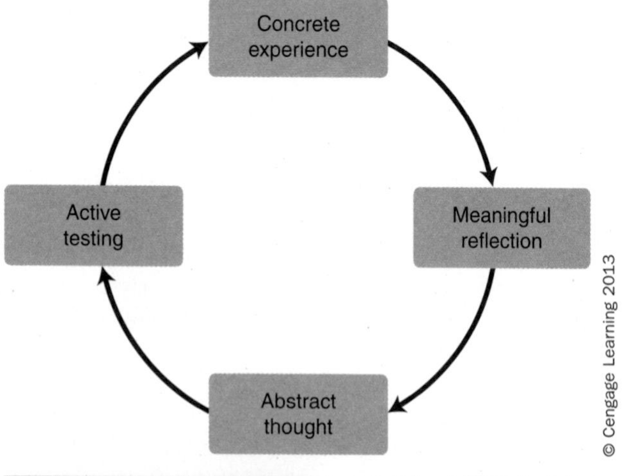

Figure 3.5

Experiential Learning—concrete experience, meaningful reflection, abstract thought and active testing.

The instructor plays an important role as facilitator to promote learning in experiential situations. Developing challenging scenarios using simulation with standardized patients or manikins and scheduling appropriate clinical and field experiences form the foundation for experiential learning in the EMS classroom. Instructors can assist students to reflect and manage emotions associated with experiential learning by debriefing, discussing, or having them journal. Deliberate facilitation may be needed to help the students make meaning of the experience so they can identify how to improve performance and use their knowledge in new or different situations. During this phase, the instructor may suggest or lead the students to other ways to solve the problem in the future, or identify areas in which additional skill practice or knowledge is needed. Effective coaching promotes students' confidence to test their new problem-solving skills or knowledge in new situations.

Context-Based Learning (Situated Cognition)

Context-based learning, or *situated cognition*, a type of experiential learning, assumes that information is more easily learned if it is taught within the environment where it will actually be used by the student.

Research Behind the Theory

Lave and Wenger state that effective learning manifests as a function of the activity, context, and culture in which it occurs—*the situation*.[24] This contrasts with most traditional classroom learning theories where learning activities are most often presented in an abstract form and out of context. For example, most EMS educators learned about starting an intravenous line in a lecture with screen projections and some demonstration bags of solutions, administration sets, lines, sterilizing wipes, gauze, and tape. Then, the drip rate was calculated on a blackboard and on sheets of paper. In context-based learning, a realistic environment and social interaction are critical components of learning. Today, students learn about starting intravenous lines in realistic laboratory settings. They are presented with a series of realistic scenarios that require responses that lead to learning. For example, the student is presented with a dehydrated patient in shock. They must determine what must be done, how it must be done, and then they must do it.

Students become experientially involved in a "community of practice." The community is made up of experts and novices. Experts are identified as individuals with real-life experience that reflects the content, whereas novices are those who wish to learn the content but have minimal or no practical experience. The community, which comprises both experts and novices, creates a dynamic learning environment.

Situated learning is usually unintentional, or incidental, rather than deliberate. Lave and Wenger call the process "legitimate peripheral participation." Content is learned, and value is "assigned" to it by the students when they have the opportunity to interact in the same environment as experienced practitioners.[25]

Practical Application of the Theory

Educators should strive to make every case scenario and workshop as realistic as possible. This can be achieved through carefully crafted scripts and a realistic environment. If a lab can be made to appear like a home living room or a real motor vehicle collision, learning will be enhanced. As an example, many EMS programs today are installing realistic patient-transport compartment labs in classrooms.

Lave and Wenger provide an analysis of situational learning in five different settings: Yucatan midwives, native tailors, Navy quartermasters, meat cutters, and alcoholics.[25] In all cases, the researchers observed a gradual acquisition of knowledge and skills as novices learned from experts in the context of everyday activities. In EMS, students who have opportunities to observe and practice their skills with real vials, needles, and syringes in real-life environments with interaction with field providers benefit greatly. Although formalized internships may not be practical for every EMS class at every level of training, the opportunity for students to participate in patient scenarios in well-scripted and environmentally realistic laboratory settings provides a reasonable alternative **(Figure 3.6)**.

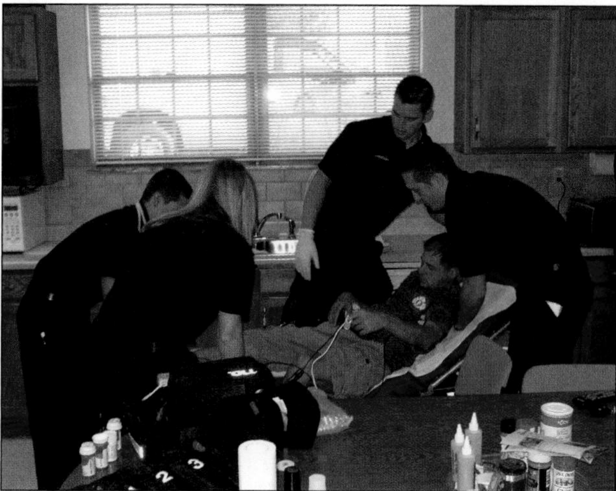

Courtesy of St. Charles County Ambulance District

Figure 3.6

Students who participate in real-life environments are more likely to be successful learners.

CASE IN POINT

The students were nearing the end of their didactic training and were beginning to transition into the "putting it all together" phase of the program, during which they would spend time in the field setting with preceptors from the ambulance service. The primary instructor, clinical coordinator, medical director, and field preceptors were meeting to finalize the details of their rotations. The primary instructor was nervous because he felt the students' skills were weak, and that this would reflect poorly on his teaching abilities. This was his first time as the primary instructor. During the final practical skills evaluations, several students scored as "marginal" or "average," and one even failed the evaluation totally and would have to complete a remediation cycle before he would be allowed to attend any clinicals. The clinical coordinator reminded everybody that the students were novices, and that the preceptors needed to work closely with them to develop their skills in all three domains of learning: cognitive, affective, and psychomotor. After the first couple of weeks of clinical rotations, the primary instructor noticed that the students were performing very well on in-class scenarios and simulations. He could not understand why they had suddenly improved so dramatically in their performance. During a mentoring session with the program medical director, he began to understand how the theory of contextual learning was affecting his students' performance. He even decided to try and include more practical application exercises in his future courses.

Summary

In conclusion, principles applied in the teaching of adult learners vary from those used for teaching children. The differences must be taken into account if success is to be achieved with the adult learner. The educator must also become familiar with the physiologic and psychological variables common to adult learners. Moreover, the major theories of adult learning highlighted in this chapter and the corresponding examples will aid educators in applying them in practical ways to help students succeed. EMS educators will have a greater capacity for tailoring classroom activities effectively and successfully when they attain a fuller understanding of how adults learn.

Glossary

andragogy The art and science of teaching adults.

autonomy Independence.

context-based learning (situated cognition) A learning strategy that places the lesson within the actual situation in which it will be used.

experiential learning Learning by doing.

Maslow's Hierarchy of Needs A theory that identifies an incremental series of human needs. Individuals must satisfy the lower level needs to achieve the higher levels.

pedagogy The art and science of teaching children.

problem-centered learning Learning placed in the context of a real-life situation. It requires application of knowledge from many subjects.

self-directed learning Learning without instructor presence.

Theory of Margins A model that examines the relationship between power (ability) and load (demands on learner).

transformational learning A learning theory centered around creating change in perception and thought.

References

1. Knowles, M. (1988). *Andragogy not pedagogy!* New York, NY: Associated Press.
2. Brookfield, S. (1988). Developing critically reflective practitioners: A rationale for training educators of adults. In *Training education of adults: The theory and practice of graduate adult education*. New York, NY: Routledge.
3. Imel, S. (1988). *Guidelines for working with adult learners*. ERIC Digest #77. Syracuse, NY: ERIC Clearinghouse on Adult Career and Vocational Education.
4. Imel, S. (1999). *New views of adult learning*. Trends and Alerts No. 5. Syracuse, NY: ERIC Clearinghouse on Adult, Career and Vocational Education.
5. Brookfield, S. D. (1986). *Understanding and facilitating adult learning: A comprehensive analysis of principles and effective practice.* Milton Keynes, UK: Open University Press.
6. Wlodkowski, R. J. (2008). *Enhancing adult motivation to learn: A comprehensive guide for teaching all adults* (3rd ed.). San Francisco, CA: Jossey-Bass.
7. Fernandez, A. R., Studnek, J. R., & Margolis, G. S. (2008). Estimating the probability of passing the National Paramedic Certification Examination. *Academic Emergency Medicine, 15*(3), 258–264
8. Mendler, A., & Moody, R. (2001). *Motivating students who don't care: Successful techniques for educators.* National Educational Service.
9. Brockett, R. G., & Hiemstra, R. (1991). *Self-direction in adult learning: Perspectives on theory, research and practice*. London and New York: Routledge.
10. Kidd, J. R. (1973). *How adults learn*. New York Association.
11. Moore A., *et al.* (2003, Spring). EMS stress-training concept "Kobayashi Moru" scenarios. Domain 3. *National Association of EMS Educators.*
12. Knowles, M. (1968). *Andragogy not pedagogy!* New York, NY: Associated Press.
13. Langenbach, M. (1988). *Curriculum models in adult education*. Malabar, FL: Krieger Publishing.
14. McClusky, H. (1963). The course of the adult life span. In: W. C. Hallenbeck (Ed.), *Psychology of adults*. Chicago, IL: Adult Education Association of USA.
15. McClusky, H. (1974). Education for aging: The scope of the field and perspective for the future. In S. M. Grabowski & W. D. Mason (Eds.), *Learning for aging*. Washington, DC: Adult Education Association of the USA, 324–355.

16. McClusky, H. (1970). An approach to a differential psychology of the adult potential. In S. M. Grabowski (Ed.), *Adult learning and instruction*. Syracuse, NY: ERIC Clearinghouse on Adult Education (ERIC Document Reproduction Service No. ED 045 867).
17. Day, M., & James, J. (1984). Margin and the adult learner. *Mountain Plains Adult Education Association Journal of Adult Education, 13,* 1–5.
18. Mezirow, J. (1981). A critical theory of adult learning and education. *Adult Education Quarterly, 32,* 3–24. Retrieved September 24, 2001, from ERIC database EJ253326.
19. Mezirow, J. (1997). Transformative learning: Theory to practice. *New Directions for Adult and Continuing Education, 74,* 5–12.
20. Clark, M. C. (1993). Transformational learning. *New Directions for Adult and Continuing Education, 57,* 47–56.
21. Baumgartner, L. M. (2001). An update on transformational learning. *New Directions for Adult and Continuing Education, 89,* 15–24. Retrieved September 24, 2001, from http://www.esd.edu/~knorum/learningpapers/transform.htm
22. Zull, J. E. (2002). *The art of changing the brain*. Sterling, VA: Stylus.
23. Merriam, S. B., Caffarella, R. S., & Baumgartner, L. M. (2007). *Learning in adulthood* (3rd ed.). San Francisco, CA: John Wiley & Sons.
24. Lave J., & Wenger, E. (1988). *Cognition in practice: Mind, mathematics, and culture in everyday life.* Cambridge, UK: Cambridge University Press.
25. Lave J, & Wenger, E. (1990). *Situated learning: Legitimate peripheral participation*. Cambridge, UK: Cambridge University Press.

Additional Resources

Anderson, J. A. (1988). Cognitive styles and multicultural populations. *Journal of Teacher Education, 39,* 2–9.

Boud, D., *et al.*, (Eds.) (1985). *Reflection: Turning experience into learning*. London: Kogan Page.

Jarvis, P. (1994). Learning. In *ICE301 Lifelong learning.* Unit 1(1). London: YMCA George Williams College.

Kolb, D. A. (1984). *Experiential learning.* Englewood Cliffs, NJ: Prentice Hall.

Kolb, D. A., & Fry, R. (1975). Toward an applied theory of experiential learning. In C. Cooper, (Ed.) (1975). *Theories of group process.* London: John Wiley.

Krzyzewski, M., & Phillips, D. (2000). *Leading with the heart: Coach K's successful strategies for basketball, business, and life.* New York, NY: Warner Books.

Schwenk, T. L., & Whitman, N. A. (1987). *The physician as teacher.* Baltimore, MD: Williams and Wilkins.

Tennant, M. (1997). *Psychology and adult learning* (2nd ed.). London: Routledge.

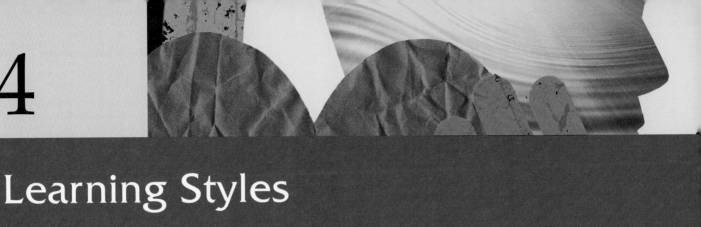

4 Learning Styles

Any training that does not include the emotions, mind, and body is incomplete; knowledge fades without feelings. — ANONYMOUS

When an educator walks into a classroom, he or she faces a group of learners—each with specific levels of intelligence, experience, aptitude, maturity, and interest. The educator's job is to convey knowledge, skills, and attitudes to each student. In doing so, one of his or her greatest challenges is to determine the most appropriate means or process for facilitating that learning. In addition, the educator must strive to make learning a meaningful, pleasant, and rewarding experience for the learner—one that promotes knowledge acquisition and retention that results in a change in practice. Therefore, the educator must appreciate that each learner has a unique means of taking in, processing, and retaining knowledge and skills. This is referred to as a **learning** or **thinking style**.

CHAPTER GOAL: This chapter explains how educators can identify different types of learners according to their learning style, and how they can use that information as a tool for enhancing learning and for guiding instruction.

Learning and the Senses

The senses are the main conduit through which a learner experiences and interacts with the learning environment. The types and numbers of senses involved in learning experiences determine how individuals learn and what they retain. It is generally understood that seeing is the main sense of learning, with hearing a distant second and much smaller amounts of learning accounted for by smell, touch, and taste.

When sensory stimulation involves more than one sense, learners retain information better. Many educational resources note that up to 90 percent of information can be retained when a learner says what he or she is doing while performing an activity—just saying something aloud or writing it improves retention by 70 percent. The combination of seeing and hearing, such as with an illustrated lecture, improves retention by 50 percent; seeing alone provides 30 percent, hearing 20 percent, and reading 10 percent toward retention.[1] While the exact origin and accuracy of these specific numbers have been called into question, there remains strong support for the general belief that a variety of sensory stimuli should be used within a continuum of classroom activities to promote the greatest student learning.[1] This sensory involvement explains why it is common practice to supplement instruction with visual and auditory aids, such as slides and audiotapes. The educator must reach out to learners through as many senses as possible, in attempting to appeal to individual learning styles.

Experiential learning provides the benefit of involving all of the senses in an active learning process. Edelman and Tononi state it simply as "doing precedes understanding."[2] Additionally, experience can involve an emotional reaction, which results in a change of body state (COBS).[3] COBS helps by involving the hippocampus in quickly creating a durable memory store of the experience which includes all of the individual's senses.

What is A Learning Style?

Learning styles involve the use of a schema. *Merriam Webster's Dictionary* defines *schema* as:

1. A diagrammatic presentation; broadly, a structured framework or plan.
2. A mental codification of experience that includes a particular organized way of perceiving cognitively and responding to a complex situation or set of stimuli.

If a person is given a list of things to remember, for instance, a shopping list, he or she can use a schema to help remember the list. The person can make the list into a story, relate it to a song, or develop a visual map or mental picture. One can even develop a routine of physical movement to help recall the items. The nature of the schema chosen may be directly related to the person's learning style or preference. For example, the person who develops a mental picture likely has a preference for visual learning; the person who uses a song prefers auditory learning; and the person who develops a pattern of body motions tends toward kinesthetic learning. Because learning involves the intake, processing, and recall of information, presenting information in a way that is consistent with a learner's style makes the teaching–learning process more effective and efficient.

Types of Cognitive Learning Styles

This section describes the following learning styles, as well as strategies for facilitating their learning experiences:

- **Auditory**
- **Visual**
- **Kinesthetic**
- **Analytic**
- **Global**
- **Social**
- **Independent**

Auditory Learners

Persons who learn best by hearing information are considered **auditory learners**. They benefit from oral presentation of information, discussion, listening, and verbalizing. They are comfortable listening to a taped lecture or an audiotape. Auditory learners can be reached through the use of phrases such as, "I hear you," and, "Listen up, class." These learners absorb didactic material best when it is taught through lectures, oral presentations, and class discussions.

When learning new skills, auditory learners must hear the instructions and any noise or tones produced by the equipment. When electrocardiogram (ECG) recognition is used as an example, this student would be best taught speaking out the rhythms, such as, "Beat, beat, complex, beat, beat, complex" for a second-degree block. He or she would also be inclined to "talk his or her way through" the ECG strip-analysis process. In practice, an auditory learner would want to turn on and listen to the cardiac monitor tone while treating a patient **(Figure 4.1)**.

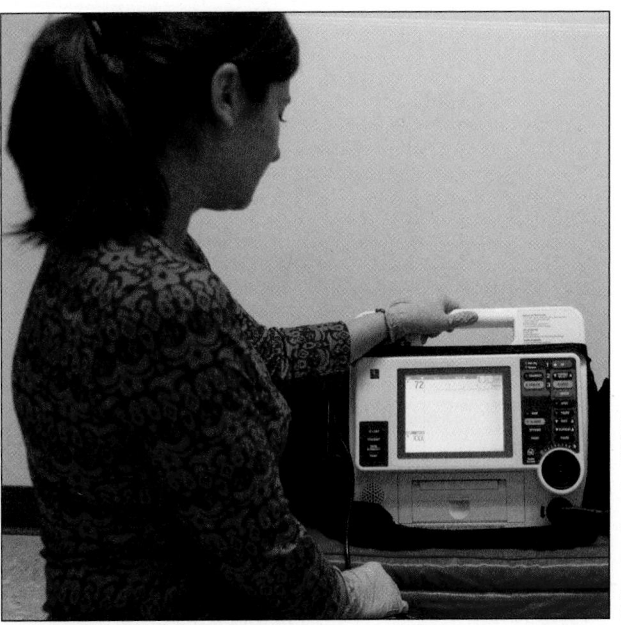

Figure 4.1

Auditory learners may benefit from listening to a cardiac monitor tone while treating a patient.

> **Teaching Tip** >> *For auditory learners, talk out everything. For example, in addition to listing the steps of a procedure on a blackboard, say the steps aloud. Also, encourage auditory learners to audiotape lectures and other presentations and to play them back when studying.*

Visual Learners

Individuals who need to see what they are learning are considered **visual learners**. They benefit from the visual presentation of material and learn best when they can look things up, write things down, and watch the performance of a skill. Educators can help these learners "see" the words by using, for example, handouts, videotapes, slides, overheads, illustrations, posters, radiographs, X-rays (**Figure 4.2**), and moulage. These individuals may speak in terms of "seeing you around" and "try to picture this." Returning to the ECG example, visual learners will need to study an ECG strip and perhaps mark intervals to help determine the rhythm. They will tend to watch the monitor whenever possible.

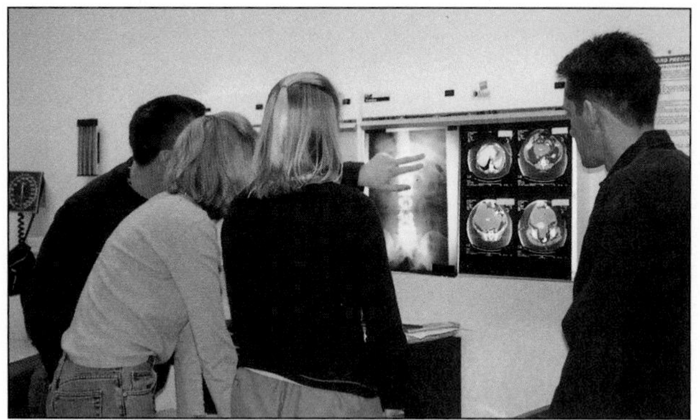

Figure 4.2

Visual learners may benefit from relating anatomy classes to X-rays.

Teaching Tip >> *Always ensure that visual aids (e.g., slides, overheads, flipchart notes) are correct. The visual learner will remember the information as he or she saw it the first time, almost as looking at a photograph.*

Kinesthetic Learners

Persons who learn with their bodies are considered **kinesthetic learners**. They prefer to associate movement and tactile experiences with learning. Educators can enhance learning for kinesthetic learners by providing opportunities for students to take things apart, make things work, and use their hands for tactile stimulation **(Figure 4.3)**. For example, when teaching the anatomy of the heart, the educator could pass around an anatomic model so students can feel the structure. Kinesthetic learners may speak of "catch you around," or, "let's get going." Laboratory sessions, scenarios, and role-playing are all effective learning activities for kinesthetic learners. They can also benefit from "air writing," in which terms, formulas, and other key statements are written in the air with the hand or finger.

Teaching Tip >> *When skills are taught, a kinesthetic learner will benefit from having the technique demonstrated on him or her. This type of learner discovers a great deal by the procedure applied to him or her.*

Analytic Learners

Persons who are logical thinkers process information logically, sequentially, and in small parts that build toward a whole. These individuals are considered

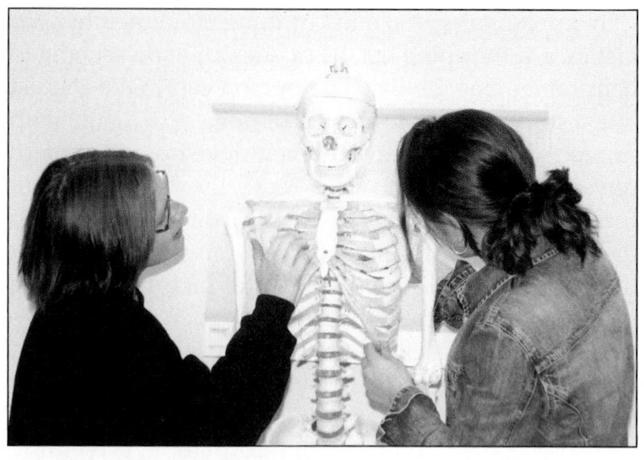

Figure 4.3

Touching and feeling things such as a skeleton can help the kinesthetic learner to understand and retain information.

analytic learners and are often described as "left-brained." Using the analogy of "the forest from the trees," the analytic learner separates the forest from the trees. He or she will look at every tree in the forest before feeling certain enough to conclude that it is a forest.

Analytic learners work comfortably by following a protocol or algorithm. They are well served by lectures that follow outlines, reading assignments, and multiple-choice questions on exams. They typically enjoy spelling, numbers, thinking, reading, analysis, and speaking. According to the ECG example, the analytic learner will look at an ECG strip and immediately begin a systematic analysis: Is it regular or irregular? Fast or slow? Is there a P wave?

CASE IN POINT

During an ECG interpretation lesson, the educator notices a paramedic student struggling with the material. The student has been studying strips and rereading textual material, but continues to misinterpret rhythms. Because this particular student tends to be physical (i.e., very active, uses hands to gesture when talking), the educator decides to implement strategies used for kinesthetic learners. He works with the student to trace ECGs with her fingertips, then to tap out the rhythms of various tracings with her feet. After running through several strips, the student seems to experience a breakthrough in understanding. She even begins to use her arms and legs to mimic a tracing in an impromptu "dance," which the class enjoys.

When learning a skill, analytic learners will benefit from detailed steps of the procedure provided in written and visual materials. These students are most comfortable mastering steps and specific information, and they need encouragement to learn judgment and global, applied concepts.

Structure, in terms of both educational process and material presented, is important to analytic learners. They may get frustrated, for example, to discover inconsistency between what is said in class and what their books say, or between what is taught and what they have been taught in the past. They may also be uncomfortable with learning that is out of sequence, or when the order of learning has been changed or rearranged. For the analytic learner, it is important to present a consistent message.

Teaching Tip >> *When a guest lecturer or secondary instructor is used, it is important to ensure consistency with the material and approach to which students have become accustomed. Analytic learners, in particular, will have trouble processing any differences. Make sure, for example, to supply the guest educator with objectives to teach from, as well as an awareness of any controversial or potentially problematic content areas. If possible, observe the class, so you can clarify points or fill in gaps later.*

Global Learners

Persons who think in terms of the big picture and who need to see the whole before the parts are considered **global learners**. They are often described as "right-brained." Returning to "the forest from the trees" analogy, the global learner will look at several trees, quickly declare it a forest, and then begin to see individual trees.

These learners tend to be creative, artistic, imaginative, emotional, and intuitive. They may be less likely to follow protocol, preferring to treat patients based on outcome, rather than on process. Global learners can also process information simultaneously; thus, they may easily move back and forth between activities and tasks. A common example of the global learner is the student who can be engaged in a task while giving instructions to others or interacting with students who are doing other tasks.

When teaching the global learner, it is important for the educator to start with an overview of the lesson, so the student knows where he or she is going. These students are most comfortable focusing on the global concepts and intuition, and they need encouragement to learn specific steps and the theory behind applications.

Teaching Tip >> *Global learners can quickly become frustrated if paired with an analytic partner, and vice versa. However, they may complement one another in the total learning experience. The educator can work with students who approach material differently by helping them to understand the differences and to value both approaches.*

Global learners enjoy working in teams. If the pace of instruction lags or is too tedious, they may become bored or distracted because they have already moved ahead to the conclusion. Techniques appropriate for these learners include mental imagery, drawing, maps, metaphors, and experiential learning.

Teaching Tip >> *Skills practice provides an opportunity for the educator to incorporate varying sensory activities and social interactions. However, specific strategies are needed to address the needs of analytic and global thinkers. Some ideas for reaching these students include the following:*

- *Use of scenarios rather than simple practice of an isolated skill*
- *Use of algorithms or protocols that students can follow*
- *Proper balance between procedure and desired result (Are other methods acceptable to accomplish the desired outcome?)*
- *Having students put skills in context by relating activity to patient-assessment findings*

Social Learners

Persons who process information best when engaged in multiple tasks in busy environments with other learners are considered **social learners** **(Figure 4.4)**. They tend to enjoy study sessions, group projects, and cooperative learning. Educators should provide opportunities for group work in class, classroom discussions, study groups, and skills groups. For social learners, background noise in the classroom or practice area, such as music or a radio, is not necessarily distracting and can even be helpful. Social networking media can be used to facilitate learning for these individuals.

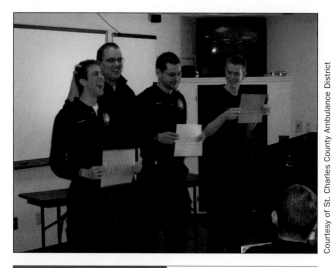

Courtesy of St. Charles County Ambulance District

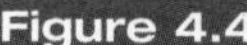
Figure 4.4

Social learners usually enjoy group projects and teamwork activities.

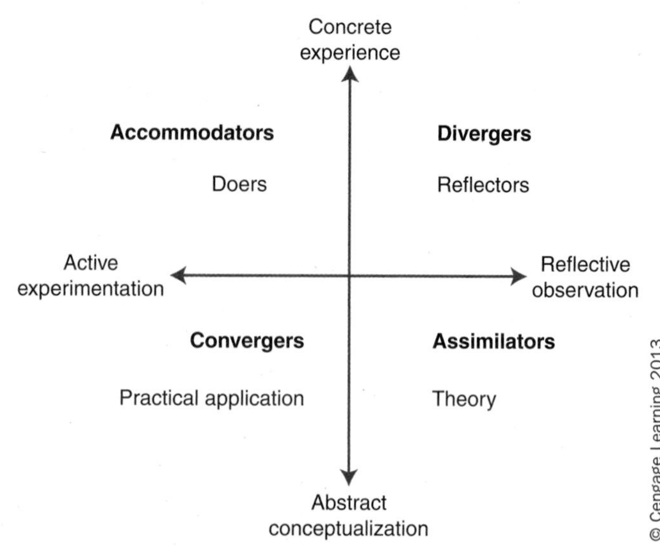

Figure 4.5

Experiential learning styles.

Independent Learners

Individuals who prefer to process information independently, isolated from other learners, are considered **independent learners**. They will seek quiet, undisturbed study environments. They react well to reading assignments, written exams, and reports. Independent learners may feel uncomfortable in "touchy-feely" classroom situations led by an educator who encourages social interaction through group exercises and projects. The response and demeanor of independent learners should not be mistaken by the social educator as lack of enthusiasm or disdain for the content; rather, the student may be uncomfortable with the presentation style.

Teaching Tip >> *When students are placed into groups, it is important for the educator to mix social and independent learners within groups. Otherwise, some groups will be gregarious, whereas others may be inhibited.*

Experiential Learning Styles

In addition to cognitive learning styles, educators need to be aware of their students' experiential learning styles.[1] This is especially true when considering practical experiences both in the field and in the classroom. Experiential learning styles are broken into four components; *convergers, divergers, assimilators,* and *accomodators* **(Figure 4.5)**.

Convergers

The converger has dominant abilities in abstract conceptualization and active experimentation. A converger favors the practical application of ideas. When teaching convergers, they will strive to find the reasoning of why a new concept or skill matters before they are willing to try something new. Ideas without obvious practical applications, such as microbiology, may be difficult for them to grasp unless the connection to practice is made.

Divergers

The diverger brings together concrete experimentation and reflective observation. Divergers are reflective and like to think through their experiences. They are skilled observers and often would prefer to watch something done first before they have an experience. Often they will reflect on an experience long after it occurred, even if they were not directly involved.

Assimilators

A combination of abstract conceptualization and reflective observation defines the assimilator, who is apt at creating theoretical models. Assimilators like to understand the theory before they put something into practice. Assimilators tend to believe that, without understanding the theory completely, they cannot treat a patient. For example, they need to understand why a medicine or procedure works before they try it.

CASE IN POINT

During a simulation, the accommodators will often be the first to volunteer. The divergers want to watch the accommodators have the experience first before they try it. Assimilators want to understand the theory first. The convergers need to understand the practical application before they have the experience.

Accommodators

Accommodators are the doers and often the first to volunteer for a new experience. The accommodator is an individual who adapts to the circumstances at hand, usually through plans and experimentation, and represents the union of concrete experience and active experimentation. Accommodators will often jump into a new experience, even if they have not learned the new concept, just to "try it out." Accommodators do not see the reason for learning theory when they can just do it.

Addressing Various Learning Styles

Learning styles are multidimensional, that is, they involve sensory input, context, experience, and environment. Because of this, the learning styles of students vary both within individual students and within the group. An educator may have to simultaneously reach learners who are visual, analytic, and independent, as well as those who are kinesthetic, global, and social—and all variations in between.

An important point to remember is that adult learners, although they have a learning preference, can adjust to other learning styles and use different styles for learning different types of material. Adults are capable of learning in almost any situation. However, the efficiency and enjoyment of the learning process for each student will vary, depending on how closely it matches his or her preferred learning style. For example, a visual learner may be required to listen to an podcast as part of a class assignment. Although he or she may not find this experience as pleasurable as seeing an illustrated lecture on the same topic, and may need to listen to the audio recording repeatedly to master the material, the student can ultimately learn from the exercise.

Educators commonly remark that they have students who are "book smart" but cannot seem to grasp practical skills (these students are often assimilators or convergers). Other learners can memorize a long list of facts but cannot seem to put them all together to develop a coherent plan of patient care. In such cases, the problem is not that these learners lack intelligence; rather, they learn some material more easily when it is presented in a style that matches their learning preference. Likewise, students may struggle with material that is presented in a style that is not congruent with their preferred method of learning.

In addition to learners who have a preference for sensory processing of new material, some regard as important the context in which information is presented. For example, some learners can easily grasp theoretical concepts presented verbally or in writing, whereas others can learn the material only when it is presented through concrete examples.

Assessing Students' Learning Styles

Before developing an instructional plan that addresses variations in student learning styles, the educator may assess the learning styles of the persons in the group. Because those who pursue a particular profession often have similar learning styles, an assessment can allow the educator to focus on the predominant learning style of the group of students.

An educator can assess students' learning styles informally in various ways, including talking with them and getting to know them; observing their behavior individually and in groups when different teaching strategies are employed; and analyzing their success in learning and retention, given different teaching strategies. For example, when an educator is talking with a student, if the student uses gestures or moves about, the educator can assume that the student is a kinesthetic learner. If the educator notices that a student speaks the words to himself while reading, then the student most likely is an auditory learner. If, after material is presented by lecture only, the student does more poorly on a quiz than he or she had done with previous material presented via video, the student is probably a visual learner. Educators can also assess students through a formal assessment process, or a standardized test, which can occur as part of a program entrance-exam process, or at the beginning of an individual course.

Remember that standardized tests are designed to assist the learner and the educator in evaluating the potential for academic and clinical success. These assessment methods should not be used as "gatekeepers" to determine which students will be allowed into a particular course. The educator is also cautioned against using test results to "prejudge" learners. Many factors beyond learning-style preference, such as innate intelligence, motivation, and previous learning success, contribute to learning and student success. Finally, even if the class appears to have a dominant learning style, the educator must continue to vary the instructional approach to stimulate as many senses as possible.

Although many standardized tests for learning styles exist, those that are most commonly used in health professions education include the Learning Styles Inventory, the Health Occupations Basic Entrance Test, and the Myers-Briggs Type Indicator.

Learning Styles Inventory

The concept of determining an individual's learning style was pioneered by Kolb, with the introduction of Kolb's Learning Style Inventory.[4] The inventory is completed by answering a series of questions that identify a person's preference for learning in four areas: concrete experience, reflective observation, active conceptualization, and active experimentation. Kolb refers to these four areas as "learning cycles." By adding together scores for the various learning cycles, four types of learners are identified; converger, diverger, assimilator and accommodator (as discussed earlier).

In addition to Kolb's Inventory, other measures of assessing learning style have been developed. The Learning-Style Model by Rita Dunn and Kenneth Dunn is one of the most researched and tested learning-style inventories.[5] This model breaks learning styles down into five stimuli that are made up of several elements **(Table 4.1)**. The learner completes a Learning Style Inventory, which asks questions related to the five stimuli and their elements. From the information gleaned about the elements, a learner can categorize his or her preference for learning in terms of the five main stimuli. This inventory gives the learner more information about how he or she *likes* to learn than is provided by the cognitive information–processing model of Kolb, which tells the learner *how* he or she learns. The Dunn and Dunn model also provides more information on learning preferences that is of value to the educator.

Table 4.1 The Learning-Style Model[3]

Stimuli	Elements
Environmental	Lighting Sound Temperature Seating arrangement
Emotional	Motivation Persistence Responsibility Structure
Sociologic (i.e., how people learn)	Alone or with peers Authoritative adult or collegial colleague Variety in learning or routine pattern
Physiologic	Perceptual skills Time-of-day energy levels Intake (eating) Mobility
Psychological	Hemispheric Impulsive or reflective Global or analytic

Damasio, 2000

Myers-Briggs Type Indicator

The Myers-Briggs Type Indicator (MBTI) is designed to determine a person's personality type.[6] It is based on the theory of personality characteristics and types developed by the psychoanalyst Carl Jung in the 1900s. The MBTI determines preferences on four dichotomies:

1. *Extraversion–Introversion*: Describes where people prefer to focus their attention and get their energy—from the outer world of people and activity, or their inner world of ideas and experiences
2. *Sensing–Intuition*: Describes how people prefer to take in information—focused on what is real and actual, or on patterns and meanings in data
3. *Thinking–Feeling*: Describes how people prefer to make decisions—based on logical analysis, or guided by concern for their impact on others
4. *Judging–Perceiving*: Describes how people prefer to deal with the outer world—in a planned, orderly way, or in a flexible, spontaneous way

Combinations of these preferences result in 16 personality types, which are represented by a four-letter acronym. For example, "Type INTJ" would be an introvert who uses intuition and thinking, as well as judging, to define his or her personality. The MBTI is useful in that it identifies differences among "normal" individuals that can lead to conflict and stress with individuals who are of different types. Strategies for addressing and avoiding these conflicts are provided. Various versions of the MBTI exist, including short versions that can be taken online. However, to be most useful, test results should be interpreted by professionals who have been trained in the administration and use of the MBTI.

Assessing the Educator's Learning Style

In addition to the impact of individual styles on a student's learning experience, the effects of the educator's personal learning style must also be considered. Educators tend to teach the way they like to learn; thus, an educator runs the risk of focusing on a particular method of instruction and possibly neglecting the needs of learners who require an alternative method of instruction.

Educators may also have difficulty understanding "problem" students owing to a difference in learning styles between the learner and the educator. For example, a learner may seem disruptive because he fidgets or moves about during class, but in actuality, he is a kinesthetic learner who feels confined in a strictly visual and auditory classroom.

Educators can use any of the common learning inventories previously mentioned to determine their own personal styles. Some educational institutions and instructor-training programs have developed "teaching style inventories" that are based on learning-style theory and research. The Myers-Briggs Type Indicator is a useful tool for determining differences between educators and students. For example, an instructor who is an extrovert may be perceived by an introverted learner as overbearing. Because of diversity within the classroom, it is important for educators to know their own learning styles and to make strong efforts to reach out to learners who use different styles or approaches to learning.

Caution on Learning Style Assessments

Caution must be taken in "labeling" a student (either by the teacher or themselves) with a particular learning style. Students will often want to know if their style is "correct," even if it only represents a preference to one method or another. No particular learning style is "better" than the other. Each has its own inherent strengths and weaknesses, and any assessment is only good for showing these particular characteristics.

The job of the educator should be to help students understand how they learn and strategies to help their learning. Educators should also try to reach as many styles as possible, but realize it may be impossible to meet everyone's personal learning style. Learning styles should not be used as a crutch or excuse, but they can help learning if identified and treated as a tool. The biggest impact of learning-style assessments may actually be in helping students foster metacognition and awareness of their learning process. The result is a process of "learning how to learn" that will help students throughout their careers. Some educational experts suggest that teaching to a particular learning style is not well supported by evidence.[7]

Using Learning Styles to Enhance Teaching

It has been said, "Variety is the spice of life." The same holds true for the classroom, especially when it comes to supporting the various learning styles of students. The simplest way for an educator to reach most learners is to vary teaching styles throughout the course and within each lesson. Variety does not necessitate jumping around and changing techniques just for the sake of change; however, a concerted effort should be made to present material and experiences in different ways to reach more learners through different senses.

The educator can use a basic instructional format, such as lecture, and supplement it with aids and activities that appeal to other learning styles. The illustrated lecture is a good example. With this method, the educator lectures (auditory) and uses projected media or writing boards (visual) or models (kinesthetic) to emphasize key points. Something as simple as a handout of the lecture outline can provide additional stimulation to help learners perceive and retain information. Workgroups can be formed or discussion begun to explore new material or solve problems; this meets the needs of social learners. Scenarios, because of their broad perspective, appeal to both global and analytic learners.

Reaching out to learners with varying learning styles is an achievable goal when the educator has a solid understanding of learning styles, basic principles of adult learning, and the various teaching strategies that are appropriate for different material and situations. Even traditional classroom activities can assist educators in providing varied presentations of the same material.

Use of diverse instruction methods ensures that each student will receive at least a small portion of the lesson through his or her preferred method of learning (**Figure 4.6**). This prevents disillusionment and frustration on the part of the learner. In addition,

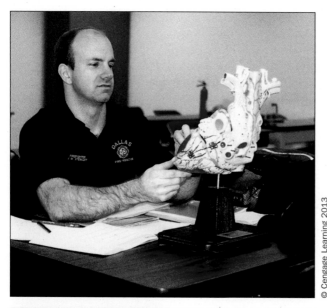

Figure 4.6

Diverse instructional methods can help ensure that each student has the opportunity to efficiently comprehend material.

it provides an opportunity for the learner to more efficiently and enjoyably comprehend the presented material. For some students, these periods of "learning comfort" (i.e., times when the material is presented in a manner consistent with the student's preferred learning style) may prevent inappropriate classroom behavior. By periodically spacing changes in presentation style throughout a lesson, the educator is able to refocus learners and stimulate their interest.

Diversity in presentation style also helps learners develop alternative learning styles and sensory preferences. For example, a visual learner may find use of an auditory mnemonic helpful. Or, an auditory learner can benefit from "going through the motions" of a procedure with the hands before taking a test. Because teamwork is so important in health care and in EMS in particular, practical sessions in which learners work in teams will promote the development of social learning preferences in independent learners. Similarly, algorithms will help global learners to become more analytic. Most learners are able to adapt to different learning styles.

CASE IN POINT

An educator is planning a lesson on musculoskeletal injuries to meet the EMT objective: "List the major bones or bone groupings of the spinal column, the thorax, the upper extremities, and the lower extremities." How might the educator enhance his or her traditional lecture to meet a variety of learning styles? Here are some ideas he or she might incorporate:

- As the opening attention getter, play the song "Them Bones" (". . . the thigh bone is connected to the hip bone . . ."). Ask students to follow along by touching each of their own bones as the song progresses.
- Show a human skeleton, and review aloud the functions and types of bones, asking students to point to their own bones as types are mentioned.
- Using slides, illustrate the key points of the lecture, with important points bolded and color coded.
- When discussing bone structure, pass around a model of a vertebra for students to examine and touch.
- When introducing new terms, ask students to repeat each term aloud as a class.
- Using blocks of wood of varying sizes with a hole in the center, have students label each appropriately sized block as a vertebra, then place it on a wire coat hanger to build a spinal column.
- Break the class into small groups, and give each group the assignment of developing a poem, song, or mnemonic for remembering the major bones of the body.
- Pass around a model of a joint for students to examine and manipulate.
- Show a short video clip, perhaps of an orthopedic operation, that shows a joint or bone type.
- Show orthopedic X-rays for guided review.
- Present a display with models or diagrams that explain the physics of joint movement and muscle involvement. This could include mathematical equations that explain the forces involved.
- During presentation of new material, make sure to relate the new to the old and to the overall context of the lesson.

Multiple Intelligences

Thus far, this chapter has described a traditional approach to learning styles, which have been discussed in terms of perception, receipt of information, and processing of information. But is there more to learning and the broader idea of intelligence? Some researchers think so. Howard Gardner of Harvard University has proposed that individuals have varying degrees of ability in eight areas, which he refers to as *intelligences*.[8] These intelligences are grouped into three broad categories: object-related, object-free, and person-related **(Table 4.2)**.

Table 4.2 Multiple Intelligences[8]

Category	Type of Intelligence	Meaning
Object-related	Logical–mathematical	Ability to work with equations and expressions, to think and process information in a logical way
	Spatial	Ability to think in three dimensions, to use and manipulate images, to apply graphic information
	Bodily–kinesthetic	Physical ability; ability to **manipulate objects**
	Naturalist	Understanding of natural and man-made systems; ability to identify and classify
Object-free	Linguistic	Ability to use words for thinking and expression
	Musical	Sensitivity to pitch, melody, rhythm, and tone
Person-related	Interpersonal	Ability to relate to others
	Intrapersonal	Ability to understand oneself and direct one's life

Gardner, 1985.

Instructor's Lesson Guide Sample[9]

COURSE: PARAMEDIC

Session Reference: 6-5

Topic: Heart blocks

Level of Instruction: Cognitive

Time Required: 3 hours

References: Paramedic ECG Textbook based on Education Standards

PREPARATION

Attention: Instructor provided

Motivation: Instructor provided

Objective: At the conclusion of this lesson, the student will be able to identify the three degrees of cardiac conduction blocks, given a real or simulated ECG tracing, without assistance, to a written test accuracy of 75 percent.

Overview:

- Anatomy and physiology of the heart
- Supraventricular conduction system
- 1st-degree block
- 2nd-degree blocks
- 3rd-degree block

LEARNING ACTIVITIES

Linguistic

In pairs, students read, discuss, and question textbook information.

Visual-Spatial

Learners identify on a heart model the location of the sinoatrial (SA) and atrioventricular (AV) nodes, the internodal pathways, and the nodal blood supply.

Musical

Learners compose a percussion piece that mimics the flow of the electrical pulse through a heart with each of the blocks.

Intrapersonal

Individually, learners identify life events that involved a delay or blockage of communications with another person.

Mathematical-Logical

In small groups, learners develop flow charts of the conduction pulse moving through the heart.

Bodily-Kinesthetic

Using paper and soda straws, as well as glue and scissors, learners construct models of the heart's conduction system.

Interpersonal

Learners role-play patients with each degree of heart block and share symptoms with each other.

Naturalist

Learners create lists of events in nature that are similar to the underlying pathophysiology of heart blocks.

SUMMARY

Review

- A&P of the heart
- Supraventricular conduction system
- 1st-degree block
- 2nd-degree blocks
- 3rd-degree block

Multiple Intelligences Toolbox[10]

LOGICAL/MATHEMATICAL

- Abstract symbols/formulas
- Calculation
- Deciphering codes
- Forcing relationships
- Graphic/cognitive organizers
- Logic/pattern games
- Number sequences/patterns
- Outlining
- Problem solving
- Syllogisms

MUSICAL/RHYTHMIC

- Environmental sounds
- Instrumental sounds
- Music composition/creation
- Music performance
- Percussion vibrations
- Rapping
- Rhythmic patterns
- Singing/humming
- Tonal patterns
- Vocal sounds/tones

BODILY/KINESTHETIC

- Body language/physical gestures
- Body sculpture/tableaus
- Dramatic enactment
- Folk/creative dance
- Gymnastic routines
- Human graph
- Inventing
- Physical exercise/martial arts
- Role playing/mime
- Sports games

VERBAL/LINGUISTIC

- Creative writing
- Formal speaking
- Humor/jokes
- Impromptu speaking
- Journal/diary keeping
- Poetry
- Reading
- Storytelling/story creation
- Verbal debate
- Vocabulary

INTERPERSONAL

- Collaborative skills teaching
- Cooperative learning strategies
- Empathy practices
- Giving feedback
- Group projects
- Intuiting others' feelings
- Jigsaw
- Person-to-person communication
- Receiving feedback
- Sensing others' motives

INTRAPERSONAL

- Altered states of consciousness practices
- Emotional processing
- Focusing/concentration skills
- Higher-order reasoning
- Independent studies/projects
- Know thyself procedures
- Metacognition techniques
- Mindfulness practices
- Silent reflection methods
- Thinking strategies

VISUAL/SPATIAL

- Active imagination
- Color/texture schemes
- Drawing
- Guided imagery/visualizing
- Mind mapping
- Montage/collage
- Painting
- Patterns/designs
- Pretending/fantasy
- Sculpting

NATURALIST

- Archetypal pattern recognition
- Caring for plants/animals
- Conservation practices
- Environment feedback
- Hands-on labs
- Nature encounters/field trips
- Nature observation
- Natural world simulations
- Species classification (organic/inorganic)
- Sensory stimulation exercises

Each individual person has varying strengths of each intelligence, and each person combines these intelligences in a personal way that defines his or her overall intelligence. For example, a person may have the ability to play the piano beautifully, but may struggle in mathematics. Another individual may be adept at understanding himself or herself, but weak at understanding others. These are examples of different intellectual strengths or combinations of strengths possessed by individuals.

Similar to the more traditional concept of one intelligence, Gardner's multiple intelligences follow a developmental sequence and emerge at different times in a person's life. They also consist of a series of subintelligences. Overall, Gardner's theory provides an expanded view of what it means to be human.

Psychologists and educators have criticized Gardner's theory saying that these "intelligences" are merely talents and personal abilities and traits, and that no empirical data supports his theory. But for the educator, it appears that curricula should be developed that appeal to these eight intelligences or personality traits. Just as it is important in the more traditional approach to learning styles to vary the presentation of material, so too should the educator plan activities that help the learner to develop his or her dominant intelligences. The text boxes on pages 63 and 64 contain strategies for each of the eight intelligences.

Summary

Each learner brings to the classroom a preference for the way he or she perceives, receives, and processes information. To maximize learning, the educator must be aware of these differences, must employ a variety of teaching strategies, and must provide a variety of learning activities that will reach all students. Similarly, educators must be sensitive to the fact that they, too, have a preference for learning that influences their teaching style and their interaction with students.

The traditional approach to learning styles has been to describe them in terms of sensory perception and social interaction. New theories, such as Gardner's multiple intelligences, are expanding the view of learning styles and challenging educators and curriculum developers to introduce new and varying ways of presenting material.

Glossary

analytic thinking Processing information in a logical, sequential manner.

archetypal pattern recognition Traits, behavior, or symbolic pattern recognition.

auditory learning Learning through sounds.

experiential learning An active learning process that engages all senses.

global thinking Processing information by seeing the whole before the parts.

independent thinking Processing information alone.

kinesthetic learning Learning through touch.

learning style A preferred method of learning.

social thinking Processing information effectively while multi-tasking in a group setting.

syllogism A type of argument in logic that contains a major and minor premise and a conclusion.

thinking style The method by which an individual prefers to make decisions.

visual learning Learning through imagery.

References

1. Lalley, J. P., & Miller, R. H. (2007). The learning pyramid: Does it point teachers in the right direction? *Education, 128*(1), 64–79.
2. Edelman, G., & Tononi, G., (2000). *A universe of consciousness: How matter becomes imagination*. New York, NY: Basic Books.
3. Damasio, A., (2000). *The feeling of what happens: Body and emotion in the making of consciousness.* New York, NY: Harcourt Brace.
4. Kolb, D. A., Ru*bin, I. M., &* *McIntyre, J. M. (1979). Organizational psychology: A book of readings* (3rd ed.). Englewood Cliffs, NJ: Prentice-Hall. (pp. 543–549).
5. Dunn, R. *S., & K. J. (1978). Teaching students through their individual learning styles: A practical approach.* Reston, Va: Reston Publishing.
6. Myers, I. B. (1980). *Gifts differing*. Palo Alto, CA: Consulting Psychological Press.
7. Pashler, H., McDaniel, M., Rohrer, D., & Bjork, R. (2008). Learning styles: Concepts and evidence. *Science in the Public Interest*, *9*(3), 106–116.
8. Gardner, H. (1985). *Frames of mind: The theory of multiple intelligences.* New York, NY: Basic Books.
9. Campbell, L. Campbell, B., & Dickinson, D. (1999). *Teaching and learning through multiple intelligences.* Needham Heights, MA: Allyn and Bacon.
10. Lazear, D. (1999). *Eight ways of knowing: Teaching for multiple intelligences* (3rd ed.). Arlington Heights, IL: Skylight Professional Development.

5

Diversity

Tolerance implies no lack of commitment to one's own beliefs. Rather it condemns the oppression or persecution of others. —JOHN F. KENNEDY

Individuals view life through a unique set of perspectives, shaped by years of accumulated experiences and interactions with the world. They absorb and reject the thoughts, opinions, and ideas of others as they see fit. Within the Emergency Medical Services (EMS) classroom, educators should allow and even encourage the presentation of conflicting viewpoints. Instructors have the ability and power to provide the information and setting necessary to promote better awareness and understanding of diversity among students, both within the classroom and later outside of the classroom, when students enter the field as interns and finally as practitioners.

The United States consists of one of the most diverse populations of people, ideas, and cultures in the world. Most people have heard the United States referred to as a "melting pot." Population data bear that out, reflecting great diversity in age, race, and religion throughout the country.[1] Many EMS instructors and providers understand the complexities involved in caring for patients and working in a diverse society. However, EMS could improve the elements of diversity seen in its curricula and in its practitioners. The Longitudinal Emergency Medical Technician Attribute and Demographic Study (LEADS) indicated that approximately 72 percent of those registered with the National Registry of EMTs are male and 70 percent are white.[2] Because there appears to be a disparity between the diversity of the general population of the nation and that of EMS, it is important that the instructor work toward including elements of diversity throughout the curriculum. This chapter cannot and should not serve as the only guide in that effort. It will, however, identify key concepts (1) to better prepare EMS providers to treat patients within a diverse population, and (2) to improve diversity within the profession, beginning with a culturally aware educational environment **(Figure 5.1)**.

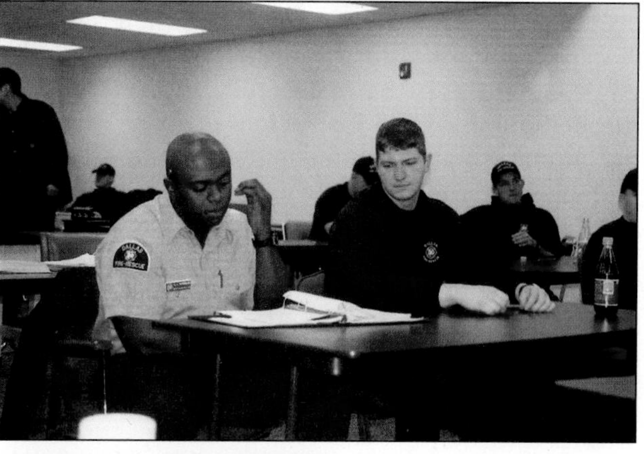

Figure 5.1

Instructors have the ability to promote understanding of diversity among students and patients.

CHAPTER GOAL: The goal of this chapter is for the educator to explore strategies to teach effectively in a diverse classroom.

Instructor, Know Thyself

All human beings are susceptible to having biases. This is not a value statement; it is simply fact. The 2003 *Merriam Webster Dictionary* defines **bias** as "an unreasonable judgment." For example, an instructor may *unreasonably* believe that all women are too weak to perform many of the tasks commonly required in EMS. That instructor might be seen often rushing to assist the female students in the class, regardless of their capabilities or requests not to be "treated special" during lifting and carrying exercises. This instructor's judgment is obviously not based on any reasoned discourse.

Biases can take many forms. Examples include biases against particular ethnicities, genders, ages, socioeconomic classes, religions, political persuasions, and sexual orientations. The *Case in Point* (below) gives an example of a person who held multiple biases, which created a negative synergistic effect on his attitude and behavior toward others. In this case, the instructor has a bias against a Latina woman's ability to understand and excel in math.

Biases become dangerous when they are manifested as behaviors. An instructor's behavior in the classroom can and will affect the probability of success for many students. An instructor who believes students can succeed makes that prospect more likely than one who believes they will fail. Students' sense of self-efficacy (i.e., their sense of "I can do it!") is directly related to the classroom environment and the instructor's expectations of those students.[3] EMS instructors must be aware of the impact their attitudes may have on students, and they should remain diligent to prevent their own biases from negatively affecting the perceptions of those students.

CASE IN POINT

It was the second day of the "med math" section of the pharmacology unit, and the instructor was busy working with the paramedic students, trying to convey the basic concepts of proportion and cross-multiplication to the group. The instructor noticed that a Latina woman seemed to be grasping the concepts easily, and she was using them to solve a complex dopamine drip problem. Later, he noticed her working with several other students. During a break in the session, the instructor approached the student, patted her on the shoulder, and said, "I am pleased that you were able to grasp the concepts quickly, especially considering your background. I appreciate that you are helping out the other women in the class."

The student appeared puzzled. "Why are you surprised?"

The instructor responded, "I figured that being female and *all,* that you probably were not really prepared in your high school for mathematics."

Silent for a moment, the student finally sighed and replied, "I'm not sure why you would think that. Actually, I excelled in math. Furthermore, I resent the idea that I could help only other women, especially since I helped three male students as well!"

To deal with or reduce bias, one first has to acknowledge its existence. Performing a critical self-reflection and recognizing one's own personal biases are ways to begin a process of self-discovery and a greater awareness of one's own potential biases. Instructors should try to see lessons and other course materials through the perceptions of others, and should consider enrolling in cultural diversity classes offered through a local college or university. For the instructor who has already critically examined and dealt with any such issues, it remains incumbent upon him or her to challenge students to do the same.

Teaching Tip >> *Ask a colleague to review exams and lesson plans for possible cultural bias.*

Diversity in the Classroom

A tremendous amount has been written about **cultural competency** within a variety of environments, including the worksite and the classroom. Earlier efforts in EMS education focused on identification of the unique traits of specific groups, based on gender, ethnic, and religious lines.[4] Although those who made these attempts meant well, the truth is that the very act of defining group characteristics can reinforce the very stereotypes that such efforts are designed to minimize. Instructors who try to modify their teaching practices based on "laundry lists" of such characteristics will quickly run into issues associated with any "one-size-fits-all" approach, namely, that not all members of a specific group of individuals are completely alike. Stereotyping assumptions will likely cause discomfort for the student and the instructor. This discomfort may rise to a level of anger and open frustration that disrupts the class.

Students within the classroom may include representatives from a wide variety of groups. Alternatively, the instructor may be faced with a group of culturally similar students, and may find him- or herself in the minority. How many ways can a single group of students be dissimilar?

- Age (younger versus older, nontraditional students)
- Appearance (e.g., hair length, hygiene, tattoos, piercings)
- Disorders (e.g., physical, emotional, and psychological/psychiatric disabilities)

- Gender identification (e.g., female, male, bisexual, transgender)
- Generational (e.g., Baby Boomers, Gen X-ers, Gen Y-ers, In-betweens, Millenials)
- Learning ability (e.g., attention deficit disorder, dyslexia, underprepared educational background)
- Language ability (e.g., speaking non-English as first language, using poor grammar, depending heavily on slang)
- Marital status (e.g., cohabitating, divorced, married, single, widowed)
- Parenting (e.g., no children, older or younger children, stepchildren, or older, dependent parents)
- Political views (e.g., conservatism, liberalism, libertarianism)
- Race/ethnicity (alphabetical categories listed here are from the U.S. Census Bureau[1] and are used on most federal and state forms: American Indian, Alaska Native, Asian, Native Hawaiian or other Pacific Islander, Black or African American, Hispanic or Latino, and White)
- Religion (e.g., Buddhism, Christianity, Islam, Romany, Wicca)
- Sexual orientation (e.g., bisexual, heterosexual, homosexual)
- Socioeconomic status (e.g., indigent, poor, middle class, wealthy)

Careful review of this list should lead to the realization that even apparently homogeneous students can be different in many ways. This should not be surprising, as it reinforces what is commonly known: Each student is an individual and does not deserve to be limited to being seen as a "representative" of any one group. Students should be seen as complex beings with much to offer the class. Each possesses experience and knowledge that can add to the richness of the classroom experience for other students and for the instructor.

Generational Learning: Is There Really A Difference?

Much has been said, discussed, and debated about the role of generations and the ways people learn. There are many labels that the general media has used over the years to describe certain age groups; a simplified way to describe these differences is as follows:

- *Baby Boomers:* Individuals born sometime between the mid-1940s and mid-1960s; born in the era that included the post World War II boom period in the United States and prior to the general mistrust of U.S. government involvement in Vietnam.
- *Gen-Xers*: Short for Generation X, a term first used by Douglas Copeland in a novel describing teenage lifestyles in the 1980s,[5] the birth dates of this generation span roughly from the mid-1960s to the early 1980s.
- *Millennials*: Sometimes coined "Generation Y," "Net-Gen," or the Digital Generation, their birth dates span from the 1980s to the late 1990s.

At the time of this publication, the "postmillennial" generation is just beginning to enter the primary educational system.

A web search produces literally millions of popular articles, blogs, and opinions on the similarities and differences of perception, values, and judgments among the different generations. Yet there is little scientific data that supports specific educational methods, geared toward apparent generational traits, actually improve learning outcomes.[6] For example, it would be a mistake to believe that a Millennial generation student would learn better with technology-based tools, simply because he or she uses social media sites easily, or possesses a smartphone, or sends text messages without a second thought. Rather, it has been suggested that the "Net-Gen" individual, while adept at being an end user of Internet technology, has a shallower base of knowledge about how the technologies work than previous generations.[7]

As it is with any other label, the use of a generation descriptor as simply a method of choosing specific learning tools would be superficial at best. Keeping the information relevant, interesting, and appealing to the student's intrinsic values is the teacher's best tool to excellent teaching.

Power in the Teaching Relationship

The relationship between student and instructor can be a powerful one, although not in the sense of *power* meaning "strength." Rather, in this case, **power** refers to the *control* that an instructor exerts upon the relationship with the student. For example, the instructor sets the teaching schedule, grades the tests, assigns the clinical rotations, and designs the curriculum, just to name a few obvious tasks. The student usually has little or no control over these areas. Another aspect of that control is the ability to decide what is taught in the classroom. The instructor may, knowingly or not, taint the material that is being taught by injecting elements of bias into lessons. Effects of bias can be seen in individual lessons and even throughout an entire curriculum. For example, although many major publishers have worked to minimize this, not all EMS textbooks equally portray individuals from ethnic minority groups and women in positions of authority.[8] The images and the *feel* of a textbook can influence an entire course. This is not to say that diversity is the only element to consider when one is choosing a text; however, it is something that should be evaluated closely.

Teaching Tip >> *When selecting a textbook, the instructor must be fully aware of the level of diversity (and equity) demonstrated in that text. It can be as straightforward as examining the number of images showing diversity of patients and EMS personnel, or the use of gender-specific pronouns such as "he" or "she."*

Instructors should not be afraid of embracing diversity. Some instructors may be tempted to ignore student diversity when it could in fact contribute to the learning environment, not only of those individuals but also of the whole group. For example, an instructor may have students from a rural, agricultural community who could directly speak to the hazards of farm machinery. Their unique cultural experiences could help to make the material more relevant for the entire class.[9] It would be tragic to ignore this wealth of information and to rely solely upon textbooks.

Opportunities to Integrate Classroom Diversity

There are many ways for an educator to create an environment that takes advantage of a classroom's diversity, rather than minimizes it. Not all approaches will work with every instructor. Instructors should decide which of the following suggestions might work for them, based on their background and comfort level. Then, they should try these suggestions or develop their own ideas; they may find these efforts to be surprisingly interesting and effective.

Instructional Materials

Attention to details influences the tone of the classroom. A small effort to include diversity in the names and characteristics of patient models, scenarios, printed materials, and visual aids goes a long way toward making students feel comfortable and valued in their learning situations.

Ethnicity and Gender

Spoken and written language should be ethnically/racially and gender nonspecific or used with equal frequency. Contrived or forced neutrality (e.g., using "he/she") should be avoided. The instructor can use "he" or "she" in alternating scenarios and test questions, or can use generic phrases such as "the patient" and "the doctor." Scenarios can be used to challenge misperceptions and to strengthen positive role models. For example, a scenario might be written in which the nurse is male and the EMS supervisor is female. By challenging traditional perceptions, these scenarios help to expose students to greater possibilities, so they can develop an openness to incorporating those possibilities into their practice.

Identifying the ethnicity or gender of patients in written scenarios is not always necessary. In general, this information can be legitimately omitted, allowing students to focus on the *real* issues at hand. However, there are times when these characteristics are significant elements of a person's medical history (e.g., when genetic disorders such as sickle cell or Tay–Sachs disease are considered). When needed, ethnic and gender identifiers should be used. Care should be taken, however, to avoid reinforcing negative—and unfounded—stereotypes. Cite accurate statistics and frame these concepts against the broad background of medicine. It can be helpful to discuss the contributions of different ethnic groups to the field of medicine as part of the curriculum and not spotlight it as a side topic. A reference librarian can serve as an excellent resource.

Printed Material and Visual Aids

The educator should ensure that models and simulated situations reflect a wide variety of cultural backgrounds. For example, computer images of people of different genders and from various ethnic, cultural, and/or religious backgrounds can be used. Scripted scenarios should also incorporate a wide range of socioeconomic factors. Frequent reviews of textbooks by instructors for issues of equity and diversity will help to ensure not only the quality of the text but also the degree to which it encourages diversity. Feedback from students will be helpful as well.

Instructional Strategies

Instructors who provide variations in teaching and learning strategies in their classrooms help assure that they will meet the needs of a diverse group of students. Further, taking steps to assure fair assessment of student learning reduces the risk for instructor bias to creates situations where evaluation is not fair for everyone.

Presentation

Rather than using only one type of presentation format (e.g., lecture), the educator should use a variety of teaching strategies. The student body within any given classroom community is likely to represent a wide range of learning styles. The use of multiple methods of instruction will help to enhance the learning of the class. Examples of teaching methods include small group exercises, take-home case studies, debates, large group discussions, web-based lessons, and role playing. As information-sharing technology and social media continue to evolve and be integrated into everyday tasks, instructors can take advantage of the different platforms and provide even greater access to their educational material. For the generation of students who are growing up not knowing the era when the Internet did not exist, the 24/7 availability of learning resources is not only useful, but even expected.

Assessment

Instructors must be aware of their own biases when they are evaluating a student's performance. It may be helpful to have students identify all written assignments with a code name or only a portion of their social security number, so their identities are shielded during grading. Multiple instructors may videotape or observe practical scenarios and role playing to establish an "average" score. (*Note:* If these scores vary greatly, it may be appropriate to discount the highest and lowest scores, averaging the remaining middle scores.) These safeguards work in two ways: They help students by ensuring that they are not unfairly penalized, and they help instructors to avoid favoritism.

Student-Educator Relations

Learning is more likely to occur when an instructor creates a safe classroom climate. It is an important aspect of an instructor's role to take concrete steps to create that climate.

Awareness

One must recognize that students come from diverse and complex backgrounds. Nothing about them should be assumed. For example, comments about social activities that assume all students are heterosexual, middle class, or Christian should be avoided. One must not assume that the most obvious perception of a student's ethnicity (or even gender) is correct (e.g., a person who might be thought of as Hispanic American may self-identify as white American). As the nation becomes increasingly diverse, the percentage of people who identify with a multiplicity of heritages (and races) also increases. Students must be permitted to explain who and what they are and how they want to be identified.

Terminology

The educator must be sensitive to changing terminology. For example, Asian Americans may not want to be referred to as Oriental, Hispanic Americans may prefer to be called "Chicano" or "Latino," and persons from diverse families may wish to be referred to as "multiracial." If it is *necessary* to categorize, ask which labels are comfortable or preferable.

Spotlighting

One must not force a student to be the spokesperson for any group. For example, when describing the higher frequency of alcoholism or diabetes within a particular group, the instructor must not single out a member of that group to be its spokesperson. However, students may volunteer to share firsthand information about their community. This type of contribution should be encouraged.

Knowledge

The instructor should get to know his or her students **(Figure 5.2)**. Office hours, class "down time," and any other lull in activity can be used to find out about personal background and learning styles. The educator can become better informed about different cultures by researching, reading, and participating in culture-specific activities. Students should be encouraged to write scenarios for the class that are based on personal experiences. This approach helps to validate students' lives for the group, and it shows that the instructor values what is shared.

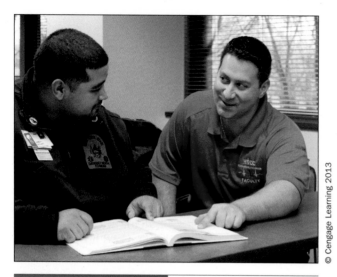

Figure 5.2

Getting to know students as individuals enables the instructor to better understand their backgrounds and values.

Behavior

One must lead by example. The instructor should exhibit the actions desired in his or her students. If comments are made in the classroom that focus on negative stereotypes, the instructor should take time to discuss and counter them with accurate information. If the instructor does not have the information available at the time, he or she should reach out to *key informants* in the community for help. Typically, these people are well known and highly respected members of a community who are eager to help share information about their community.

Environment

The educator must create a classroom environment that is a safe haven for discussion and exploration. Distasteful or abusive remarks, even if spoken in jest, must not be tolerated. It is important to remember that what is humorous to some may be hurtful to others.

Acceptance

Many elements of everyday behaviors are influenced by cultural rules. For example, some cultures may consider eye contact between an elder (the instructor) and a child (the student, regardless of age) to be disrespectful, whereas many in our society view such contact as just the opposite. The instructor who is aware that such *cultural disconnects* exist can avoid embarrassing and even infuriating moments.

Preparing Students to Incorporate Diversity Awareness into their Practice

Open communication is an essential element to any successful group endeavor. Instructors must foster clear dialogue within their learning setting to promote learning and develop a collegial group experience.

Culture

When the word **culture** is mentioned, images of racially or ethnically based differences often come to mind. Many social scientists, however, define *culture* as an amalgamation of customs, experiences, languages, and beliefs common to a defined group. For example, various regions of the nation are described as having uniquely identifiable cultures with predominant characteristics for that area (e.g., Southeastern states, Appalachia, inner-city urban areas). The same can be said for regions of the world (e.g., Central America, South Pacific, Middle East).

Social scientists define *culture* as a group of people who share experiences, language, and values that permit them to communicate knowledge not shared by those outside the culture. An example of a culture is EMS itself. How many providers have used the jargon of the profession ("10-8," "code 3," "ALS") in a conversation with people outside the industry, only to have someone look quizzically at them—when EMS providers get together and begin talking, they should take pity on the non-EMS person who tries to keep up with the discussion. Any person who is looking from the outside in would likely be very confused about what is being said and meant. This lack of "getting it" is an example of low *cultural competency.* It is possible that students in the EMS classroom come with culturally specific elements in their communication. The EMS instructor must be aware of this potential challenge and should build tools to overcome it. One strategy would be to invite students to write down a list (with definitions) of the slang words they commonly use. Another strategy would be to simply ask students what they mean any time an unknown word is noted in the classroom.

CASE IN POINT

It was early Monday morning, and an EMT instructor was just about to begin her class. About half of the students were in the classroom; some were reviewing their textbooks, while others were reading the newspaper. As the instructor came into the room, she noticed that a few students were congregated toward the back of the room. One animated student was relating to a group of students the details of an EMS call he had observed the previous day. The instructor overheard a few laughs but did not really pay any attention to the conversation. Soon, the class came to order, and the day's lesson on cardiac emergencies began.

During lunch, a student came to see the instructor in her office. This student was visibly angry and obviously needed to talk. Concerned, the instructor closed the office door and listened carefully to her. Apparently, the conversation that the animated student was leading earlier involved a patient who was suffering from end-stage AIDS, necessitating an urgent call for EMS. The student had described how he had been riding along as an EMT observer with the crew. The student who was currently upset had overheard the other student saying comments such as "homosexuality is a sin" and "AIDS is what you get when you're gay." Even though she was not part of the discussion, this student was angered by the comments, especially because her sister had died of AIDS only six months earlier.

The instructor asked the student if she said anything to the other student about his comments. She shook her head—no; she felt very uncomfortable talking to him directly. Angrily, the student said, "I just want him to know that not all AIDS patients are gay, and even those who are do not deserve to suffer like that!"

FOLLOW-UP

After the upset student left the instructor's office, the instructor spent the remainder of her break finishing her lunch and thinking about how she could manage the situation. Despite her own discomfort and anger about what the other student had said to his classmates, she knew she had to intervene to try to turn a tense situation into a learning experience for all involved. In her conversation with the instructor, the upset student had indicated that she was not seeking an apology from the other student, nor did she want to get him "into any trouble."

The instructor decided to implement the following plan:

1. At the next break, she would pull aside the student who had made the negative comments and determine what he had actually said during the discussion. She would advise him that the comments, if stated as reported, were hurtful to another student and would not be considered professional behavior in her class. The instructor would also provide the student an opportunity to express his feelings about what was said and about how another person perceived his comments. However, she would make sure that he understood that the comments he had made were inappropriate, and that he should avoid making similar ones in the future. Later that day, she would document her conversations with both students, possibly having each student sign a copy of the respective incident reports.
2. At the next class, she would engage the class in a short discussion about verbal behavior in the classroom, as well as in the clinical setting. She felt it would be important to reinforce to the entire class how critical it is to be mindful of other people's feelings and perceptions, in case a conversation is accidentally overheard. She would be careful to avoid "shutting down" the student who had made the comments and would make sure that he continues to feel valued as a member of the classroom community.
3. Later in the semester, she would provide additional information about HIV and AIDS through handouts, Internet links, and discussions in class.
4. She would schedule clinical rotations with a local AIDS hospice. Each student would be required to submit a written summary of his or her experiences and to share those experiences with the entire class in a discussion or presentation.

Transcultural communication can open doors to greater understanding, but it can also lead to misunderstanding. Misunderstanding, often caused by ignorance, can make or break the medical management of an event. The following section provides some suggestions on how to reduce the occurrences of misunderstanding; ways to implement a culturally aware medical curriculum are discussed.

Developing A Culturally Sound Teaching Curriculum

Instructors expect to follow specific steps for students to learn skills such as airway management. It is equally important to design purposeful strategies to promote their skills related to cultural awareness.

Needs Assessment

Not all areas of the nation are similar in terms of the cultures that exist there. For example, the incidence of homelessness may be greater in an urban, inner-city area than in a sparsely populated, rural area. A needs assessment, or evaluation, should be conducted by the EMS instructor for the purpose of ascertaining which terms, customs, and other cultural elements should be introduced into the curriculum to best serve local, regional, and national needs.

Sometimes what is needed is evident. For example, the rapid influx of an ethnically based population, for whom English is not the primary language, may necessitate a specific training effort to educate the EMS system about basic practices and traditions within that population. Many texts are available to learn more about the theory of evaluation techniques. (For more information, see the works of Guskey, Tyler, and Scriven in the Additional Resources section of this chapter.)

Research

This can often be the most labor-intensive step of developing a culturally sound curriculum. What information is needed during preparation of the lesson plan that will deliver the concepts? Often, the information cannot be found in traditional EMS textbooks. However, it can be found in many places, including libraries, the Internet, journals, and textbooks. (For more information, see Sue and Sue in the Additional Resources section of this chapter.) Other sources may provide more accurate and relevant information to EMS than can be found in published writings. One such source consists of those persons identified as community leaders or key informants within the population in question.

Other Resources

Local service agencies often focus on specific groups within a community and can offer a wealth of information about their clientele. Many such agencies are more than happy to share their expertise with anyone who wishes to become more enlightened. For example, a local council on aging might offer an entire presentation on the psychosocial issues the elderly face when living alone, or they might help to arrange for elderly persons to serve as patients during presentation of a unit on Geriatrics.

In addition to local resources, many helpful sources of information are available at the federal and national levels. Organizations such as the American Medical Association (AMA) and the American Association of Medical Colleges (AAMC) have released compendiums of references on the needs and resources of specific populations. The American Association of Universities and Colleges (AAUC) has compiled resource information on culturally aware teaching practices. (Some of these sources can be located in the Additional Resources section of this chapter.)

Instructional Strategies

Many cultural concepts can be integrated directly into the medical curriculum that is being taught. In doing so, the instructor must take the time needed to develop and establish the "ground rules for a safe environment." These rules must include statements assuring all students that they will have the opportunity to speak and to be heard. Students must know, however, that there are limits to this free speech. This limit in the classroom, as in society, means that *one person's right to expression stops at the next person's nose.* That means students may speak, they may be honest, and they may disagree; they may not, however, attack one another. So, although *ideas* may be torn apart (i.e., with the use of reasoned arguments, or *discourse*), *people* may not be. The instructor must present these rules to the class and must ensure that all participants understand and agree to abide by them. Students should be given an opportunity to read and add to or argue against the specifics of the list of rules, but in the end, they must all sign a contract of agreement with the final document.

Instructors can incorporate diversity into a classroom community by employing a variety of educational methods, including some of those discussed in the following paragraphs.

Case Studies

These scenario-based lessons tell students about an event, the actions taken, and the outcomes. For example, students may be given a written exercise that contains a short scenario about an elderly woman who was found "down" in her apartment by neighbors. The case proceeds to detail what the responding crew found, how they treated the patient, and how the patient responded. These types of scenarios may be created to include a wide variety of diverse elements.

Guest Presentation

If the community of interest is a particular religious group, a member of the local house of faith could be invited to present a lecture to the class. This lecture might include a brief history of the group, an explanation of its core beliefs, and any special information that would be particularly useful during an emergency (e.g., perhaps members of this faith do not accept blood products or medications, or perhaps they permit female patients to be touched only by female caregivers). Students should be encouraged to ask questions, and the presenter must be made to feel welcome, even when his or her beliefs seem strange or extreme.

Community Outreach

Students often engage in community-minded projects, such as staffing first aid stations, providing blood pressure checks, and giving bicycle safety lectures **(Figure 5.3)**. It could be helpful for the instructor (or the program) to sponsor such efforts in targeted communities. Students could set up a health education booth at a community center in an ethnic minority neighborhood, or they may provide free cardiopulmonary resuscitation (CPR) classes for a low-income, single-parents group. The communities that receive these services may, in turn, share intimate knowledge about the group. Students may be invited to attend local festivals or events, an opportunity that would further their understanding and appreciation of that culture.

Group Discussions

An open forum is best supported by clear guidelines and goals. If some students in the class identify themselves as members of the community of interest, they should be invited (not compelled) to share their thoughts and experiences. Other sources of information are local community leaders (e.g., ministers, business owners, and instructors). The instructor must begin such discussions with a brief outline of

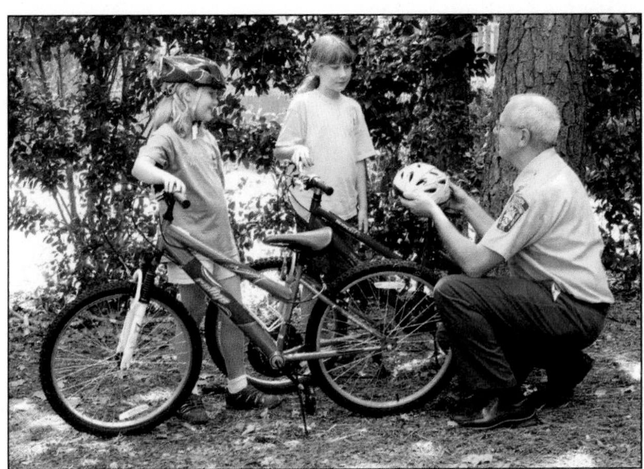

Figure 5.3

Injury-prevention activities sponsored by the educational program can be educational for the community, as well as for school-age students.

CASE IN POINT

"Uh oh, what did I do now?" the instructor thought to herself as she walked into her supervisor's office. Everyone knows just how unpleasant "visits" like these can be. No notice, no warning—she was getting dressed for shift in the locker room when the overhead page requested her presence on the second floor.

She was a bit surprised when she entered the office. In addition to her supervisor, an elderly man was sitting in the room. Smiling, her supervisor introduced her to the director of the senior citizen assistance office of the county health department.

"Remember when you were talking about the number of hip fractures you were handling at the elder care high-rises downtown?" her supervisor asked.

"Uh huh," the instructor replied. (She was actually ranting and raving about how ambulance resources were being used to handle these cases. It seemed like a city rig goes to a report of a "person found down" once or twice a week!)

"Well," the supervisor said, "by chance, I was talking to the director here about another issue, when I mentioned this might be a problem. He has offered to listen to your complaint and offer some assistance." The three began a discussion about identifying the nature of the problem.

FOLLOW-UP

First, the instructor established a common ground with all interested parties—everyone involved in this case understands the serious effects of a fractured hip for elderly patients. Next, the three discussed the possibility of performing a risk analysis to determine what factors increase or decrease the likelihood of a fall. The county's public health office probably has a tool for gathering such information. Those data could be used in the design of a safety program that eliminates hazards (e.g., loose carpeting replaced with a nonslip version, hand rails added to all rooms) and teaches residents how to monitor their personal risk index. Lastly, the instructor decided to establish a ***train the trainer*** model by which she would prepare her staff to go out into the community and educate the staff at the elder care centers.

the rules for the event. These rules must establish that ideas are welcome but attacks are not. Each student must feel safe if open and frank discussions are to occur. The instructor should function as the facilitator, guiding the discussion but not controlling it. The instructor will be *the guide on the side—not the sage on the stage.*[10]

CASE IN POINT

During a recent class discussion, the instructor presented information about initial scene assessment (the global survey). He stated that some EMS agencies provide bullet-resistant vests for their personnel. One local agency does this, and they allow the employees to wear the "over the shirt" type of vest whenever the employees believe it is justified. A student asked why most of the EMS personnel she knows wear the vests only when they get a call to go to areas of town that are primarily populated by ethnic minorities. The class immediately began a debate about the "facts" that these parts of town have more calls that are violent, and that EMS is more likely to be threatened in these areas. Some members of the class describe this as a reasonable precaution. Others describe it as racial profiling. They turn to the instructor and look for guidance. What does he do?

FOLLOW-UP

First, the instructor distills the arguments on both sides to their most salient points (e.g., crime rates, number of past EMS assaults, overall violence in the areas). Then, he gets each side to do some research to back up their beliefs. They could examine publicly available statistics and invite local community leaders to discuss the issue. He asks that each side bring their results back into class and present them to one another. This case is based on local practices, so it would be appropriate to bring in a representative of the local EMS to explain the reasoning that went into the policy's creation and implementation.

Practical Skills

Ideally, an actor is brought into the skills laboratory for each practical scenario. The actor must be prepared to play his or her role. Care should be taken to create scenarios that inform students and even challenge perceptions. For example, a scenario about a pregnant teenager should not always include a person of one particular racial/ethnic or socioeconomic group. If actors are not available, students can be coached to take on the patient roles, and to conduct the research necessary to perform the role accurately. Although they may be labor intensive, such exercises can stimulate alternative learning opportunities for all students involved.

Clinical Rotations

Clinically oriented rotations can be supplemented by limited observations in nontraditional settings. For example, if the community of interest includes severely intellectually disabled patients, students may be assigned clinical rotations with a center that specializes in the care of these patients. Such rotations could provide students with expert opinions and a chance to put a face on the disorder, thereby making it more meaningful to them.

Identity

Instructors and students make assumptions about others. These assumptions include labels of ethnicity, religion, disability, and more. One strategy that is useful for challenging such potentially erroneous assumptions is known as the "identity game." During this type of exercise, students might be asked to elaborate (by writing on an index card) on how they see *themselves* (e.g., "heterosexual, Christian, male"). Each student could label his or her card using a code name known only to the instructor. These completed cards would be turned in to the instructor, who would then randomly assign the cards to other members of the class. Each student's assignment would be to try to identify the classmate whose card he or she was given. The class would be polled to see how many students were able to identify the author of their card.

Role Playing

Students are asked to identify a group (e.g., ethnic, gender, religion) that is different from their own. They are then assigned to play parts in a patient care scenario based on their new identity. For example, a Christian female student may play the part of an elderly Jehovah's Witness male patient, or an ethnic minority male student might play the part of the nonminority male firefighter. This exercise has been used in EMS classrooms with great success. However, a degree of caution must be issued here. These portrayals can be full of stereotypes and clichés. Some will break down walls and use humor to demonstrate the ridiculousness of such beliefs. Others may cause needlessly hurt feelings and have the potential to create disharmony within the classroom community. It is recommended that this exercise be used in classrooms in which there is a tradition of open dialogue, and one in which the instructor feels comfortable that a safe environment will be maintained.

Communication Games

Through games, students can learn the importance of communication and ways that it can be affected. One example of such games would be to split students into two groups. Group A would be asked to leave the classroom and go into the skills laboratory to prepare equipment for spinal immobilization. Once in the lab, this group would be told to reverse the meanings of their words (e.g., they will say "more" when they mean "less," or "right" when they mean "left"). When Group B enters the lab, they would be told to partner with those persons already there. The ensuing confusion can be humorous. It can also demonstrate how communication, although usually taken for granted, can lead to misunderstanding and can even be counterproductive.

Using the Critical Incident Questionnaire in Diverse Classrooms

Stephen Brookfield (2006) feels that the Critical Incident Questionnaire (CIQ) classroom assessment technique is particularly helpful to use in diverse classrooms. The tool is simple. Students are asked to anonymously jot down the answers to the following questions at the end of a class period:

1. At what moment in class this week did you feel most engaged with what was happening?
2. At what moment in class this week were you most distanced from what was happening?
3. What action that anyone (teacher or student) took this week did you find most affirming or helpful?
4. What action that anyone took this week did you find most puzzling or confusing?
5. What about this class surprised you the most? (This could be about your own reactions to what went on, something that someone did, or anything else that occurred.)

The instructor informally summarizes the results and shares common areas of concern with the class. There are many uses and benefits of the CIQ. In diverse classrooms, the CIQ may alert the instructor to teaching strategies that are meeting the diverse learning needs of the class, or to classroom activities that are seen by some students as unfair or alienating. This tool contributes to a sense of inclusivity within the classroom and permits students to express sensitive concerns in a non-threatening manner so they can be addressed.[11]

Summary

Although the United States is often referred to as a *melting pot,* perhaps a better analogy is that of a *stew-pot,* in which distinct elements are blended together to make up a delicious concoction that is far greater than its parts. By supporting and celebrating diversity in the EMS classroom, students can become better prepared to deliver care with greater empathy for, and understanding of, the many cultures and groups they will encounter. These future health care providers may become more attuned to the diversity of the EMS profession itself and, where needed, they may even improve it.

Glossary

bias Unreasonable judgment.

culture Amalgamation of customs, experiences, languages, and beliefs common to a defined group.

cultural competency Awareness of beliefs and customs of cultures.

power Control.

References

1. U.S. Census Bureau, (2010). USA quickfacts from the U.S. Census Bureau. Available at: http://quickfacts.census.gov/qfd/states/00000.html. Accessed December 31, 2010.
2. Gibson, G., National Registry of Emergency Medical Technicians. Data from the LEADS data project. Personal communication, December 28, 2010.
3. Bandura, A. (1997). *Self-efficacy: The exercise of control.* New York: W. H. Freeman.
4. Honeycutt, L. (1997). Cultural diversity: Essential education. *Journal of Emergency Medical Services, 39.*
5. Copeland, D. (1991). *Generation X: Tales for an accelerated culture.* New York, NY: St. Martin's Press.
6. Reeves, T. C. (2007). *Do generational differences matter in instructional design?* Athens, GA: University of Georgia.
7. Oblinger, D., & Oblinger, J. (Eds.), (2005). *Educating the Net Gen.* Washington, DC: EDUCAUSE.
8. Hunter, S. L. (2003). Defining and valuing diversity in EMS. *Emergency Medical Services: Journal of Emergency Care and Transportation. 32,* 88–89.
9. Cole, H. (1997). Stories to live by: A narrative approach to health behavior research and injury prevention. In *Handbook of health behavior,* vol. 4, Relevance for professionals and issues for the future. pp. 325–349.
10. Collison, G., Elbaum, B., Haavind, S., & Tinker, R. (2000). Facilitating online learning. Madison, WI: Atwood Press.
11. Brookfield, S. D. (2006). *The skillful teacher: On technique, trust, and responsiveness in the classroom* (2nd ed.). San Francisco, CA: Jossey-Bass.

Additional Resources

Guskey, T. R. (1958). Does it make a difference? *Educational Leadership. 59*(6), 45–51.

Guskey, T. R. (1998). The age of accountability. *Journal of Staff Development. 19*(4), 36–44.

Scriven, M. (1967). The methodology of evaluation. In R. W. Tyler, R. M. Gange, M. Scriven, (Eds.), *Perspectives of curriculum evaluation* (pp. 39–83). AERA Monograph Series on Curriculum Evaluation. No. 1. Chicago, IL: Rand McNally.

Sue, D. W. & Sue, D. (2002). *Counseling the culturally diverse: Theory and practice.* (4th ed.). New York, NY: John Wiley & Sons.

Tyler, R. W. (1949). *Basic principles of curriculum and instruction.* Chicago, IL: University of Chicago Press.

PART III

Education Essentials

Like a building whose integrity is only as strong as the foundation it rests upon, your teaching is strengthened and supported by a clear understanding of core concepts in education. This part of the text explains the learning domains, shows how to address them in goals and objectives, describes how to create effective lesson plans, and provides useful information about pertinent legal issues, as well as the technical tools that enhance your presentation.

Although the foundation of a building may not be as glamorous or attention getting as the architectural details found on its facade, it provides the stable platform from which those details shine. So should be your teaching. Your ability to convey ideas and concepts in a brilliant way depends first on your ability to integrate the domains of learning into a comprehensive, deliberate lesson plan. Your strong implementation of that plan in a supportive learning environment is the rich architectural detail that your students will notice and appreciate.

Return to these chapters from time to time to reacquaint yourself with the material. With additional experience, you may be able to more readily apply the information and reevaluate what you are doing—and why.

6

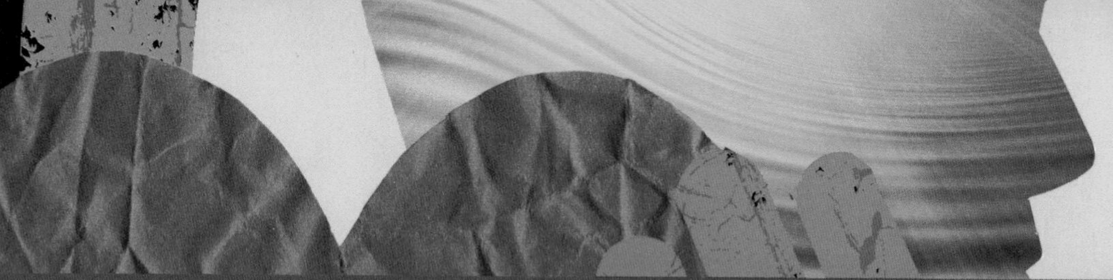

The Learning Environment

Liberty without learning is always in peril; learning without liberty is always in vain.
— John F. Kennedy

Being an educator involves much more than simply imparting knowledge and anecdotes. An effective educator is responsible for ensuring student success by providing an appropriate learning environment.[1] According to *The American Heritage Dictionary of the English Language,* the term *environment* is defined as, "The combination of external or extrinsic physical conditions that affect and influence the growth and development of organisms" and "The complex of social and cultural conditions affecting the nature of an individual or community." A learning environment is an environment designed with the students' learning in mind.[2] When used to describe an educational setting, the term "environment" can be associated with positive or negative feelings of the student or the instructor. A positive learning environment is one that allows for a free exchange of ideas and information, one in which students feel safe asking questions and the educator has or acquires the necessary tools to answer those questions. It is one in which the atmosphere is supportive and students are encouraged to concentrate on academic success. Additionally, a positive learning environment is one that consistently demonstrates respect for students, as well as for the instructor. A negative environment prohibits or interferes with learning, and students may feel inadequate or may believe that their ideas do not matter or cannot be expressed.

Abraham Maslow published his theory regarding human motivation and developed a hierarchy of needs in 1943. According to this theory, all individuals have needs that must be met, from basic survival needs to the need of self-actualization and transcendence—helping others to self-actualize. Once these needs are met in systematic order, the individual is motivated to realize his or her true potential and self-fulfillment can occur. This is a crucial step, because motivation effects engagement, and engagement is required for learning.[3]

In 1970, Malcolm Knowles reintroduced the concept that the environmental climate surrounding learning could affect learning, an idea that had been explored for many years by early educational theorists. Since that time, research has shown that a multitude of physical, psychological, and social factors can affect learning.[1,4,5,6,7,8] Physically, the environment needs to be comfortable and conducive to learning. Psychologically, students need to feel safe and respected in the classroom, free from ridicule, and able to ask questions. Socially, positive relationships established in the classroom can enhance the learning experience.

CHAPTER GOAL: This chapter explores how EMS educators can effectively set and maintain an appropriate physical and psychological learning environment in order to achieve student learning.

The Welcome

A student's introduction to the learning environment can make a lasting impression, greatly affecting the learning that takes place thereafter.[1] Sights, sounds, smells, atmosphere, and rapport with the instructor established on the first day of class can potentially establish the culture for the remainder of the class or course. Each classroom, each school, develops its own culture—a blending of external and internal experiences. The culture developed gives meaning to the learning process that occurs in the class. Thus, the educator needs to give special attention to the first day of class to ensure a positive learning experience can occur **(Figure 6.1)**.

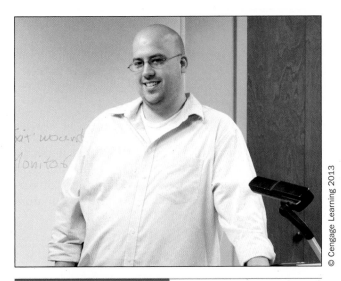

Figure 6.1

A warm and friendly smile from the instructor can go a long way toward setting a positive learning environment.

Something as simple as learning the names of students and helping them to learn one another's names can quickly break the ice, as a first step in creating a positive learning environment. Further, it reinforces that the educator values his or her students as individuals and expects that they value one another.[9,10]

Teaching Tip >> *On the first day of class, an educator can play a "name game," which can take many different forms. One suggestion is to make a class rule that a person needs to use another person's name every time he or she speaks. Another game is to start at one end of the room and have the first student say his or her name out loud. The next student has to repeat the first student's name, then add his or her name. The third student has to repeat the first and second students' names, then add his or her own, and so forth, until the last person in the classroom has to recite the entire class of names. It is important that these types of games be presented in a nonthreatening manner so that a student feels safe to "mess up" or forget a name.*

Housekeeping

A fundamental part of creating a comfortable learning and teaching environment is assurance that the basic needs of both the student and the educator are met. This includes giving directions about where the restrooms and refreshments can be found, and providing adequate break times so that students have time to visit the restroom or relax for a certain amount of time. A general rule of thumb is to schedule breaks approximately every 1 to 1.5 hours. Breaks should be regular, so a student knows when to expect them. Most institutions use the 50-minute class hour, which consists of 50 minutes for instruction and a 10-minute break.

The class may also include handicapped students who need special consideration. Instructors must make sure that students have the opportunity to discuss their needed accommodations with a disability resource so that the instructor makes appropriate accommodations.[9] (See Chapter 10: Legal Issues for EMS Educators, and Americans with Disability Act, for further information.)

Setting Expectations

Students enter the classroom from a variety of cultures and backgrounds and with a variety of preconceptions of learning. The educator should recognize this and immediately set the standard of expected behavior and achievement. By setting a standard, the educator maximizes each student's chances for learning success.

The Syllabus

The syllabus or student handbook represents a written learning contract between the educator and the student. This contract clearly outlines the learning expectations of the course and evaluation of course work, but it should also contain information about appropriate behaviors and consequences of unacceptable behaviors. This document protects the educator and the student and provides a consistent place at which students can review class expectations. (For more information about the course syllabus, see Chapter 24: Administrative Issues.)

Accountability

The educator plays the role of the recognized leader in the classroom. As the leader, he or she is responsible for setting and enforcing the norms of conduct and for being the role model for those norms of conduct. This means that the instructor must clearly identify the expectations of the student during the course. Behavioral expectations should be included in the syllabus and discussed during the first day of class. If inappropriate behavior does occur, it is important that the matter be discussed with the student in a consistent and fair manner.[6,11,12] The instructor must also follow behavioral requirements set forth for students.

Students enrolled in classes have the right to expect a safe environment and appropriate behavior on the part of fellow classmates, as well as from professional educators in the classroom, lab, or clinical setting. Immature and disruptive behavior on the part of students deters serious academic students from enrolling in future courses. Moreover, such disruptive behavior adversely affects the learning environment of all students enrolled in the course, and it distracts the educator from his or her role as instructor and facilitator.

Even though EMS educators are usually teaching adults in an adult setting, educators must engage in some type of discipline at some time. It is important that educators recognize disruptive behavior and actions that have the potential to create an unsafe environment. Moreover, they must learn techniques by which to maintain adult classrooms that are conducive to quality learning. EMS instructors teaching high school students may need to be more tolerant; however, professional behavior should still be an expectation. (For more information, see section on Special Student Consideration in this chapter.)

The Physical Environment

The physical component of the learning environment can vary greatly depending upon the nature of the course. In the past, all classes were conducted in a classroom; but with the expansion of technology, this is no longer a requirement. The physical environment can include a classroom, library, laboratory, informal space, and virtual space.[13] Regardless of where a class takes place, the educator needs to ensure that the environment contributes to a positive learning experience.

In this modern era, students expect certain components within the physical classroom—adequately functional furniture and lighting, instructor-smart podiums, available student computers in libraries, and wireless access everywhere. The physical facilities are the visual component of the learning environment. As a result, students consider the physical environment an important factor in their selection of a school.[14] Ensuring that all physical resources within the environment are working well and fit the needs of the student is the responsibility of the educator.

Room Temperature

The temperature in the classroom should be at a comfortable setting for the task at hand. This may mean having the heat turned down a little for skills days when the students are actively moving around. Students should also be advised that they might wish to bring a sweater to class if they are normally cold, as the environment will be controlled to ensure the comfort of the majority.

Lighting

The lighting should be adjustable so that it can be dimmed to make best use of audiovisuals but light enough for demonstrations or taking notes, or perhaps completely off to simulate a nighttime environment for a scenario.

Distractions

Distractions such as noise, bright sunlight, and interruptions can also affect the learning environment.[3] Although some sources of distraction are out of the educator's immediate control, anything that can be done to minimize distractions will improve the learning environment. For example, the educator should ask that students shut off pagers and cell phones, or turn them to vibrate and accept only emergency calls. The instructor should set an example by putting his or her electronic devices to vibrate also. When conducting outside simulations, the instructor should hold the class in a discrete area that prevents pedestrian traffic from coming through.

Physical Safety

Rules for classroom safety should be explicitly stated by the educator and listed in the course syllabus. Students should exhibit appropriate behavior around special equipment and with other class members to prevent harm to anyone in the classroom. Universal precautions should be followed at all times in an effort to minimize the risk of exposure.

Seating Arrangements

Ideally, an educator should be able to configure and reconfigure a classroom in a variety of ways to accommodate the instructional strategy for that session. Furniture that can be rearranged is preferable. Furniture should be comfortable and should fit students and the classroom well. If 8-hour class sessions are planned, padded seats are essential. If class will not last longer than two hours, padded seats may be optional. The physical comfort of the seats should be taken into account, as well as the arrangement of the seats in light of the focus of the instruction.

A variety of classroom setup strategies are possible, depending on the instructor's goals. A few examples are the following:

- *Traditional.* The traditional classroom setup is ideal for a large number of students. This style is not recommended, however, for small group work or for psychomotor skill development. This structure may allow students to "hide" behind others, and it can be difficult for some students to see over others. The educator at the front of the room may also have difficulty seeing all the students in the room and may focus only on the first row.
- *Theater.* The theater classroom setup is optimal for a very large number of students. In this type of configuration, the seats rise from the front to the back, allowing better visibility of the educator and any instructional media or demonstrations. In addition, this arrangement allows the educator to have better eye contact with the group as a whole. This style is not recommended for small group work.
- *Circle, square, and rectangle—open.* This style places the educator in the center of a U-like shape. The educator may sit with the group or may enter the center area. This can be an ideal setup when all students are expected to participate in a discussion, as it allows them to see one another. It can also work well for a psychomotor demonstration. It does not work well, though, for a lecture scenario, as someone will ultimately end up sitting with his or her back to the presenter.
- *Circle, square, and rectangle—closed.* This classroom setup places the educator either sitting or standing off to the side after instructions are provided. It can be an ideal setup for a larger discussion group when all students are expected to participate, as it allows students to see one another. Similar to the open version, this type of setup is not recommended for lectures or presentations, because the focus may not be on the educator but on the person sitting across the way.
- *Round table.* With this classroom setup, small groups are arranged around different round tables or workstations. The focus of instruction is within the space of each individual table or station. It is important with this style that the educator circulates around the room, or that additional educator facilitators assist in monitoring the work at the individual stations. This setup allows some privacy between workstations. Visualization of each station may not be an issue, but it can be controlled with partitions or room dividers. It is important to maintain adequate room between stations or tables to allow for movement and to reduce the noise level. Groups can be working on the same activity simultaneously (but independently), or they can be working on different activities. With this setup, the educator balances between monitoring and allowing students to direct their own learning. This setup is not as useful for lectures or presentations, as inevitably some of the students' backs will face the presenter **(Figure 6.2)**.

Extra Considerations

The instructor should be able to evaluate the class and answer such questions as the following:[1,3, 8,10,15,16]

For a positive learning environment:

- Is the room of adequate size?
- Is there adequate space for each student to sit, take notes, and view the reference materials?
- Can each student see and hear the instructor and any audiovisual presentations?
- How can the lighting be changed so that there is adequate light for skills, lecture presentations, or discussion activities?
- If the classroom has windows, how can natural light be blocked or adjusted to achieve optimal lighting for audiovisual presentations?
- How can environmental controls be adjusted if it gets too hot or too cold?
- Where is the space for breaks that allows for eating and drinking?
- Where are the emergency exits?
- Where are the restrooms?
- Where is the equipment stored? Is it accessible to students?
- Is the classroom space accessible to students with a variety of physical abilities, such as the need to use a wheelchair?
- How can distractions from the outside environment be minimized (e.g., closing doors or windows to minimize interfering noise)?
- Is lighting/security for the parking area adequate when dark?

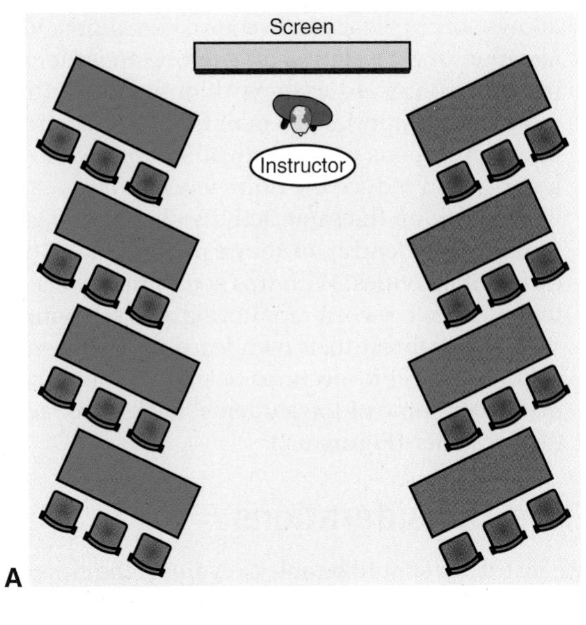

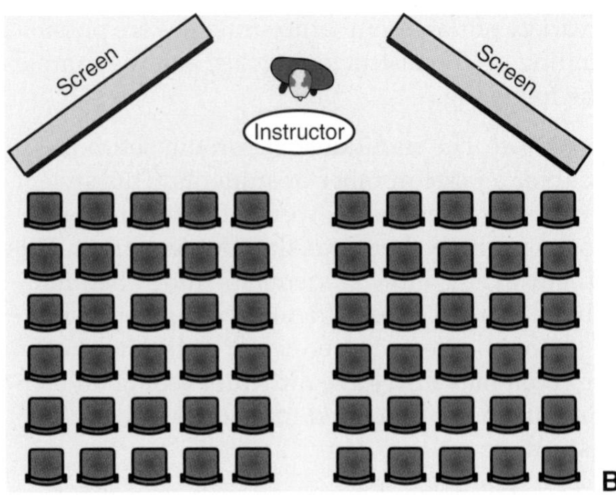

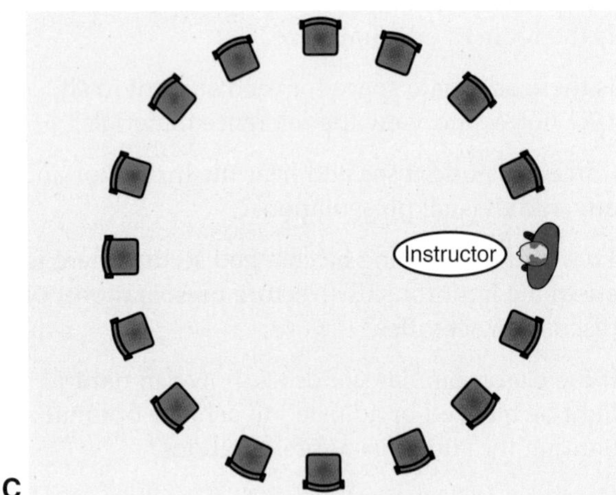

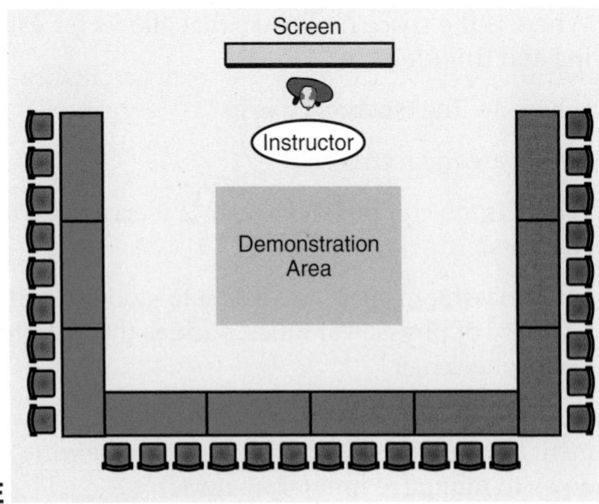

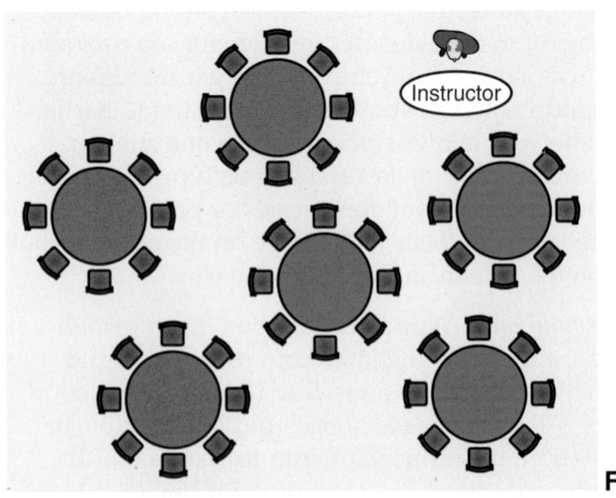

Figure 6.2

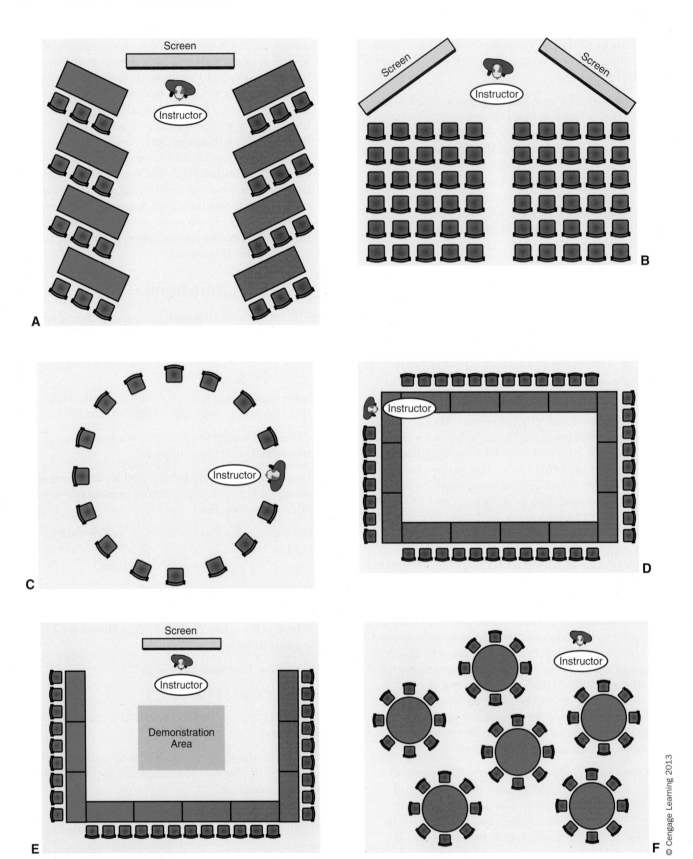

Types of classroom arrangements. A. Traditional. B. Theater style. C. Open circle. D. Open square. E. U shape. F. Round table.

For clinical settings:

- Have patients provided consent for student participation?
- Do the faculty understand their role in the experience?
- Is there adequate space and clinical experiences for all students?
- Are there adequate safety requirements (gloves, masks, sharps containers, etc.)?
- How much time is available for student experiences?

Audiovisual Equipment

As part of the physical environment of the classroom, the educator must ensure that audiovisual equipment is in working order and that a backup is planned and available. (See Chapter 16: Using Technology to Enhance Classroom Learning for more information on audiovisual equipment.)

The Psychological Environment

The effective educator sets the psychological tone of the learning environment by establishing the psychological parameters of behavior. It is essential that the expectations of the course be thoroughly discussed on the first day, and be a component of the syllabus. It is the educator's responsibility to create a psychologically safe environment, in which students can make and learn from their mistakes. Psychologically safe environments exist in an atmosphere of mutual respect, shared responsibility, and safety. The relationship between student and educator is extremely important, and it has been directly related to student academic satisfaction.[17] The following are some strategies that can be used to establish and maintain an effective learning environment.[4,11,18,19]

Mutual Respect

One should strive to establish positive adult-to-adult rapport with students. The educator should treat each student as an adult whose life experiences can contribute to his or her learning and the learning of the entire class. The rapport between student and faculty is a powerful component of the learning environment, impacting the level of student engagement, quality of student learning, and behavioral issues. In positive environments, educators express enthusiasm for learning, are respectful, use appropriate humor, and voice expectations that all students can learn.

Shared Responsibility

A participatory environment should be fostered, wherein students share responsibility for their own learning. The educator's role should be one of guide or helper in the pursuit of knowledge. The learning environment should encourage intellectual freedom and creativity. It should promote trial and error with positive feedback and represent an interactive learning agreement between students and educators. Students value a supportive environment, one in which the student perceives the educator is making sincere efforts to assist them in the learning process.[17] Student-centered learning activities are important to encourage shared responsibility for learning. (See Chapter 11: Introduction to Teaching Strategies for additional information on student-centered learning.)

Safety

Creating a safe place for students to learn without fear of ridicule is extremely important in the creation of a positive learning environment. In a safe environment, a deeper aspect of learning is possible and true assessment can be achieved by the educator. The goal of adult education is to generate change. Abraham Maslow found that growth requires change, and change results from a sense of inner safety.[15] A positive learning environment must be safe and free of coercion by fellow students, the instructor, or the administration. Further, students should be able to develop a trusting relationship with the educator. The federal Safe School Act employs a zero tolerance for behaviors that threaten safety. (See Chapter 10: Legal Issues for EMS Educators and more information on the safe learning environment laws.)

Learning requires an environment in which the student is at ease and is able to experiment without fear of making a mistake. As a general rule, in a safe and positive learning environment, the following can be expected:[4,7,10,11,20,21]

- Students are free from harm.
- Students are free from discrimination.
- Students are free from sexual harassment.
- Students are free from teasing.
- Students and educators exhibit tolerance and acceptance.
- Students and educators encourage new ideas.

CASE IN POINT

The new cohort of EMT students consists of a group of employees from an EMS agency. They are friends and know one another well. They tend to joke and laugh and promote a casual yet highly competitive learning environment in the classroom. The instructor has allowed the casual atmosphere and believes that it can promote a positive learning environment. However, there are two students who are not doing well in class. The instructor suspects that these two students may be intimidated by the other students in class. They do not ask questions, and when they do, the instructor notices nonverbal clues that appear to be somewhat condescending from the other students. These two students seem reluctant to practice during skills sessions and seem to lack confidence. The instructor talks to the class about the class environment and the importance of respect for all students in the class. If improvement is not noted, the educator might find a way to pair the two students with more aggressive students in the class who have good leadership skills and will serve as mentors for these students. Or, the offending students could be talked to individually, and discipline procedures will be implemented, if necessary. Whatever the best solution, the plan for improvement likely requires an improvement in the psychological environment of the class. Both individuals and groups of individuals must be held accountable for expected behavior and must be encouraged to contribute to a safe and positive learning environment for everyone involved.

Teaching Tip >> *It is easier for an instructor to lighten up on class control than to start with less control and attempt to tighten up.*

It is important for an educator to establish a classroom culture that accepts mistakes as part of the normal part of learning. Trial and error should be encouraged, and students should not feel that they will be punished for errors. It is important for an educator to realize that his or her response to student mistakes is critical. The instructor can acknowledge that the incorrect answer may seem plausible under the circumstances, and then discuss the correct answer with an explanation as to why it is correct. The instructor should find something positive to say about the answer before explaining why it is incorrect. Every attempt should be made to have a positive reaction to mistakes.

Discussion of a student's poor performance should always be conducted in private. Providing a safe environment for learning is essential. The student must feel comfortable enough to "get it wrong" if the student is to progress to a point where he or she can "get it right."[1,11,22]

Intellectual Challenge

Research shows that there is increased interest in learning and stimulation when students are challenged to think and react just above their current threshold of learning and understanding.[4,10] Setting a challenging pace, even sometimes to the point of discomfort, is an important aspect of creating a positive learning environment. This pace must be set accurately so it does not overwhelm students and cause them to give up, but it also should not be so easy that nothing is accomplished or learned by the experience.

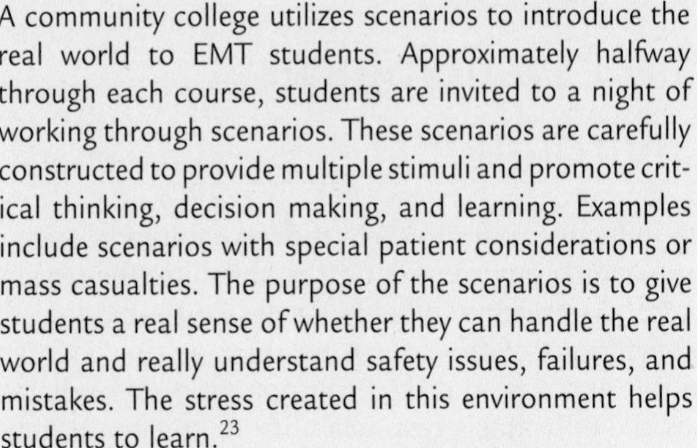

CASE IN POINT

A community college utilizes scenarios to introduce the real world to EMT students. Approximately halfway through each course, students are invited to a night of working through scenarios. These scenarios are carefully constructed to provide multiple stimuli and promote critical thinking, decision making, and learning. Examples include scenarios with special patient considerations or mass casualties. The purpose of the scenarios is to give students a real sense of whether they can handle the real world and really understand safety issues, failures, and mistakes. The stress created in this environment helps students to learn.[23]

Conflict

Conflict is a fact of life in higher educational classrooms and can be dealt with constructively. Effective educators are not afraid of conflict, and realize the moment presents an opportunity for them to manage the situation, and for students to deepen their level of understanding. The best educators realize this and learn how to manage conflict in an effort to bring positive and fair outcomes for all involved. Positive conflict is constructive and can be helpful in keeping the class energized and creative. It is the educator's responsibility to build and maintain an environment that encourages all students to become equal participants in the learning process.[11]

In an effort to keep the conflict positive in the classroom, the educator is faced with the challenge of managing the behavior appropriately.[3] The student grapevine moves quickly, and the manner in which the instructor manages the conflict will be remembered, and sets the tone for future discussions in the classroom. Attention should be focused on how to make the conflict a constructive learning experience for the students.

There are three steps to effective classroom management:[24]

1. Clarify the problem—ask questions in an effort to clearly understand the issue at hand. After receiving feedback from students, the educator should restate the problem. This step identifies the students involved and clarifies the issue so that all are under the same understanding.
2. Identify a workable solution—have students offer suggestions for solutions, and work together to identify an agreeable solution. All parties should work together with positive attitudes and identify ground rules and criteria for the solution.
3. Application of the solution—have students work together to develop a plan of action and ensure the implementation of the agreed upon solution.

Negative behaviors such as foul language, loud voice, angry tones, and disrespect are disruptive and should not be permissible in the classroom. Students should understand that differences of opinion are normal and acceptable in the classroom culture, and that everyone in the room needs to be treated with respect.

The Social Environment

It is important for the educator to remember that the learning environment is dynamic. As a group of individuals gets to know one another, the social interactions between them may change. This can create an evolving learning environment, which can be positive. For example, if everyone is speaking up and asking questions and learning from one another because they feel safe to do that within the group, that is obviously a positive change. Even a case in which two students have become friends, and discuss questions among themselves, can lead to a positive learning environment. The key is to establish mutual respect and classroom expectations, so that the classroom relationships are not disruptive to the other members of the class.

At a fundamental level, the classroom experience can be thought of as a social arrangement. At the center of the social participation is the educator, who may possess a high degree of expertise in an academic discipline but may not be as skilled at promoting the positive social environment needed for effective learning.[11] It is important that the educator set the tone and keep the tone even as class dynamics change. Studies have shown that learning increases when there is a positive rapport between students and educator.[25]

The instructor is the primary role model in the classroom. To act appropriately as a role model, he or she might clearly identify the behaviors that students should exhibit. By modeling appropriate conduct, the instructor stands the best chance of developing the desired behaviors in students.

Encouraging Teamwork

A career in EMS will involve many team activities; therefore, teamwork skills are essential. Group projects are a wonderful way to teach students about working in a team, and can be an important tool for learning. The optimal group size consists of less than five students; this size allows for individual student contribution and at the same time prevents the more industrious student from doing the majority of the work. Although the instructor may encounter students who have already developed excellent team skills, he or she is more likely to find students who need coaching on teamwork and group dynamics.[11] For educators, a basic knowledge of how groups form and function is important for promoting positive team activities.

As groups form, there is a predictable dynamic to the growth of the team. Different stages may take varying amounts of time to evolve. Awareness of team stages seems to shorten their duration, as team members have an awareness of what will occur and know the language to describe group dynamic problems that they encounter.

The first step is the **forming** stage, wherein team members encounter one another for the first time. The dominant theme of this stage is that members attempt to define the task assigned to them, and they start to determine the future course. Because the group has not worked together before, there are no set ground rules or expectations. Expectations must be clarified before the team can progress. This can result in impatience, as some members seek to jump into tasks before consensus on goals and expectations has been reached.

As the group begins to establish goals and expectations, invariably, conflicts arise. This leads to the second stage—**storming**. The dominant theme of this stage is the jockeying for position by team members, as they struggle to define the team's leadership. This struggle can cause arguing and conflicts among team members, even when there is agreement on the real issue. In some cases, this conflict is externalized to the educator.

As conflicts are settled and a leadership system for the team emerges, the team progresses to a point at which interpersonal relationships grow more important than the team goal. This is the third stage—**norming**. The dominant theme of this stage is emphasis on getting along, even when disagreements and open discussions are necessary. A sense of cohesion develops, and the team has now established and is maintaining ground rules.

This gives rise to the fourth stage—**performing**. During the performing stage, the team balances interpersonal relationships with the team's needs, and results begin to occur. By the time this stage is reached, the team has developed the ability to work through group problems.

Although it is difficult to observe teams going through this process, it is important for the educator to realize that the process itself is what allows students to learn teamwork skills. The role of the educator in team development is to guide students through these phases, pointing out landmarks and assisting them in working through obstacles.

Special Considerations

Much of the education in EMS courses occurs outside a traditional classroom. Instructors who pay careful attention to detail when planning activities in these settings maximize the students' ability to learn.

The Laboratory and Clinical Environment

An essential part of EMS education is learning and practicing skills in a laboratory or clinical environment. The clinical environment in most EMS courses includes hospital, ambulance, and field clinical situations. As with any instructional activity, preparation and environment are important aspects of the overall experience. The necessary equipment, supplies, and teaching aids should be identified and secured. An instructor should never assume that the equipment and materials needed to conduct the skills lab will be available in the classroom. This is especially true in multiple-use facilities, where different instructors and different classes may meet.

When setting up a skills learning environment, the educator should consider the following:[9,10,26]

- *Safety.* Safety should be considered not only in terms of practice by learners **(Figure 6.3)**, but also in terms of any inherent danger associated with demonstrating the skill **(Figure 6.4)**, or any potential danger to the patient, if one exists. For example, caution is needed when defibrillation is demonstrated. Electrical shocks can be dangerous to nonfibrillating hearts. The educator should clearly define what is safe and should enforce it. Additionally, the educator must ensure safety with appropriate knowledge and practice of universal precautions, proper disposal of sharps, immunizations, proper body mechanics, and all aspects of a safe physical environment. All skills must be competently and consistently demonstrated prior to doing skills on patients. The educator must advocate for the patient as well as the student in this situation.

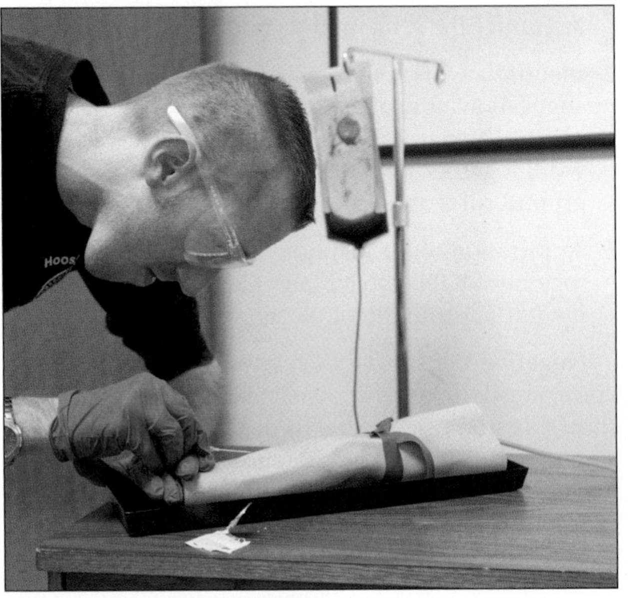

Figure 6.3
Safety in the clinical area is more likely if it is practiced in the classroom and laboratory.

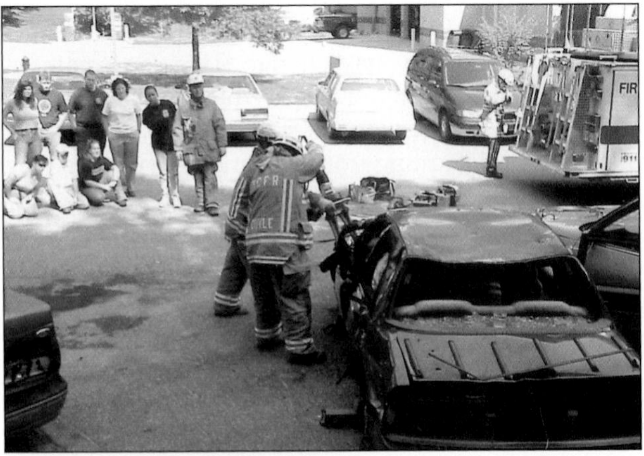

Figure 6.4
Special precautions may be necessary when students are introduced to certain exercises.

- *Visibility.* For the learner to model and imitate a skill, he or she must be able to first see all aspects of the process. It is, therefore, important that the educator provide visibility. This may involve moving learners and using special, large-scale models or cameras and video projectors.
- *Rehearsal.* Regardless of how many times or how well an educator can perform a skill, it is always prudent for the educator to practice the skill before class. This is especially true when a special model or equipment is used that is different from what the educator routinely uses.
- *Practice space.* If the learners will practice the skill, the educator must ensure that sufficient space is provided, as well as equipment, at each skill practice arena.
- *Encourage self-learning.* Set the expectation that learning, especially skills learning, is not dependent on an educator. After an instructor demonstrates a particular skill, he or she should expect that students will watch one another, go through a detailed skills checklist, and work through their mistakes before asking the instructor to watch them perform the skill. This type of self-learning practice encourages lifelong learning.
- *Simulate real environments.* Where possible, an educator should use "real" props to simulate an actual working environment. For example, moving a patient off of a sofa is different from moving someone off of a classroom chair.
- *Appropriate dress.* Students should be advised about when they will be performing psychomotor tasks so that they may wear or bring appropriate clothing—for protection and to prevent embarrassment. This applies to the instructor as well.

Nontraditional Environments

In EMS education, typical learning environments include the classroom, laboratory, hospital setting, or the field. As settings become more complex, they integrate higher levels of thinking skills and psychomotor skills. No longer is simple knowledge adequate for performing a task; the student must function at the application level or problem-solving level to perform in this different environment. (See Chapter 7: Domains of Learning.) When psychomotor skills are taught, students in clinical settings must apply these skills to a patient situation. For example, it is one thing to recite the steps for cardiopulmonary resuscitation (CPR) in class, but quite another to recognize that a patient is "down" at a scene, and then manage the situation and the patient. A change in learning environments can be an effective tool for improving performance.[10,23] Increasing the complexity of the learning environment may promote critical thinking or, conversely, simplifying the environment by removing complicating factors may restore student confidence and enhance performance.

The learning environment can also be specific to location. For example, a student who has come from a rural area may be very comfortable transporting patients for 30 to 60 minutes, but is failing to get all treatments done in a timely fashion in the urban setting, where transport times are less than 10 minutes. The problem in this case is likely the change in the environment, and not the student's knowledge base. Skill training around efficiency, multitasking, and delegation may provide keys to this student's success. An EMT student who has worked for a private ambulance provider for 3 years may have a level of discomfort during his internship at a large, urban fire department. His emotions and stress may be interfering with his ability to recall information and perform skills adequately. Acclimating to the fire service will do more in this situation to improve his performance than any amount of studying; therefore, the plan for improvement should include activities to increase his comfort level at the station and with station personnel. His best option for adjusting may include additional observation time provided before patient care tasks are added to his assignment.

Students entering a clinical environment for the first time, where they are introduced to staff members and oriented to the facility, feel more comfortable and are set up for more successful learning.[22] However, as each new environmental element is introduced to a student, previous feelings of comfort and safety are challenged.[6,12]

Using New Technologies

The Internet, computer-based teaching and learning tools, and satellite education are just some examples of technologies that can be used to enhance the learning environment.[10,26,27] Use of technology to create a simulated "real environment" for students may result in successful practice and, ultimately, in learning.[27] In addition to simulations, examples of using technology in the classroom include such innovations as an online library database or computer-generated "Jeopardy-like" games. The use of different types of technology can create a dynamic and fun environment that facilitates learning. This also allows the instructor to evaluate learning and student responsiveness in a more stressful and competitive environment. Technology can be used to create a fun place for learning.

Special Student Considerations

Although a caring classroom and a positive instructor foster a better learning environment and improve discipline, the fact is that there are students who will challenge the instructor. Following are a few of the trials that every instructor will face.

The Late Comer

This is the student who regularly comes to class or lab late. Fellow students watch the offending student arrive late week after week, and silent frustration begins to build in the classroom setting.

- The educator can start the class with a quiz or other classroom assignment that will encourage everyone to show up on time. A missed quiz could negatively affect the student's grade and should be a strong deterrent to coming in late.
- The educator can pull the student aside and counsel him or her regarding the tardiness. Has the student encountered any problems that have kept him or her from coming to class on time? Most EMS students are holding down a job while attending class and may have run into a particular problem. Have the student put together and sign a plan that will solve this problem, now and for the future.

The Bored One

This is the student who appears to be bored by the class either through body language or lack of participation. These actions of this student could be the result of a variety of issues. The lack of interest could be related to the pace of the class, the lack of group activity, the fact that the student may be lost in the material, or the simple preoccupation of a student with work or family responsibilities.

- The instructor can create an opportunity for the student to participate by allowing the student to present a portion of the material at a later date. Actively engaging students makes them stakeholders in the learning process and creates active learners.
- The educator could visit with the student in an effort to identify the underlying issue. The problem may be a personal issue that has nothing to do with the instructor or the material that is being presented. The pace of the class may be too slow or too fast, a fact that can be discovered in talks between the educator and the student. Once the issue is identified, the instructor and student can write a corrective plan of action together.

The Social Butterfly

These students tend to spend more time visiting with everyone as opposed to learning. They tend to hold side conversations and seem more interested in the socializing that occurs, causing problems during the instructor's presentation. A few students may even be using the classroom as a potential dating pool. Although the instructor wishes to encourage a friendly and interactive environment, clear rules and guidelines must be in place to create boundaries that both the instructors and the students have mutually agreed upon.

- This type of student may require a job assignment in class that will allow him or her to put his or her people skills to work. The instructor can channel this type of student in a positive manner that can add rather than detract from the classroom experience.
- A brief discussion with the student focusing on the effects of their behavior to the class may be in order.

The Introvert

Every classroom has a few introverts, who are more comfortable avoiding discussion. These students are more like tourists than active participants. They remain distant and are not interested in becoming part of the tour, keeping themselves invisible in the group.

- These students need to become involved in the learning process. Traditionally, instructors were taught to bring these students out by putting them on the spot through Socratic questioning in the classroom. However, this may cause further isolation and may lead the student to drop the class, feeling that he or she is being singled out. A better strategy is to have the student lead a small group discussion or group activity. By scaling down classroom interaction to a few members and allowing the student to take a more active role, the instructor can promote a sense of belonging and ownership within the process.
- Encouraging these students to take chances is another strategy that can work to their advantage. Small risks can lead to bigger risks that are safe

and that will allow these students to pull out of their shell. The instructor must be careful not to put this type of student in a position that he or she cannot handle.

The Domineering One

As future health providers, allied health students need to be assertive in their nature. However, in the classroom, a dominant student can be disruptive to the learning environment.

- Small groups with other students serving as the leaders can help to direct energy in other areas. Students in the group will, if carefully selected, be able to manage this personality type.
- Assign a project to the student if too many questions are asked. The educator can complement the student on being inquisitive, and ask the student to research the topic and report to the class during the next meeting.
- If the behavior is consistently disruptive, the educator should confront the student and explain how the student can participate positively in the classroom. Explaining how their behavior affects the learning of other students can help the domineering student realize the outcomes of such behavior.

The Sleeper

EMS students usually work a job in addition to taking classes, and this lifestyle can be exhausting for the student.

- Calling on the student to answer questions verbally asked in the classroom is a good way to encourage involvement.
- Ensure that students have a break every hour.
- Involve students in learning activities other than the traditional lecture format. Group activities can work wonders in keeping students engaged in the learning process. Changing the presentation style can keep students interested and is a necessary part of teaching the adult learner.

The Confused One

This is an interesting student who may have problems in grasping the material. He or she may exhibit this by not engaging the instructor or other students, or by asking a tremendous number of questions. The latter can slow down the instructor's presentation style and may lead to palpable frustration among the student's peers.

- The educator should provide students with clear expectations and a detailed plan on how to accomplish the goals of the class. This may require the instructor to begin by outlining the classroom lecture for the day or for the week, so that the student can have a picture of how instruction will proceed.
- Group projects can help reinforce theory to this student, and establish a social network upon which academic assistance can occur. Peer support can be a powerful, nonthreatening, and reassuring strategy.
- Tutoring can also be arranged by faculty at prearranged times to help clear up any confusion.

The Hostage

Those who deal with fire agencies or companies who require their employees to attain a mandatory EMS certification have had to deal with this group. These students shuffle into the classroom and strike an almost defiant pose for the instructor. For the new instructor, this is one of the most difficult groups to deal with and to teach. Even seasoned instructors may develop a sense of dread knowing they have to motivate these students.

To manage this type of student, instructors must recognize that motivation results from an interrelationship between the students' internal factors (the value they put on the learning goals and their belief that they are capable of achieving those goals—called "expectancy"). These intrinsic factors interact with how the students see the environment as being either supportive or unsupportive. So a disorganized classroom, or one the learner feels is unfair, will quickly dissolve positive attitudes.[28] Establishing a positive classroom environment from the first class day is critical. Clearly articulate how each step of the learning process is important to help the students achieve their individual learning goals to focus on their success.

The educator can take clues for dealing with this type of student from the Motivational Framework for Culturally Responsive Teaching developed by Wlodkowski and Ginsberg[29,30] The framework identifies four components:

1. *Establish inclusion*: This element includes developing a safe classroom community where each student's opinion is valued and one in which others in the group have their best interests in mind. Involving students in meaningful group activities can enhance their feelings of self-worth and their engagement in the learning process.

2. *Develop attitude*: Students desire to learn because they believe the material is relevant. This fosters curiosity and interest that is necessary to establish intrinsic motivation to learn. Instructors should harness the fact that these students must achieve licensure to maintain employment by coaching them in a positive manner toward that goal. Fernandez, Studnek, and Margolis found that the need to pass the licensure exam to retain employment is associated with increased success on the exam.[31]
3. *Enhancing meaning*: Learning experiences engage and challenge the students and include the learner's perspectives and values. Allow students to apply information in contexts that simulate real life so they see how the pieces of their education fit together to permit them to succeed in real-life patient situations.
4. *Engendering competence*: Most students are capable of learning material they believe is valuable, and they also want to be proficient at relevant tasks. Providing the opportunity to demonstrate mastery of tasks and providing frequent positive feedback promote feelings of success and further motivate the learner.

It is important that all disruptions and breaches of classroom behavior be documented, so that if and when disruptions become persistent, a record of noncompliance is available to support the instructor's actions. A concise written statement of the behavior, including its impact on others and the intervention provided, is an important part of record keeping. These behaviors should be documented on the affective (professional behavior) evaluation.

Additionally, the educator may ask the student to formulate a plan to stop the disruptive behavior by suggesting alternatives. Students may need help in determining appropriate alternatives to disruptive behaviors. The plan for improvement should be short and concise, and should have a high probability of success. This plan can be either written or verbal, but it should be reasonable and doable. Behavioral contracts or plans should be negotiated in a neutral, nonjudgmental tone. The educator should assist the student in moving forward and in planning for a better approach to classroom citizenship that will help him or her to succeed.

Although most classroom issues can be dealt with in conversations with the student, it is sometimes necessary for the instructor to deal with the issue in accordance with a formal discipline system. Instructors should check their organization's policies for the specific requirements. Formal discipline processes should be explained in the student handbook and during the first class session.

Summary

The environment in which learning is expected to occur is an important aspect of education that must be taken into consideration. An effective educator makes every effort to create a physically, psychologically, and socially safe environment, where students can feel free to make mistakes and learn from one another, the educator, and different situations. It is a place that creates positive feelings, and in which the educator and students are free to focus on academic success. The tactics and resources needed to foster an environment that promotes positive learning may change with each new class of students. Instructors should continually evaluate each situation and each new group of students and should review all acquired information, then devise a plan that will promote a positive learning environment for the given situation.

Glossary

forming stage Team members encounter one another for the first time, attempt to define the task assigned to them, and start to determine the future course.

norming stage Team establishes and maintains ground rules.

performing stage Team develops the ability to work through group problems, and results begin to occur.

storming stage Team members jockey for position as they struggle to define the team's leadership.

References

1. Imel, S. (1996). Inclusive adult learning environments. Retrieved from *ERIC Digest No. 162*. Available at http://www.ericdigests.org/1996-2/adult.html. Accessed 2010.
2. Jackson, G. A., & Deal, T. E. (1985). Technology, learning environments, and tomorrow's schools. *Peabody Journal of Education, 62*(2), 93–113.
3. Hutchinson, L., Cantillon, P., & Wood, B. F. (2003). Educational environment. *British Medical Journal, 326*(7393), 810–812.
4. Billington, D. D. (2002). Seven characteristics of highly effective adult learning programs. *New Horizons for Learning*. Available at: http://www.newhorizons.org/lifelong/workplace/billington.htm. Accessed 2010.
5. Biswalo, P. (2001). The systems approach as a catalyst for creating an effective learning environment. *Convergence, 34*(1), 53–67.
6. Cleave-Hogg, D., & Rothman, A. I. (1991). Discerning views: Medical students' perceptions of their learning environment. *Evaluation & the Health Professions, 14*(4), 456–474.
7. Diamantes, T. (2002). Improving instruction in multicultural classes by using classroom learning environment. *Journal of Instructional Psychology, 29*(4), 277–283.
8. Magolda, M. B. B. (2000). Teaching to promote holistic learning and development. *New Directions for Teaching & Learning, 82*, 88–99.
9. Davis, B. G. (2001). *Tools for teaching*. San Francisco, CA: Jossey-Bass.
10. Simplicio, J. S. C. (1999). Some simple and yet overlooked common sense tips for a more effective classroom environment. *Journal of Instructional Psychology, 26*(2), 111–116.
11. Anderson, J. A. (1999). Faculty responsibility for promoting conflict-free college classrooms. *New Directions for Teaching & Learning, 77*, 69–76.
12. Morris, W. (Ed.) (1976). *The American heritage dictionary of the English language*. Boston, MA: Houghton Mifflin, p. 438.
13. Lippincott, J. K. (2009). Learning spaces: Involving faculty to improve pedagogy. *EDUCAUSE Review, 44*(2), 16–25.
14. CDW Government (2008, October). *The 21st century campus: Are we there yet?* Available at http://www.cdwg.com/21stcenturycampus. Accessed 2010.
15. Mann, K. V. (2002). Thinking about learning: Implications for principle-based professional education. *Journal of Continuing Education in the Health Professions, 22*(2), 69–77.
16. Streibel, B. J., & Joiner, B. J. (1988). *The team handbook*. Madison, WI: Joiner Associates
17. Winteler, A. (1981). The academic department as environment for teaching and learning. *Higher Education, 10*, 25–35.
18. Imel, S. (1988). Guidelines for working with adult learners. Retrieved from *ERIC Digest No. 77*. http://www.ericdigests.org/pre-929/working.htm. Accessed 2010.
19. Imel, S. (1989). Teaching adults: Is it different? Retrieved from *ERIC Digest No. 82*. Available at: http://www.ericdigests.org/pre-9211/teaching.htm. Accessed 2010.
20. Backes, C. E. (1997). The do's and don'ts of working with adult learners. *Adult Learning, 8*(3), 29–32.
21. Robins, L. S., *et al.* (1997). A predictive model of student satisfaction with the medical school learning environment. *Academic Medicine, 72*(2), 134–139.
22. Newble, D. I., & Hejka, E. J. (1991). Approaches to learning of medical students and practicing physicians: Some empirical evidence and its implications for medical education. *Educational Psychology, 11*, 333–343.
23. Moore, A., *et al.* (2003). EMS stress-training concept "Kobayashi Moru" scenarios. Domain 3. National Association of EMS Educators.
24. Holton, S. A. (1999). After the eruption: Managing conflict in the classroom. *New Directions for Teaching and Learning, 77*, 59–68.
25. Sutliff, M., Higginson, J., & Allstot, S. (2008). Building a positive learning environment for students: Advice to beginning teachers. *Strategies*, 31–33.
26. Firebaugh, F. M., & Watkins, D. O. (1997). The college embraces technology for education. *Human Ecology Forum, 25*(4), 1.
27. Dwyer, C. A. (1999). Using emerging technologies to construct effective learning environments. *Educational Media International, 36*(4), 300–310.
28. Ambrose, S. A., Bridges, M. W., Lovett, M. C., DiPietro, M., & Norman, M. K. (2010). *How learning works: Seven research-based principles for smart teaching*. San Francisco, CA: Jossey-Bass.
29. Wlodkowski, R. J. (2008). *Enhancing Adult Motivation to Learn* (3rd ed.). San Francisco, CA: Jossey-Bass
30. Wlodkowski, R. J. (2004). Creating Motivating Learning Environments. In M. W. Galbraith (Ed.), *Adult Learning Methods: A Guide for Effective Instruction* (3rd ed.). Malabar, Fl: Krieger Publishing Co.
31. Fernandez, A. R., Studnek, J. R., & Margolis, G. S. (2008). Estimating the probability of passing the National Paramedic Certification Examination. *Academic Emergency Medicine, 15*(3), 258–264.

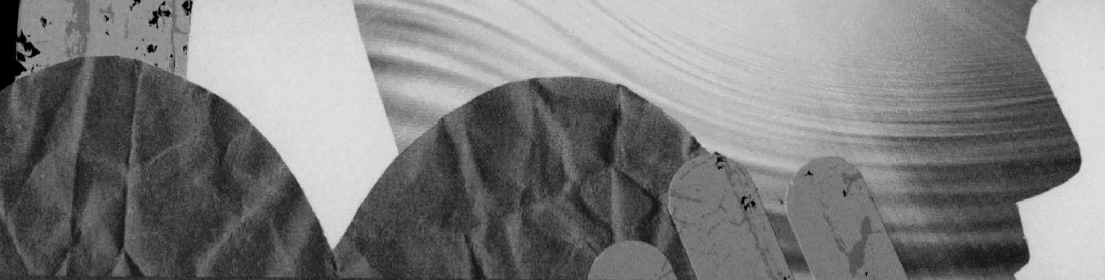

7 Domains of Learning

Meaning making involves thinking, feeling, and acting, and all three of these aspects must be integrated for significant new learning, and especially in new knowledge creation. —J.D. Novak

For many years, researchers have identified different domains, or categories, of learning that educators use in several ways in their practice of teaching. In the instructional design process, the **domains of learning** are always considered when goals and objectives are established and written. Educators also identify student knowledge and behaviors that exemplify the domains of learning. In the context of a medical event, these domains are targeted in the lesson plans and choices regarding the teaching strategies that will be used. Finally, educators consider each domain when formulating evaluation criteria and methods. The domains of learning lie behind every stage of the learning and teaching processes.

This chapter will assist instructors to recognize how to integrate each domain of learning into their teaching practice. Adopting these strategies will promote student acquisition of the knowledge, skills and professional behaviors essential for practice in EMS.

CHAPTER GOAL: The intent of this chapter is to provide the traditional perspective of the three predominant domains of learning.

Categorizing The Domains

Dr. Benjamin Bloom and a team of researchers first categorized the domains of learning in 1956.[1] Bloom and colleagues described three distinct domains of learning: cognitive, affective, and psychomotor.

Bloom chose the term "domain" to describe the major divisions of his concepts because a domain is a related collection of things or items. Collectively, his work is known as **Bloom's Taxonomy**.

Since the time of Bloom's original work, other researchers have built upon his concepts and have developed several other strategies of classification and additional categories of learning domains. However, because Bloom's strategy is commonly used in the medical field, this is the only strategy described in this textbook.

Cognitive Domain

Simply put, the **cognitive domain** describes learning that takes place through the process of thinking; it deals with facts and knowledge. For example, a student who reads a textbook and learns the contraindications of administering a certain medication is operating in the cognitive domain. Much of what we accomplish in the medical profession is based upon the ability to acquire knowledge and use it for the greater good of patient care.

Affective Domain

The **affective domain** describes learning in terms of feelings, emotions, attitudes, and values. For example, a student who participates in case scenarios and learns to appreciate how vulnerable patients can feel when they are sick or injured is operating in the affective domain. This domain is essential to all education, but in the education of health care professionals specifically, it is of utmost importance that aspects from the affective domain be embedded into the instructional process.

Psychomotor Domain

The **psychomotor domain** describes learning that takes place through the attainment of skills and bodily, or kinesthetic, movements. For example, a student who physically practices in a skills station will achieve competency in how to properly perform the skill and thus meet the needs associated in the psychomotor domain.

It is important for educators to understand that, although Bloom and his colleagues described learning processes that take place within three distinct categories, learning seldom takes place solely within one category without at least some aspects of the other two. For example, for a student to properly perform a psychomotor skill, he or she must possess cognitive, affective, and psychomotor knowledge. An Emergency Medical Technician (EMT) who performs cardiopulmonary resuscitation (CPR) effectively must first know the correct sequence of the steps for CPR (cognitive domain), must then make a decision regarding whether or not to begin resuscitation efforts through the application of ethical and moral values dictated by protocol or standing orders (affective domain), and, once the decision to treat has been made, must correctly and efficiently perform the skills (psychomotor domain).

Domain Levels

Each domain is structured into distinct divisions, or levels, that reflect the increasing depth and breadth of understanding an individual achieves progressing through the domain. Several systems of categorizing these levels are applied within each domain, and these systems are classified as either formal or informal. Of the two types, formal systems provide a greater amount of structure. Therefore, formal systems are typically used by the instructor for greater precision in determining how much content to cover on a given topic, and in identifying the appropriate depth and breadth of content for evaluation purposes.

Bloom's Taxonomy

Bloom and his associates originally identified and described five levels within each of the three domains of learning. After 1956, a sixth level ("evaluation") was added to the cognitive domain **(Table 7.1)**. It should be noted that specific action verbs can be used to describe behavioral characteristics required within each level. A partial listing of some of the action verbs that are appropriate for each level is found in Chapter 8: Table 8.1.

Cognitive Domain Levels

Level 1: **Knowledge** focuses on memorization and recall of information.

Level 2: **Comprehension** focuses on interpretation and understanding of the meaning behind information.

Level 3: **Application** deals with relating classroom information to real-life situations and experiences. At this level, students should be able to identify subtle differences between concepts and should begin to see how those differences can be used in practical application. They will still, however, require assistance from instructors in thinking through these ideas.

Level 4: **Analysis** requires that the student be able to separate whole concepts into individual, smaller parts to analyze their meaning and understand their importance.

As students progress to Level 5: **Synthesis**, they are able to combine pieces of information into new and different whole ideas. They are beginning the process of combining seemingly unrelated ideas together and can use logic to defend why they have made certain choices.

In Level 6: **Evaluation**, the student has attained cognitive mastery of the concepts and is able to make judgments and decisions about information. The evaluation level represents metacognition (thinking about thinking), in which the thought process is scrutinized as closely as the outcome.

Table 7.1 Bloom's Taxonomy of the Domains of Learning[1]

Levels	Cognitive Domain	Affective Domain	Psychomotor Domain
1	Knowledge	Receiving	Imitation
2	Comprehension	Responding	Manipulation
3	Application	Valuing	Precision
4	Analysis	Organizing	Articulation
5	Synthesis	Characterizing	Naturalization
6	Evaluation*		

*Note that the level of evaluation, the sixth level in the cognitive domain, was added a few years after Bloom's original work was completed in 1956.

Bloom, 1956

CASE IN POINT

A paramedic student first learns the contraindications of administering a specific medication and is able to list them (Level 1: Knowledge). Next, the student comprehends the adverse effects of the medication on a patient for whom it is contraindicated (Level 2: Comprehension). In Level 3: Application, the student can explain the physiologic principles behind why and how the adverse effects occur. Next, given a specific patient scenario, the student is able to determine whether or not the medication would be contraindicated (Level 4: Analysis). Moving one step farther, the student, having made the determination that the medication is contraindicated, makes a decision concerning the next appropriate treatment step (Level 5: Synthesis). Finally, in Level 6: Evaluation, the student accurately and efficiently runs through such a patient scenario in a skills practicum and performs with minimal assistance from the instructor.

Affective Domain Levels

Level 1: **Receiving** occurs as the student acquires awareness of the value or importance of learning information and expresses a willingness to learn. At this level, students may not agree with or value the actual concepts, but they are open to listening.

Level 2: **Responding** expands upon level 1 as the student actively participates in the learning process and begins to derive satisfaction from it.

Level 3: **Valuing** is the level in which the student individually perceives that the behavior has worth or value. If the concept or idea was previously a part of a student's value system, this is the level at which he or she begins within the affective domain.

Level 4: **Organizing** integrates new, refined, or different beliefs into the student's existing value system and reconciles differences between old and new beliefs. Students should also begin to replace preexisting values that conflict with the newer ones being adopted.

Level 5: **Characterizing** is the most sophisticated level in the affective domain. It requires the development of one's own value system that governs behavior and, like Level 6 (Evaluation) in the cognitive domain, it involves a degree of metacognition as the student scrutinizes the processes used in deriving his or her values, beliefs, and opinions.

CASE IN POINT

A 17-year-old student expresses a reluctance to work with elderly patients. After discussing this matter with him, the student's instructor determines that he has had limited exposure to elderly individuals and arranges for the student to spend time visiting with residents of an independent living community (Level 1: Receiving). The student develops a relationship with one of the residents and begins to visit him regularly (Level 2: Responding). The student begins to understand the importance and value (Level 3: Valuing) of geriatric patents. The student continues to visit elderly patients. The student even becomes a geriatric EMS course instructor so that he might teach other EMS providers about geriatric patients, and structures his opening presentation around the value of elderly people (Level 4: Organizing and Level 5: Characterizing).

Psychomotor Domain Levels

Level 1: **Imitation** occurs as students repeat and mimic demonstrations given by an instructor.

Level 2: **Manipulation** occurs as students practice the skill and begin to create their own styles of performance. Because students lack sophistication at this point, experimentation and trial and error are expected and should be encouraged by the educator.

Level 3: **Precision** is the point at which the skill should be performed without mistakes. Students should also begin to transfer its use to other situations or circumstances. However, this will be done with a high degree of error in performance, necessitating resumption of the trial-and-error process (but with a new emphasis on exploring "what if" concepts).

Level 4: **Articulation** occurs as students become proficient and competent in the performance of the skill, adding their own style or flair. At this level, students should be able to modify the performance of the skill in appropriate ways and defend their choices and decisions.

Level 5: **Naturalization** is the mastery level of skill performance. In contrast to the cognitive and affective domains, this level is attained when the student performs the skill seemingly without any cognition required. This level is sometimes referred to as "muscle memory," or "automatic memory." True naturalization occurs when skill performance is correct despite the environment or circumstance in which the skill is performed.

CASE IN POINT

When students begin the skill of bag valve mask (BVM) ventilation, there is a process of building through the five phases of the Psychomotor Domains Levels. The first time these concepts are presented, the instructor acts out the steps needed to properly use the BVM. Students are first encouraged to watch and do what the instructor does with a BVM on a manikin. Seal the mask correctly over the nose and mouth as well as properly squeeze the bag (Level 1: Imitation). The students practice with the BVM, demonstrating various techniques of squeezing the bag as well as various techniques of securing the mask on the nose and mouth of the manikin (Level 2: Manipulation). As the students gain confidence in performing the proper methods of ventilating a manikin with a BVM, the instructor begins to introduce "what if" scenarios into the airway management simulation, causing the students to react and make appropriate adjustments in their treatment plans (Level 3: Precision). The students react appropriately in most scenarios and, when questioned, can defend their treatment choices with logical reasoning. This includes the ability to select different types of BVM device (bags as well as masks) and still achieve success in securing and properly ventilating the manikin (Level 4: Articulation). When the students are presented with various scenarios in a variety of skills stations, the students automatically demonstrate their competence, regardless of the type of bag or mask, and achieve success in the proper ventilation of the manikin (Level 5: Naturalization).

Addressing The Domains in Goals and Objectives

The domains of learning are used in the instructional design process for writing goals and objectives. Educators must understand the language of an objective or goal and must discern specific meaning from the verbs used to write them. (See Chapter 8: Goals and Objectives.) This enables the educator to plan instructional and evaluative processes that assist students in meeting the objectives and provide a means of measuring their achievement.

In the knowledge level of cognition, the following terms are useful: *arrange, define, describe, identify, label, list, name, match, memorize, order, recall, recite,* and *repeat.* The analysis level of the cognitive domain uses such action verbs as *analyze, calculate, compare and contrast, differentiate, and examine.* In the psychomotor domain, Level 1: Imitation employs terms such as *repeat, mimic,* and *follow,* whereas Level 4: Articulation uses *demonstrate proficiency* and *perform without assistance.* In the affective domain, terms such as *accept, attempt,* and *willing* are appropriate for Level 1: Receiving, and *join* and *participate* are found in Level 5: Characterizing. Goals and objectives are more explicitly addressed in Chapter 8.

Addressing The Domains in Teaching Strategies

Learning within one domain is often interdependent on learning in another domain. For example, cognitive knowledge and concepts are required for the hands-on practice of psychomotor skills to be most effective. Students will achieve mastery of endotracheal intubation more quickly if they can identify the necessary equipment, understand the indications for the skill, and recite the sequence of events required for completion of the skill before they ever attempt to perform it.

At the same time, mastery of knowledge in one domain does not imply mastery in the other domains. For example, a student who can answer multiple-choice exam questions about the procedure for spinal immobilization is not necessarily able to fully immobilize a patient without compromising the spine.

As educators plan learning, they should consider the level of learning that has taken place within each domain and how it relates to their instructional objectives. This process of building new learning upon previous learning is called "scaffolding." In the building trade, scaffolds allow an individual to move from one floor, or level, to another. They are often fragile structures that depend on firm attachment to multiple points below them. Learning scaffolds are also highly dependent upon successful performance at lower levels **(Figure 7.1)**.

To properly scaffold learning, teaching strategies and evaluation methods must target the top of the level in which students are learning. To do this, the instructor should review objectives from the course, unit, or lesson to determine the appropriate depth and breadth at which to teach the material. To determine depth and breadth, one of the two formal strategies should be used to identify the level of the objective.

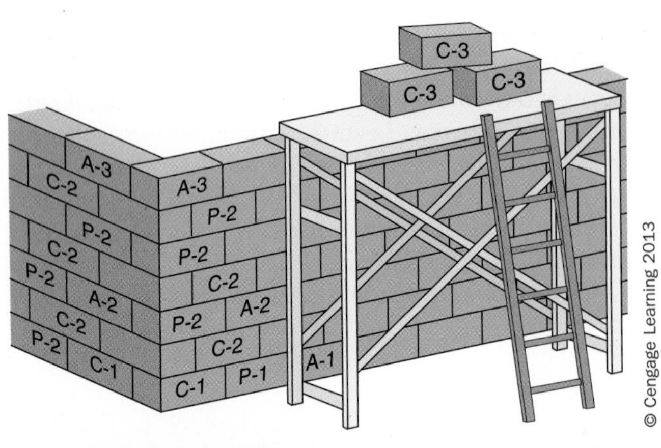

Figure 7.1

The process of building new learning upon previous learning is called *scaffolding*. In the building trade, scaffolds allow an individual to move from one floor, or level, to another. They are often fragile structures that depend on firm attachment to multiple points below them. Learning scaffolds are also highly dependent upon successful performance at lower levels. To properly scaffold, teaching strategies and evaluation methods should target the top of the level at which students are learning.

Depth and breadth examples:

- Objective A states that the student should take a supplied list of names of seven organs and label those organs on a manikin.
- Objective B states that the student should draw a human skeleton and label all the major bones from memory. (Objective A deals with cognitive domain Level 1: Knowledge, whereas Objective B deals with cognitive domain Level 5: Synthesis.)
- Objective C states that the student should be able to take an empty oxygen cylinder and switch the regulator to a full tank. If an instructor demonstrates this skill, but only some (not all) of the students mimic her, it is unlikely that the entire class will be successful in an evaluation of this skill. Skill demonstration and practice are Level 1 activities, whereas performance of a skill for testing purposes with confidence and proficiency is a Level 5 activity.
- Objective D states the student should be able to list the Five Patient Medication Rights. If, in reviewing what was taught in a lesson, the instructor realizes that he stressed only four of the rights, it is unlikely the students will be able to successfully test on this objective based on their classroom lessons alone.

Clever educators can devise methods for integrating learning across several domains to enhance both depth and breadth of knowledge. This is accomplished by engaging as many senses as possible to enhance retention. For example, use of multimedia, class discussion, and role-playing are all ways of successfully engaging the students' senses. Studies on retention suggest that, as more senses are engaged in the learning process, more learning takes place. Additional studies show that greater retention occurs as concepts are revisited and reviewed.[2,3]

Teaching Tip >> *A common strategy used to assist students in attaining mastery of depth and breadth is to account for memory degradation by teaching one level beyond that required by the objective. However, if time is at a premium (which it often is), this may not be possible.*

Individual student learning styles and preferences magnify the interdependence of the different learning domains. (See Chapter 4: Learning Styles). Students who are strongly kinesthetic (hands-on) in their learning preference may have difficulty understanding cognitive concepts until they are able to experience their psychomotor application. On the other hand, students who identify most strongly with global tendencies may be more attuned to feelings than are analytic individuals and therefore may require more (or less) attention to the affective domain.

Teaching Tip >> *Chapter 4 contains information on learning styles and preferences. While reading that chapter, an instructor should consider how this information influences the domains of learning.*

The application of learning domains to teaching strategies is more explicitly discussed in Chapters 12 to 19 of this text.

Addressing The Domains in Evaluation Methods

Educators must devise evaluation strategies that determine the progressive mastery of each level in every domain. Educators who assume competency and fail to evaluate students will quickly learn the importance of doing so. In addition, evaluation should occur to ensure that students retain concepts from the previous level(s).

Teaching Tip >> *An instructor can take a quick look at the course grading policy to ensure that a program places equal emphasis on each domain of learning.*

Written and oral exams are useful for evaluating the cognitive domain. Class participation, demonstrated leadership, and peer supervision are useful for evaluating the affective domain. Skill competency exams and evaluation within the clinical setting are useful for evaluating the psychomotor domain. The application of learning domains to evaluation methods is more explicitly covered in Chapters 20 to 22 of this text.

Summary

Ultimately, students must achieve proficiency in all three domains of learning if they are to be competent health care providers. The domains of learning levels are scientific tools that instructional designers and educators use to craft objectives, identify the appropriate depth and breadth of content to plan lessons and teaching strategies, and effectively evaluate learning and retention. Savvy educators recognize their importance and know how to use them in practicing and honing the art of teaching.

Glossary

affective domain Learning in terms of feelings, emotions, attitudes, and values.

analysis The cognitive domain level that requires separation of whole concepts into individual, smaller parts to analyze their meaning and understand their importance.

application The cognitive domain level that relates classroom information to real-life situations.

articulation The psychomotor domain level that occurs when proficient and competent performance of the skill, with personal style or flair occurs.

Bloom's Taxonomy A description of the domains of learning developed by Dr. Benjamin Bloom.

characterizing The affective domain level that requires development of one's own value system that governs behavior.

cognitive domain Learning that takes place through the process of thinking; it deals with facts and knowledge.

comprehension The cognitive domain level that focuses on interpretation and understanding meaning.

domains of learning Categories of learning that include cognitive, affective and psychomotor.

evaluation The cognitive domain level where mastery of cognitive concepts is achieved to allow judgments and decisions about information.

imitation The psychomotor domain level that occurs as students repeat and mimic demonstrations.

knowledge The cognitive domain level that focuses on memorization and recall.

manipulation The psychomotor domain level that occurs as students practice a skill and begin to create their own styles of performance.

naturalization The psychomotor domain level that represents skill performance mastery.

organizing The affective domain level where the learner integrates new, refined, or different beliefs into their existing value system.

precision The psychomotor domain level when the skill is performed without mistakes and transfer to other situations or circumstances begins.

psychomotor domain Learning that takes place through the attainment of skills and bodily, or kinesthetic, movements.

receiving The affective domain level that occurs as the student acquires awareness of the value or importance of learning information and expresses a willingness to learn.

responding The affective domain level where the student actively participates in the learning process and begins to derive satisfaction from it.

synthesis The cognitive domain level that combines pieces of information into new and different whole ideas.

valuing The affective domain level in which the student perceives that a behavior has worth or value.

References

1. Bloom, B. S., *et al.* (1956). *Taxonomy of educational objectives, cognitive domain.* New York, NY: Longman.

2. Cicchetti, G. (1990). *Cognitive modeling and reciprocal teaching of reading and study strategies.* Watertown, CT:

3. Mayer, R. E. (1998). Cognitive, metacognitive, and motivational aspects of problem solving. *Instructional Science. 26,* 49–63.

Additional Resources

Adult Education Resource and Information Service (ARIS) Information Sheet, (2000). Learning to learn. Melbourne, Australia.

Hodell, C. (1997). Basics of instructional systems development. The American Society for Training and Development*(ASTD) Info-line,* Issue 9706.

8

Goals and Objectives

Objectives are not fate; they are direction. — Peter F. Drucker

More often than not, goals and objectives are considered to be the backbone of the instructional process. They provide the educational framework for instruction by identifying what educators should teach and what students are expected to learn. This chapter presents how the various taxonomies of the domains of learning categorize learning into discrete levels. This chapter then builds on that concept by using those levels in the process of writing goals and objectives.

During instructional planning, educators use goals and objectives to determine the appropriate depth and breadth of content required to teach a given topic, including differentiating between necessary and unnecessary content. This planning helps to ensure that instruction is targeted to specific goals. Goals and objectives are also used in the test item writing and evaluation processes to effectively evaluate student learning. Finally, these tools are useful for measuring the effectiveness of the educator's teaching activities.

Through goals and objectives, students are positioned to focus their learning and begin to differentiate important content from unimportant content. Students should be able to track their individual progress in a course of instruction by evaluating their ability to perform (by answering questions, exhibiting professional behaviors or demonstrating skills) required class objectives and to meet the course goals. Instructors should ensure that students have course goals and objectives and use them to focus their studying.

Although several strategies for writing goals and objectives may be applied, this chapter focuses on a single, generic technique for writing that uses two tiers: goals followed by objectives. Educators should determine whether their specific department uses a different strategy. If that is the case, this chapter will still be helpful, as the concepts explained here are similar to those associated with other objective- and goal-writing methods.

CHAPTER GOAL: This chapter describes how the instructor can use the levels within the domains of learning to guide their process of writing goals and objectives.

Teaching Tip >> *Although an entry level educator may not be required to write objectives, it is important that the educator understand how goals and objectives relate to the planning and evaluation of instruction.*

What are Goals and Objectives?

Educators can make the best use of goals and objectives when they have acquired a keen understanding of exactly what these instructional tools are and can identify the differences between them. The words "goal" and "objective" are often used interchangeably and without regard for their actual meaning, which can lead to confusion. In this textbook, a two-tiered system is described wherein the term *goal* is used only to describe the uppermost level of instruction and the term *objective* is used to describe the subordinate level.

A great deal of support is available for use of this method. In many instructional materials, goals and objectives are presented in two distinct levels, with objectives being subordinate to goals. The first level (which is generally the goal) identifies the overall intent of instruction for the course or specific instructional event. Confusion arises when this tier is called a "terminal objective" instead of the "primary goal of instruction."[1]

Objectives are always subordinate to the goal. In completing each objective, a student makes progress toward meeting the overall goal. Sometimes, objectives are called "enabling objectives." This terminology is common when goal statements are named "terminal objectives." Every goal statement should have at least one objective that relates to it, and every objective should relate to at least one goal. The content of the lesson (sometimes called the "declarative material") should relate to the goals and objectives, and should not contain information that does not relate to the goals and objectives (see the section Performance Agreement later in this chapter for further details).

Teaching Tip >> *Another strategy for writing goals and objectives applies three tiers of distinct goals and objectives. In this strategy, the "goal" is the upper tier. The second tier is often called the "terminal objective," and the last tier is called the "enabling objective." In this strategy, various enabling objectives are grouped together under a single terminal objective that directly relates to the goal. Completion of the enabling objectives leads to completion of the terminal objective. Completion of several terminal objectives leads to completion of the goal. This strategy of classification is useful when one is describing a program with multiple class sessions that are offered over a certain length of time. It can also be used to break down each block of instruction for a semester-long course.*

Goals

Goals are philosophical statements about what learning is intended to produce. They are often broad, generalized, and overarching with no specific information on how learning is to be accomplished or measured. Goals are similar in nature to mission or vision statements. For example, an educator may establish goals for an entire course, a learning module, a 1-hour skills practice, or a single case scenario.

Examples of goal statements include the following:

- The goal of this chapter is to explain the concepts of basic airway management.
- Students who attend this cardiopulmonary resuscitation (CPR) course will perform all required CPR techniques correctly on a manikin.
- Upon the completion of English 203, the student will be able to compose essays using a technical writing style.

Objectives

For a goal to be accomplished, specific and measurable **objectives** must be identified. The word *objective* literally means "observable." Objectives are expressed statements of expected learning outcomes, which include products or behaviors that students are required to exhibit. As with goals, an educator may establish objectives for a course, a particular lesson, a skills practice, or a single classroom exercise, just to name a few examples. Some instructors use the SMART mnemonic used to describe essential characteristics of an objective: objectives should be specific, measurable, achievable, realistic, and timely.

An objective should be detailed enough to encompass the aspects of "who, what, when, where, and how" of the behaviors appropriate for accomplishing that goal. To provide this information, an objective should clearly identify four distinct items:

1. Target audience
2. Expected behavior
3. Condition under which that behavior will be performed
4. Measurement tool or strategy used to evaluate the objective for successful completion (or outcome)

Each of these elements must be expressed in a manner assuring that anyone who reads the objective will clearly understand the "pass/fail points" for each objective and will know exactly what behavior is expected.

This format describes the **ABCD model** (*A*udience, *B*ehavior, *C*ondition, and *D*egree) for writing objectives. This generic strategy is basic to most behavior-based goal and objective models. Examples of complete objectives include the following:

- The students will use their own words to correctly define at least five of the following six terms pertaining to respiratory emergencies: dyspnea, apnea, eupnea, hyperpnea, tachypnea, and bradypnea.
- Upon completion of this module, the students in this Advanced Emergency Medical Technician program will be able to demonstrate insertion of a supraglottic airway to 80% accuracy and with no critical errors as indicated on the skill checklist.
- Given a series photographs of skin rashes, the student will identify all photographs that show a vesicular skin rash.

Performance Agreement

The link between goals and objectives is established through an evaluation process called a **performance agreement**. Performance agreement is the process of critically evaluating the goals, objectives, and declarative content for the purpose of validating their logical relationships to one another, and to ensure that they adequately support one another. For performance agreement to exist within a body of planned instruction, each goal statement must be supported by one or more objectives that link directly to it. At the same time, each objective should link to at least one goal. The declarative content should provide the depth and breadth described by the verbs written in the objectives. (Refer to the previous chapter for a discussion of the levels of sophistication for each domain of learning.)

Any goal or objective within the block of instruction that does not have a clear link should be evaluated further for appropriateness. These "unlinked" goals or objectives may represent omissions of the content required for the lesson. They may also highlight unnecessary material that should perhaps be moved into another lesson or deleted from the section altogether **(Figure 8.1)**.

For the educator, the exercise of looking for and validating performance agreement is useful for identifying unnecessary instruction or any voids in a lesson plan. It helps to ensure that the content found within the lesson plan (which may or may not have been developed by the same educator) and the content presented in the classroom match the goals stated for the lesson in the curricula. In general, educators can focus on teaching only the necessary and appropriate content when they evaluate performance agreement.

Teaching Tip >> *When performance agreement is assessed before instruction is provided, adjustments can be made before mistakes are made in the classroom. When performance agreement is assessed after instruction has been provided, content omissions or areas requiring remediation or reteaching can be identified.*

Performance Agreement	No Performance Agreement
Topic: Method to Assess Pulse *Objectives:* On a written test, to 90% accuracy, the student will be able to: 1. Explain how a pulse is generated. 2. Label a diagram with four locations commonly used to assess the pulse. 3. Outline the technique to assess the pulse. *Presentation Content:* A. Pulse generation 1. Heart rate 2. Arterial blood flow B. Pulse locations 1. Carotid 2. Arms 3. Legs C. Pulse assessment technique 1. Measuring rate 2. Other pulse characteristics *Performance agreement is attained. Each objective has associated content and there is no content that is not related to an objective.*	*Topic: Method to Assess the Pulse* *Objectives:* On a written test, to 90% accuracy, the student will be able to: 1. Explain how a pulse is generated. 2. Label a diagram with four locations commonly used to assess the pulse. 3. Outline the technique to assess the pulse. *Presentation Content:* A. Pulse locations 1. Carotid 2. Arms 3. Legs B. Pulse assessment technique 1. Measuring rate 2. Other pulse characteristics C. Abnormal pulse findings 1. Fast or slow rate 2. Irregular pulse 3. Weak pulse *Performance agreement is not achieved. There is no content related to objective 1. In addition, the content about abnormal pulse findings is not related to any objective. An objective for this content could be "Recognize implications of abnormal pulse findings."*

Figure 8.1

Performance Agreement (good example) versus No Performance Agreement (poor example).

CASE IN POINT

An educator is reviewing his lesson plan for his next presentation on the topic of interpreting 12-lead electrocardiograms (ECGs). He begins by reviewing the goals and objectives for the session. He notes that all four of the goals listed are covered by at least one of the objectives, and each objective is linked to at least one goal. He then reviews the content for the presentation and discovers two places that lack performance agreement, because there is a disconnection between the goals, objectives, and declarative content. The first error he discovers is that two of the objectives listed do not seem to be covered in the declarative section of the lesson plan; so, he adds the necessary material to make certain that he has covered all objectives. The second problem he notes is that a section of the material is not described in either the goals or the objectives for the lesson plan. As he reviews this material, he decides it is not really appropriate for this lesson, but should be covered in the next. He moves this information to the next lesson after discussing his findings with his mentor. He updates this lesson plan with these changes so that the next time this plan is used, it will be more complete. His mentor compliments him on his plan and on finding the problems before attempting to teach the material.

Whenever possible, an educator should conduct a postpresentation evaluation for performance agreement. This should occur immediately after instruction has been provided for the purpose of reviewing what was taught and identifying whether any omissions, sidetracks (superfluous content), or other deviations from the lesson plan occurred. One method for conducting this type of performance agreement is to ask students to summarize the lesson or to provide their impressions of the key points covered. Another method of conducting this assessment is through the use of post-tests. Omissions identified during this performance agreement assessment can be made up during future teaching sessions or through alternative learning opportunities outside of the face-to-face meeting.

Teaching Tip >> *The postpresentation evaluation for performance agreement provides an excellent time for the educator to draft exam questions or select questions from a test-item bank. Once an instructor has determined performance agreement exists and this review is fresh in her mind, then she can select test items that most closely reflect the content delivered.*

Checklist for Writing Objectives

- All four parts of the *ABCD* behavioral objective are present
  - Audience
  - Behavior
  - Condition
  - Degree
- Accurate terminology is used to reflect the domain of learning level
- Expected outcome is clearly articulated and measurable
- Expected outcome is written in terms of behaviors to perform or observe
- The scoring method for pass/fail is clearly articulated
- A measurement tool is discussed or described
- Objective supports overarching goal (performance agreement)

Components of an Objective

Many methods, models, and templates are available for teaching an educator how to write objectives. The generic ABCD model, which is commonly used, lists the parts of a behavioral objective, where ABCD indicates the required elements of information. In this model, A = Audience, B = Behavior, C = Condition, and D = Degree.[2] Objectives need not be written in the ABCD order, but should contain each of these four elements.

Two simple models to follow in constructing the order for an objective include:

1. The (Audience) will (Behavior) under (Condition) to (Degree).
2. Given (Condition), the (Audience) will (Behavior) to (Degree). This format is more often followed and referred to as the CABD format for writing objectives.

Audience

The *audience* describes the receiver (student) of the instructional activity **(Figure 8.2)**. When reviewing objectives before providing instruction, the educator should ensure that the intended audience matches the actual audience for the instruction. If, for example, the intended audience for the lesson is identified in

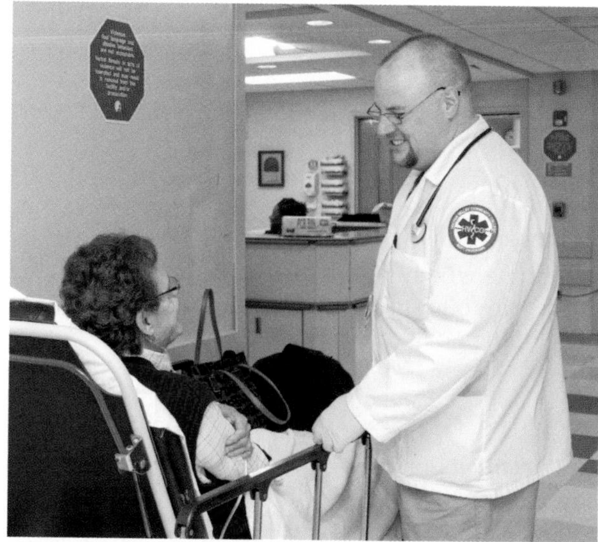
A

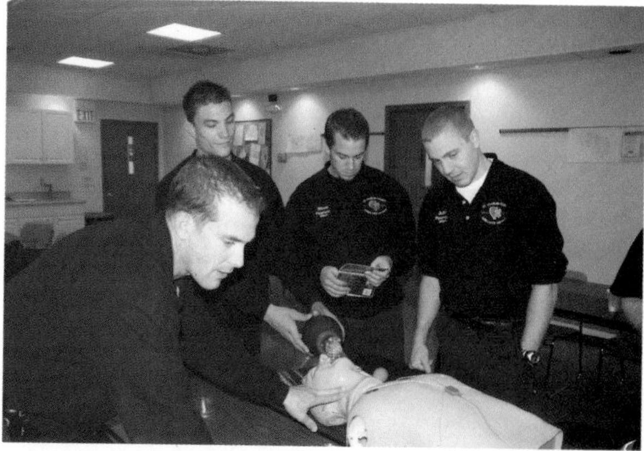
B

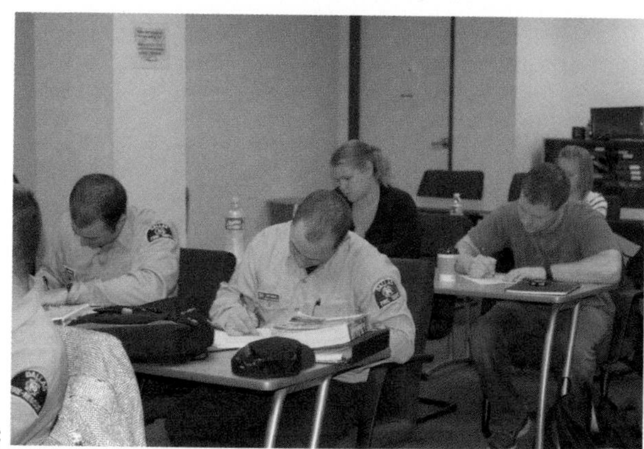
C

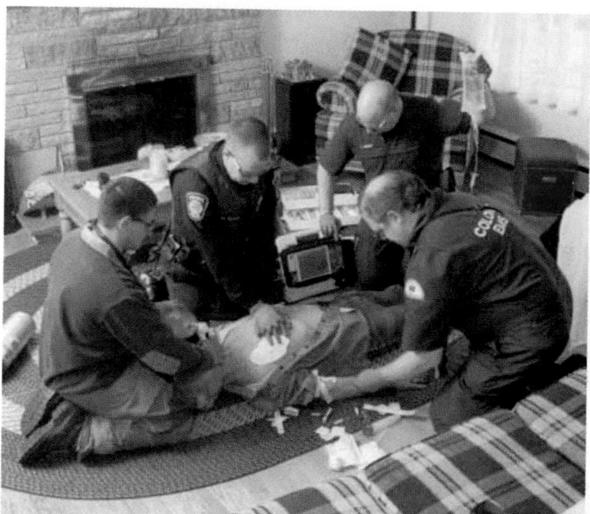
D

Figure 8.2

The audience (students) may be in A. the hospital B. the skills lab, C. the classroom, or D. the field.

the objective as advanced life support (ALS) providers, but the educator is using it for basic life support (BLS) providers, she will need to compensate for the disparity. In this case, the educator could supplement the lesson with additional material or, if appropriate, expand the presentation over a longer time period to account for deficits in the BLS provider's depth of knowledge.

In another situation, the audience identified in the objective may have significantly different prerequisites from the audience the instructor is about to teach, or may be at a different intellectual level. In this circumstance, the educator could plan additional learning opportunities, make adjustments in timing, or rearrange the lesson entirely to suit the new target audience.

Because the audience remains constant throughout a series of objectives in, for example, the same lesson plan, textbook chapter, or block of instruction, the audience statement is often limited to the goal or first objective found in that series. In this case, the educator can assume the stated audience carries through for the remainder of the objectives in that section.

Examples of audience statements include:

- The Columbia Community College freshman student
- The paramedic refresher-course participant
- The cadets attending this seminar

Behavior

The *behavior* statement describes the expected outcome or capability the learner should exhibit after the instructional event has occurred. Robert Mager, a behavioral theorist, is credited with the concept that goals and objectives should be tied to measurable outcomes.[3] The term he used to describe this relationship was "concrete." That is, any statement, or objective, tied to measurable behavioral outcomes is concrete; those not tied to measurable behavioral outcomes are called "fuzzy," meaning they are immeasurable statements. Mager believed objectives should always be written in terms of performance so that learning can be measured. This concept is the foundation for the process of writing objectives. If an objective is written so it can be measured or observed, it becomes concrete enough to form the basis of evaluation. The relationship between goals, objectives, and evaluation is explored at the end of this chapter.

Review the following two objectives. According to the criteria established by Mager, Objective 1 is not measurable, and Objective 2 is measurable.

- Objective 1: The student will identify equipment used to immobilize a patient to a long backboard.
- Objective 2: Given a BLS ambulance stocked with all the required equipment and supplies identified by the state protocol, the student will identify every piece of equipment used to immobilize a patient to a long backboard.

Objective 1 states the audience and behavior, but does not articulate any conditions or degree. It does not state how or what equipment will be used in the test, nor does it state the required score for successfully satisfying this objective. Thus, it would be difficult for an instructor to perform an evaluation of this objective. Objective 2 tells both the instructor and the student that they will be required to identify all required equipment and supplies, and that they will be working with an ambulance stocked according to an established standard. Therefore, objective 2 leaves little room for subjectivity in interpretation.

If objectives are observable and measurable, a tangible product or outcome that can be scrutinized and evaluated should be the result. This product or outcome can take the form of demonstrated knowledge, performance of a skill, or expressed or modeled feeling or emotion. It can come from any of the domains of learning (cognitive, affective, or psychomotor) and can be written to correspond to any of the levels of sophistication within a domain. It should be a realistic behavior related to the real-life scope of practice for the student.

Examples of behavior statements include:

- Describe the steps used to initiate a peripheral IV.
- Demonstrate how to put on sterile gloves.
- Challenge statements that do not support professional behavior and conduct.

Verbs such as "understand," "know," and "think" are not measurable and should be avoided in writing objectives.

In some educational settings, the terminology used to construct the behavioral statement carries legal connotations. In this case, there is a significant difference between phases such as "should be able to" and "will be able to." It is important for the instructor to determine whether such a circumstance exists, and if it does, to follow the requirements accordingly when developing goals and objectives.

Condition

The *condition* portion of the ABCD objective describes any circumstance that influences the performance of behavior. It may include a list of tools or equipment that may or may not be used in completion of the behavior; it may describe environmental or weather conditions or identify specific locations or situations, such as time of day or season of the year. Time limits may also be imposed as a condition of the performance of a skill.

Examples of condition statements include:

- . . . in swift-running river water with class II rapids . . .
- Given a table of assorted splinting equipment, . . .
- . . . within 1 minute . . .

Take this example of a measurable objective for a trauma lesson: The EMT student will perform a trauma patient assessment on a simulated patient placed in a difficult-to-access location, without committing any critical errors. In this case, critical errors should be defined on the performance checklist or rubric. (See Chapter 22: Other Evaluation Tools, for more information about rubrics.) The conditions affecting the performance (in this case, the skill of trauma patient assessment) of this objective are the use of a simulated patient (necessitating the finding of predetermined signs or symptoms) and a challenging environment. Because the condition is well articulated, both the instructor and the student can determine what behavior is expected and how it should be tested. This leaves little room for surprises during testing and helps create realistic expectations for both students and instructors.

Degree

The *degree* portion of the objective provides the standard of accuracy required for acceptable performance. It describes the actual measurement tool used to assess the student's performance and clearly identifies the point at which the student will be successful in her performance. Objectives can be measured by both **quantitative** and **qualitative** criteria.

Quantitative criteria identify behaviors through conditions that impose or describe limitations (e.g., the lowest acceptable passing score, time limits, or limits on number of attempts) and provide this information as a percentage or point value. Qualitative criteria include non-numerical observations that show underlying dimensions or patterns of relationships (e.g., expressing the value or acceptance of a concept or idea, defending a decision or action, or adopting a new behavior pattern). Quality standards are often more difficult to assign numeric scores, but they can be observed for performance. The use of rubrics as evaluation tools can be helpful in qualitative measurements.

What Are Rubrics?

A **rubric** is a grading tool that uses rating scales that often incorporate examples to provide a framework to score a student's performance. Rubrics are used for both qualitative and quantitative evaluations. Rubrics work well with qualitative criteria because they provide concrete examples of the expected level of behavior or content, along with the scores or grades that will be awarded if the learner meets the specifications within each category. Rubrics are also useful for more subjective evaluations because they quantify the expected outcomes. Grading of essay questions is generally considered subjective, but is made less so when graded with rubric tools that identify the desired level of performance within specified categories. These categories typically include content, organization, and process. Instructors determine criteria for each level ahead of time so both students and faculty have clear guidelines to define performance. For example, the rubric may state that the student will receive 5 points for each key concept that he or she explains in his or her essay, up to a total of 50 points. It may also include a deduction of 5 points for every unrelated concept or incorrect item that he or she includes in the answer. Another rubric may score the essay by creating a scale for punctuation and spelling errors, awarding up to 10 points for 0 to 5 errors, 9 points for 6 to 10 errors, 8 points for 11 to 15 errors, and so forth. Scoring within the rubric should allow for evaluation of each of the dimensions of the project. Students can even be provided examples of answers for each grade range. Tools for developing rubrics can be found on various websites on the Internet.

Here are several qualitative examples of degree:

- . . . using therapeutic communication strategies throughout the simulation . . .
- . . . by using all of the affective domain characteristics described in the chapter that apply to this scenario . . .
- . . . without committing any critical-fail-point errors . . .

Additional factors to consider in measuring performance according to an objective are whether steps required to perform a skill are ordered (and if this order is important), and whether any factors or steps are critical to the performance. Examples of critical factors include the wearing of gloves when one approaches an appropriate patient situation, and the performing of an assessment before one begins CPR. Such factors are often labeled "critical criteria" or "critical fail points," and failure to satisfy or perform them may result in immediate failure in the performance of an objective. Critical fail points are generally absolute, which means that failure is imposed despite an otherwise acceptable performance. For this reason, critical fail status should be reserved for extremely important steps or considerations. In the EMS domain, the psychomotor examination checkoff sheets of the National Registry of EMTs include at the bottom of each skill sheet critical criteria, called "critical fail points."

Some additional examples of degree statements include:

- . . . seven out of ten times . . .
- . . . to 80 percent accuracy . . .
- . . . for every patient care encounter . . .

It is important that the performance level be specifically stated; otherwise, an educator may assume that 100 percent accuracy is required. (Note that a performance level of 100 percent accuracy for quantitative or qualitative measures is not required for every objective.) Educators should scrutinize objectives carefully to determine the acceptable level of performance and should plan instructional time and emphasis accordingly.

Often, it is difficult to distinguish between some of the ABCD components of an objective, as there seems to be crossover between them. Take, for example, the following objective:

"Upon the completion of this lesson on trauma, the student will be able to correctly demonstrate the application of a rigid splint to a simulated open fracture of the upper extremity within 7 minutes, without committing any critical errors."

Instructors may debate whether the statement "within 7 minutes" represents a condition or a degree. They may also debate whether the words "correctly demonstrate" indicate that a score of 100 percent accuracy is required to satisfy this objective. This objective leaves little doubt about what behavior is expected of the student (apply a rigid splint to an open upper extremity fracture) and about how the student will be evaluated (it must be done correctly within 7 minutes, and the student cannot commit any critical fail errors). The word "correctly" may cause minor confusion, but most instructors would overlook this wording because the phrase about committing critical errors sets a clear boundary.

This example draws attention to the fact that the writing of objectives is not a simple task. In this case, it is important for the educator to identify the behavior portion of the objective and to place that behavior in the proper context within the domains of learning. In so doing, the instructor can identify the depth and breadth required to teach the content so that the objective is satisfied. This objective requires problem-solving behavior via Cognitive Level 3: Application, Level 4: Analysis, and Level 5: Synthesis, as well as psychomotor performance at Level 3: Precision.

Teaching Tip >> *When working from goals and objectives that have been supplied to an instructor, it is critical that the educator review the objectives to ensure completeness and relevance to the audience and situation.*

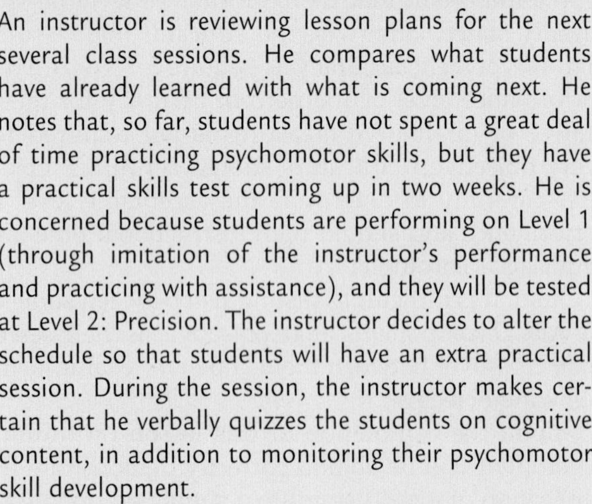

CASE IN POINT

An instructor is reviewing lesson plans for the next several class sessions. He compares what students have already learned with what is coming next. He notes that, so far, students have not spent a great deal of time practicing psychomotor skills, but they have a practical skills test coming up in two weeks. He is concerned because students are performing on Level 1 (through imitation of the instructor's performance and practicing with assistance), and they will be tested at Level 2: Precision. The instructor decides to alter the schedule so that students will have an extra practical session. During the session, the instructor makes certain that he verbally quizzes the students on cognitive content, in addition to monitoring their psychomotor skill development.

Terminology and Precision

Objectives must be written with clear, unambiguous terminology that is free of jargon. All acronyms and potentially confusing terms should be clearly defined. Statements must be written in observable and measurable terms, with careful attention to ensure that action verbs used to describe the required behavior/expected outcome reflect the desired level. **Table 8.1** provides a listing of appropriate verbs that correspond to the various levels within Bloom's taxonomy.[4]

Objectives are always results-oriented. Unlike broader goal statements, objectives describe specific expectations. When they read an objective, there should be no doubt in the student's and instructor's minds about exactly what behavior is expected. Returning to a previous example ("The EMT student

CASE IN POINT

A paramedic student meets with the primary course instructor with the intent of informing her that he intends to drop out of the program. The student tells the instructor that he is having trouble with medical terminology, and feels that he cannot possibly memorize all the terms the instructor went over in class in preparation for the upcoming test in three weeks; he feels he will be unable to keep up in the program because of this event. The course is 18 months long, and this lesson occurred during the second week of the program. This student successfully passed two semesters of anatomy and physiology at the community college and has one year of experience as an EMT. He is in his late thirties and has a bachelor's degree in finance. He left a successful career in banking and is becoming a paramedic because of his desire to help others. Using the objectives in the course syllabus, the instructor works with the student until he understands that he is not required to memorize all the terms covered in the lesson for the test in three weeks, but that by the end of the course, he will be required to know all these terms. She emphasizes that, for this upcoming test, the student needs to understand how to break down a medical term into its component parts (word root, suffix, and prefix) in order to properly define it. She also suggests that he begin to memorize commonly used terms, and she recommends that he create flashcards to help him study. She agrees to provide the student with a list of required medical terms for each section of the course to assist him with studying.

Table 8.1 Action Verbs Corresponding to Bloom's Taxonomy[4]

Domain	Levels	Appropriate Verbs
Cognitive	1 Knowledge	Arrange, Define, Describe, Identify, Label, List, Name, Identify, Match, Memorize, Order, Recognize, Recall, Recite, Repeat
	2 Comprehension	Classify, Discuss, Distinguish, Explain, Identify, Indicate, Locate, Review, Rewrite, Summarize, Tell, Translate
	3 Application	Apply, Choose, Compute, Demonstrate, Operate, Practice, Prepare, Solve
	4 Analysis	Analyze, Calculate, Compare, Contrast, Criticize, Diagram, Differentiate, Distinguish, Examine, Experiment, Evaluate, Relate, Separate, Select
	5 Synthesis	Assemble, Compose, Construct, Create, Combine, Design, Formulate, Organize, Prepare, Set up, Summarize, Tell, Write
	6 Evaluate	Appraise, Evaluate, Judge, Score
Affective	1 Receiving	Accept, Attempt, Willing
	2 Responding	Challenge, Select, Support, Visit
	3 Valuing	Defend, Display, Offer, Choose
	4 Organization	Judge, Volunteer, Share, Dispute
	5 Characterization	Consistently, Join, Participate
Psychomotor	1 Imitation	Repeat, Mimic, Follow
	2 Manipulation	Practice with minimal assistance, Create, Modify
	3 Precision	Perform without error, Perform without assistance
	4 Articulation	Demonstrate proficiency, Perform with confidence, Perform with style or flair
	5 Naturalization	Perform automatically

Bloom, 1956

will perform a trauma patient assessment on a simulated patient placed in a difficult-to-access location, without committing any critical errors"), imagine the difficulty this student would face if, every time they practiced a trauma patient assessment, it was on a manikin lying supine on a blanket in the middle of the classroom floor. Yet, on the night of the test, the simulated patient was placed head down on the side of a dark hill outdoors.

The Relationship between the Domains of Learning and Objectives

There is a strong link between objectives and the domains of learning, a fact that is thoroughly explained in Chapter 7: Domains of Learning. As a simple review, Benjamin Bloom grouped learning into three distinct domains, or categories of related elements: cognitive, psychomotor, and affective domains.[4] These domains reflect the fact that learning can take place in a variety of ways, depending on how we feel emotionally about an issue, how we perform skills and procedures, and how we think about concepts and ideas.

Each domain is subdivided into five or six distinct sections. These sections are arranged into levels. As an individual's learning progresses within a domain, increasing sophistication (more internal processing with less reliance upon the instructor's input or guidance) is required, and greater mastery is attained. In the three-level system, Level 1 is the knowledge level, Level 2 is application, and Level 3 is problem solving. The degrees of sophistication that require less depth of knowledge (e.g., when a student defines words or matches terms with meaning) are referred to as the lower level or Level 1 objectives. Level 2 (application) objectives are at an intermediate level between Levels 1 and 3. Level 3 (problem solving) represents the highest level of learning and requires that students think critically about a topic, debate it, and understand it in depth.

Goals and Objectives and the Evaluation Process

Once the level has been identified for the goal or objective, the instructor can determine which level the evaluation tool should address. Formative evaluation tools can target any level: knowledge, application, or problem solving. Evaluation tools may be formative or summative in nature. Summative tools should focus on the higher levels of application and problem solving. They should include some assessment of verification of competency in the knowledge level, as well as at higher levels. This condition will be important in the event that the student does poorly on the evaluation, as this information can help focus the remediation process by identifying where the deficit occurred. (Chapter 20: Principles of Evaluation of Student Performance, takes an in-depth look at formative and summative evaluation tools.)

Use each of the following objectives (presented earlier in this chapter) to determine at what depth the instructor should evaluate, and to stimulate discussion of possible evaluation tools:

1. The EMT students will use their own words to correctly define at least five of the following six terms pertaining to respiratory emergencies: dyspnea, apnea, eupnea, hyperpnea, tachypnea, and bradypnea.
2. Upon the completion of this module, the students in this Advanced EMT program will be able to demonstrate insertion of a supraglottic airway to 80% accuracy and with no critical errors as indicated on the skill checklist.
3. Given a series photographs of skin rashes, the student will identify all photographs that show a vesicular skin rash.

Objective 1 asks the student to provide definitions. Bloom's taxonomy places this type of cognition in Level 1: Knowledge. Thus, a fill-in-the-blank question format would be an appropriate evaluation tool.

Objective 2 asks the student to apply advanced airway skills, so they must possess knowledge (Level 1), but must also apply techniques of airway management (Level 2). The student also may encounter problems that would require him or her to troubleshoot and use critical-thinking skills (Level 3). The student in this situation would need to operate on all three levels to satisfy this objective, but the objective concentrates on Level 2. The objective states that the student must insert a supraglottic airway (a psychomotor activity), so a demonstration of those skills is the appropriate requirement for evaluation. The evaluator should also ask knowledge questions to ensure that Level 1 has been mastered. It would not be appropriate for the evaluator to introduce problems deliberately into the examination, as the objective does not state that such a high level of performance is expected. Also, in the event of a problem, it may be appropriate for the evaluator to assist the student. It would be helpful to place this objective within the context of the overall program. If this happens early in the course, the student may not possess many problem-solving skills. However, because this is an advanced course, the student may be expected to have already mastered a certain number of problem-solving skills.

Objective 3 may appear to be of a higher level upon first glance, but it is operating primarily at Level 2: application. In this objective, the student will be shown a series of photographs, and they must apply the rules and knowledge obtained in Level 1 to make some decisions about images that do not meet the criteria. The student is not asked to defend his choices or to determine whether the rash presented represents a specific disease or not. Because the objective states that students will be given a finite grouping of photographs to look at, all they will really be doing is sorting them into one of two categories: those photographs that meet the criteria and those that do not. This involves mainly knowledge Level 1: Knowledge activities, along with some Level 2 skills, in that they are applying their knowledge of the rules. An evaluation approach that would be appropriate for this situation would be showing students a series of slides and asking them to write "yes" or "no" on an answer sheet. Another way to evaluate this objective would be to give students a pile of cards with the images on them, and to ask them to sort the cards into two piles: one showing vesicular rashes and one with images that are not.

Summary

As the backbone of instructional planning, goals and objectives clarify for the educator and for the student precisely what learning should take place and how learning will be evaluated. Educators can use the ABCD method to write complete and accurate measurable objectives that address the three domains of learning (cognitive, affective, and psychomotor). By evaluating for performance agreement, the educator can determine the appropriate depth and breadth of content that should be taught on a given topic and can determine whether lesson plan content is complete. Goals and objectives are also used in decisions about appropriate evaluation tools.

Glossary

ABCD model A model to write objectives in which the audience, behaviors, conditions, and degree required to achieve the objective are clearly defined.

goal A broad statement of instructional intent.

objective A specific, measurable learning outcome.

performance agreement Concordance of goals, objectives, content, and evaluation tools.

qualitative Non-numerical observations that show underlying dimensions or patterns of relationships.

quantitative Criteria identify behaviors through conditions that impose or describe limitations.

rubric A measurement tool that establishes a framework for evaluation.

References

1. Hardt, U. H. (1977). Determining goals, objectives and strategies for the domains of learning and instructional intents. *A guide to lesson and unit planning. ERIC.*
2. Hodell, C. (1997). Basics of instructional systems development. The American Society for Training and Development *ASTD Info-line*, Issue 9706.
3. Mager, R. F. (1972). *Goal analysis.* Belmont, CA: Fearon Publishers.
4. Bloom, B. S., *et al.*, (1956). *Taxonomy of educational objectives. Book I: Cognitive domain.* New York, NY: Longman.

Additional Resources

Gronlund, N. E., & Brookhart, S. M. (2009). *Gronlund's writing instructional objectives,* (8th ed.). Upper Saddle River, NJ: Pearson Merrill Prentice Hall.

Nooman, Z. M., Schmidt, H. G., & Ezzat, E. S., (Eds.) (1990). *Innovation in medical education.* New York, NY: Springer Publishing.

Novak, J. D. (1977). *A theory of education.* Ithaca, NY: Cornell University Press.

Smilkstein, R. (1993). Acquiring knowledge and using it. *Gamut, 16,* 41–43.

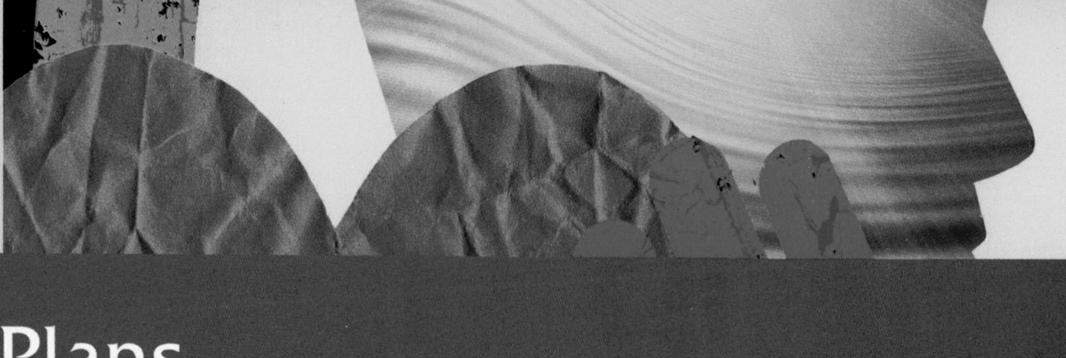

9 Lesson Plans

The whole art of teaching is only the art of awakening the natural curiosity of young minds for the purpose of satisfying it afterwards. — Anatole France

The process of education can be described as a journey. As with any journey, the traveler or student has to know where he or she is going and the path he or she will take. Along the way, various waypoints will indicate the progress that is being made. In an educational journey, the final destination is indicated by the course or terminal objective. Waypoints along the way correspond to the student performance objective, and the map that keeps the learner, and the instructor, on track and heading toward the final destination is the lesson plan. Thus, it can be seen that the lesson plan plays a key role in the educational process.

CHAPTER GOAL: This chapter discusses how to develop effective lesson plans.

Overview of Lesson Plans

The lesson plan is a valuable teaching tool on many levels. In addition to keeping the instructional process on track, it serves a variety of other important functions. For the instructor, it provides the basic information needed to teach as well as to prepare the lesson. A properly formatted lesson plan includes not only the materials needed to meet the lesson objectives, but also the introductory material needed to prepare the lesson. It provides information and guidance on the development and use of instructional aids. And, because it is tied to the lesson objectives, it serves as a basis for, and even provides, student evaluation.

Lesson plans assist the instructional process and directly help the instructor. Lesson plans explain the depth and breadth of the lesson and tie together the student objectives. And, perhaps as important as the assistance they lend to the instructor, lesson plans ensure continuity and consistency in instruction. So, even if multiple instructors are involved in an educational program, the lesson plan serves as the "common map" that guides the course instruction.

For the new instructor, or even the seasoned instructor, who is moving into a new content area, the lesson plan takes on increased importance. In such cases, the instructor will most likely not be the one developing the lesson plan. Standardized courses, such as Advanced Cardiac Life Support (ACLS), typically use lesson plans provided by the sponsoring agency. Institutions providing Emergency Medical Technician and paramedic education may produce standardized lesson plans for their program or institution. The availability of prepared lesson plans frees the instructor to concentrate on the instructional process and not on course and lesson development. Although advanced instructor-training programs teach ways to develop lesson plans, the knowledge and process awareness needed to develop plans may be beyond the scope of the typical Emergency Medical Services (EMS) instructor. However, even the rookie instructor should be familiar with the required components of a lesson plan, and should be able to evaluate a plan for completeness and appropriateness, and make modifications when necessary.

Purpose of a Lesson Plan

The lesson plan is truly a multipurpose tool. It serves a number of functions in the educational process, including the following:

- Ties all lesson objectives into a coherent plan of instruction
- Provides a structure or framework from which the lesson is presented
- Ensures that important material is covered and learning objectives are met

- Plans classroom time management to determine what content should be read outside of class by students and what content should be reviewed in class and how to reach application and synthesis
- Helps the instructor prepare to teach the lesson
- Matches declarative material with each objective
- Provides a basis for the development of student evaluative activities
- Serves as a means by which instructor performance can be evaluated
- Helps to keep the instruction on track and on schedule
- Assists substitute or secondary instructors and instructional assistants
- Provides consistency across multiple sections of a course
- Ensures adherence to institutional goals, objectives, and standards

Sources of Lesson Plans

Lesson plans are available from a variety of sources, ranging from the course instructor to outside agencies to textbook publishers. Some common sources of lesson plans include the following:

- *State EMS offices.* State agencies may develop lesson plans for EMS courses in their state.
- *Primary or senior instructors.* Instructors who have been teaching a course for some time most likely will have modified existing lesson plans or developed their own. These instructors may be adept at writing lesson plans, thus serving as a lesson development mentor for new instructors. However, instructor-modified lesson plans can be very personal and should be tailored to a particular instructor's style and preferences in teaching. Therefore, each instructor should carefully review and modify a lesson plan before it is used.
- *Lesson plans for nationally recognized courses are frequently obtained from publishers.* Publishers of textbooks often provide not only lesson plans, but also complete instructional support packages to supplement their texts. One must remember that these lesson plans and accompanying materials are designed for a wide audience and may be biased toward a particular product or approach. They often need modification and must frequently be tailored if they are to address local system issues. Instructors should avoid relying totally on these instructional packages; they must be sure to invest sufficient time in their own lesson preparation and delivery.

  Often, packaged lesson plans are prepared to meet minimal objectives. They may not incorporate higher learning objectives or include activities designed to synthesize information and encourage problem solving and critical thinking.

  The instructor should not assume that a packaged lesson plan addresses all of the education standards at the appropriate level. Instructors should conduct an analysis to determine whether the lesson includes the competencies, behaviors, and judgments essential to the standard. Instructors should consider customizing objectives by cross referencing with required standards and also list the standard number with the relevant objective. This may involve including activities that integrate information from early lessons to reinforce and build on earlier learning at each step of the program.
- *Several national organizations and groups produce specialty courses that cover a specific topic in detail.* Examples of these "alphabet soup" or "boutique" courses include Advanced Cardiac Life Support, Pediatric Advanced Life Support (PALS), and International Trauma Life Support (ITLS). Lesson plans provided for these courses vary in complexity. However, most are very basic and are designed to follow closely an accompanying PowerPoint presentation. Lessons are planned around a specific time frame and evaluation process. Because of the administrative control associated with many of these courses, instructor variation through tailoring of lesson plans is limited. Instructors must follow the lesson plans and schedule closely because they are often one of a cadre of instructors who have been assembled to teach such courses.
- *One of the activities of the National Association of EMS Educators (NAEMSE) is to prepare and disseminate model curricula on various topics.* Produced as packages for the instructor, these curricula contain lesson plans designed to be modified and customized by the EMS instructor.
- *Institutions and agencies such as fire departments and EMS services may produce their own lesson plans to ensure consistency and uniformity in instruction.* This is usually the case with in-house and procedural training courses, especially when instruction is scheduled to occur at various geographically separated locations. A trainer or central office staff may prepare lesson plans for distribution to instructors at various locations.

Teaching Tip >> *An instructor who is selecting lesson plans must make sure that the source is appropriate for the students. An instructor would not want to use a lesson plan on the cardiovascular system at the paramedic level to teach a citizen CPR course. Note that some commercial lesson plans have costs or restrictions associated with them. Proper permission to use a lesson plan must be obtained.*

Teaching Tip >> *Class time is precious! Consider assigning students to read the appropriate text chapter before class time and use class time more strategically. The instructor can spend time clarifying any complex content and then applying the content to patient situations.*

Parts of the Lesson Plan

As has been stated, lesson plans can come from numerous sources and may be written in a variety of formats. The instructor may have little control over how a lesson plan is constructed. However, most standard lesson plans consist of the following:

- Audience description
- Lesson goal(s)
- Cognitive objectives
- Psychomotor objectives
- Affective objectives
- Recommended list of equipment and supplies
- Recommended schedule
- Suggested motivational activity or anticipatory set
- Content outline and instructor notes
- Summary
- Evaluation
- Next assignment/lesson
- References

The format of lesson plans varies greatly according to the source. However, as a rule, most lesson plans include these listed parts in some form. If the selected lesson plan does not comprise all of these parts, missing sections should be added. If the instructor is inexperienced with curriculum development, he or she should seek help in preparing more complicated parts of the lesson plan.

Front End

The first few parts of the lesson plan comprise what can be called the "front end," which contains administrative details and information. This section should contain a title for the lesson or some other scheme by which the lesson can be identified and sequenced. Specific parts of the front end are as follows.

Audience Description

The audience description is just what the name implies. It is a statement describing who the intended audience is for the lesson. In a certification course, this description may be the same for all lesson plans. An example would be "Entry level EMT students." For a more advanced course, the description might be "Senior paramedic with command responsibility."

Lesson Goal

Course designers develop an instructional goal for the entire course, as well as a goal or goals for each particular lesson. This is presented as a broad statement of what will be accomplished during the lesson. For example, "At the conclusion of this lesson, the student will be able to identify and describe the functions of the endocrine system." The lesson objective is supported by the listed affective, cognitive, and psychomotor objectives that follow. The action verb used in the lesson goal determines, to a large extent, the instructional approach and corresponds to Bloom's taxonomy. (See Chapter 7: Domains of Learning, and Chapter 8: Goals and Objectives.) A goal that uses verbs such as "identify," "describe," and "discuss" will most likely be pursued through a lecture or presentation format. A goal that identifies "demonstrate" as the desired outcome behavior will be addressed as a practical session. The same applies to design of the evaluation method. Lesson goals that are predominantly cognitive will be assessed through paper tests, such as multiple choice and short answer. Psychomotor goals will be evaluated by methods such as observation or a skills check sheet.

Lesson Objectives

The lesson objectives portion of the lesson plan is a listing of student performance objectives that support the lesson goal. Objectives are categorized according to the three domains of learning: affective, cognitive, and psychomotor. Depending on the lesson plan format or the institutional preference, objectives may be assigned a numeric sequencing. This allows the objective to be referenced on tests and other course materials without the need for the instructor to write out the entire objective. Similar to the lesson goal, lesson objectives should be reviewed with students, so they know in greater detail what will be covered in the lesson. This is especially important for concrete and field-dependent learners.

Teaching Tip >> *Students should be given a complete list of objectives for each lesson of a course. That way, they know what material will be covered. Objectives also make a good study guide.*

Recommended List of Equipment and Supplies

Classroom success for the instructor is most often ensured by careful preparation. This preparation process includes reviewing the material, refreshing knowledge and skills, preparing the learning environment, and preparing instructional materials. The lesson plan contains a list of equipment and supplies needed for the lesson to be taught effectively **(Figure 9.1)**. This list may include such items as instructional models, audiovisual materials and equipment, handouts, student practice materials, and practical training equipment. This list is also useful at the completion of the lesson as a checklist to ensure that materials are accounted for and returned to their proper storage locations.

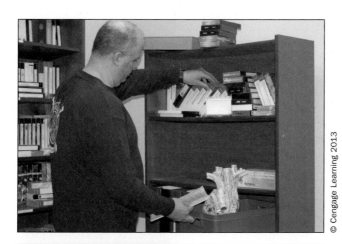

Figure 9.1

An equipment list is an important part of the lesson plan that should not be overlooked. Equipment should be kept updated and in working order.

Teaching Tip >> *Instructors should not forget to prepare the basic "tools of instruction," such as whiteboard markers, erasers, a laser pointer, and a podium.*

If any part of a lesson is going to fail, it most likely will be the part that is related to or dependent on equipment or technology. For this reason, the instructor should begin by becoming familiar with all material and aids to be used. Instructors should not assume that they know how something works. Instruction manuals are an excellent source of information and usually contain additional facts worth presenting to learners. Because of this, instructors should arrive well in advance of the class start time and should check and review all equipment. The instructor should not assume that because a particular audiovisual device or piece of equipment was in the classroom during the last session, it still is available. Also, instructors should know whom to contact if assistance is needed with equipment. The complexity and costs of current educational technology preclude replacement or repair by the average instructor.

The instructor must have a backup plan in the event of equipment failure or other such problems that can occur with technology-dependent lessons. The backup plan may involve alternative aids to accomplish the lesson, material to be presented, or an entirely different lesson to replace the intended one. The good instructor always has one or two lessons "in the can" in the event of an unforeseen problem.

Teaching Tip >> *If a planned lesson cannot be presented and no backup lesson is available, the instructor can always conduct skills practice or discuss patient scenarios. Even at the beginning of a course, the instructor can review prerequisite skills. He or she should never waste a lesson by canceling class. Practice and review are always needed.*

An area of concern in EMS education is the quality and amount of equipment available for training. Too often, outdated or broken equipment is relegated to training, or the amount of equipment is insufficient for active student participation. This sends a negative message about the service and its appreciation of training for the learner. It also violates basic educational principles in that learners are not receiving the most realistic experience during the learning process. Behavioral modeling may have as great an impact on learner development as what students are taught by the instructor. The lack of equipment identical to that used in the student's practice also requires that the provider must be trained again before he or she can begin functioning in the field setting. If he or she is participating in a field internship, the provider may become confused and frustrated because of differences in equipment and procedures between the classroom and the field site.

The use of realistic simulators has become common in EMS education. Although a very valuable teaching tool, the use of such simulators requires specialized training on the part of the instructor as well as proper set-up. Often, a dedicated simulation lab with assigned staff is used, requiring the instructor to arrange lab time in advance and to work with the lab staff to make sure the proper objectives and skills are covered. Again, preplanning for instruction becomes a critical concern for the instructor as well as a backup plan in the event of equipment failure or other unforeseen problems. (For more information on the use of simulation, see Chapter 18: Tools for Simulation.)

Teaching Tip >> *A lesson plan may be designed to "teach" a particular model or type of equipment. This is especially true of lesson plans provided by equipment manufacturers. The instructor must make sure that what he or she is teaching matches the equipment the students will be using for practice.*

If the instructor is teaching students who provide a mixture of services, he or she can ask students to provide an inventory of equipment available to them. In this way, the instructor can determine whether students will be using different or unusual equipment in the field. If the instructor does not have a specific piece of equipment in his or her training cache but students may benefit from instruction on it, he or she can make arrangements to borrow equipment from the service for a single class session.

Recommended Schedule

This is the estimated time needed for the instructor to teach the lesson. For a practical session, it may include a schedule for practice activities. If the number of learners in a class is variable, this section may list time frames in terms of a set number of participants. For example, each group of five students will require 20 minutes to cycle through the skills stations. The recommended schedule may include information on planned breaks.

Teaching Tip >> *As a rule of thumb, an instructor should plan three hours of preparation time for each hour of instruction.*

Suggested Motivational Activity

Learner motivation can vary greatly over the duration of a course. In the beginning, learners are often highly motivated in anticipation of the course. This is especially true for courses leading to a certification level. However, as the course progresses, motivation may wane. Even the most dynamic instructor would find it hard to keep paramedic students motivated after three weeks of cardiology. Thus, instructors must continually motivate learners at the beginning of each class session. Lesson motivation also serves to increase learner interest in the material of each individual lesson. Most importantly, it establishes the environment, or what is also called the "anticipatory set," in which learning occurs.

The suggested motivational activity should be designed to appeal to as many learner motivational needs as possible. It should serve to move the learner mentally from the external environment to the lesson. It should both peak and focus the learner's attention. Some motivational activities include the following:

- Show a picture and pause for reflection. The instructor may show a picture or a video clip related to the lesson topic and follow up by asking the learners how this picture affected them.
- Play a dispatch tape of an actual 911 call. The instructor may ask the learners whether they feel ready to respond to such a call.
- Tell a "war story" about a personal experience.
- Invite a survivor or former patient to address the class. Depending on the topic and the class length, this may not be practical for short lessons.
- Engage the students in an "icebreaker" activity that relates to the class topic.
- Invite a provider to tell about a significant experience that would be motivational to the learners.
- Administer a pretest (ideally with an audience response or classroom feedback system) to evaluate how much the students think they already know (or whether they have done the required reading).

Regardless of the technique used, instructors must be cautious of two things: patient confidentiality as required by the Health Insurance Portability and Accountability Act (HIPAA) guidelines, and overstimulation of learners to the point that a negative emotional response may be created. An example of the latter would be use of an event that may have emotional and personal ties to the learners.

Body of the Lesson Plan: Content Outline

The sections covered thus far form the front end of the lesson plan. Once the instructor and learners are prepared and motivated, it is time for the instructor to present the actual material that will allow learners to meet the lesson goal and objectives. To do this, the instructor must have a complete understanding of the lesson objectives and of the depth and breadth of material to be presented. Is material being presented for awareness or for **mastery**? This can be determined by the action verbs used in the course goal and objectives. Each domain of learning has a hierarchy that determines the required level of learning or mastery. The cognitive domain, for example, comprises six levels of mastery: knowledge, comprehension, application, analysis, synthesis, and evaluation. These six levels can be grouped into the following three levels of understanding:

1. *Basic.* The learner acquires new information or develops a new skill with instructor feedback. It includes objectives that demonstrate knowledge and comprehension (Level 1). This new information may be obtained by the learner on his or her own by reading the book. The instructor would need to verify students have learned this information without holding up classmates.
2. *Intermediate.* Learners connect the knowledge learned in the basic level with knowledge gained through experience. It includes objectives that demonstrate application (Level 2).
3. *Advanced.* Learners move toward learning why events occur as opposed to how to perform a skill. The instructor serves as a facilitator in a coaching or mentoring role. It includes objectives that require analysis, synthesis, and evaluation (Level 3).

Often, instructors or institutions assign a level code, similar to these for the cognitive domain, to each objective. This helps the instructor know which level of mastery is required for each objective.

Teaching Tip >> *The instructor should teach Level 1 material before Level 2 information is presented, and Level 2 before Level 3. Students should be evaluated for mastery before they are permitted to move on to the next level.*

Once the level of instruction is known for each lesson objective, an actual teaching outline is developed. Objectives are arranged and grouped in the order in which they will be taught. This teaching cycle is used to integrate affective, cognitive, and psychomotor objectives. The actual ordering of objectives can be based on a number of different schemes that will determine the order in which declarative material is presented. This will be the actual order of instruction during the class. It is important that the declarative material be presented in a coherent fashion that supports learner understanding and retention. Some examples of schemes include the following:

- Whole-part-whole
- Procedurally from beginning of a procedure to end
- Chronologically
- As specified in protocol
- Body or organ system based
- Simple to complex
- Small to large
- Algorithm based
- ABCs
- Head to toe
- Dispatch to return to service
- Known to unknown
- Following textbook content

However, in another way, a simple plan is to "tell 'em what you are going to teach 'em, teach 'em, and then tell 'em what you taught 'em." More specifically, explain the importance of the lesson, deliver the content, allow students to apply or practice the material, gather feedback, provide remediation, and evaluate performance. An easy way to do this is to open with a quick overview of lesson material and close with the same overview used as a summary.

The lesson plan developer has chosen a level of specificity for the content portion of the lesson plan. The specificity of the outline, that is, the number of levels used in the outline, varies according to the complexity of the material being presented and the instructor's teaching ability and familiarity with content. A primary instructor may simply need "B. Start IV" and be able to teach the entire process. A new instructor, however, will want the lesson broken down to list the various knowledge points and skills necessary to start an IV. The extent of the outline is really a matter of personal preference. However, a lesson plan that is developed for use by various instructors must be adaptable to various levels of instructor expertise; toward that goal, sufficient declarative material must be included. When one is teaching skills, it is especially important to provide sufficient detail to the learner. An experienced practitioner may be so comfortable doing a procedure that he or she may not realize the many small steps and nuances important to its successful completion; thus, he or she may not emphasize or share these with new learners. It is also good practice to include in the lesson outline formulas and drug names to ensure that they are properly presented to the new learner.

As shown in **Figure 9.2**, a good format for a lesson plan is the use of two facing pages with the right page divided into two sections. The left page contains the declarative material in outline form. The first column of the right page includes notes for the instructor. This format allows lesson plans to be easily personalized by different instructors. In the notes space, the instructor can include notes and comments that he or she wants to cover in class, additional information that may be needed to answer student questions, drawings to be written on the board, and questions and answers. If teaching formulas or problems, the instructor should include the solving methods and correct answers in this area. This format is especially helpful for new instructors who might become flustered or confused during a lecture. The far right column is used to list audiovisual aids, handouts, or activities that support the declarative material. Again, it is easy for even the experienced instructor to get off track and forget to use a teaching aid. This format also provides a complete and integrated lesson plan that can be used easily by substitute instructors.

Teaching Tip >> *An instructor can place the pages of his or her lesson plan in clear sheet protectors. This not only protects the pages, but it allows the instructor to write class-specific notes and comments on the page protectors with a transparency-marking pen. Notes can be wiped clear for use with another class. Additionally, other material such as instructions or protocols can be tucked between the sheets for easy access if needed during class.*

Back End

The remaining parts of the lesson plan constitute the back end, which contains sections that pull the lesson together, check student understanding, and prepare learners for the next lesson.

Lesson Plan Title

Audience:

Lesson Goal: *After completing this lesson, the student will be able to...*

Objectives:
Affective
Cognitive
Psychomotor

Equipment & Supplies:

Schedule:

Motivational Activity:

Lesson Content

Overview

Outline

Summary

Evaluation
Assignment
Next Session

Instructor Notes	References and Aids

Figure 9.2
Sample lesson plan.

Summary

Regardless of the format used or the complexity of the material presented, the instructor must provide closure to the lesson. Just as the motivational activity sets the stage for the lesson, the summary brings it together for closure. A simple summary involves using the overview that began the presentation of the declarative material. It is even possible for the motivational activity to be used again, if it is a simple one such as a picture or video clip; this allows students to appreciate the importance of the lesson material and relate it to reality.

Evaluation of Learning

To ensure that learning has taken place during a lesson, the instructor must evaluate learner mastery of the material. Various approaches may be used to conduct such an evaluation, and discussion of each is beyond the scope of this chapter. More information on this can be found in Part V: Student Evaluation. However, the instructor should specify in the lesson plan an evaluation method that will be used to determine learner mastery of the material presented. This may be as simple as a few questions asked at the conclusion of the lesson to gauge learner understanding, or student self-assessment undertaken to determine whether a particular objective has been mastered. **Classroom feedback** or **audience response systems** or mini whiteboards are a great way to obtain formative feedback throughout the lesson to determine whether students have "got it." Conducting scenarios that relate to the lesson is another way to see if they can integrate content and apply it in context. Or, it may take the form of an announcement that a 20-question, multiple-choice quiz on the material will be given at the beginning of the next session.

The evaluation section concludes the formal parts of a lesson plan. However, a few additions to the end of the lesson plan that may be helpful to the instructor and to the learners include assignments, the topic for the next session, related readings, and additional references. If the instructor has planned any "homework" for the learners, this can be assigned or distributed at this time. The next lesson topic serves as a reminder to the learners to prepare for the next session and reinforces any required readings or preparative assignments. The end of the lesson is also an opportunity for the instructor to announce any schedule changes and to remind students to bring special equipment, such as turnout gear, to the next session. Finally, the instructor can come to class prepared with a list of references, websites, or other sources that may be of interest to learners or that may provide greater detail or explanation of the material already presented. If learners have questions or concerns, they can be referred to this reference list.

Lesson Plan Evaluation

Once the institution or instructor has developed a lesson plan, the development process does not stop there. In addition to initial evaluation of its effectiveness, the lesson plan must be reviewed again periodically for timeliness, correctness, and applicability to the overall curriculum and learner needs.

If an instructor is teaching a new course with newly developed lesson plans, he or she may be involved more closely in the evaluation process. The initial evaluation process involves a formative evaluation that is ongoing and begins while the lesson plan is being constructed. The instructor should constantly compare the overall goals of instruction, lesson objectives, and content to determine whether performance is in agreement. Tests, audiovisual materials, student materials and activities, and reference materials should be evaluated as well for relevance to the instructional goal.

> **Teaching Tip** >> *It is handy for an instructor to have a pad of "sticky notes" while teaching. If an instructor finds a problem with a lesson plan or class, he or she can jot down a quick note and stick it on the lesson plan. This is also helpful if he or she needs to find additional material to answer a student's question, or for noting areas that need remediation.*

Even established and published lesson plans should be periodically evaluated throughout their life span. Often, lesson plans are produced according to a certain standard or medical protocol that may change over time. This can be seen in lesson plans that accompany ACLS, which change according to changes in American Heart Association (AHA) Guidelines. A summative evaluation of lesson plans is used to determine the effectiveness of the teaching strategy and to provide information on ways that future performance of the same strategy and related material can be improved. Again, tests, audiovisual materials, student materials, and reference materials should be evaluated as well.

Lesson Plan Troubleshooting

Regardless of who creates a lesson plan, or where it comes from, the potential for problems always exists. Problems usually fall into two broad categories: structural and factual.

CASE IN POINT

THE LAST-MINUTE LESSON PLAN

An instructor has just finished teaching a session of EMT to new hires at a commercial ambulance company. As she is walking back to her office, the director of training comes rushing up to her. She informs her that another instructor who teaches the company's paramedic course is tied up on a long critical care transport and will be at least an hour late for his class that starts in an hour. She asks the instructor to fill in for the absent instructor until he gets back. The instructor hesitates, then says okay. The instructor asks the director if she has a copy of the class lesson plan. The director says that she does not, but she is sure the other instructor has all his lesson plans in his office. The two walk to the instructor's office, and the director lets both of them in. To put it mildly, the other instructor is not the most organized person! Papers, books, teaching materials—everything is strewn about the office. The two cannot even find a place to begin looking for lesson plans. After a quick search, the instructor realizes it is hopeless and that time is getting short before class begins. She knows the lesson topic—obstructive pulmonary disease. At least that is the topic listed on the schedule the director had on file. What should she do to prepare for the lesson?

At this point, the fill-in instructor has two major problems. First, she does not know the instructor's plan for that night's class. Are the students expecting a quiz or another activity? She also does not know the level of the students, or which topic is scheduled to be covered. Are the students ahead of schedule? Or, are they behind schedule and not ready for this lecture? Her second concern is that her paramedic course lesson plans are at her home because she has been teaching only EMT classes.

What should the instructor do? To help her plan a class that is on schedule, the instructor can:

- Try to reach the absent instructor;
- Check to see if the training director's office or human resources department keeps copies of attendance rosters—these rosters may list the topics covered in each class session, or the training director may be able to provide a list of students and their contact information; someone can call students to find out what was planned;
- Go to the classroom or another nearby area early to try to intercept a student who is arriving early;
- Begin class by explaining the situation and finding out what was planned—she could work with the students to conduct a meaningful lesson, even if it is a review session of knowledge and skills taught previously;
- Give the students a brief assignment that they can complete on their own, and leave the classroom for 15 minutes to prepare a quick teaching outline.

Now that the instructor knows the content scheduled for the class, how can she teach without a lesson plan? She can do the following:

- Ask students if they have an outline for each course lesson. If not, do they have a list of objectives? Any handout materials?
- Use the textbook to create a "down and dirty" lesson plan. Use the chapter heading as the main point, subheadings as secondary points, and so forth. For each heading of the "outline," she can try to think of important facts or ideas to convey. She can jot down these ideas as they come to mind, then skim the text for key points. This approach usually works best if the instructor is familiar with the material and has taught it before. The "lesson plan" will not be extensive or eloquent, but it will provide a rough organizational framework.
- Use the same approach for class objectives. This is more difficult without textual material for elaboration. The same holds true if the instructor has access to a PowerPoint presentation on the lesson topic.
- Use the National Highway Traffic Safety Administration (NHTSA) website (www.ems.gov) to download appropriate parts of the online copy of the Paramedic Education Standards. Accompanying materials include instructional guidelines; however, care will need to be taken to identify new and updated information.
- Check the *Trading Post* on the NAEMSE website to see if a lesson plan or pictures are available.
- Depending on the topic, she can use her EMT lesson plan as a basis for instruction.

The take-home message from this case study is that many options are available by which instructors can quickly produce a basic lesson plan for an instructional crisis. The instructor must be creative and should be sure to be honest with students about "winging it" and needing their cooperation. Who knows? This lesson may turn out to be better than one that was developed with proper preparation time.

CASE IN POINT

LESSON PLAN DISCONNECT

An instructor has been assigned to teach a paramedic refresher course at the local hospital. The class is made up of experienced paramedics. The instructor is teaching the course because he must obtain instructor certification as a requirement for promotion to supervisor. For maintenance of standardization throughout the institution, he is required to teach from a lesson plan that has been developed and approved by the EMS training officer. While preparing to teach the unit on cardiac emergencies, he finds that the lesson plan contradicts current ACLS guidelines. He also notes that, although a protocol is in place for handling cardiac patients, he and most other paramedics in the hospital use a slightly "modified approach" rather than strictly adhering to the protocol. Because he knows his audience so well, he knows that they will give him a hard time if he tries to teach the material as outlined in the lesson plan. However, he does not want to "make waves" with the training officer because he is coming up for promotional review. What should he do?

This is a situation that involves dynamics beyond the scope of educational instruction. It is also a management issue. For the purposes of this chapter, the alternatives must be examined from an educational delivery perspective. In other words, how should the instructor handle this disconnect in the classroom? Possible approaches include the following:

- Teach the lesson directly as outlined in the lesson plan, and ignore any questions or criticism from the class. Such an approach would ruin credibility and could lead to loss of class control. This outcome would not make the instructor look like supervisor material.
- Present the material in the lesson plan and state that this is institutional policy. Then, ask the class if they have any other approaches to handling such situations. This should lead to discussion about how things are actually done in the field setting.
- Take a reverse approach to presenting the material. Give the class a scenario in which the responders treat the patient as is really done in the field setting, then ask them to contrast this with the institutional protocol.

An instructor can use these and similar strategies to handle disconnects between the lesson plan and textbooks, protocols, guest lecturers, or other instructors. Regardless of an instructor's approach, he or she should not use the instructor's podium as a "bully pulpit" to complain or attack others. If an instructor must address a controversy, he or she should present both sides of the argument impartially so that students can analyze the situation and come to their own conclusions.

Structural problems have to do with the delivery of the lesson material. When structural problems occur, the material to be presented in the lesson plan is correct and up to date, but something is wrong with the delivery of the material. Examples include using in a 3-hour session a lesson plan designed for a 2-hour block of instruction, or working alone to teach a skills lesson designed for a four-instructor team. In most cases, the instructor can remedy the problem by keeping the lesson material but rewriting the lesson plan into a more usable format. However, the instructor must be aware of how this lesson fits into the overall scope of the course so as not to disrupt future lessons. Shrinking a 4-hour lesson into a 2-hour session may be possible, but what are the consequences? If enrolled in a certification course, students may be required to have a minimum number of instructional hours in a topic, and this change could affect their eligibility for certification.

Structural problems can often be easily corrected if they are detected in advance of the lesson. However, factual and timeliness issues are more complex. First, the problem has to be discovered. Then, the instructor has to research to find the correct information and make changes as needed. This may seem straightforward, but a problem may arise with making changes. If a standardized curriculum is being used, the instructor may not be authorized to make changes. If the program is being taught with other instructors, or if the course is being taught in multiple sections, the lesson plan will have to be changed for *all* instructors. In addition, many programs require that the medical director approve all lesson plans—a requirement that adds another level to the process. To make matters more complex, some medical practices and procedures are not embraced by all medical professionals or groups. Such research must be verified and studied in greater detail. However, the instructor may find himself or herself standing in front of a class teaching the basics of a "traditional" CPR class that has just read in the local newspaper about a study advocating that mouth-to-mouth does not need to be performed.

Summary

The lesson plan is a valuable and essential tool of effective and successful EMS education. It provides the map that guides the learner through the educational journey. It also serves to tie together the instructional goal, the course objectives, and the teaching strategy. Moreover, it is a helpful tool that allows the instructor to present the course material in an organized and confident manner, thus ensuring learner success.

Glossary

audience response systems A system whereby the instructor receives feedback from the audience or class to specific, posed questions through an electronic device that tallies the responses.

classroom feedback systems See definition for audience response systems.

mastery Achieving goals and objectives established for a specific knowledge area.

Additional Resources

Gagné, R. M. (1974). *Essentials of learning for instruction.* Hinsdale, IL: The Dryden Press.

Gagné, R. M., & Briggs, L. J. (1979). *Principles of instructional design* (2nd ed.). New York, NY: Holt, Rinehart and Winston.

Mager, R. F. (1975). *Preparing instructional objectives* (2nd ed.). Belmont, CA: Fearon Publishers.

Mager, R. F., & Beach, K. M. Jr. (1967). *Developing vocational instruction.* Belmont, CA: Fearon-Pitman Publishers.

Mayer, R. E. (2011). *Applying the science of learning*. Boston, MA: Pearson.

Tyler, R. W. (1949). *Basic principles of curriculum and instruction.* Chicago, IL: University of Chicago Press.

10

Legal Issues for EMS Educators

No man is above the law and no man is below it; nor do we ask any man's permission when we require him to obey it. —Theodore Roosevelt

Since the enactment of the Highway Safety Act in 1966 (23 U.S.C. §§ 401 *et seq.* [2010]) and the formal beginning of EMS, the goal of EMS systems has been to reduce avoidable death and disability.[1] While this goal has remained constant, the public's expectations of emergency response may not necessarily reflect the reality of EMS.[2] The reality of 15,000 EMS systems, upwards of 800,000 EMS providers (emergency medical technicians, firefighters, first responders, law enforcement officers, paramedics, and other emergency services personnel), responding to more than 16 million transport calls annually is that the public's expectations for successful prehospital interventions are not always met.[3] The expectations for emergency care along with the likelihood of lawsuits have increased, as have the expectations of EMS students and the number of lawsuits filed by them. Those who deliver emergency care first must be properly trained. Those who teach emergency medical care must be knowledgeable of both the legal issues related to the delivery of patient care, and the legal issues associated with teaching.

This chapter is not provided as a substitute for legal advice or training. When legal questions arise, EMS educators should seek the service of competent attorneys with expertise in health law and educational law.

While many people consider America to be a litigious society, all citizens have a fundamental right to file meritorious lawsuits and seek the redress of their legitimate **grievances**. However, no one has the right to abuse the process by filing frivolous lawsuits, and attorneys are legally and ethically responsible for screening suits to make sure they have merit. Still, baseless lawsuits are not always preventable. The best way for EMS educators to avoid being sued is to have a sound understanding of basic legal concepts and terminology, and an appreciation for the facts and circumstances that caused others to be sued. Such an understanding begins with a brief overview of America's legal system.

CHAPTER GOAL: The goal of this chapter is to help course coordinators, EMS educators, and others involved in EMS education understand the basic legal issues associated with educating emergency medical providers and avoid the circumstances that give rise to lawsuits, as well as limit the potential for liability and damages should a suit be brought.

Hierarchy of Laws

In the American legal system, there are three levels of government: federal, state, and local. Each level of government is commonly made up of three branches: legislative, executive, and judicial. At their most basic level of functioning, the legislative branch creates the laws, the executive branch enforces the laws, and the judicial branch interprets the laws.

Congress is the federal government's legislative branch, and enacts laws called statutes. Each state has a legislative branch that can enact state statutes. Localities may adopt ordinances.

Within the executive branches of government, administrative agencies exist that are authorized to create regulations, which are methods of enforcing the law created by the legislative branches. The Occupational Safety and Health Administration (OSHA) is an example of a federal agency that develops regulations that affect EMS educational programs. Similarly, state EMS agencies generate regulations that govern EMS education and delivery in the state. Localities may elect officials or committees in order to effectuate ordinances.

The judicial branch of government interprets and applies laws in the context of cases. A court's ruling in a case can establish a particular interpretation or application of the law by setting a precedent, but precedent may evolve over time as courts continue to interpret the meaning of laws.

Generally speaking, there are four primary sources of law:

1. Constitutions (federal and state) and charters (local)
2. Statutes (federal and state laws) and ordinances (local government laws)
3. Regulations (laws created by federal, state, and local government agencies)
4. Common law and case law (precedent)

The U.S. Constitution is the supreme law in the United States. State constitutions represent the highest law in each state, subject only to the U.S. Constitution. No law may supersede or contradict the U.S. Constitution, not even international law.

The judicial branch, from local courts up through the U.S. Supreme Court, is responsible, among other things, for ensuring that all laws and governmental actions are compliant with the U.S. Constitution.

Areas of Law

The American legal system can be divided into two broad categories: criminal law and civil law. Criminal law refers to public wrongs, or crimes that violate laws at the state or federal level. Criminal cases are prosecuted by an attorney for the government on behalf of the citizens, such as a district attorney, state's attorney, or attorney general. Violation of criminal laws can result in fines, imprisonment, or both, among other sanctions.

Civil law involves private matters (e.g., contracts, business transactions, wills, and domestic relations, among other types of actions) between persons or legal entities such as corporations. In civil cases, the injured party (called a plaintiff) seeks recovery of money or other forms of relief for an alleged act or omission. This claim is made against another person or entity (called a defendant). A defendant who claims to have been injured by a plaintiff may also file a counterclaim against the plaintiff as part of the same lawsuit. In other types of civil cases, the parties may seek the court's assistance in determining their rights, without necessarily alleging any wrongdoing, such as in a suit to determine the wrongfulness of an injury or death.

Tort Law

A **tort** is a private or civil wrong or injury, other than a breach of contract, for which the law allows a remedy. It is an act committed by one party, in either an intentional or negligent manner, against another party that causes personal injury or property damage. A claim of medical negligence, or professional malpractice, is a tort action, as are **assault**, **battery**, **defamation**, and **misrepresentation**, among many others.

Teaching Tip >> *EMS educators should be alert to high-risk activities in the classroom, lab, clinical setting, or field that could result in a tort claim. For example, special precautions or safeguards should be in place when students are lifting and moving live patients on backboards. Spotters, lab instructors, or safety officers should be in place to observe for proper techniques and focus on safety issues.*

Assault and Battery

Although assault and battery are frequently discussed in combination as if they were a single phenomenon, they are actually separate torts. An assault occurs when one person places another person in reasonable fear of immediate harm or physical contact. For example, if a student raises his fist in a menacing manner toward an instructor as if about to strike the instructor, causing the instructor fear of being struck, the student has assaulted the instructor. Verbal assault occurs when a person states the intent to harm another person. Nonverbal assault occurs when a person creates an atmosphere of intimidation, such as when brandishing a weapon or advancing toward another person.

Battery is the physical, unlawful touching of another person without consent. It is important to ensure students understand that even well-intentioned treatment can later be the subject of a battery claim. For example, some religions forbid the use of blood transfusions, and doing so on a patient of that persuasion may constitute battery if no defenses are available. However, instructors must also be aware that any physical contact they may have with a student that is not consented to could give rise to a claim for battery.

Consent is a defense to any claim for assault or battery. It is always advisable to obtain a person's consent prior to making physical contact with them. This includes when making physical contact with a student for demonstration purposes in a classroom setting. Students must be taught when and how to obtain consent to treat patients, even in an emergency situation, and even in some situations when the patient may be unconscious.

Defamation

Defamation can be the intentional or reckless making of a false statement, or the sharing of true, but private, information that injures the reputation of another. Libel is the written or printed form of defamation. Slander is the spoken or oral form of defamation. Truth is one potential defense to a claim of defamation; it is, however, not a defense when private, sensitive information is willingly shared without permission.

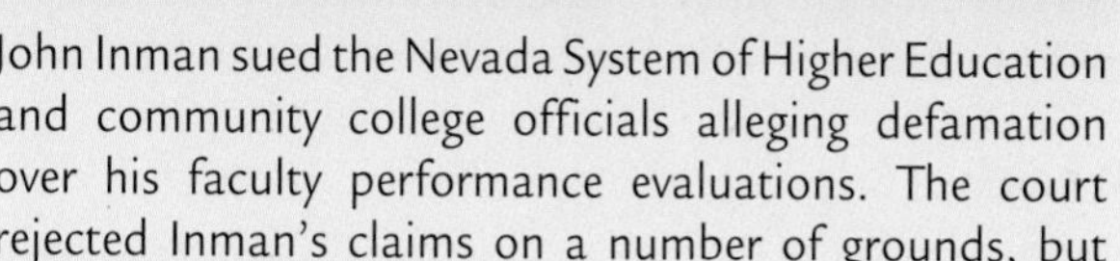

John Inman sued the Nevada System of Higher Education and community college officials alleging defamation over his faculty performance evaluations. The court rejected Inman's claims on a number of grounds, but most importantly because the evaluations contained statements of opinion and not fact. As such they could not be false.

Inman v. Thawley, 297 Fed.Appx. 683 (U.S. Circuit Court of Appeals for the 9th Circuit 2008) (unpublished).

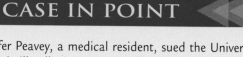

CASE IN POINT 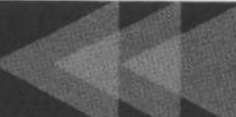

Jennifer Peavey, a medical resident, sued the University of Louisville alleging, among other claims, that her supervisors' statements to the Federation of State Medical Boards regarding her eccentricity constituted defamation. The court found that the defendant was not liable because its opinion was based on truth, namely that: 1) Peavey telephoned a hospital executive at home and inquired about a nurse who had been fired; 2) Peavey discussed the nurse's termination at work with other nurses; 3) Peavey's supervisors were contacted and told she was difficult to work with; 4) Peavey told a hospice patient that he could stay in the hospital for six months; 5) Peavey was not able to accept feedback or constructive criticism from her supervisors and the University's professors, all of which tended to prove she displayed eccentric behavior. This, in conjunction with other academic shortfalls, resulted in Peavey's dismissal from the program, which was upheld by the court.

Peavey v. University of Louisville, 2011 U.S. Dist. LEXIS 75786 (U.S. District Court for the Western District of Kentucky, Louisville Division 2011).

Misrepresentation

Misrepresentation is the making of a false statement with intent to deceive, that causes actual harm to someone who reasonably relies upon it. It is a polite way of saying "**fraud**." In education, misrepresentation could occur when marketing material for a program indicates that it is something other than what it is. For instance, if a marketing brochure indicates that a program is accredited by certain organizations, when it is not, someone who attends the class may have a cause of action for misrepresentation. An emerging trend in lawsuits against schools focuses on schools' misrepresentations on the number of students who are employed upon graduation, whether those students are employed within their fields of study, and the salaries of graduates.

Negligence

Negligence is the failure to exercise the care that a reasonably prudent person would have exercised in a similar situation that causes damages to another. In our everyday lives, we are all held responsible to act as the fictional reasonably prudent person would act under similar circumstances. This applies when we are driving our cars, cooking a meal, or engaging in normal activities.

However, people who have specialized skills and training, such as doctors, nurses, paramedics, and EMTs, are held to a higher standard of care when acting in their respective professional capacities. A professional is held to the standard of care that the reasonably prudent professional of like skill and training would exercise under like circumstances. As such, a paramedic is held to the standard of the reasonably prudent paramedic, and an EMT is held to the standard of the reasonably prudent EMT.

Negligence claims must establish four elements:

1. A legal duty
2. Breach of the requisite standard of care
3. Injury or damages
4. The resulting injury or damage was caused by the breach of the standard of care

A claim of medical negligence brought against EMS would likely be brought in conjunction with a claim for professional malpractice; the elements are the same, with the caveat that the EMS defendant is a professional held to the higher standard of care exercised by other similar professionals under like circumstances. In many states, expert testimony is required in order to establish that the elements of professional malpractice have been met. In such states, a suit based on the negligence of a professional cannot legally be successful without the testimony of an expert. In some states, the suit may not even be filed without an expert's certification that the suit has merit. This is because a baseless accusation of professional negligence has serious repercussions against the professional's career and reputation; in some instances the professional could even countersue the plaintiff for defamation. *Experts* are generally defined as persons who, through education or experience, have developed skill or knowledge in a particular subject, so that they may form an opinion that will assist the judge or jury in assessing a dispute.

CASE IN POINT

In this hypothetical case, Able is teaching a class on patient lifts and carries. A student, Baker, is asked to serve as a patient and is seated on a stair chair as two other students attempt to carry him down a flight of stairs. Able does not instruct the students to secure patients to the chair using the attached straps, and in fact observes the students lift Baker and start to carry him with the straps dangling. One of the students steps on a strap, causing Baker to fall and injure his back and neck.

An analysis of these facts follows in light of the elements of negligence:

1. Able, as an EMS instructor, has a legal duty to his students to exercise reasonable care.
2. Able very likely breached the standard of care by (a) failing to properly train his students before allowing them to engage in a dangerous activity, and (b) failing to stop the students from engaging in a dangerous activity even though he observed an obvious safety risk. It would be up to a jury to determine what the reasonably prudent EMS instructor would have done, and if Able's conduct met or failed to meet that standard. The jury would be instructed to compare Able's conduct to that of other EMS instructors in like circumstances.
3. Baker was injured.
4. Able's breach of the standard of care caused the injuries to Baker.

Duty

The first element of any negligence claim, legal duty, is usually undisputed in actions against EMS providers because the duty exists by virtue of the providers being on the job and responding to a call for emergency assistance. However, duty to act is actually a challenging area of the law. Duty to act often becomes an issue for off-duty personnel who come upon an injured person.

As a general rule in the United States, no one has a legal duty to come to the aid of another person, absent some special relationship. Relationships that create a duty to act include parent to child, spouse to spouse, and teacher to student. Thus a teacher would have a legal duty to come to the aid of a student who is stricken or injured during a class. A teacher would also have a legal duty to take reasonable precaution to protect students from foreseeable, preventable harm.

Breach

The second element of a negligence claim, breach of the standard of care, asks what a reasonably prudent person, or professional, would have done in the same or similar situation.

Teaching Tip >> *EMS educators have an affirmative legal duty to take reasonable protections to protect students from foreseeable, preventable harm.*

Evidence of the applicable standard of care may come from any of the following sources, among others:

- Expert witnesses
- Authoritative books
- Industry wide standards
- EMS agency operating procedures, policies, and rules
- Federal and state laws
- State and local protocols for emergencies
- U.S. Department of Transportation's educational standards

The term "standard of care" is commonly used in two different senses. In one sense, it refers to prevailing or routine practice patterns; in another sense, it refers to what is regarded as best practice in view of current knowledge of emergency medicine and expert opinion. In any event, the totality of the circumstances is always taken into consideration. For example, EMS responders likely would not be required to place themselves in danger in order to care for a trauma victim, even if that meant the victim's injuries would worsen without immediate treatment.

Injury

The third element of negligence, injury or damages, is required in order to pursue a claim of negligence. A breach of the standard of care that does not produce appreciable injury or damages, will not give rise to a negligence claim. Some states do not allow recovery for injuries that are purely psychological, such as emotional distress, in the absence of some physical symptom. In some cases, damages may not be allowed for a purely economical loss.

Causation

The final element of negligence, causation, requires that the negligent act or omission be the legal cause of the damages or injuries to the plaintiff.

A lack of causation is often raised as a defense in negligence cases. For example, just because a patient dies en route does not mean that EMS committed negligence, or that the death was the result of a careless act or failure to act. One common causation defense to a medical negligence or professional malpractice claim is to assert that even if treatment was performed perfectly by the book, the patient still would have died. Another common causation defense is to assert that there are two or more acceptable ways to treat a certain medical condition, and that it was reasonable for the provider to choose one course of treatment over the other. Still another common defense is to assert that the patient contributed to the negative outcome, such as by ignoring the provider's advice, as discussed in the following section.

Defenses to Negligence

There are three common defenses to negligence claims:

1. Assumption of risk
2. Release of risk
3. Contributory or comparative negligence

Assumption of Risk

The assumption-of-risk doctrine generally indicates that individuals who willingly participate in an activity known to involve risk (such as EMS clinical education) cannot recover damages resulting from injury due to the materialization of risks generally associated with that activity. It cannot, however, always be assumed that individuals have accepted the inherent risks involved in a particular activity.

Release of Risk

Educational institutions frequently require students (or parents/guardians) to sign release or waiver-of-risk forms. This is done to establish the assumption-of-risk doctrine. The signed release form is evidence that the student was aware of, and assumed, the risk involved with the activity.

EMS educators should be cautious in the creation of release-of-risk and waiver-of-risk forms. These forms should be clearly written and in compliance with federal and state laws. Minors may be considered by the courts to be owed a greater duty of care than adult students, and in addition may not be legally able to sign a waiver for themselves. It is vitally important that legal counsel review any proposed release and waiver forms before they are used by an EMS educator. An EMS educator must never simply take another organization's release or waiver and adapt it for his or her own needs.

Contributory or Comparative Negligence

Up to this point we have focused on liability concerns when one person was totally at fault for another person's injuries. What happens if the victims themselves bore some responsibility for their own injuries? This is known as "contributory negligence."

Contributory negligence was a legal theory in many states, stating that individuals cannot recover for an injury if they, themselves, were negligent. If there was contributory negligence, individuals were completely barred from any recovery if the injury suffered was even only partly their fault.

Today, nearly all states have abandoned contributory negligence in favor of a doctrine known as "comparative negligence." Under comparative negligence, an individual's damages are reduced in proportion to their degree of fault in causing their own injury. For example, if an individual was found to be 30 percent at fault for an injury, their award of damages would be reduced by 30 percent.

Let us consider an example in a classroom setting: A and B are engaged in horseplay that results in severe injuries to B. If a jury determines that each was 50 percent responsible for the injuries, then B could only recover 50 percent of her damages from A. If we take this same scenario a bit further, suppose B sues A and the EMS instructor claiming the instructor's negligent supervision played a role in her injuries. The jury could find that A, B, and the instructor were liable and apportion fault accordingly, keeping in mind that if B was partially at fault, B cannot recover 100 percent of damages from A and the instructor.

Risk Management

Risk management is the process of preventing, or at least minimizing, harm or loss to a business, organization, or person. The discussion of risk management fits into this discussion of tort law because by following sound risk-management principles, liability exposure can be reduced.

While reducing liability is an important consideration in risk management, there is also a more important factor: safety. Risk-management steps taken to prevent lawsuits and liability have the additional advantage of enhancing safety.

Consider the risk-management value of a driver-training program. By training drivers to a standardized curriculum, liability exposure to the organization is reduced. In the event of a lawsuit stemming from a vehicle collision, it can be proven that all drivers have met a minimum level of training and competence, which may prove valuable in limiting liability and monetary damages against the educational institution. But just as importantly, the workplace is made safer by ensuring drivers are better trained and less likely to get into a preventable collision.

Whenever an injury occurs, the victim may likely attempt to place blame and seek compensation. Risk management helps to focus EMS educators on preventing such injuries from occurring, and mitigating the liability costs associated with injuries when they do occur.

Methods of Risk Management

There are two principal methods of risk management that EMS educators should consider. The first method, risk control, is the process of reducing the rate and intensity of potential harm. This is a preventive process in which safety methods are employed to modify potential activities or equipment that could lead to institutional or personal liability. The second method of risk management is risk transfer. Waivers, releases, and insurance policies are all forms of risk transfer.

EMS educators should be actively involved in risk management in their classrooms and clinical-education settings. Based on the very nature of the EMS profession itself, safety is of critical importance. Safety education should be an initial component of any EMS curriculum. Safety tests should be given to students, and a high level of success should be required to continue in the program. The results of safety exams should remain on file with the educational institution. Record keeping is critical for establishing a strong defense against litigation when the institution is sued under a vicarious liability theory. Two examples of high-risk, high-frequency activities that warrant risk-management attention by EMS educators are stretcher handling and sharps handling.

Student Supervision

There are no laws that directly govern the supervision of students while engaged in classroom, laboratory, hospital or field work. EMS educators must therefore be guided by considerations of what the reasonably prudent educator of like skill and training would be expected to do under similar circumstances.

EMS educators should adhere to all applicable institutional or state policies. Educators should consider students' level of maturity, safety education, and type of activity before leaving students unsupervised.

EMS educators should be alert for a student who may have mental health or behavioral problems that are not properly controlled and that may affect the student's ability to competently and effectively perform EMS tasks. In such a situation, the EMS educator should follow the school's protocol when documenting their observations and referring the student to mental health assistance, keeping in mind the student's right to privacy.

For classes that are not affiliated with an educational institution, the EMS educator should seek assistance from the sponsoring agency.

Emergency Protocol Procedures

It is doubtful that anyone is more familiar with the value of emergency protocol procedures than EMS educators. Educators should be familiar with emergency procedures at each teaching venue, and be able to implement them quickly and properly. This includes how to summon help, the address of the venue, and the location of available implements such as defibrillators.

Hazardous Events in Clinical Education Whenever students are placed at risk in an educational situation, special care should be taken by EMS educators. Students are owed a duty of protection from reasonably foreseeable dangers that are known to exist in their assignments. Programs that require students to drive emergency vehicles should be particularly cautious given the high-risk nature of operating emergency vehicles. Other areas of concern include exposure to infectious diseases and helicopter transports.

Blood-borne Pathogens and Infectious Diseases EMS personnel are at occupational risk of exposure to blood and other bodily fluids that might contain hepatitis B virus, hepatitis C virus, or human immunodeficiency virus (HIV), among other infectious diseases.

Students should be fully trained in infection control as required by OSHA regulations before being potentially exposed to blood-borne pathogens and infectious agents. EMS educators should also ensure that students are provided with, and are required to use, appropriate protective barriers (such as gloves, gowns, aprons, masks, or protective eyewear) during time spent in labs, hospitals, or ambulances.

Training records should document that students have been trained in proper procedures and counseling should be documented when deviations occur.

Teaching Tip >> *EMS educators should require students to employ standard precautions when exposed to blood, other bodily fluids containing visible blood, semen, and vaginal secretions, as well as to tissues and cerebrospinal, synovial, pleural, peritoneal, pericardial, and amniotic fluids, as advised by the Center for Disease Control and Prevention (CDC). This includes exposures during lab work in addition to field work.*

All occupational exposures should be considered urgent medical concerns to ensure timely management and administration of postexposure prophylaxis. Students should be given a written, easily accessible policy concerning what to do once they have an exposure and to whom they should report. Hospital and field personnel should also be clear about the process to follow for their students. In addition, consultation with local experts and the National Clinicians' Postexposure Prophylaxis Hotline (1-888-448-4911) is advised.

Helicopter Emergency Medical Service (HEMS) Flights

HEMS flights carry certain inescapable risks, causing many EMS educators to question the advisability of unnecessarily exposing students to this activity during their clinical education **(Figure 10.1)**. The risks versus benefits of such training must be evaluated by each educational program.[4] Because HEMS flights are inherently dangerous,[5] EMS educators might consider restricting students to accompanying patients on flights to emergency care institutions only in situations where other methods of EMS transportation are impractical, if not impossible.[6]

Site Selection

EMS educators should be cognizant of inherent dangers when selecting educational sites for clinical

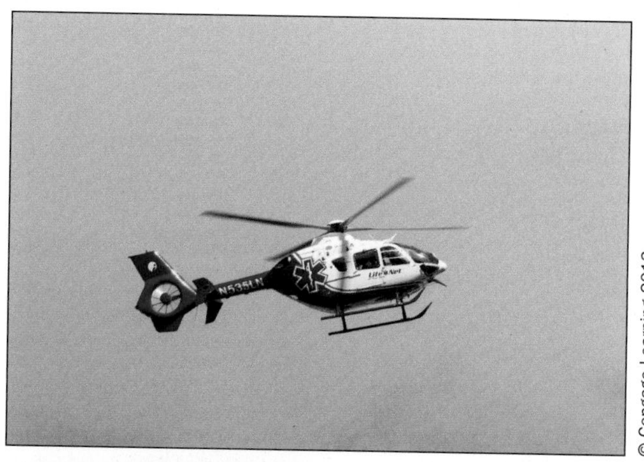

Figure 10.1

Helicopter EMS flights are inherently dangerous and educators should carefully consider alternatives prior to assigning students to this activity.

affiliations. Although no guarantee may be made to ensure students' safety as they complete clinical rotations, educators should be aware of potential risks based on site selection, such as where reductions in EMS services leave insufficiently trained or supervised staff to provide proper student supervision.

Civil Rights and Nondiscrimination Laws

The U.S. Constitution, federal laws, and state laws prohibit discrimination in a variety of settings, including the work place, public spaces, and educational institutions. EMS educators should be familiar with the ethical, legal, and practical considerations of discrimination and civil rights laws, and in particular with the specific applications of these laws to their classroom and clinical programs.

Teaching Tip >> *EMS educators must ensure students understand their obligation to promote universal respect for, and observance of, all human rights and freedoms without distinction as to disability, language, race, gender, or religion. The best way to do this is by consistently modeling the appropriate behavior. Educators must also be mindful that as role models they cannot condone others who demonstrate a lack of respect for the rights of others in their classrooms. An instructor who observes discriminating behavior in the classroom and does not stop it, condones it.*

Federal Constitutional Protections

The U.S. Constitution prohibits any level of government from violating the constitutional rights of individuals. Congress has enacted a law, 42 U.S.C.A. § 1983, that allows persons to sue a governmental actor who violates their constitutional rights. EMS educational institutions and instructors may be considered governmental actors if they receive government funding or are contracted by the government; other factors may also be considered in determining whether EMS educators or students are acting under the color of the law.

To the extent that EMS educators and fellow students are governmental actors, they can be sued in their individual capacities for violating constitutional rights of others. While aggrieved individuals face significant obstacles to successful litigation, constitutional mandates serve as an important guide for EMS educators and discrimination lawsuit victories do occur.[7]

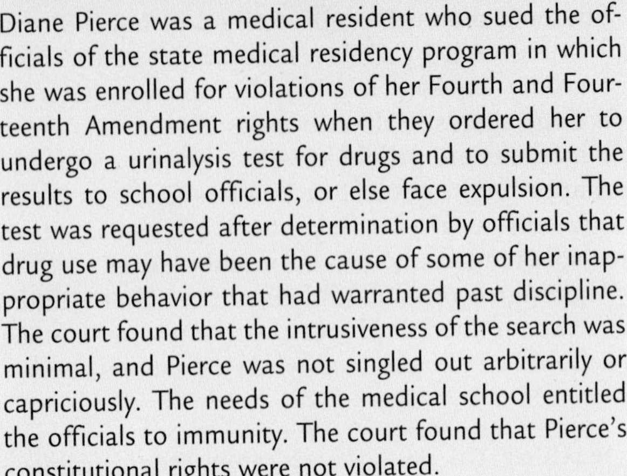

CASE IN POINT

Diane Pierce was a medical resident who sued the officials of the state medical residency program in which she was enrolled for violations of her Fourth and Fourteenth Amendment rights when they ordered her to undergo a urinalysis test for drugs and to submit the results to school officials, or else face expulsion. The test was requested after determination by officials that drug use may have been the cause of some of her inappropriate behavior that had warranted past discipline. The court found that the intrusiveness of the search was minimal, and Pierce was not singled out arbitrarily or capriciously. The needs of the medical school entitled the officials to immunity. The court found that Pierce's constitutional rights were not violated.

Pierce v. Smith, Binder, and Texas Tech University Health Science Center, 117 F.3d 866 (U.S. Court of Appeals for the 5th Circuit 1997).

Search and Seizure Clause of the Fourth Amendment

The Fourth Amendment provides that individuals have the right to be free against unreasonable searches and seizures by the government (U.S. Constitution Amendment IV). Generally, the treatment and transportation of patients is not considered custody for purposes of the Fourth Amendment (*Jackson v. Schultz,* 429 F.3d 586 [U.S. Circuit Court of Appeals for the 6th Circuit 2005]). However, Fourth Amendment violations may arise when EMS providers acting in a governmental capacity restrain patients in order to effectively administer medical attention.

Search and seizure laws commonly come up in an educational context with regard to locker searches. The Fourth Amendment's protection against unreasonable searches and seizures applies to any location where a person has a "reasonable expectation of privacy." Courts have found that students and employees may enjoy a reasonable expectation of privacy in locations such as lockers, desks, backpacks, and briefcases.

What can an EMS educator do if informed by a student that another student has illegal drugs in their locker? Would it matter if it was a handgun?

Governmental institutions and agencies are well advised to address these concerns proactively by adopting policies that inform employees and students that they have no expectation of privacy in locations such as a locker. Such a policy should clearly indicate that the entity reserves the right to search areas such as lockers at any time. The existence of a well-written and well-known policy thereby shapes and alters the expectation of privacy that employees and students may reasonably have.

Due Process and Equal Protection Clauses of the Fourteenth Amendment

The Equal Protection Clause of the Fourteenth Amendment provides that people have the right to equal protection of the laws, while the Due Process Clause provides that no person can be deprived of their "life, liberty, or property, without due process of law" (U.S. Constitution Amendment XIV § 1).

Federal Nondiscrimination Laws

While the U.S. Constitution prohibits government from violating the civil rights of individuals, Congress has gone a step further by enacting federal laws that prohibit various types of discrimination. Although this list is not all-encompassing, these five federal nondiscrimination laws impact educational institutions and EMS educational programs:

- Americans with Disabilities Act of 1990, 42 U.S.C.A. §§ 12101 *et seq.* (2009)
- Title VI of the Civil Rights Act of 1964, 42 U.S.C.A. § 2000d0200d-7 (1986)

CASE IN POINT

Horowitz, a student at the University of Missouri–Kansas City Medical School, was dismissed by school officials for failure to meet academic standards. She sued, alleging that officials had not accorded her due procedural process prior to her dismissal. The reasons Horowitz was dismissed included erratic attendance and a lack of concern for personal hygiene. For these she was put on probation, and while on probation, she received unsatisfactory ratings for her clinical performance. The U.S. Supreme Court found that the school had not deprived her of a liberty or property interest, that she had been informed of the school's dissatisfaction with her progress, and the decision to dismiss her was careful and deliberate, all of which was sufficient under the Due Process Clause of the Fourteenth Amendment. The Court found that less stringent procedural requirements are necessary when a student is dismissed for academic reasons than when a student is dismissed for violation of valid rules of conduct. Moreover, academic due process is less formal than judicial due process and does not always require a hearing.

Board of Curators of the University of Missouri et al. v. Horowitz, 435 U.S. 78 (U.S. Supreme Court 1978).

- Equal Employment Opportunity Act of 1972, 42 U.S.C.A. §§ 2000e *et seq.* (1991)
- Pregnancy Discrimination Act of 1978, 42 U.S.C.A. § 2000e(k) (1991)
- Title IX of the Education Amendments of 1972, 20 U.S.C.A. § 1681 *et seq.* (1990)

Americans with Disabilities Act (ADA) of 1990 and the Rehabilitation Act of 1973

The ADA was enacted in 1990. Before that time, the key piece of legislation addressing persons with disabilities was Section 504 of the Rehabilitation Act (29 U.S.C.A. § 794 [2002]). Both Section 504 and the ADA prohibit disability-based discrimination. The ADA states, "No covered entity shall discriminate against a qualified individual on the basis of disability in regard to job application procedures, the hiring, advancement, or discharge of employees, employee compensation, job training and other terms, conditions, and privileges of employment." (42 U.S.C.A. § 12112 [2009]). Several terms with which EMS educators and students should be familiar are defined in **Table 10.1**.

Table 10.1 Americans with Disabilities Act (42 U.S.C. §§ 12101-12213) Terminology

Term	Definition	Comments
Qualified individual with a disability	Any individual with a disability who, with or without reasonable accommodation, can perform the essential functions of the employment position that he or she holds or desires . . .	The term "handicapped" has been replaced by "disability," which is the politically correct term to use. Alcohol and illegal drug abuse do not qualify.
Reasonable accommodation	Making existing facilities used by employees readily accessible to and usable by individuals with disabilities; job restructuring, part-time/modified work schedules; acquisition or modification of equipment or devices; appropriate adjustment or modifications of examinations, training materials, or policies; provision of qualified readers or interpreters, and other similar accommodations . . .	An interactive process involving the EMS educational institution representatives and the disabled student determines student accommodations to be provided.
Undue hardship	Nature and cost of accommodations; overall financial resources of the facility, etc.	Financial burden may be respected in light of establishing undue hardship for the educational facility.
Major life activities	Functions such as caring for oneself, performing manual tasks, walking, seeing, hearing, speaking, breathing, learning, and working . . .	To qualify for disabilities, individuals must have substantially limited activity or activities . . .
Substantially limited	Unable to perform a major life activity that the average person in the general population can perform . . .	Factors to consider in determining whether an individual is substantially limited include nature and severity of impairment, duration of impairment, and permanent or long-term impact of impairment.

Teaching Tip >> *It is important for EMS educators to understand that the ADA and Rehabilitation Act establish a dual mandate of nondiscrimination and accommodation. These laws not only prohibit discrimination, but also mandate that affirmative steps be taken to accommodate the needs of individuals with disabilities.*

This dual commitment is particularly important in the context of situations where students with special needs may require certain accommodations in order to fulfill their educational requirements.

Mentally and physically challenged students face many hurdles when seeking to establish a *prima facie* ADA case in which their evidence is strong enough to create a presumption that a disability exists. To prevail in any litigation, students must be able to demonstrate the following:

- They are disabled within the meaning of the ADA.
- They are otherwise qualified to perform the essential functions of a job or educational activity with or without reasonable accommodations.
- They suffered an adverse decision with regards to education due to the disability.

See 42 U.S.C.A. § 12112 (2009).[8]

While disabilities are interpreted in a broad and inclusive manner, students with alcohol and illegal drug abuse problems are not considered disabled under the ADA (42 U.S.C.A. § 12114 [2009]). Otherwise, the definition of disability under the ADA is construed in favor of the broadest coverage (42 U.S.C.A. § 12102[4][A] [2009]).

CASE IN POINT

ZsaZsa Millington, a third-year student, sued Temple University alleging discrimination under the ADA. Millington was given numerous accommodations but was ultimately dismissed from the university. The courts held in favor of the university since Millington was dismissed based on poor academic performance, which occurred before and after the alleged onset of her disabilities. Moreover, the university was not required to approve requests for accommodation, which would fundamentally alter its academic program.

Millington v. Temple University School of Dentistry, 261 Fed.Appx. 363 (U.S. Circuit Court of Appeals for the 3rd Circuit 2008), cert. denied, 129 S.Ct. 419 (U.S. Supreme Court 2008).

The National Registry of Emergency Medical Technicians offers reasonable and appropriate accommodations for the written component of the registration examination for persons with documented disabilities. Persons who present documentation of a learning disability in reading, decoding, reading comprehension, and/or written expression are permitted to take the standard format of the examination but receive an extended time in which to complete the exam.

Title VI of the Civil Rights Act of 1964

Whereas the ADA and Rehabilitation Act protect individuals with disabilities from discrimination, Title VI of the Civil Rights Act prohibits discrimination based on race, color, or national origin by any program receiving federal funding. The law prohibits educational institutions and EMS educational programs that receive federal funds from engaging in discrimination on the basis of race, color, or national origin.

Equal Employment Opportunity Act of 1972

Under Title VII of the Civil Rights Act (42 U.S.C.A. §§ 2000e *et seq.* [1991]), it is illegal to discriminate in the hiring or terminating of employees, or in any other act of employment, such as in EMS educational programs, based upon age, race, color, religion, sex, or national origin. Students, as well as applicants to an EMS program, are afforded the same rights as employees **(Figure 10.2).**

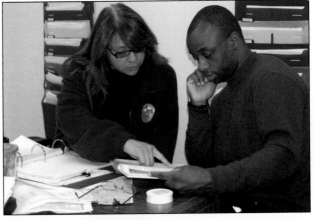

Figure 10.2

EMS education is enriched by diversity, and EMS instructors should be clear about providing the same opportunities to all without bias based on age, race, color, religion, sex or national origin.

Pregnancy Discrimination Act of 1978

Pregnancy discrimination has been a longstanding problem. What makes it particularly challenging is that some well-intentioned efforts to "protect" pregnant women, have the "effect" of discriminating.

Pregnant women cannot be categorically excluded or restricted from work or training programs based upon their pregnancy. The Pregnancy Discrimination Act (42 U.S.C.A. § 2000e[k] [1991]) requires educational institutions and EMS educational programs to provide to pregnant women the same accommodations they provide for other temporarily disabled workers with similar levels of incapacity.

Teaching Tip >> *Educators should be aware that female students who become pregnant during their EMS education may need to delay some educational experiences (hospital or field) if recommended by the individual's physician. The ultimate decision rests with the student and her doctor, not the educator. Educators may wish to include special provisions addressing pregnancy in release and waiver forms.*

Title IX of the Education Amendments Act of 1972

Title IX of the Education Amendments Act provides that individuals may not be excluded from participation in, be denied the benefits of, or be subjected to discrimination by any educational institution or clinical-education program receiving federal funding on the basis of their gender (20 U.S.C.A. § 1681 [1990]). Gender discrimination cases are frequently filed under Title IX, Title VII (Equal Employment Opportunity Act), or a combination of these two laws. EMS educational programs that receive federal funds may not discriminate in admission, dismissal, or any other way based upon gender. Even though not required by law, EMS educational activities that are not federally funded would be wise to follow the same nondiscriminatory practices.

Public Health and Safety Laws

Various federal and state workplace and environmental regulations require EMS educators to assess and improve the adequacy of the equipment and clinical education provided to students who work with organic hazardous waste materials (such as bodily fluids and tissues), as well as understand how to respond to situations involving chemical hazardous waste. Workplace safety cases are being prosecuted with increasing frequency and success,[9] so it is critical that federal, state, and local regulations be clearly understood. As with any type of EMS activity, response is much more effective if potential problems are examined beforehand and procedures are developed, such as by having an emergency protocol in place for chemical or bodily fluid exposure.

Federal Health and Safety Laws and Affirmative Duties

On both the federal and state levels, environmental laws are increasingly being used in combination with workplace safety regulations whenever death or serious injury occurs due to inadequate safety equipment or protocols. Environmental regulations, unlike the relatively modest penalties of traditional workplace regulation, carry the possibility of substantial financial penalties, as well as felony convictions and lengthy incarceration. This regulatory interplay is of particular consequence to EMS educators dealing with hazardous substances, because even routine safety incidents may subject educational institutions and EMS educators to increased scrutiny in both the workplace safety and the environmental spheres.[9] Fit testing for N95 masks and ensuring latex-allergic students can obtain nonlatex gloves are some examples of how the educator can make sure the students' environment is safe.

Occupational Safety and Health Act of 1970

The Occupational Safety and Health Act, enacted in 1970 to ensure safe and healthful working conditions, is overseen by the Occupational Safety and Health Administration (OSHA) (29 U.S.C.A. §§ 651 *et seq.* [2010]); Congress enacted federal OSHA legislation upon a finding that personnel injuries and illnesses arising out of work situations impose a substantial burden upon the economy in terms of the following:

- Disability compensation payments
- Lost production
- Medical expenses
- Wage loss

For four decades, this situation has been addressed by OSHA by the following:

- Encouraging employers and employees to reduce the number of safety and health hazards at the workplace
- Ensuring that employers and employees share in this responsibility
- Establishing and enforcing occupational health and safety standards
- Encouraging labor and management to jointly reduce employment injuries and disease

EMS educators should be familiar with all OSHA guidelines that impact emergency medical interventions.[10] While the safety of students must always be considered, EMS educational programs also must do the following:

- Acquire and inspect relevant safety gear to be used by students
- Conduct applicable safety education
- Routinely inspect potential sources of health hazards

While OSHA regulations are not legally binding on students per se, they do apply to anyone who is an employee. That would include instructors and it may include students where the educational program is being delivered to employees. In any event, EMS training programs are wise to implement OSHA's policies, whether mandatory or not.

OSHA is authorized to investigate, with no advance warning, suspected safety hazards and violations of its regulations. Harsh penalties and restrictions may be imposed for safety violations. Workplaces cited for safety violations may be fined, those found guilty of second offenses may face more substantial fines, and a third offense could put programs under OSHA's oversight with the federal government determining what safety steps must be taken.

Occupational Safety and Health Act of 1970

Congress enacted the Occupational Safety and Health Act upon finding "that personal injuries and illnesses arising out of work situations impose a substantial burden upon, and are a hindrance to, interstate commerce in terms of lost production, wage loss, medical expenses, and disability compensation payments" (PL 91-586). This situation is to be relieved in the following ways:

- Encouraging employers and employees to reduce the number of occupational safety and health hazards at the workplace
- Assuring that employers and employees share in this responsibility
- Creating an Occupational Safety and Health Commission
- Advancing initiatives to provide safe and healthful working conditions
- Providing occupational safety and health research
- Exploring the relationship between diseases and environmental conditions
- Providing medical criteria for safe and healthful working conditions
- Providing training programs
- Establishing occupational health and safety standards
- Enforcing standards
- Encouraging states to assume fullest responsibility for administration and enforcement of OSHA policies
- Creating appropriate reporting procedures
- Encouraging labor and management to jointly reduce employment injuries and disease (*id.*)

Emergency Planning and Right-to-Know Act of 1986

The Emergency Planning and Right-to-Know Act (42 U.S.C.A. §§ 11001–11050 [1986]) gives employees and members of the community the right to better understand that risks that are posed by chemicals and toxins present in a given workplace. EMS educators are required to obtain Material Safety Data Sheet information on all applicable toxins or chemical hazards present in the workplace, and provide training to students so that they understand the need for gloves, face shields, masks, or even respirators to protect themselves when exposed to such products. EMS educators should also include this information on waivers and releases signed by students.

State Public Health, Safety, and Education Codes

Each state has a lead agency that has overall responsibility for public-sector occupational safety and health. Although OSHA is a federal law that applies to private-sector employers, states have been offered the opportunity to accept responsibility for administration and enforcement of OSHA policies. Nearly half of the states assume this responsibility.[11] In such a state, all entities, both public and private, must comply with federal OSHA regulations.

EMS educators should be familiar with their own state's OSHA requirements for compliance.[9]

EMS Standards of Education

Besides the state agency responsible for managing occupational safety and health, states have assigned responsibility for addressing EMS-related oversight to a state agency. Some states assign responsibility for EMS to the state health department, while others assign it to the state fire marshal. EMS educators should be familiar with the licensure, certification, and instructional regulations that the applicable state agency has issued. In this regard, state EMS offices are an important source of regulatory and administrative rules for EMS educators.

For example, some states require students to have a current state EMT license to participate in hospital clinicals as paramedic students. States may also regulate what students can or cannot do when working as a student versus what that student can do when employed. For example, typically, paramedic students can perform advanced skills under specific circumstances during their hospital or field clinical experience but cannot perform any advanced skills when functioning in an employment situation as EMTs.

Paramedic educational programs accredited by the Commission on Accreditation of Allied Health Education Programs (CAAHEP) and the Committee on Accreditation of Educational Programs for the Emergency Medical Services Professions (CoAEMSP) reflect meeting a minimum national level of educational standards. In following state guidelines, educational institutions may establish standards of instruction required of all EMS educators. Frequently, EMS educators must hold teaching certifications or credentials. It is critical that EMS educators meet or exceed the minimum standards for both the EMS and teaching professions established by accrediting bodies and states.

State Immunity Laws

In order to encourage EMS educators and students to participate in educational and clinical-education programs, most states have enacted broad general immunity laws for EMS educators. Nevertheless, immunity generally is not granted for gross negligence and willful misconduct.

CASE IN POINT

Tanya McAlexander, a student in an EMT training class offered by the college, filed suit after suffering injuries during a rope-training exercise. McAlexander alleged that the instructor's negligence caused her injury. The court found California's immunity law granted immunity to the instructor based on the law's express intent to promote the development, accessibility, and provision of emergency medical services and to encourage training regarding the same. McAlexander claimed the rope training was beyond the scope of EMT training, but the court found it was appropriate training for situations requiring extrication and mountain rescues. Instructors were permitted to develop training programs based on geographic challenges students might encounter in their respective environments. McAlexander further claimed the instructor was not properly qualified in rope techniques, but the court found liability on that basis would defeat the law's intent to provide immunity for instructors. The court found the college was immune from liability for personal injury and further that the law does not violate due process because it applies to all students, not just EMT students.

McAlexander v. Siskiyou Joint Community College, 222 Cal.App.3d 768 (Court of Appeal of California, 3rd Appellate District 1990).

Program Clinical Affiliation Agreements

EMS is a highly complex system, and **affiliation agreements** to educate students should account for this complexity. Educational institutions should have agreements with all clinical sites involved in clinical-education activities. A standard affiliation agreement should be clearly written and approved by legal counsel. Clinical sites may also require that documents be reviewed by their legal counsel.

Emergency Protocols and Procedures

Affiliation agreements establish guidelines that are mutually acceptable to both the educational institution and clinical sites. Well-written agreements identify obligations required by educational institutions, by students, and by the clinical sites. Emergency protocols and procedures to be followed should be clearly defined. In the event that policies conflict, the agreements should indicate which should be followed. Addressing this information in the agreements before students are assigned to clinical sites is helpful in addressing potential conflicts before they arise.

Framework for Clinical-Education Agreements

To minimize litigation potential, affiliation agreements should contain basic components that are delineated below. There are several other important clauses to include within a contract; the components discussed below are particularly important for an affiliation agreement. Legal counsel should be consulted in drafting any agreement.

Introductory Clause

Affiliation agreements should clearly identify the parties involved. At a minimum, the parties would include the educational institution and the clinical site. The introductory clause also often includes the date of the agreement.

Dates

Affiliation agreements should identify the starting and terminating dates of the contract. Multiple-year agreements are generally advantageous in that they eliminate the need for annual renegotiations. The parties, in consultation with their legal counsel, should determine if agreements should be developed on a case-by-case basis or as multiple-year contracts.

Performance Objectives

Affiliation agreements should provide measurable student achievement-based objectives (knowledge, skills, and judgment). In this way, each party will be aware of its duties in the hospital or field education of students. Where student achievement falls short of the learning and performance objectives, the agreement should define who evaluates the student and how the student is remediated.

Student–Employee Relationships

Affiliation agreements should define the student–employee relationship with the clinical sites. In most cases, students do not receive remuneration for their clinical experiences. EMS educators should be aware of federal, state, and accreditation policies and should clearly identify these in the agreements. CAAHEP requires that educational programs not substitute students for paid personnel.

Liability Expectations

This section of the affiliation agreement is designed to define the liability responsibilities and expectations of each party. Indemnification information should identify who has a duty to remediate any loss, damage, or liability incurred. Inherently dangerous educational activities should be addressed such as the protocols that students should follow when dealing with blood-borne pathogens and infectious disease exposures.

Mutual Obligations

This part of the affiliation agreement should be specific as to the exact steps necessary to ensure compliance with the agreement itself. Generally, this part addresses obligations of the educational institution to students and to cooperating clinical sites, as well as obligations of the clinical sites to students and to the educational institution.

Key Contacts

Names, titles, mailing addresses for formal notifications, and contact numbers for both the educational institutions and the clinical sites should be included. All parties to the contract should have immediate access to their counterparts.

Signatures

Signatures are required on affiliation agreements. Because these agreements are considered legal documents, only authorized persons should affix their signatures. Educational institutions should determine who this individual is and should notify EMS educators. State law varies as to whether signatures need to be witnessed and/or notarized in order to make the contract valid. State law also varies as to how the signature block is to be formatted such that the entities that are party to the contract are held liable for any breach, and that the individuals who signed on behalf of the entities are not held personally liable.

Curriculum Issues

EMS educators should establish a curriculum that is in compliance with the U.S. Department of Transportation's educational standards and federal and state laws, and that adheres to accreditation standards.[12] Beyond that, EMS educators have the right to adapt the curriculum within their programs to meet local needs.

Student Issues

Student issues in EMS educational programs are similar to those of most educational programs. Common student issues include, among others, the following:

- Institutional relationships
- Enrollment and dismissal
- Background checks and drug screening
- Discipline in the classroom
- Professional appearance
- Academic dishonesty
- Bullying (including cyber-bullying)

The issues identified in this chapter provide merely a brief overview. EMS educators should become familiar with all local, state, and federal regulations under which their program operates. It is vital that educators have access to appropriate support by administrators and/or legal counsel to avoid being placed in positions of potential liability.

Institutional Relationships

Student–institution relationships are among the most critical and most challenging components of any educational system. Establishing a positive student–institution relationship is critical to the success of programs and their graduates. Documents, including but not restricted to catalogs, handbooks, course syllabi, and advertising materials, play an important role in promoting a positive relationship between institutions and students. All information should be correct, current, detailed, and readily available to the public.

Catalogs

Catalogs, electronic or otherwise, are perhaps the most enduring document of the student relationship with educational institutions. Information generally provided in catalogs includes the following:

- Institutional data
- Academic requirements
- Enrollment and dismissal rules and regulations
- Student support services

Student Handbooks

Depending on the size and type of the EMS educational program, students may receive a variety of handbooks that provide rules, regulations, and information pertinent to their educational endeavors. Some programs combine general student handbooks with the educational institution's handbooks. Traditionally, student handbooks are broad in scope and include information pertinent to the entire EMS program.

EMS educators may develop handbooks specifically for students in their educational program. This handbook may provide specific information on the following:

- Attendance guidelines
- Curricula
- Uniform or dress code
- Code of conduct

EMS educators may also create handbooks that provide rules, expectations, and guidelines relevant to activities in the hospital and field settings. (See Chapter 24: Administrative Issues, for more on syllabi, handbooks, and policies.)

When developing program policies, EMS educators may establish standards that are stricter than those of the general-education institution. No policies should be established that are less stringent or that conflict with institutional or governmental policy. EMS educators should have their suggested policies approved by their institution or their institution's legal counsel before the time of publication.

Related Printed Documents

EMS educators may use printed documents for recruitment or related activities. All published documents may provide information that, when interpreted by the reader, may lead to litigation and should first be approved by the educational institutions. The Higher Education Resources Act (20 U.S.C.A. §§ 1001 *et. seq.* [2010]; 42 U.S.C.A. §§ 2751 *et seq.* [2010]) requires all educational institutions that participate in federal financial aid programs to provide key information to all prospective and current students. Materials must include information on the following:

- ADA support
- Confidentiality of records
- Descriptions of educational programs
- Financial assistance opportunities
- Nondiscrimination policies
- Refund policies
- Program costs
- Veterans' benefits

Challenges to Printed Documents

In today's educational system, catalogs and handbooks are perceived by students as legal documents that create a binding, inflexible obligation on the part of the institution. Many educational institutions include disclaimer statements to protect themselves from potential litigation. Printed documents are where many of the current misrepresentation lawsuits, discussed in this chapter, originate. Many students view these printed documents as containing promises made to them by the educational institution which they expect to be fulfilled, particularly when they have taken out sizeable student loans in order to undertake an educational institution's program.

Courts have established that students have rights and do not lose their basic constitutional freedoms when they enter an educational institution. EMS educators should be careful not to violate students' constitutional rights when making programmatic changes. Students' constitutional rights include the following:

- Freedom from discrimination
- Freedom of assembly
- Freedom of speech

Enrollment and Dismissal

The enrollment process in EMS educational programs begins with recruitment. All applicants and students should be treated equitably and according to published guidelines. The ultimate goal is to see students successfully complete the programs and become gainfully employed. However, on some occasions, students must be dismissed from EMS programs. When this occurs, students should be treated in a fair and equitable manner so potential litigation can be avoided.

Recruitment

When recruiting students, EMS educators should be certain that unlawful discrimination does not occur. Printing a nondiscrimination statement on all recruiting documents is a good starting point. However, policies should go beyond written statements and should be implemented and strictly enforced. The two most common areas of litigation involving recruitment are breach of contract and misrepresentation or fraud.

The relationship between an educational institution and a student is essentially based upon a contract. The institution agrees to provide an educational opportunity, and the student agrees to pay a fee and attend courses.

However, there are numerous subtle details between the parties that also exist and become part of the agreement: that the student will obey the rules; that the institution will hold the classes that the student needs; that the student will attend classes; that the institution will hold the classes at the place and time scheduled, and so on.

When EMS educational programs do not meet a written or implied expectation of a student, it may be considered to be a breach of contract.

Misrepresentation may occur when an EMS program intentionally provides false or misleading information to students to induce their attendance. In cases of misrepresentation, students must prove:

- A false statement of material fact
- Known by the EMS program to be false, or uttered with reckless disregard for the truth or falsity of the statement upon which the students reasonably relied
- Resulted in damages to the students

EMS educators should be extremely careful in determining the factual accuracy of all printed material that will be used for recruitment and enrollment of students, particularly regarding employment and compensation rates of graduates. Nonaccredited and provisionally accredited programs should clearly acknowledge this fact. For instance, paramedic students should be advised that they may not be able to be certified or licensed if they attend an educational program that is not fully accredited by the Committee on Accreditation of Education Programs for the Emergency Medical Services Professions (CoAEMSP) and the Commission on Accreditation of Allied Health Education Programs (CAAHEP) after January 1, 2013.

Acceptance

Once accepted, students have a right to know what is expected of them, not only in the general EMS program, but also in specific clinical courses. Also, once accepted, students should be asked if accommodations are necessary to meet essential functions. Student handbooks may provide most of this information. During the first session of each class, EMS educators should provide students with course syllabi. Each syllabus should be clearly written and adhere to institutional guidelines. All course expectations and grading criteria should be set forth unambiguously. Well-written syllabi limit students' ability to threaten or pursue successful litigation.

Dismissal

EMS educators like to see their students succeed. Occasionally, however, students fail to meet the published educational standards, and for that, or for other reasons, must be dismissed from the program. This is a difficult situation that should be handled carefully. Attention should be paid to fully documenting the entire situation. Just as with other aspects of student–institution relationships, fair treatment is critical. If EMS educators follow their own rules, the courts are likely to uphold their academic judgments.

Student dismissal is similar to employee dismissal. In terms of student issues, litigation may result if EMS educators fail to do the following:

- Regularly and objectively document student behavior
- Provide educational experiences, both academic and practical, directed toward success
- Keep evidence of both positive and negative completed student work
- Maintain fair and objective student evaluations
- Communicate as though every word, written or spoken, would be broadcast in public
- Treat all students the same and objectively
- Maintain students' confidentiality before, during, and after the educational experience

Most EMS educators recognize the importance of careful documentation. As educators, EMS professionals should adapt the ability to document to their classroom and clinical-education activities. Again, it is critical that all students be treated equitably, and it is vital that this equitable treatment be documented.

CASE IN POINT 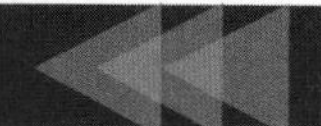

Lue Ella Rogers, a second-year nursing student, sued the Tennessee Board of Regents, alleging denial of procedural and substantive due process rights after she was dismissed from a community college for receiving an unsatisfactory grade on her clinical performance evaluations. Rogers claimed she was not given a chance to correct deficiencies that led to her dismissal. The court held for the Board of Regents since Rogers was afforded sufficient procedural process to appeal her dismissal, and her interest in higher education was not protected by substantive due process.

Rogers v. Tennessee Board of Regents, 273 Fed.Appx. 458 (U.S. Circuit Court of Appeals for the 6th Circuit 2008).

Background Checks

EMS educational programs may require students to pass criminal background checks, including fingerprinting that screens for violent criminals and registered sex offenders, and review of tracking systems for incidents of child abuse and neglect.

Without screening and background checks, clinical sites might be exposed to claims that they did not sufficiently vet students. Such claims could be brought under the existing tort liability doctrine of negligent hiring and retention, which could subject EMS educational programs to liability if they fail to gather or act on relevant information indicating someone was a dangerous fit for EMS.

Criminal Convictions

The Joint Commission on Accreditation requires criminal background checks on anyone who provides EMS care when required by state law, regulation, or clinical-education site policy. Student failure to disclose a felony conviction often results in dismissal from EMS educational programs, as well as suspension from a current job, license, or certification. Felony convictions must generally be disclosed to state EMS agencies within 30 days of entry of final judgment; a failure to disclose results in a temporary suspension of a license or certification.[13] Some felony convictions may prohibit student participation in hospital or field experience and prevent EMT state licensure.

Screenings for Illegal Drug Use

EMS educational programs may require drug tests for illegal drug use. Test results may be validated by asking about lawful drug use or possible explanations for the positive results other than illegal use of drugs. However, disability-related questions are prohibited and students who take drugs under medical supervision should not be compelled to disclose their medical condition unless it affects their ability to safely participate in the program or serve in the EMS profession.

Therefore, while follow-up questions in response to a positive drug test are permitted, there are specific limitations on the types of information that can be elicited by someone other than a medical officer. For instance, a student who is taking antiseizure or antiretroviral drugs should not be compelled to disclose that he or she is epileptic or HIV-positive unless such disclosure is made to a medical officer. The medical officer then must make a determination if the medical condition is one that might be dangerous in an EMS setting. No one other than a medical officer should ever be present during this follow-up questioning of students.[8]

Social Networking and Credit Record Screening

Neither social network screening nor credit record screening is recommended; it risks claims of unfair discrimination based upon embarrassing but otherwise legal behavior. Other pitfalls include violating equal opportunity employment laws like the ADA or Title VII, and could implicate fair credit-reporting standards that require an opportunity to respond to any damaging information a background search could produce.[14]

> **CASE IN POINT**
>
> Edward Senu-Oke, a student, sued Jackson State University after he was dismissed for failing to attend orientation or giving a reason for his absence. The student filed suit to be let back into the university. The court held for the university, finding that educational institutions are better suited to evaluate the suitability of students than courts.
>
> *Senu-Oke v. Jackson State University*, 283 Fed.Appx. 236 (U.S. Circuit of Appeals for the 5th Circuit 2008).

Discipline in the Classroom

One of the most common problems faced by EMS educators is addressing student misconduct in the classroom, clinical, and field settings. There are two primary pathways for dealing with problems related to student conduct. One path is academic and the other is disciplinary. Courts have traditionally supported educational institutions in dealing with professional conduct issues as academic issues rather than disciplinary issues, provided that student rights are not violated.[15,16]

Academic requirements should include specific professional behavioral expectations and evaluation, which in EMS are identified by the National EMS Education Standards and include the following behaviors: integrity, empathy, self-motivation, appearance and personal hygiene, self-confidence, communications, time management, teamwork and diplomacy, respect, patient advocacy, and careful delivery of service. These characteristics should be evaluated during each course and verified that they are adequate or the student will not pass. Any specific problem with one of the above should indicate a need for an additional evaluation to point out and direct the student to appropriate behavior. Failure of that evaluation at whatever point is identified, would result in failure of the course.

Students who fail their affective or professional behavior requirements are entitled to the same grievance for that failure as they would be for a failure of any examination or course. The courts have generally supported academic decisions by instructors as long as they are not arbitrary or capricious.

The disciplinary process is the other pathway to deal with behavioral issues. It is up to each educational institution to develop its own disciplinary process. With the disciplinary path, for instance dismissing a student for cheating, the institution might not be able to immediately dismiss the student unless there is a specific threat for the student to be in the classroom or other educational setting. That will of course depend upon the institution's specific disciplinary policy and procedure.

Due process must often be provided in disciplinary dismissals at major institutions prior to the student being dismissed. Due process may also be an issue if the institution is a public agency. Due process can be rigorous in terms of hearings and the various levels of appeals that must be followed. Consequently, it is generally to a program's advantage to use the academic pathway rather than go down the disciplinary path. The disciplinary path should be determined by the written grievance policies provided to students, and each progressive step along this path should be fully documented and supported should the student turn to litigation after dismissal.

Professional Appearance

EMS educators and students are traditionally held to a higher standard of professional appearance than the general public. The appearance of EMS personnel not only establishes a level of professionalism, it also is a matter of hygiene and safety. Educators should expect students to adhere to dress codes as approved and provided by the educational institution. Dress code policies may address the following:

- Body piercings
- Fingernails
- Hairstyles, including facial hair
- Jewelry
- Tattoos
- Uniforms
- Other related personal hygiene issues

Policies regarding student uniforms and personal hygiene should be established in accordance with input from advisory committees, and they should be written in compliance with clinical-education expectations. If clinical sites have dress codes or personal hygiene policies that are stricter than those of the educational institution, EMS educators may enforce such guidelines, provided that such requirements are reasonable.

Policies should be clearly presented to students in their handbooks and/or syllabi. EMS educators should not assume that students know what acceptable appearance is. If students are required to wear identification badges or name tags, it is the educator's responsibility to notify students of this. If stethoscopes and bandage scissors are part of the uniform, students should know this in advance.

Depending on the EMS program, students may be required to be in uniform at all times. It is also possible that they may be assigned to wear uniforms only during time spent in the hospital or field education. Again, it is important that students are provided this information as early in the educational process as possible. By informing students, the EMS educator has clearly identified the standards and has established a basis for expectations.

Although student appearances may be perceived as problematic, EMS educators should use caution in dealing with issues such as clothing and hairstyles. Courts have allowed educational institutions to establish dress codes to restrict clothing or other appearances deemed to be unsafe, offensive **(Figure 10.3)**, or unsanitary.

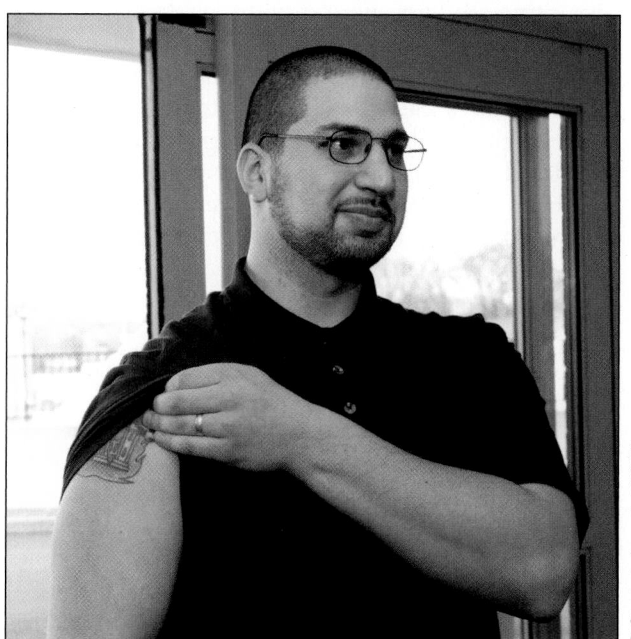

Figure 10.3

Students with offensive tattoos can be required to cover them before being allowed in the hospital.

While observing health and safety practices regarding hairstyles, EMS educators also should be cognizant of prohibitions that may be deemed unconstitutional. Ethnic hairstyles have been protected by the courts, even when they violate professional dress codes.

Academic Dishonesty

Academic dishonesty in the classroom is not a new concept. It is, however, on the rise with the increase in the uses and capabilities of technology. Printed information in catalogs, handbooks, and syllabi should contain clearly established policies on academic dishonesty. Such policies should be made available to students upon enrollment and should be reinforced at the beginning of each course. In the event that academic dishonesty does occur, students will have already received the institutional policy and will know the related penalty. The courts generally support educational institutions in matters of academic dishonesty. The most common current form of academic dishonesty is plagiarism.

Bullying

Educational institutions should have a strict policy that prohibits hazing and bullying of fellow students and coworkers. This policy should be broad enough to include hazing and bullying in all of its various forms, including cyber-bullying.

It is important for the institution to adopt a formal policy on hazing and bullying. In the absence of such a policy, it is likely that an offender may successfully claim a First Amendment right to use the Internet. It is also important to recognize that such a policy may not extend to all online hazing and bullying activities, only those that impact a fellow student at the institution, or a coworker.

Grievance Policies

Every educational institution should have a published formal grievance policy for both their employees and students. Although policies may differ according to the nature of the institutional relationship, the concepts are the same. Paramedic educational programs accredited by the Committee on Accreditation of Educational Programs for the Emergency Medical Services Professions are required to have a defined and published policy and procedure for processing grievances.

Students

Grievance policies should be made readily available to all students upon enrollment in EMS educational programs. Many educational institutions elect to publish the grievance procedure in their institutional catalogs or program handbooks. When disciplining students, EMS educators should attempt to resolve issues at the lowest possible level. If unable to resolve student issues, educators should be certain that the steps in the student grievance policy are carefully followed and documented. Failure of educators to adhere to their institution's published policies may enhance student opportunities for successful litigation.

Educators

EMS educators should also have published grievance policies relative to their employment. Just as students do not sacrifice their constitutional rights when they enroll in EMS educational programs, educators should be afforded the opportunity to respond when their rights appear to have been violated. These rights, however, have limitations.

Where EMS educators might have a constitutional claim under the First Amendment for an adverse job action their employers have taken based on their speech, this right is restricted if their words are uttered or their deeds done in the course of their employment duties (*Garcetti v. Ceballos*, 547 U.S. 410 [U.S. Supreme Court 2006]). In particular, where a public employee is acting as a spokesperson for her employer, the employee does not enjoy complete First Amendment protections (*Foley v. Town of Randolph*, 598 F.3d 1 [1st Cir., 2010]). Employers may lawfully discipline educators who publicly voice concerns about issues such as fraud, mismanagement, misuse of funds, student discipline and discrimination practices if they fail to clearly establish that they are speaking as a private citizen.[17]

Safe Learning Environment Laws

While safe environments are established on the basis of laws and consistent enforcement of safety programs, Virginia Tech University awakened American society in 2007 to real and potential campus violence. Educational institutions were once considered secure. However, when a student at Virginia Tech killed 32 students and faculty, injured 17 more, and then took his own life in the deadliest campus shooting in U.S. history, it became clear that educational institutions are not free of violence.[18]

Federal Safety Laws and Directives

EMS educators should strive to provide safe learning environments for their students. Among the federal laws requiring safe environments with which EMS educators should be familiar are the following:

- Safe and Drug-Free Schools and Communities Act (20 U.S.C.A. §§ 7101 *et seq.* [2002])
- Gun-Free Schools Act (20 U.S.C.A. § 7151 [2002])
- Jeanne Clery Disclosure of Campus Security Policy and Campus Crime Statistics Act (20 U.S.C.A. § 1092[f] [2009])

Safe and Drug-Free Schools and Communities Act of 2002

The Safe and Drug-Free Schools and Communities Act (20 U.S.C.A. §§ 7101 *et seq.* [2002]) introduced zero-tolerance policies with regard to any type of disruption into educational environments, including hate speech, harassment, fighting, and inappropriate attire. Consequently, strictly speaking, EMS educators are responsible for safeguarding students from activities occurring outside their gates that ultimately have an impact inside their gates, such as cyber-bullying.[19] Whether EMS educators choose to severely punish disruptive students who disrupt academic achievement is a question that must be answered by individual educational institutions. It is uncontroverted that educators have the legal authority to do so.

Through this law, educational institutions were mandated to establish clear and consistent programs of school drug and violence prevention, education, and rehabilitation referral for students. This law also encourages the sharing of disciplinary records of students who transfer between educational institutions.

Gun-Free Schools Act of 2002

Despite the prevalence of zero-tolerance policies for disruptive behavior by students, it is a deadly legal fiction to assume educational institutions are free of guns.[20] While some states apply the federal Gun-Free Schools Act (20 U.S.C.A. § 7151 [2002]) to higher education, most state laws allow gun possession if allowed by the educational institution. While some state laws restrict guns in educational institutions, almost all states explicitly permit adult students to have firearms in locked cars; other states allow licensed guns to be stored in student dormitory rooms.

Jeanne Clery Disclosure of Campus Security Policy and Campus Crime Statistics Act of 1990

In 1990, the Jeanne Clery Disclosure of Campus Security Policy and Campus Crime Statistics Act (Clery Act) was adopted by Congress (20 U.S.C.A. § 1092[f] [2009]). The name is in memory of a Lehigh University freshman in Pennsylvania, who was sexually assaulted and murdered in her residence hall in 1986. Her murderer was another student whom she did not know. After investigation, Jeanne's parents learned that 38 undisclosed crimes had occurred on the university's campus during the three years before Jeanne's death.

Today, all higher education institutions receiving federal funds are required to publish annual reports on crime statistics. Within this document, three years of statistics must be reported. The report must be provided to all current students and employees. Additionally, this information may be provided to prospective students and employees, as well as the public upon request. Crime statistics must include data from all campus and local law enforcement agencies, and they must include incidents that occurred on the campus and in public areas surrounding the campus.

Educational institutions are also required to issue annual statements of current policies regarding immediate emergency-response and evacuation procedures. The policy statement must articulate procedures that will be used to notify the campus community upon confirmation of a significant emergency or dangerous situation involving an immediate threat to the health or safety of students occurring on the campus. EMS educators may want to review or even reconsider whether their campus emergency-response efforts are sufficiently coordinated for maximum effect.[21]

Crime Categories to be Reported Under the Clery Act

- Aggravated assault
- Arson
- Burglary
- Manslaughter (negligent)
- Murder and non-negligent manslaughter
- Motor vehicle theft
- Robbery
- Sex offenses (forcible)
- Sex offenses (nonforcible, incest, and statutory rape)
- Other hate crimes involving bodily injury

Negligent Referrals

Educational institutions and EMS educators should be aware of potential litigation that may result from **negligent** or inaccurate **referrals**. Any educator who writes letters of recommendation owes a duty to not misrepresent the qualifications or character of students if such action could result in harm to prospective third parties; this is especially the case when students have a known history of actions that may put others at risk.[22]

Workers' Compensation and Other Public Benefits Laws

Workers' compensation and other public benefits laws usually supplant tort litigation as a method of resolving disputes over workplace injuries. Workers' compensation laws have been established to determine who will be eligible for benefits such as the following:

- Family support
- Medical expenses
- Wage loss

Workers' compensation is a type of strict liability, no-fault insurance in the event of injuries or illnesses related to EMS educational activities. In such cases, the EMS program does not admit fault for the injury and the injured student agrees to receive benefits without litigation. Workers' compensation benefits are not generally provided for injuries resulting from intentionally harmful conduct, horseplay, alcohol, or illegal use of drugs.

Coverage

Each state determines workers' compensation coverage. Because penalties against employers who fail to provide workers' compensation insurance can be severe, EMS educators should check and monitor the coverage of clinical sites.

Since EMS educational programs have the potential for injury, educators should be aware of institutional policies and should follow procedures exactly.

In many cases, injury or incident reports must be completed within a specified time frame. Injured individuals may be required to visit a physician who has contracted with the educational institution or state workers' compensation insurance.

EMS educators also should be familiar with the status of students in their programs in regard to workers' compensation coverage. Some states may cover students in clinical education; other states may provide no workers' compensation coverage for students under any circumstances.

Fraud

Misrepresentation of injuries might result in charges of fraud. Because workers' compensation benefits are determined by physicians' reports, injured parties should be sure to provide accurate and detailed information. Most states have laws that require employers, insurance carriers, and the public to report suspected cases of workers' compensation fraud. States frequently allow the informer to remain anonymous. Fraudulent workers' compensation claims may be subject to criminal proceedings.

Health and Malpractice Insurance

Traditionally, students who are enrolled in a university-based program must show proof that they have personal health-insurance coverage. If unable to provide such proof, students may be required to purchase health insurance through the educational institution. Some students may be employed by an EMS provider and covered under their plan as an employee. In addition to personal health coverage, most institutions, clinical affiliations, and certification boards require that students carry malpractice insurance in the event that students cause injury to third parties. EMS educators should comply with institutional expectations in advising students regarding health and malpractice insurance.

EMS Instructor Malpractice

Malpractice insurance is generally not a covered benefit, so EMS educators should determine the necessity of carrying such insurance themselves. In some institutions, EMS educators are required to carry malpractice insurance. The value of carrying malpractice insurance is that it protects the EMS educator's certification, registration, or licensure in the event of injury to another person.

Confidentiality and Data Privacy Laws

Based on their medical experiences, EMS educators are already familiar with the privacy rules of patient confidentiality. As educators, the rules of data privacy and confidentiality extend to the their students and their activities.

Federal Privacy Laws and Directives

The three most important federal laws regarding data privacy are the following:

- The Family Educational Rights and Privacy Act of 1974 (**FERPA**) (20 U.S.C.A. § 1232g [2002])
- The Health Insurance Portability and Accountability Act **HIPAA** Privacy Rule (42 U.S.C.A. § 1320d-6 [2010])
- The Freedom of Information Act (FOIA) (5 U.S.C.A. § 552 [2009])

Family Educational Rights and Privacy Act of 1974

Popularly known as the Buckley Amendment, based primarily upon the efforts of New York Senator James Buckley, FERPA was enacted in response to concerns that personal information was being maintained and disseminated by the government. FERPA prohibits the release of a student's personally identifiable information to anyone without a legitimate educational interest in the information. All educational institutions that receive federal funds are required to comply with FERPA.

FERPA Guidelines

The Family Policy Compliance Office in the U.S. Department of Education interprets and enforces FERPA and publishes advice letters to clarify the Act. FERPA guidelines, established to protect the confidentiality and handling of student records, clarify the following:

- Student records must be kept confidential, with access provided to outside third parties only with parental consent or with the consent of adult-aged students.
- They must be accessed on request by the student's parents/guardians (for minors) or adult-aged students.

- They may be challenged by parents or adult-aged students who think that the records are misleading, inaccurate, or a violation of their privacy rights.

Under federal law, educational institutions must inform students or their parents of FERPA guidelines. Students under 18, the legal age of full responsibility, are generally considered minors, and their parents or guardians have legal access to their educational records. Once students turn 18 or enroll in higher education institutions, they are considered adults under FERPA; at this point, parents and guardians have no legal right to access student information.

Educational records

Documents maintained at an educational institution that specifically relate to students are considered educational records. These records may take the form of written documents, video or audiotapes, films, photographs, or computer files. Five types of documents are excluded from FERPA regulations:

- Sole possession notes (instructor's notes) that are not accessible or revealed to any other person (such as grade books)
- Medical records of adult-aged students (such as letters from physicians, psychiatrists, or psychologists for the purpose of treating students)
- Law enforcement records
- Student employee records
- Alumni records unrelated to their attendance as students (34 C.F.R. pt. 99 [2010])

While the definition of educational records has been the subject of significant litigation, the courts have broadly defined the term to cover disciplinary records.[23]

Disclosure Policies and Practices

Single acts do not violate FERPA; instead, educational institutions and EMS educational programs must have a policy or practice of permitting unauthorized release.[24] Thus, FERPA does not govern every single disclosure that might constitute an unauthorized release of educational records. Instead, FERPA forbids only policies or practices that condone such releases.

According to FERPA regulations, student records may be disclosed in only three ways:

- To students directly
- To third parties with written permission of students (or parents/guardians)
- To third parties without written consent

Under the following circumstances, educational records may be released without previous written consent:

- Directory information (unless a written request denying the publication of this information is provided by the student or parent)
- Information required by a school official who has a legitimate educational interest (Educators should be careful to demonstrate the legitimate educational interest, or they could be in violation of FERPA.)
- Information requested from an educational institution into which the student plans to enroll
- Financial aid documentation
- Documents necessary for accrediting bodies (It is best to remove student identification whenever possible.)
- Information necessary for studies on behalf of the institution regarding financial aid, testing, and other related research (Again, if possible, it is best to remove any personal identification.)
- Health and safety information necessary to protect other persons in the event of an emergency
- Documents or data required under lawfully issued subpoenas or orders

EMS educators should understand the circumstances under which educational records have been requested and should be certain to comply with federal regulations. For instance, law enforcement may obtain student health data only with a court order (34 C.F.R. § 300.535[b][1] [2006]).

Legitimate Educational Interests

Student records may be obtained by EMS educators who have legitimate educational interests. While student records may be accessed for information pertinent to employment, each situation should be handled individually and on a need-to-know basis.

HIV/AIDS Status FERPA does not allow EMS educational programs to disclose the HIV status of students solely for the promotion of general health and safety (20 U.S.C.A. § 1232g[b][1][A] [2002]). EMS educators have to decide whether HIV status poses a special health risk in EMS clinical education. The courts, including the U.S. Supreme Court, usually insist that only a narrow set of deserving individuals with HIV-positive status qualify for confidentiality protection under state confidentiality laws (see

Bragdon v. Abbott, 524 U.S. 624 [U.S. Supreme Court 1998]). Individuals with HIV-positive status are continually failing to present evidence to obtain protection from discrimination.[24] The courts point to two facts for this lack of general protection: there is no cure for HIV/AIDS (Acquired Immune Deficiency Syndrome) at this time and widely disseminated preventive vaccines or curative medicines are likely years away.[25,26]

Student Health Emergencies FERPA allows for parental notification, without student consent, in cases of health emergencies where knowledge of the information is necessary to protect a student (20 U.S.C.A. § 1232g[b][1][I] [2002]). While such emergencies often involve potential suicides,[27] it is not clear what constitutes a health emergency and whether hospitalization is required before parents/guardians may be notified.[28]

A second exception is rare infectious outbreaks such as methicillin-resistant staphylococcus aureus (MRSA).[29] Such outbreaks are clearly covered by the health emergency exception to FERPA (20 U.S.C.A. 1232[g] [2002]).

Employee Reimbursement Disclosures It is common in the EMS profession for employers to pay for employees' education. In return, employers expect to remain informed about student academic standing. This is a contractual issue between the employer and the student employee. It is the student employee's responsibility to provide this release. EMS educators should not release information to employers, without the student's (or parent's) written permission.

Moreover, reimbursement contracts should be established with employers before students enroll in EMS programs. These contracts should clearly identify the expectations of both parties and should be signed and dated. For instance, employers might agree to pay for tuition, books, supplies, and all related educational expenses. In return, students may be expected to provide records of attendance and/or transcripts at the completion of each grading session.

Challenges to Educational Records

Students have no enforceable right to sue to enforce provisions of FERPA, which prohibits the federal funding of educational institutions that have a policy or practice of releasing educational records to unauthorized persons (*Gonzaga University v. Doe*, 536 U.S. 273 [U.S. Supreme Court 2002]). Under FERPA, only parents/guardians and adult students have the right to review and challenge educational records. Such a request must be made in writing, and EMS educators or institutional representatives must respond within 45 days. Parents' financial records and confidential letters of recommendation are not subject to this review.

HIPAA Privacy Rule

The HIPAA Privacy Rule requires EMS educational programs to safeguard patient privacy in a variety of ways (42 U.S.C.A. § 1320d-6 [2010]). For instance, with some exceptions, EMS must do the following:

- Obtain a patient's permission before speaking to third parties about the patient's medical condition (45 C.F.R. § 164.510 [2009])
- Distribute privacy notices containing information concerning use and disclosure of patients' health records (45 C.F.R. § 164.520[a] [2009])
- Allow patients to inspect their health records and request that they be modified or used restrictively (45 C.F.R. §§164.520 [2009]; 45 C.F.R. § 164.522 [2009])

Oversight

The Office for Civil Rights in the U.S. Department of Health and Human Services is responsible for enforcement of HIPAA. As the first federal legislation to protect medical privacy, HIPAA established the norm to be used throughout the nation. No state may be less restrictive than the national law; however, states may be more restrictive.

EMS educational programs should establish written policies and procedures to adequately segregate and protect patient health information that may be received inadvertently on student assignments. Collecting any patient-identifiable information should be avoided in student assignments as much as possible, and any sensitive personal information collected with other information should be destroyed.

Notice of privacy practices

EMS training educational programs that provide direct patient care are required to develop a Notice of Privacy Practices in accordance with HIPAA regulations. This document should inform patients about how their medical records will be used both within and outside the program. Records that include protected health information should be released only in accordance with HIPAA.

Teaching Tip >> *EMS educators should ensure students diligently strive to protect patients' privacy.*

Federal and State Freedom of Information Acts

Federal (5 U.S.C.A. § 552 [2009]) and most state FOIAs require EMS records and reports to be available upon request to law enforcement officers investigating criminal conduct. Such requests may be made under federal or state public records law, and may also be made for civil litigation purposes. What information requests will be honored is not clear;[30] but see *Hill v. East Baton Rouge Parish Department of Emergency Medical Services*, 925 So.2d 17 (Court of Appeal of Louisiana, First Circuit 2005), writ denied by 927 So.2d 311 (Louisiana Supreme Court 2006) exempting 911 records from public view.

Closed Circuit Television Programs

EMS educators should be knowledgeable of any closed circuit television (CCTV) program policies in the municipalities where their students have their clinical education. CCTV programs in Baltimore and Washington, DC are garnering significant attention as this practice spreads across the United States.[31] CCTV programs increasingly place government-owned cameras in public areas of the community and stream the cameras' video feeds to an observation room, where employees view multiple screens and see multiple areas of the municipality at the same time. By monitoring video feeds, EMS educators could use CCTV information to review student clinical activities and assist students in making the best decisions.

Practical issues as well as constitutional issues arise when balancing security, privacy rights, and EMS program transparency. For an effective, efficient CCTV program, EMS educators should clearly articulate their end goal in education as well as the means for which they plan to use CCTV technology for their students. Citizens may request recorded CCTV footage, and attorneys may subpoena either recordings or governmental employees who watched an incident unfold on a CCTV monitor (5 U.S.C § 552 [1966]). Students should be made aware of the possibility that the treatment they are delivering in a public place is being recorded, and could possibly be used in any subsequent litigation.

Legal Research

Because this chapter provides limited information on legal issues for EMS educators, additional research may be of value. When completing legal research, EMS educators should be cognizant of copyright laws and intellectual property.

Federal Copyright Laws and Protection

Copyright protection is afforded to original works of authorship fixed in any tangible medium of expression (17 U.S.C.A. § 102 [1990]). Most individuals think of printed materials when they hear the term copyright; however, works published on the Internet are also fully protected and subject to the same qualifications and limitations as nondigital works. Copyright protection extends to any original work of authorship in physical or electronic format, including ideas, procedures, processes, systems, methods of operation, concepts, and principles. This includes written and recorded classroom or clinical site lectures, including PowerPoints, as well as videos of classroom or clinical sites. Copyright protection,

Works Subject to Copyright Protection

According to federal law (17 U.S.C.A. §§ 101–102), works of authorship that are afforded exclusive rights as copyrighted works include the following, among others:

Category	Examples
Literary works	Textbooks, journals, reference materials, research CD-ROMs
Musical works, including accompanying words	Printed music, musical CDs, videos
Dramatic works, including accompanying music	Plays, dramas, videos, movies, musicals
Pantomimes and choreographic works	Dramatic performances, dances
Pictorial, graphic, and sculptural works	Art, statues, logos, identity marks
Motion pictures and other audiovisual works	Movies
Sound recordings	Music, radio broadcasts
Architectural works	Buildings, bridges

while going through a fundamental rethinking, endures for the following terms:

- General works (single author): the life of the author plus 70 years after the author's death
- Joint works: the life of the last surviving author plus 70 years after the last surviving author's death
- Anonymous works, pseudonymous works, and works made for hire: for 95 years from the year of the work's first publication, or a term of 120 years from the year of its first creation, whichever expires first (17 U.S.C.A. § 302 [1998])

Fair Use in Education

While many exceptions exist, U.S. copyright law provides no definitive legal standard for the acceptable scope of copyright exceptions and limitations. While the fair use doctrine, which is the first listed and best known of the exceptions listed in the Copyright Act (17 U.S.C.A. § 107), and surrounding case law provide some guidance on how exceptions can be crafted to permit beneficial and reasonable uses without causing undue harm to rights holders, fair use is a difficult concept to master. Fair use is fact specific and unique to any given situation, with a court reviewing four factors in particular when determining if the exception will apply.

With the increased number of distance-education programs now available, EMS educators should be cognizant of copyright issues. It may be tempting to copy sections of text into Web-based courses or for distribution via interactive video. However, educators should be aware that the same potential copyright violations apply to distance education as to the traditional classroom. When determining whether permission is needed for making copies of copyrighted material, it is best to err on the side of caution.

Fair Use Factors: 17 U.S.C.A. § 107

Fair Use Factor	Generally Accepted
Purpose and character of use	Nonprofit, educational, and/or personal use
Nature of work to be used	Fact-based research and publication
Amount and substantiality of material	Small amounts of copyrighted information
Effect on the potential market	No concrete response as it stands alone; depends on the nature of the previous three factors

Digital Millennium Copyright Act of 1998

The Digital Millennium Copyright Act (DMCA) (17 U.S.C.A. §§ 512, *et seq*. [2010]; 28 U.S.C.A. § 4001 [1998]) amended copyright law to address the issues raised by the emergence of the Internet and digital communications technology. Among other things, the DMCA helps protect the integrity of copyright-protected content while creating processes to permit Web-service providers, such as educational institutions, some modicum of assurance that good-faith posting of content will not be held against them. Note that the "safe harbor" provisions of the DMCA that limit service provider liability do not extend to the original poster of infringing content; individual educators still must ensure that their use of others' materials complies with copyright law.

Legal Resources

The primary legal resource for any EMS educator should be the institution's attorney or risk-management office. Those who are working for public or private EMS providers should have access to their city or county attorney or corporate attorney for private entities. The greatest single access to printed legal resources is found in public law libraries, but not every educator has such a library near where they live or work. Electronic legal research is also valuable. Remembering that educators are not always experts in the field of law, EMS educators should first and foremost rely upon formal legal counsel for advice and direction.

Summary

Legal issues affect EMS educators on a daily basis. Educators may not even be aware of the impact that federal or state laws have. Nonetheless, educators need to gain a basic understanding of the legal system and should know how to access appropriate information. Because they are rarely legal experts, educators should not become involved in legal matters without the knowledge and support of their administrators and legal counsel.

Laws, rules, and regulations may be established at the federal, state, or local level. The U.S. Constitution is the supreme law of the land, and no laws may be in conflict with it. Although federal laws establish a basis for national legal standards, state laws may be more restrictive. At no time are state or local laws allowed to be in conflict with or allow for lower expectations than federal laws.

Standards for EMS education should uphold the integrity of the profession. EMS educators should be familiar with nondiscrimination laws. Students should be treated fairly and in a nondiscriminatory manner from the time of initial recruitment through graduation. All EMS program information should be accurate and reflective of what actually exists. Students have the right to access and challenge their educational records in compliance with FERPA guidelines. Every EMS program is required to have formal, published grievance policies in place for EMS educators and students.

Tort law is especially important to EMS educators. Care should be taken to avoid assault and battery, defamation, misrepresentation, and negligence situations. The best protection against tort liability is to implement effective risk-management practices. Some of these practices include waivers and releases, safety instruction, student supervision, and careful clinical site selection. Affiliation agreements should be developed and should include all necessary components.

Educational programs should be as safe as possible. Federal laws, such as the Safe and Drug-Free Schools and Communities Act, the Gun-Free Schools Act, the Clery Act, and OSHA provide direction in establishing and maintaining safe educational environments.

EMS educators should become familiar with their own states' and institutions' rules on workers' compensation insurance. Printed information should be available regarding who and what is covered under workers' compensation. False claims of workers' compensation are considered fraud and punishable by law. It is also important for EMS educators to know which health and malpractice insurance is provided for them, or whether they are expected to provide their own coverage. The same is true with regard to students.

Confidentiality is critical in both the EMS profession and education. FERPA and HIPAA clearly define federal guidelines and standards in the areas of educational and health confidentiality.

Copyright issues should always be reviewed with students. EMS educators involved in research and publications should comply with all copyright laws. EMS educators should not reproduce material from other sources without appropriate permission when required.

Wise EMS educators should be familiar with legal issues that affect their programs. Although educators are not expected to be legal experts, a basic knowledge of legal concepts and an ability to apply them are critical in alleviating potential litigation, as is the ability to identify situations in which their institution's legal counsel should be consulted.

Glossary

affiliation agreements An agreement between the academic or educational institution and a clinical facility.

assault Occurs when one person places another person in reasonable fear of immediate harm or physical contact.

battery A physical, unlawful touching of another person without consent.

constitutional protections The U.S. Constitution prohibits any level of government from violating constitutional rights. Congress has enacted a law, 42 U.S.C.A. § 1983, that allows persons to sue a governmental actor who violates their constitutional rights. EMS educational institutions and instructors may be considered governmental actors if they receive government funding or are contracted by the government.

copyright protection Protection afforded to original works of authorship fixed in any tangible medium of expression.

defamation The sharing of true but private information that injures the reputation of another, or the intentional or reckless making of a false statement. There are two types of defamation: libel and slander.

FERPA Family Education Rights & Privacy Act of 1974 that prohibits release of a student's personally identifiable information except under certain circumstances.

fraud Misrepresentation, or the making of a false statement with intent to deceive, that causes actual harm to someone who reasonably relies upon it.

grievance A wrong considered as grounds for a complaint and potential lawsuit.

HIPAA The Health Insurance Portability and Accountability Act, which protects the medical privacy of patients.

misrepresentation Fraud, or the making of a false statement with intent to deceive, that causes actual harm to someone who reasonably relies upon it.

negligent referral The inappropriate recommendation of an individual that misrepresents qualifications or character.

risk management The process of preventing, or at least minimizing, harm or loss to a business, organization, or person.

tort A private or civil wrong or injury, other than a breach of contract, for which the law allows a remedy.

Notes

1. Legal documents may appear complicated until EMS educators become familiar with the legal system and have a basic understanding of them. As with any educational concept, legal concepts and terminology and an awareness of current litigation surrounding emergency-care practices become easier to understand the more one is aware of the issues facing EMS professionals.

   Case citations: Case citations are standardized as to the information they provide. Each citation indicates the name of the case, the title of the publication in which it is printed, the court and jurisdiction where it was decided, the decision date, and relevant, subsequent legal history, if any.

   - The plaintiff was an individual named Stephanie Peete, who brought suit against the defendant, Metropolitan Government of Nashville. The name of the case is always printed in italics; hence, *Peete v. Nashville.*
   - The number 486 indicates the volume number of the legal publication, also known as the "reporter," in which the case is published. This case was published in the *Federal Reporter* (F.) Third Series (3d). The second number, 217, represents the page of the *Federal Reporter* on which the case begins.
   - This case was decided by the Sixth U.S. Circuit Court of Appeals in the year 2007.
   - The petition for certiorari, a hearing before the U.S. Supreme Court, was denied in 2008, as reported on page 1032 in volume number 553 of the U.S. Reports.

   Statutory citations: Laws are also generally cited in a standard format, whether enacted by Congress or state legislatures. An instance of a federal nondiscrimination law is the Americans with Disabilities Act of 1990, 42 U.S.C.A. §§ 12101 *et seq.* (2009).

   - The name of the law is the Americans with Disabilities Act, otherwise known as the ADA.
   - Congress originally enacted the law in 1990.
   - The number 42 represents the title number of the U.S. Code (U.S.C.) in which the law is officially recorded. Federal law is organized into Codes, such as the Criminal Code or the Bankruptcy Code; each Code has its own title number. The U.S. Code Annotated (U.S.C.A.) is an unofficial publication that contains notes on the law, short summaries of relevant cases, and citations to other authorities on the law. It is what most attorneys prefer to use, especially because it is published and updated more frequently than the official U.S.C.
   - The symbol § identifies the cited section of the Act; when two § symbols are used the citation is referring to multiple sections.
   - The designation *et seq.* means "and following." It means that the entire law is contained in multiple sections of the title number, often too numerous to list individually. When this is the case, the number for the section given, here 12101, refers to the section of 42 U.S.C.A. in which the citation begins before continuing in other sections.
   - The year of this law's latest amendment is 2009. When different sections of the law were enacted or amended in different years, the current year is instead given because that is the year of the publication's copyright.

   Laws are originally assigned public law numbers based on the session of Congress in which they were enacted. For instance, HIPAA was initially enacted in 1996 as Public Law No. 104-191. The designation P.L. 104-191 indicates that this was the 191st law to be enacted during the 104th Congressional session.

2. All definitions in this chapter are derived from *Black's Law Dictionary* unless cited otherwise.[32]

References

1. National Highway Traffic Safety Administration (NHTSA) (2009). *A leadership guide to quality improvement for Emergency Medical Services (EMS) systems.* Washington, DC: U.S. Department of Transportation/NHTSA.
2. Cox, M. A. (2009). Laryngoscopes, lidocaine, and liability: The absence of immunity protection for prehospital providers in Indiana. *Indiana Health Law Review, 6,* 77–105.
3. Gundlach, J. (2010). The problem of ambulance diversion, and some potential solutions. *New York University Journal of Legislation and Public Policy, 13,* 175–217.
4. National Transportation Safety Board (NTSB) (2008). *Most wanted transportation safety improvements: Aviation, improve the safety of emergency medical service flights.* Washington, DC: NTSB.
5. NTSB (2006). *Special investigation report on emergency medical services operations,* Washington, DC: NTSB, p. vii.
6. Federal Aviation Administration (FAA) (2009). *Fact sheet, helicopter emergency medical service*

safety. Washington, DC: U.S. Department of Transportation/FAA.

7. Hoffman, S. (2009). Preparing for disaster: Protecting the most vulnerable in emergencies. *University of California Davis Law Review*, *42*, 1491–1547.
8. Danaher, M. G. (2010, February 26). Non-disabled individual can support claim of "improper medical inquiry" under the ADA. *Attorneys Journal*, *12*, 7–11.
9. Riesel, D., & Chorost, D. (2005). When regulatory universes collide: Environmental regulation in the workplace. *New York University Environmental Law Journal*, *13*, 613–645.
10. Occupational Safety & Health Administration (OSHA) (2004). *Principal emergency response and preparedness: Requirements and guidelines*. Washington, DC: U.S. Department of Labor/OSHA.
11. Institute of Medicine (IOM) (2006). *Emergency medical services at the crossroads*. Washington, DC: IOM.
12. NHTSA (2009). Emergency medical technician—basic: National standard curriculum. Washington, DC: U.S. Department of Transportation/NHTSA.
13. Daniels, T. B. (2008). Kentucky's statutory collateral consequences arising from felony convictions: A practitioner's guide. *Northern Kentucky Law Review*, *35*, 413–476.
14. Ho, K. K. (2009, Winter). Think twice before you tweet: Practicing restraint in a twittering, Linkedin, Facebook world. *San Francisco Attorney*, 24–27.
15. Zirkel, P. A., & Covelle, M. N. (2009). State laws for student suspension procedures: The other progeny of Goss v. Lopez. *San Diego Law Review*, *46*, 343–354.
16. Chouhoud, Y., & Zirkel, P.A. (2008). The Goss progeny: An empirical analysis. *San Diego Law Review*, *45*, 353–382.
17. Stuart, S. P. (2008). Citizen teacher: Damned if you do, damned if you don't. *University of Cincinnati Law Review*, *76*, 1281–1342.
18. Chapman, K. (2009). A preventable tragedy at Virginia Tech: Why confusion over FERPA's provisions prevents schools from addressing student violence. *Boston University Public Interest Law Journal*, *18*, 349–385.
19. Kerkhof, E. K. (2009). Myspace, yourspace, ourspace: Student cyberspeech, bullying, and their impact on school discipline. *University of Illinois Law Review*, *2009*, 1623–1624.
20. Kopel, D. B. (2009). Pretend "gun-free" school zones: A deadly legal fiction. *Connecticut Law Review*, *42*, 515–584.
21. Griffin, O. R. (2009). Constructing a legal and managerial paradigm applicable to the modern-day safety and security challenge at colleges and universities. *Saint Louis University Law Journal*, *54*, 241–270.
22. Strong, A. J. (2009). "But he told me it was safe!": The expanding tort of negligent misrepresentation. *University of Memphis Law Review*, *40*, 105–164.
23. Schulze, Jr., L. N. (2009). Balancing law student privacy interests and progressive pedagogy: Dispelling the myth that FERPA prohibits cutting-edge academic support methodologies. *Widener Law Journal*, *19*, 215–276.
24. Gupta, B. (2005). Occupational risk: The outrageous reaction to HIV-positive public safety and health care employees in the workplace. *Journal of Law & Health*, *19*, 39–73.
25. International AIDS Vaccine Initiative (IAVI) (2006). *Imagining a world without AIDS: A history of the International AIDS Vaccine Initiative*. New York, NY: IAVI.
26. DeGroat, D. M. (2009). When students test positive, their privacy fails: The unconstitutionality of South Carolina's HIV/AIDS reporting requirement. *American University Journal of Gender, Social Policy & the Law*, *17*, 751–783.
27. Blanchard, J. (2007). University tort liability and student suicide: Case review and implications for practice, *Journal of Law & Education*, *36*, 461–477.
28. Zirkel, P. A. (2010). Counterpoint introduction: Student suicide: Dying for university liability? *Journal of Law & Education*, *39*, 221–244.
29. Wiley, L. F. (2010). Adaptation to the health consequences of climate change as a potential influence on public health law and policy: From preparedness to resilience. *Widener Law Review*, *15*, 483–519.
30. Cameron, C. J. (2009). Jumping off the merry-go-round: How the federal courts will reconcile the circular deference problem between HIPAA and FOIA. *Catholic University Law Review*, *58*, 333–358.
31. Xenakis, A. B. (2010). Washington and CCTV: It's 2010, not nineteen eighty–four. *Case Western Reserve Journal of International Law*, *42*, 573–593.
32. Garner, B. A. (Ed.) (2009). *Black's law dictionary* (9th ed.). Eagan, MN: West Thomson Publishing (owned by Thomson Reuters, parent company of Delmar Cengage Learning).

Additional Resources

Ahronheim, J. C. (2009). Service by health care providers in a public health emergency: The physician's duty and the law, *Journal of Health Care Law & Policy*, *12*, 195–233.

Beebe, R., *et al.* (2010). *Fundamentals of basic emergency care.* (3rd ed.). Florence, KY: Cengage Learning (offers EMS educators an overview of National EMS Education Standards).

Centers for Disease Control & Prevention (CDC) (2009). *Advisory Committee on Immunization Practices: Influenza vaccine workgroup considerations*. Atlanta, Georgia: U.S. Department of Health & Human Services/CDC.

Cornett, L. J. (2009). Remembering the endangered "child": Limiting the definition of "safe haven" and looking beyond the safe haven law framework. *Kentucky Law Journal, 98*, 833–854.

Cvetanovich, B., & Reynolds, L. (2008). Recent development: Joshua Omvig Veterans Suicide Prevention Act of 2007. *Harvard Journal on Legislation, 45*, 619–640.

Gifford, D. G. (2008). Impersonating the legislature: State attorneys general and *parens patriae* product litigation. *Boston College Law Review, 49*, 913–969.

Grafft, J. A., & Grafft, K. K. (2011). *Essentials for the emergency medical responder*. Florence, KY: Cengage Learning (offers EMS educators an overview of National EMS Education Standards).

Grossman, J. L. (2010). Pregnancy, work, and the promise of equal citizenship. *Georgetown Law Journal, 98*, 567–628.

Hamner, J. C. (2009). Regulating safety: Can the National Transportation Safety Board and the Federal Aviation Administration improve the safety of EMS flights? *Journal of Air Law & Commerce, 74*, 597–626.

Khoday, A. (2009). Prime-time saviors: The West Wing and the cultivation of a unilateral American responsibility to protect. *Southern California Interdisciplinary Law Journal, 19*, 1–53.

Marks, C. M. (2010, July 3). Free speech in question when talking out of school. *Wall Street Journal*, p. A-3.

May, C. (2009). "Internet-savvy students" and bewildered educators: Student Internet speech is creating new legal issues for the educational community. *Catholic University Law Review, 58*, 1105–1141.

Nelson, C. A. (2010). Racializing disability, disabling race: Policing race and mental status. *Berkeley Journal of Criminal Law, 15*, 1–64.

Novogrodsky, N. (2009). The duty of treatment: Human rights and the HIV/AIDS pandemic. *Yale Human Rights & Development Law Journal, 12*, 1–61.

O'Brien, K. J. (2008). Federal regulation of state employment under the commerce clause and "national defense" powers: Constitutional issues presented by the Public Safety Employer–Employee Cooperation Act. *Boston College Law Review, 49*, 1175–1211.

Olick, R. S., *et al.* (2009). Recent developments in New York law: Taking the MOLST (medical orders for life-sustaining treatment) statewide. *Pace Law Review, 29*, 545–559.

Occupational Safety & Health Administration (OSHA) (2009). *Best practices for protecting EMS responders during treatment and transport of victims of hazardous substance releases*. Washington, DC: U.S. Department of Labor/OSHA.

Propper, V. H. (2010). One treatment, two individuals: An analysis of health economics and the Age Discrimination Act of 1975 in the context of a public health emergency event. *Journal of Medicine & Law, 14*, 215–247.

Smith II, G. P. (2009). Reshaping the common good intimes of public health emergencies: Validating medical triage.*Annals of Health Law, 18*, 1–34.

Sonderling, K. E. (2009). POLST: A cure for the common advance directive: It's just what the physician ordered. *Nova Law Review, 33*, 451–480.

Stanger, K. C., *et al.* (2008). Consent for health care under Idaho law: A primer. *Idaho Law Review, 44*, 379–420.

Stelter, J. D. (2008). The IRS's classification settlement program: Is it an adequate tool to relieve taxpayer burden for small businesses that have misclassified workers as independent contractors? *Cleveland State Law Review, 56*, 451–481.

Wang, H. E., *et al.* (2008). Tort claims and adverse events in emergency medical services. *Annals of Emergency Medicine, 52*, 256–262.

Zande, K. (2009). When the school bully attacks in the living room: Using Tinker to regulate off-campus student cyberbullying. *Barry Law Review, 13*, 103–136.

Zigmond, J. (2008, November 3). Flight plans: NTSB adds EMS flights to "most wanted" safety list. *Modern Healthcare, 33*, 44–56.

PART IV
Delivering the Message

One thing is true about the learning process: it is not static. Learning can take on many different shapes, can employ all forms of media, and may involve groups of many sizes and activities of all kinds. One must add to this the fact that Emergency Medical Services (EMS) educators and students must adapt the learning process to some of the most difficult circumstances known to education. The educator must consider the need to coach a single student on assessing pulses with a lab manikin; teach spinal immobilization to a small group in severe heat or in a very cold temperature; explain cardiac physiology during a distance education course; and model compassionate patient care during an actual call for a sick intoxicated person. In all these situations, EMS educators must tailor their instruction if the best results are to be achieved.

Variety is the spice of life, as the saying goes, and so it is with teaching and learning. Sometimes, the most *efficient* method is the least *effective* method of teaching. The tips and techniques described in these chapters are tools that you will undoubtedly find useful in your practice to maximize learning and retention. This part of the text introduces teaching strategies for individual students, small groups, large groups, distance-learning students, simulation and students in field and clinical settings.

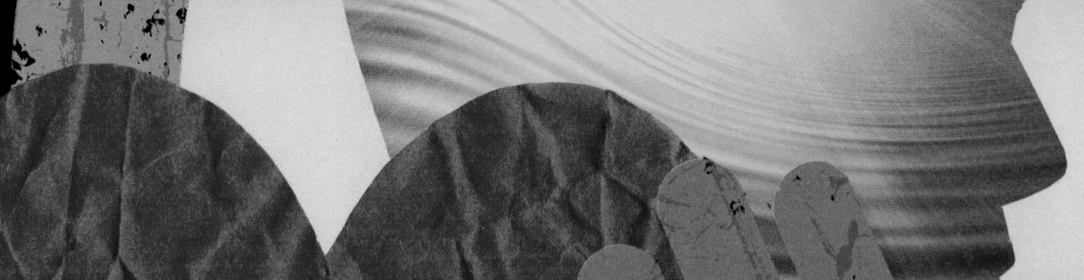

11 Introduction to Teaching Strategies

The mediocre teacher tells. The good teacher explains. The superior teacher demonstrates. The great teacher inspires. — William Arthur Ward

Teaching strategies vary depending on the setting, the students, and most commonly the instructor. We frequently teach the way we were taught, since that is often what we are the most comfortable with. However, that strategy may not be the most effective way for students to learn and to make meaningful changes in knowledge and behavior. Faculty must consciously make instructional method decisions to promote student growth in all domains of learning—cognitive, psychomotor, and affective. There are many techniques that allow the instructor to be more effective in facilitating learning.

CHAPTER GOAL: This chapter discusses the evolving teaching strategy of **student-centered learning** as well as **facilitation** and questioning techniques to enhance learning.

Traditional Education

Traditional education uses as its centerpiece the lecture format, perhaps because it is an efficient way to deliver a large amount of material to any size audience. It is said that we teach the way we were taught. Since the traditional approach to the classroom of "I teach, you listen" is likely the way most current educators were taught, it is no surprise that it is often the most common technique used by today's EMS educators.

Teacher-Centered Learning

Teacher-centered learning focuses around the teacher and lecture. Although the lecture format itself is not problematic, major reliance on this type of teaching tool can lead to problems because of its teacher-centered approach.

One problem created by the "mostly lecture" approach is that the lecture and the textbook become the major delivery system of information for students. Students are expected to listen, read, and be prepared to take and pass tests. Their success is determined by how well they can memorize the information that is presented. This type of instruction places a high value on memorization, which is usually a low-level learning task. Recall of straight facts is usually at the "knowledge" level of the cognitive domain, most likely to be forgotten, and least likely capable of being applied to other circumstances in which the student may need to use the information.

Another problem with "mostly lecture" is students become submissive in the educational process and learning is passive. When students need only to sit and listen, and perhaps take notes, they are not engaged in the learning process. Again, they are more likely to forget the information and least likely to be able to apply the information when needed, such as in an atypical patient-presentation situation. They may also fail to learn critical-thinking skills.

In classrooms where lecture is the primary delivery model, it becomes difficult to assess the *affective* component of education. A teacher-centered environment does not provide time or opportunity for the instructor to facilitate development of the whole person. The focus is too often on ensuring that students have the information needed to pass their exams, rather than developing the character and critical-thinking skills needed to apply the information to real-life challenges.

Usually in a classroom focused only on lecture, the lesson plan is prepared in advance and facilitated by use of PowerPoint. Because these presentations are predetermined, students are not allowed to be *stakeholders* in the direction and scope of their education. Instructors act as if they know best and dictate the pace and focus of students' education. Instructors who subscribe to this philosophy often believe that students who fall behind must not have the aptitude needed to master the information. However, it is possible that they are bored or have yet to be engaged in the material by a teacher who has valued the students' life experiences as they may relate to the material at hand.

Emerging Trends

As the body of evidence grows regarding memory, cognition, and how the brain receives, processes, stores, and retrieves information, all educators from kindergarten teachers to college professors are being forced to re-evaluate the traditional, teacher-centered approach to education.

Student-Centered Learning

Educators should consider the value of alternate methods of presenting information that puts the *learner* at the center of the educational event. The evidence is becoming increasingly clear: in order to reach higher-level learning goals such as synthesis and evaluation, or what many would call "application, problem solving, and critical thinking," the *learner* must *do* something with the information. The students must experience the material, relate it to their own life experiences, make judgments about it, and create meaning regarding how the information will be used. It is highly unlikely that those educational events are going to occur during a lecture, since most of what is told to students will be forgotten.

A student-centered approach uses innovative teaching strategies that create an active and exciting learning environment. This does not mean that some traditional approaches such as lecture are abandoned; rather, they are used less frequently to afford time for discussion, group work, case studies, role play, scenarios, writing assignments, games, and other activities which are known to promote collaboration, communication, and problem solving. A student-centered approach creates a shared experience wherein the student becomes a stakeholder in the educational process and introduces a sense of community to the learning process.

One characteristic of the student-centered approach is that the learning process is fluid and should be engaging for both the teacher and students. The goal is discovery of information and a shared commitment to excellence. Subjects are explored from a variety of sources inside and outside the classroom. Students present materials to the class and have some control as to the pace of instruction and the amount of material that is shared. If students have a problem understanding a module, more time can be committed to ensure mastery of a particular area. This process minimizes the artificial time constraints that are typically imposed on the learning process.

In the student-centered approach to learning, the experiences of students are respected, and the teacher becomes more of a facilitator than the focal point of instruction. Students are viewed as experts who have a wide array of life experiences that they bring to the classroom experience. The students' own experiences are woven into the instruction so that clarity can be achieved from various points of view. Students are encouraged to relate their life experiences to the material that is presented. For example, if an instructor had a fire engineer in his EMT refresher class, the instructor might relate the concept of septic shock to the student and the class by asking "what would happen if, after you have primed the line to the fire, I poked holes in the hose with an ice pick?" The student would likely answer that the line will lose pressure. The instructor would then ask him how he would try to rectify the situation so that the firefighters on the nozzle still got enough water pressure. He would likely answer by saying, "I would have to try to compensate by increasing the pressure." And so the instructor would relate the concept of distributive shock as a loss of vascular tone and pressure from fluid leaking out of the vascular space, causing hypotension and shock. While this could have been a difficult concept to grasp, by using an example that this student and likely many others in the group were familiar with from their own life experiences, the instructor engaged the students. The instructor increased the likelihood that they will be able not only to recall but to apply the concept, and even begin to problem solve how the body might compensate during times of distributive shock.

In a student-centered classroom, students are given responsibilities in the classroom, lab, and clinical setting to foster a sense of community, respect, and discipline **(Figure 11.1)**. The EMS profession requires that students be ready to accept leadership responsibilities. The seeds of leadership can be planted in the classroom by assignment of roles that allow students to practice and improve their leadership skills. The classroom experience can be enhanced by appointment of a class representative or officers, a roll taker, equipment officers, note takers, lab assistants, and team leaders on community-service projects. Another effective technique is to pair advanced students with instructional staff in the lab to help train and educate students who need more help. This cooperative educational technique is a powerful and productive tool

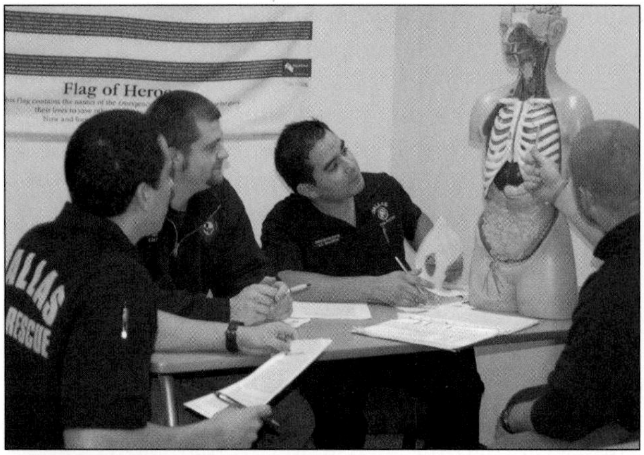

Figure 11.1
Learner-centered classes bring a sense of personal responsibility to the classroom.

for any EMS institution. Although the intended goal is to build leadership skills, the instructor will also note that many positive and powerful attributes in terms of respect, discipline, and a sense of community are realized. In the final analysis, students become a part of the learning process and are better prepared to enter the profession.

In traditional classrooms, a concerted effort is made to develop the whole student through equal emphasis placed on values and character as they relate to academic study. Too many instructors believe that the value of an education for students is measured in their success in tackling the cognitive and psychomotor domains. Very little value has been placed on the affective domain, and yet issues around the students' affect, or behavior and attitudes, are the leading cause of complaints, not only from instructors but from employers. While it is true that there is no room for incompetence, the affective domain may be more critical to the quality of patient care and what this student will contribute to the profession than all the knowledge and skills the instructors push students to master. Helping students understand their strengths and limitations in relation to their values and character can mean more to a student or an employer than has ever been previously understood. Values and feelings can impact our clinical decision making and judgment about patients and their care more than we realize.[1]

One of the goals of EMS education must be to create lifelong learners and prepare them for a career of self-discovery in a constantly changing and dynamic profession. Because medicine is a science, what they do for patients and how they practice medicine will constantly change throughout their careers. Students should not view the end of the class as the end of their education. Regular assignments that require students to read about their profession and present topics of interest to their classmates can be crucial to establishing the practice of continued education and discovery in a complex and changing profession.

The *Case in Point* on page 157 puts students at the center of the learning and places the instructor in the role of facilitating the process. Students remain active throughout the process by formulating responses, defending their position, practicing compromise, and looking at the subject critically. This student-centered, active, multidimensional approach is the very "glue" that will help reinforce the subject matter and make it stick.

Techniques to Enhance Student-Centered Learning

Several techniques and concepts are common to enhancing student-centered learning, whether this is done in individual student sessions, small groups, or large groups. These include facilitation techniques, group work, questioning techniques, and **experiential learning**.

Facilitation Techniques

Student-centered instruction places the student at the center of the learning process, and the instructor assumes the role of facilitator. Facilitation is an important teaching strategy, and a better understanding of how it is accomplished is important for the educator.

Creation of a relaxed atmosphere that is focused more on the learner constitutes the core of facilitation. In fact, *facilitate* means "to make easier." This strategy allows the educator to create an environment in which student learning is enhanced by interaction and engagement. Coaching, mentoring, feedback, and positive reinforcement represent a variety of techniques that are considered facilitative strategies for learning.

Keys to Facilitation

Facilitation has also been called "the guide on the side" by Allison King, Jon Van Ast, and other adult educational researchers. One of the key elements of facilitation is for the instructor to create action in the classroom in which students experience or do something with the information. This is done, in part, by avoiding lectures when possible and engaging learners in activities, such as writing, role-playing, and cooperative group work.

CASE IN POINT

CLASSROOM TOPIC: DRUG ABUSE

Instructor-Centered Method

The instructor tells students to read the substance abuse chapter in the assigned textbook, and then provides a lecture to support what is in the textbook. Follow-up consists of a written test on the subject.

Learner-Centered Method

The instructor gives a scenario and asks the students to decide if they believe the scenario on the board is or is not drug abuse. Perhaps the scenario is "your babysitter and her boyfriend are caught smoking marijuana in the backyard while the baby takes a nap." If students believe that this is an example of drug abuse, they must physically move to one side of the classroom. If they do not think this is drug abuse, they move to the other side, creating two opposing groups of students. Volunteers are then asked to share their rationale for their opinion. Because the teacher is asking the students' opinion, there is no right or wrong answer, and it becomes a safe place to make a decision. However, the physical act of moving to one side of the room forces the student to decide and prohibits indecision, since decision-making capability is an important skill in emergency medicine. Next, the instructor gives one or two more examples and asks the students to again move to one side of the room or the other, depending on their opinion. Another scenario might be a high school wrestler who uses speed to meet a weight requirement, or a police officer who goes to the local tavern after every shift to have a few beers and wind down.

The instructor then asks students to take out a blank piece of paper and write down in their own words the definition of "drug abuse," as they understand it. Once the students have had three or four minutes to formulate a response, they are paired with another student in the class to compare answers. Each pair must arrive at an entirely new definition based on input from both students. Once each pair of students has developed a revised definition, the instructor requests that each team pair up with another team and repeat the process. The pairing process is repeated until three or four large groups have been formed, each with its own definition arrived at through teamwork and collaboration. At the conclusion of the exercise, each team reads its definition or writes it on the board. The instructor asks the class to compare and contrast the various definitions until final agreement is reached regarding which definition is most correct given the textbook information. A short discussion can then ensue about how their own personal experiences with drugs and alcohol shaped their initial decisions about each scenario, and whether or not it was technically "drug abuse."

First, the instructor should consider the layout of the classroom (see Chapter 6: The Learning Environment for more details). The arrangement of the classroom sends a signal to students about the class session. The use of groups in facilitation may be made most beneficial when the instructor sets up tables and semiprivate work areas, so that greater interaction can take place between students and instructors. The goal of this strategy is to take the emphasis off the instructor as the "gatekeeper of information" and to place the burden of interaction with the group. This creates interaction between learners but still allows interaction with the instructor, who will manage the learning activities.

The importance of creating the expectation in learners that they are required to participate actively in the learning process cannot be overstated. Students have been conditioned to be "tourists" or visitors in the classroom. They have been conditioned to be passive observers, much like those who are on vacation. Tourists follow the tour guide, taking pictures and having minimal interaction with anyone in the museum, then move on to the next destination. Instructors must work to limit tourists in the classroom by actively seeking student participation in the learning process, which may be foreign to many. Patience, guidance, and positive reinforcement of learners are necessary as they move into this new area. As students succeed, their expectations for learning will change in very positive ways.

Promoting active participation of class members is a way educators can increase the success of facilitation in the classroom. One method of increasing participation is to have students assist in some of the day-to-day activities of the course. This may involve something as simple as having them set up the room or bring in equipment. In academic settings, class leaders are often appointed to assist the instructor in maintaining control when breaks begin and end. When not actively involved in a scenario or role-playing exercise, students can act as recorders, time keepers, and note takers. *Peer observation allows all learners to gain constructive feedback in a setting that is actively engaged.* Stronger students can serve as mentors or coaches when they study in groups or when they assist others in learning and perfecting skills.

Educators may assign roles, such as leader, scribe, and reporter, to various members in the class. Strategies used to assign roles to learners must be creative so they are as fair as possible for students. Techniques include alphabetical order, birth date, hiring date (oldest or youngest), color lottery, random numbers, and a sticker on a name tag or chair. Whichever manner is chosen, duties should be rotated equally among the student body so that favoritism is avoided.

Not everyone will agree with or like this new style of learning. Some students will continue to be passive learners despite the instructor's best efforts. The instructor must not be discouraged; it takes effort and persistence to move into the use of facilitation. As the instructor works to include the reluctant learner in the process, eventually the student may choose to willingly participate or may be coerced by fellow classmates to actively participate in the learning process. The student-centered learning approach takes more effort on the part of the student. Instructors may find students who simply do not want to exert the effort required to prepare for and participate in class. Grades for affective behavior and participation, as well as clear expectations in class syllabi, make it clear that such behavior will not be acceptable in the EMS course and will be reflected in grading.

Occasionally other, more traditional faculty will be critical of the facilitation process as facilitated classrooms are livelier, and sometimes louder, appearing as if the instructor has less control of the classroom. EMS educators moving toward facilitation and active learning may find themselves in a position to have to cite the research about how retention is more dependent upon depth of processing than how many times material is reviewed[2] or other brain-based learning principles in order to defend their more modern, more effective approach to teaching and learning.

Facilitating Discussions

Facilitation requires active learner participation; one of the easiest forms of participatory learning is discussion. This technique is effective for many different types of courses, including continuing education or refresher classes, in which concepts are reviewed and topics involving opinions are discussed. Facilitation can also be used to motivate a class start-up or a review. In order to keep all learners actively engaged in the discussion, the instructor could have small groups discuss the same idea. This is effective because all students are actively working toward the solution simultaneously without the anxiety of having to share their response with the large class. It is harder to opt-out of a small group discussion, but if some students become distracted or inattentive, they should be redirected back to the group for participation. It may also be helpful to give each group an opportunity to evaluate each other on their contributions to the group after such exercises, reinforcing the concept of accountability for participation in the group. Rubric-type evaluations can be used at the end to determine the success of the group as a whole and/or individual participation. This may help identify a group problem or weakness such as one person dominating the discussion.

The instructor can keep everyone engaged in the discussion by moving the responses from group to group in an unpredictable pattern. A prop or some other strategy, such as drawing the name of the group out of a hat, will work just fine. Facilitating takes more time to accomplish than does simply lecturing to the group.Keep in mind that it is not necessary to comment on each person's contribution; rather, it is more important that students contribute. To check for understanding of the instructor and of the learners, one might paraphrase the responses so that key points can be easily made for the entire group.

Teaching Tip >> *One way in which the instructor can ensure that students remain focused is to establish a time when the group will come together and report back on its work or progress. With these mini-deadlines in place, students know that they are responsible for giving a progress report and will more readily stay on task. For example, if a set of 10 small cases is provided for students to work through, the instructor should not request completion of all 10 at one sitting. Instead, the class should be divided into groups, with three or four cases assigned to each group. Students work on three cases, then the entire class comes together to discuss those cases. The small groups re-form to work on the next three cases. This keeps the class working together, and if one group is not working as it should, the groups can be reconfigured before they get together again. This can appear to be the instructor's initial strategy so no one has hurt feelings. This approach also allows the instructor to group students who would not usually work together.*

The instructor should compliment the student on a good comment and redirect an inaccurate or incorrect statement to the group, so students understand, stay on track, and avoid becoming confused. Sometimes many answers are heard but it can be difficult for students to determine which was the "right" answer. If a "right" answer is shared according to the objectives or what might be tested, be sure every student is clear about that answer.

Similar to diplomats, educators are often required to mediate differences of opinion in the classroom.To perform this delicate balancing act, one must try to keep the discussion going without interjecting oneself as the authority—a move that could damage momentum. Students should be encouraged to back up their statements with facts, and everyone must be reminded that differing opinions are important to an active and engaged learning community.

Close the session by summarizing what occurred in the discussion and by providing follow-up information for additional studying or reading, so that the group knows where they have been and where they are going in the future.

Facilitation is challenging for educators, and can be frustrating for students at first. When students encounter difficulty with an assignment, they may be more willing to give up and quit working than to ask for assistance. The instructor must be careful not to do students' work for them. Rather, the instructor should be ready to offer assistance to help students locate the necessary resources and should keep learners actively involved in the lesson. In short, a key element of facilitation is to help students become more resourceful and capable of problem solving, with less reliance on an instructor.

Teaching Tip >> *One way by which the instructor can maintain learner involvement is to invoke the "three before me" technique before intervening. This technique requires that when asking for help, learners must inform the instructor of at least three places where they have looked to find the information. They should be directed to the appropriate resources if they have not located enough information on their own. However tempting, it is not in the learners' best interest for the instructor to simply tell them the correct answers, even though this may appear easier.*

The goal of the educator is to assist students in becoming critically thinking professionals as they move from lower levels of learning to higher levels of learning. This is nearly impossible to accomplish if learners are not active participants in the learning process. Rarely do they argue with the results of their own learning when they discover the answers themselves. If a topic is learned by this method, students "own it."

Group Work or Collaborative Learning

In real life, EMS problems are often solved by a team approach to a situation. Not every student is comfortable working with others, but teamwork is an important goal of EMS education and included in the evaluation process. Instructors will need to create opportunities for students to learn to work effectively in teams. Some identify disadvantages of this method of learning, noting that students typically progress at varying rates and that quiet students may not feel comfortable in a team setting. Additionally, teams may inadvertently increase competition among students and some students may succumb to conformity just to fit in. Nevertheless, groups frequently devise solutions that are better than the most advanced student and learn better from each other than from the teacher.[3]

Because time is precious, classroom groups should be identified in a quick and efficient manner. Some situations dictate that groups should stay the same; others do not. EMS personnel will not always be working with the same partner or crew, and variation among members of groups, as well as among skill levels, can enhance the overall performance of individual members and of the team.

Use of randomization techniques such as counting off, drawing numbers, or some other method allows learners to maintain some control in the sorting process. If the teacher controls selection, it can be done ahead of time based on the instructor's knowledge of the group, keeping in mind student strengths and limitations.

Effective Group Management

For groups to work effectively, written ground rules must be established at the first meeting. Certain mandates should be assigned by the facilitator, including attending class sessions on time, completing all assignments before class and being prepared to discuss them, notifying other group members in advance if class will be missed, willingly sharing information, respecting the values, views, and ideas of others, and abiding by all other rules as agreed on by the group.

One of the most effective strategies for managing a group of learners in a team is to add one additional member whose sole job is to function as a peer facilitator to guide the group and help resolve conflicts. Members of each group must actively rotate roles within the group so that all students can gain experience in all areas of the activity **(Figure 11.2)**. The peer facilitator, if used, or activity leader works to

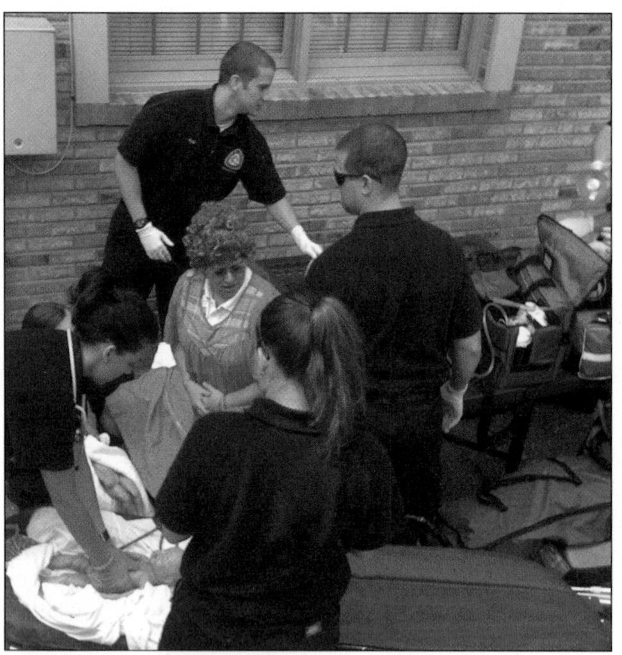

Courtesy of St. Charles County Ambulance District

Figure 11.2

Creative educators can making learning easier for students by requiring their active participation.

keep the group on track and monitors participation of group members. The recorder, or scribe, records assignments, strategies, unresolved issues, and data, and may convene the group outside of class when necessary. The reporter is responsible for reporting the group's findings to the entire class during discussions and writes a final draft of all assignments. The accuracy coach or timekeeper checks for understanding of the group, locates resources, and manages time.

Time spent in facilitated learning should be short in the beginning of the course, and then build to longer segments as students demonstrate their ability to perform appropriately and stay on task. The class must be brought together for discussion and clarification of issues at frequent intervals throughout the session. Educators may need to specifically identify which objectives were covered through the group activity or discussion to keep students from feeling like the activity "was a waste of time." In addition, the instructor should plan for individual and group assignments. The opportunity for group members to take the assignment lightly can damage the effectiveness of the strategy. The instructor must remain vigilant for behavior that might diminish the group's strength and undermine it. Peer facilitators can be used to assist both the learners and the instructor in maintaining the integrity of this strategy.

Conflict Resolution In Group Work

Not everyone in a family always gets along with one another, and members of the learning community are no different from a family. In fact, they may actually spend more time with one another than family members do. Tempers often flare when people spend a great deal of time with one another in close proximity. Several levels exist at which the instructor can reduce the likelihood that conflicts will escalate.

The first level focuses on preventing escalation of a conflict.The instructor should monitor the group for early signs of conflict such as raised voices or defensive body language and should intervene immediately to prevent additional problems. Group evaluations can assist the instructor in monitoring individual student behavior that may need correction.

The second level of conflict resolution centers on student empowerment.The instructor must listen to students' concerns and encourage them to peacefully resolve any conflicts they may be experiencing. Educators can coach students on strategies for possible resolution of conflicts. If a peer leader is involved, this person should not be undermined in front of the other students, or he or she will lose authority among them. The instructor should speak with this leader before he or she addresses the other group members to ensure s a game plan is in place for resolving the issue.

The next level of conflict requires active resolution of problems that may arise. Each participant must be allowed to present his or her point while the others actively listen. Students should be asked to define their ideas on an expected outcome, although no guarantees exist that these will be honored. The instructor's role is to facilitate the discussion of possible outcomes that may affect those involved in the conflict. If a peer leader participates, the instructor may serve as an observer while the peer leader manages the conflict.

Questioning Techniques

Another way by which the instructor can move toward a more student-centered classroom is through questioning. *Questioning* is an inquiry that invites a response. Thought-provoking questions used in the classroom can promote active thinking and stimulate higher-level learning and problem-solving skills. This technique can increase interaction between the teacher and students and assist with application in the patient care environment.

Socratic Method

The **Socratic method** of questioning is a popular method with law and philosophy professors, but can have a place in the EMS classroom too. The Socratic method of questioning uses the practice of asking, rather than telling, to arouse curiosity in the subject matter so students will arrive at their own conclusions rather than being told the "right" answer. The process uses logical, incremental questions designed to challenge assumptions and move students toward greater specificity in their answers as they apply principles on their own. The following is a description of the process: The instructor will call on a student who has presumably read the material for this class session. This method has been criticized because it could be embarrassing if a student is not prepared. However, students are allowed an "occasional pass" if they truly do not feel prepared. The instructor will ask for the student's opinion, which negates the concept that an answer is wholly right or wrong, further making the Socratic method safe to use in the classroom. Next, the student will paraphrase the concepts from the reading and the instructor asks if the student agrees or disagrees with the idea. The student is asked to defend his or her position, backing up his or her opinion with fact and logic. The instructor's role is to continue asking questions, or, some would say "playing devil's advocate," until the student is able to conclude confidently that he or she was justified in the answer based on the facts and logic explored in the questioning.

CASE IN POINT

The instructor presents the case of a 54-year-old man with a history of chronic obstructive pulmonary disease (COPD), who is short of breath, speaking in three-word bursts, sitting in tripod position, with circumoral and nailbed cyanosis. The instructor asks the class "what should we do for him?" A student answers, "Put him on oxygen." The instructor, "Yes, that's correct! Why should we put him on oxygen?" Note the strong reinforcement of the correct answer here. If the instructor fails to reinforce that the student does have the right answer, he or she is likely to change the answer, seeing it as a challenge to their thinking. Instructors and employers do not want EMTs or paramedics to waffle in their on-scene decision making. Reinforcement that they have the correct answer is essential to building confidence. The student now may answer something low-level, such as "Because he needs oxygen." Encourage the student to elaborate with more questions, such as "How can you tell he needs oxygen?" The student then replies, "Because he looks hypoxic." Instructor says, "Which signs or symptoms demonstrated hypoxia?" And so the exchange goes, reinforcing the right answer and building the student's confidence in his or her knowledge. Plus, this increases the likelihood that the student will answer again in the future.

Building Confidence in Decision Making

Because EMS professionals function in high-stress, time-pressured environments, decision-making ability is imperative to their success. Yet, frequently educators hear from preceptors and field-training officers that interns and new employees "just won't make a decision" on scene. New practitioners seem paralyzed by the choices they face and consequences of their decisions. Educators can assist students in learning to trust their decisions by reinforcing the correct choices they make in the classroom. Confidence breeds competence, and competence, or making the correct choices, breeds confidence. Essentially, instructors should make an effort to "catch" students doing things right, and reinforce their right decisions with praise and positive feedback. But, just saying "good answer" is not enough. The instructor has to help students see how they arrived at the right answer, and that their decision making is solid.

Wait Time

Wait time is an important concept in questioning techniques. It is important that students be given time to think about questions posed to them and to ponder their response. However, it is not unusual for an instructor to wait only one or two seconds for students to respond, and when nobody does, the instructor gives the answer. When the instructor simply gives the answer, students come to know the questions as rhetorical, where the instructor was not really expecting a response anyway. In these classrooms, students never bother to think about the question and attempt to formulate a response. Waiting a reasonable amount of time, which has been suggested might be anywhere from 8 to 30 seconds, before calling on a student can increase the number of students who respond and the length of their responses. Before asking a question, the instructor can insist that no one raise his or her hand to answer. This discourages the situation in which the predictable students raise their hands and others immediately quit seeking the answer. By waiting, students are more likely to consider the question. After waiting, the instructor calls on a random student or a volunteer and asks the student to answer. This method allows more students to be involved in the process.[4] The technique is known as **ask, pause, and call (Figure 11.3)**.

Other Questioning Techniques

Other questioning techniques can be used to engage students. One is the "overhead question," which is given to the whole group, sometimes embedded

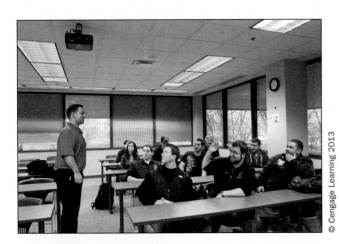

Figure 11.3

Effective questioning techniques include the use of thought-provoking questions and the "ask, pause, and call" technique.

into the PowerPoint presentation, without calling on someone in particular. After most have written down an answer on paper or a personal dry erase board, the instructor "calls for" an answer. The teacher can either ask all students to raise their boards at the same time to see how many had the correct answer, or ask for a volunteer to elaborate on the correct answer. The "relay question" involves calling on different students to add or comment on the previous student's responses until all important information has been obtained. Another technique is the "reverse question," wherein the instructor answers a student's question with another question or asks the class to respond.

Experiential Learning

Another concept important to EMS classroom and clinical educators is the use of experiential learning. Carl Rogers was a pioneering psychotherapist who wrote extensively on the concept of experiential learning.[5] He felt so strongly about the role that experience plays in how individuals learn that he distinguished learning into two distinct types: cognitive (which Rogers described as "meaningless") and experiential (which he deemed as "significant"). He wrote that "all human beings have a natural propensity to learn; the role of the teacher is to facilitate such learning." According to Rogers, learning is facilitated when (1) the student participates completely in the learning process and has control over its nature and direction, (2) it is primarily based on direct confrontation with practical, social, personal, or research problems, and (3) self-evaluation is the principal method of assessing progress or success. Rogers also emphasizes the importance of learning to learn and being open to change. As medicine relies heavily on continuing education and learning throughout one's career, being concerned with teaching students how to learn and inspiring curiosity and inquisition ought to be a primary consideration for any health professions educator.

Rogers identified the following five core elements of facilitation that are necessary for successful experiential learning:

1. Setting a positive climate for learning where students understand this to be a safe place to make mistakes. This means not allowing hazing, harassment, or teasing when mistakes are made, and giving regular, timely, honest feedback, including positive feedback for correct decisions and tasks well done.
2. Clarifying the purposes of the learner(s), such as why they are taking the class, what they hope to gain, and how they will use this information in their jobs or lives.
3. Organizing and making learning resources available, while teaching students to be resourceful. This might be access to lab equipment, helpful websites to practice ECG interpretation, or referral to a mentor in the field who can help them to navigate the social norms of the profession.
4. Balancing intellectual and emotional components of learning, such as learning to trust their instincts, to handle the stress of a bad emergency situation, or the grief of a patient who died in their care.
5. Sharing feelings and thoughts with learners but not dominating, which is similar to the concepts of facilitation used in discussion and other classroom activities already explored in this chapter.

EMS is the ideal discipline by which the benefits of experiential learning can be maximized, because so much of what is done by care providers can be recreated in the classroom through the use of patient care scenarios. In addition, most students will spend valuable time in the clinical and field settings, hoping to apply what they have learned in the classroom. Chapter 19: Tools for Field and Clinical Learning details how instructors can maximize the clinical experience for students. Following are examples of classroom scenarios that can be used to maximize the potential for experiential learning.

For the following example, a standard as been taken directly from the 2009 U.S. Department of Transportation National EMS Education Standards for the EMT.

Example 1: Fundamental Depth and Foundational Breadth of the Anatomy, Physiology, Pathophysiology, Assessment and Management of the Acute Coronary Syndrome to Include Angina Pectoris and Myocardial Infarction

It is easy enough for the instructor to ask students to read the text on cardiovascular emergencies, then discuss in class the rationale for administering a particular medication for the management of chest pain. However, use of this standard to drive a patient scenario can be much more effective.

"The process whereby knowledge is created through the transformation of experience," is how David Kolb, a leading expert in the study of experiential learning, defines learning. "Knowledge results from the combination of grasping and transforming experience."[6] **Kolb's theory** describes two ways that learners can transform experience into knowledge—reflective observation and active experimentation. Kolb believes that learners transform their previous experience into new knowledge by evaluating and building on this foundation. Many things that are easily done in the EMS classroom can serve as excellent models for these two modes of learning. In the chest pain scenario, students actively engaged in a simulated patient encounter learn through active experimentation. The simulated patient is preprogrammed to provide certain responses to help guide students in performing appropriate steps without providing obvious direction. Observers and participants benefit from reflective observation by participating in a follow-up critique of how the patient was treated.

Following is another example of experiential learning in which the instructor uses active exploration as a means of reinforcing a particular learning objective.

Example 2: Fundamental Depth and Foundational Breadth of Techniques of Physical Examination of the Neurological System

This objective could easily be approached by lecture and is generally covered quite well in the textbook with the use of illustrations. However, allowing students to experience the practice of assessing pupils and having them see and document their findings will help cement the knowledge through experiential learning.

The examples shown are just a few of the ways in which an instructor can use an alternative or student-centered method to meet common objectives. Through the process of trial and error, the instructor discovers which methods work best for certain objectives. The challenge for the EMS educator is to

CASE IN POINT

LIVE SCENARIO

Two or three students are selected to play EMTs and are asked to leave the room. Another student is selected to play the role of the patient; this student should be instructed to present with all the classic signs and symptoms of cardiac chest pain, including a recent history of angina. Additional input can be solicited from the class regarding how this patient should present. The patient is provided with a small bottle of medication labeled as nitroglycerin. Small mints or some similar candy is placed in the bottle to represent the medication. The patient is instructed to "pass out" should the EMTs decide to administer the medication before a baseline blood pressure has been established, or if the EMT fails to determine how many pills the patient has already taken, or whether or not the patient has taken sexually enhancing drugs such as Cialis or Viagra.

The primary objectives of the scenario are (1) to reinforce the need to establish a minimum blood pressure before medication is administered, and (2) to gather an appropriate history before any medication is given. Several secondary objectives may come up during the postscenario critique.

The EMTs are brought into the room with a simulated dispatch, such as "Rescue 51: respond code 3 to residence for a man with chest pain." The scenario is allowed to progress until the instructor believes it has met the stated objective and concludes with a brief critique. For example, if the students do give the nitroglycerin without first assessing a blood pressure, the simulated patient becomes unconscious and the call can be stopped. The team of responders, beginning first with the team leader, should have an opportunity to critique his or her own performance and state why he or she thinks the patient went unconscious. Self-assessment is a key element of development in experiential education and should be encouraged. Other members of the team would then be given an opportunity to comment on what went well and what did not relative to the objective of the scenario. Students who are observing are invited to critique the team's performance. The instructor's job is to steer the critique along the path toward the intended objective, encouraging students to think critically and experience the learning, rather than just hearing or reading about it.

CASE IN POINT

EXPERIMENTING WITH PUPIL REACTIONS

It is difficult for students to actually see pupil changes in a well-lit room. For this reason, it is best for the instructor to ask students to pair up and take turns assessing pupil response with a penlight or a similar light source. First, one student should document pupil size and equality on a fellow student. The lights should be turned out for no less than two minutes before students are asked to recheck pupil response with the penlight. Both eyes should be checked several times so the pupils can actually be seen to change in response to light. Students should be asked to record their results for each student in the class, then compare their results during a debriefing of the activity. Some students should be positioned in a location where side lighting may affect the readings or the ability to assess pupils. Students should be asked to lie on their backs and look up into the overhead classroom lights. When the instructor debriefs this activity, he or she should ask students how the position of the patient in the ambulance and light levels will affect their ability to evaluate pupils.

identify those objectives with the highest priority and experiment with various methods of delivery. The process of developing a more learner-centered approach to the classroom initially requires more work and adds increased risk to what the instructor does. However, the rewards for both students and instructor are immeasurable.

Experiential Tips

Following are just a few examples of experiential techniques that can help reinforce specific learning points:

- Have students feel the pulse of a person with an irregular heart rhythm.
- Use a dual-earpiece teaching stethoscope to assist students in understanding what sounds they are listening for when taking a blood pressure.
- To reinforce the importance of the physical exam, have students practice a patient assessment where there are actual simulated injuries to find, such as a bruise on the abdomen or subcutaneous emphysema on the chest made out of bubble wrap. (If students do not expose and touch the patient, they will not find all of the hidden injuries.)

Matching Teaching Strategies to Goals and Objectives

Making the conscious decision to become a more student-centered instructor is quite different from actually making it happen. It may be comforting for the instructor to know that half the battle has already been decided for EMS instructors in that the objectives to which they must teach have been defined by such documents as the U.S. Department of Transportation (DOT) National EMS Education Standards, the core content, and the scope of practice for each level of care. The challenge for the instructor is to continue to master current teaching methods while developing new and innovative methods that are best suited for the various standards.

The task of addressing during class time each and every objective included within the standards can be overwhelming. In fact, this is one of the biggest challenges for instructors, given the short duration of most Emergency Medical Responder, EMT, Advanced EMT, and Paramedic programs. The development of objectives from the paramedic Education Standards competencies, behaviors, and clinical judgments, could likely include more than 2,000 objectives that must be addressed at some time during the course of the program. Although it is true that some standards overlap, instructors still must "triage" the components of the standards and select those most worthy of focus during class time. It will be impossible to cover every standard in class. Some must be addressed in homework, reading assignments, and activities outside the classroom.

Instructors can maximize their valuable time by ensuring that they understand the instructional level required to attain the chosen objectives. Chapter 7: Domains of Learning describes Bloom's taxonomy and provides verbs used to describe the behaviors expected at various levels. For example, if an objective begins with "list the signs and symptoms of...", then the instructor knows this to be a low-level, or knowledge, or recall-level objective. Little explanation or classroom activity is likely to be required to achieve competency in this objective. A simple reading assignment may accomplish the task. However, if the objective began, "Recognize the signs and symptoms of...", then this is going to be a higher-level objective and may require photographs, video, or a live-patient demonstration in order to teach the content to this level.

The instructor must devise a teaching and evaluation strategy that provides the lower levels of understanding, then allows students to progress toward the upper levels. The old saying, "you must walk before you can run," can be applied here as well. The wisest EMS instructors know that a valuable EMS provider not only understands when to do something, but also knows when *not* to do something. This level of understanding comes only through a thorough immersion into all aspects associated with the particular concepts. Students must understand all appropriate terminology and be able to see subtle differences between similar terms. Terminology begins in the lowest levels of understanding within each domain. Terminology concepts are then applied as students begin to understand the subtle differences between words and appreciate their meaning. As students work through problems and scenarios, they use their understanding of the terminology in accurate ways to get their meaning across in words or actions.

For example, many distinct differences can be noted between "ventilation" and "respiration," and students must understand these differences as they evaluate the effectiveness of airway management and adjunct usage. However, many educators may have forgotten the differences, or they may have not learned through their educational process how to make the distinction. Students may experience frustration when they encounter an evaluation process that requires they discriminate among concepts for which they cannot recall differences. If the instructional process does not focus on students learning the difference between these two concepts, but instead focuses on the development of psychomotor skills, students will be unable to effectively problem-solve an airway management issue that differentiates between the two concepts. An example may be a patient with adequate tidal volume and respiratory rate but who remains hypoxic because, despite adequate ventilation, the fluid in his alveoli is preventing proper gas exchange or respiration.

Summary

The goals of any teacher are to convey information to students and to make a lasting change in their behavior. To do this, the educator must develop teaching strategies that result in meaningful change. Teaching is both an art and a science. Great educators must also be great performers (the art), but they must also gain expertise in facilitation techniques that involve groups of students, questioning techniques, and experiential learning. The effective educator recognizes the many teaching strategies that are available and chooses which technique will be best for a given situation.

The goal of the following chapters is to introduce both novice and seasoned EMS instructors to a variety of traditional and nontraditional teaching concepts and strategies to ensure a successful and engaging educational experience for both the student and the instructor. Achieving a practical balance between these two approaches is encouraged. It is hoped that the instructor will come away with an understanding of the importance of this balance.

Chapter 12 discusses each domain of learning, along with specific methods for promoting student learning in each one. Chapter 13 focuses in great detail on specific tools that instructors can use to promote individual and one-on-one learning. Chapter 14 discusses methods and tools most appropriate for small groups, including ways to enhance psychomotor abilities and critical thinking skills. Chapter 15 provides insight into instructional methods aimed at large groups, as well as methods used to enhance the lecture approach to instruction. Chapter 17 introduces the many tools and methods used in distance learning. Chapter 18 discusses tools for simulation experiences and Chapter 19 introduces key strategies for enhancing student field and clinical experiences.

Glossary

"ask, pause, and call" technique A questioning technique where the instructor waits for a longer time—up to 30 seconds—before allowing a student to answer a posed question.

experiential learning The concept developed by Carl Rogers who felt so strongly about the role that experience plays in how individuals learn that he distinguished learning into two distinct types: cognitive (which Rogers described as "meaningless") and experiential (which he deemed as "significant").

facilitation To make easier.

Kolb theory Describes two ways that learners can transform experience into knowledge—reflective observation and active experimentation.

Socratic method A method of questioning that uses the practice of asking, rather than telling, to arouse curiosity in the subject matter so students will arrive at their own conclusions rather than being told the "right" answer.

student-centered instruction/learning Puts the learner at the center of the educational event and incorporates innovative, active teaching strategies such as group work, case studies, role-playing, writing assignments, and so on.

teacher-centered instruction/learning Instruction that focuses on the teacher and thus, primarily, the lecture format.

wait time A concept in questioning techniques that gives time to students to think about questions posed to them and to ponder their response.

References

1. Croskerry, P. (2007). The affective imperative: coming to terms with our emotions. *Academic Emergency Medicine, 14*(2), 184–186.
2. Craik, F., & Tulving, E. (1975). Depth of processing and the retention of words in episodic memory. *Journal of Experimental Psychology: General*. Vol. 103: No. 3, 268–294.
3. Barkley, E. F., Cross, K. P., & Major, C. H. (2004). *Collaborative learning: A handbook for college faculty*. San Francisco, CA: Jossey-Bass.
4. Paulson, D. R., & Faust, J. L. (1999).Techniques of active learning. Active learning for the college classroom. Available at:http://www.chemistry.calstatela.edu/Chem&BioChem/active/main.htm.
5. Rogers, C., & Freiberg, H. J. (1994). *Freedom to learn*. Columbus, OH: Charles E. Merrill.
6. Kolb, D. A. (1984). *Experiential learning: Experience as the source of learning and development*. Upper Saddle River, NJ: Prentice-Hall.

Additional Resources

Areeda, P. E. (1996). The Socratic method. *The Harvard Law Review, 109*(5), 911–922.

Brereton, M. F., Leifer, L., Greene, J., Lewis, J., & Linde, C. (1993, September). An exploration of engineering learning. In T. K. Hight, & L. A. Stauffer (Eds.). *Proceedings of the ASME design theory and methodology conference*, Albuquerque, NM: American Society of Mechanical Engineers (ASME), Vol. 53, 195–206.

Combs, A. W. (1976). Fostering maximum development of the individual. In W. Van Til, & K. J. Rehage (Eds.). *Issues in secondary education (NSSE yearbook)*. Chicago, IL: National Society for the Study of Education.

deWinstanley, P. A, & Bjork, R. A. (2002). Successful lecturing: Presenting information in ways that engage effective processing. *New Directions for Teaching and Learning, 89*, 19–31.

Galbraith, M. W. (1991). *Adult learning methods*. Huntington, NY: Robert E. Krieger Publishing.

Johnson, D. W., Johnson, R.T., & Smith, K. A. (1998). Maximizing instruction through cooperative learning. *American Society for Engineering Education (ASEE) Prism, 7*, 24–29.

King, A. (1993, Winter). Sage on the stage to guide on the side. *College Teaching*, Vol. 41, No. 1.

National Highway Traffic Safety Administration (2009). National Emergency Medical Services Education Standards. http://www.ems.gov/pdf/811077a.pdf

Norman, G. R., & Schmidt, H. G. (1992). The psychological basis of problem-based learning: A review of the evidence. *Academic Medicine, 67*, 557–565.

Nowell, L. (1996). Rethinking the classroom: A community of inquiry. Presented at: National Council on Creating the Quality School, Norman, Oklahoma. Fort Worth, TX: Wesleyan University, School of Education, ERIC Document Reproduction Service No. ED350 273.

Reese, A. C. (1998). Implications of results from cognitive science research. [online serial]. Available at: http://www.Med-Ed-Online.

Rideout, E. (2001). *Transforming nursing education through problem-based learning*. Sudbury, MA: Jones and Bartlett.

Springer,L., Stanne, M. E, & Donovan, S. S. (1999, Spring). Effects of small group learning on undergraduates in science, mathematics, engineering, and technology: A meta-analysis. *Review of Educational Research*, Vol. 69, No.1, 21–51.

VanAst, J. (1997). Sage on the stage or guide on the side: An outcome-based approach to the preparation of community college vocational-technical faculty for the 1990s and beyond. *Community College Journal of Research & Practice, 21* (5), 459.

12

Teaching in All Domains

Education is not the filling of a pail, but the lighting of a fire. — Heraclitus

The practice of Emergency Medical Services (EMS) is a complex activity that involves teaching in multiple domains and at multiple levels. It is not enough that EMS educators prepare future providers to be highly skilled professionals who are able to perform flawlessly every skill, nor is it enough that they are able to correctly recite every treatment protocol and every drug dosage and procedure. In addition to these knowledge and psychomotor skills, the EMS provider must be a skilled communicator who demonstrates empathy and a deeper appreciation of each patient's social, family, and ethnic background honoring patients' diversity. This chapter prepares the EMS educator for the challenge of providing a comprehensive EMS education that will produce competent, compassionate care providers.

CHAPTER GOAL: This chapter discusses how to teach **critical-thinking** skills and how to apply them to the knowledge, psychomotor, and affective domains.

Teaching Thinking Skills

Widely regarded as the "father" of modern critical thinking, John Dewey defined critical thinking as, "... the active, persistent, and careful consideration of a belief or supposed form of knowledge in light of the grounds which support it and the further conclusions to which it tends." By using the term "active," Dewey contrasts this method of learning from the more passive method in which the student simply receives information or ideas from someone else. John Dewey believed that the attainment of higher-level thinking skills, sometimes called "critical thinking," could be nurtured and developed in students. Approaches to teaching that involve critical thinking require the student to think things through, raise additional questions, and explore solutions for themselves. Dewey believed that educators should pay close attention to each student's life experience and should develop curricula that connect with and extend student experiences to real world application. Dewey suggested that school should be less about preparation for life and more about life itself.[1]

It is not enough to simply assume that students will think critically all on their own. Although some do, many must be introduced to this skill in the classroom. By keeping alert to available opportunities, educators can begin to develop more meaningful lessons. In the examples given in this chapter and in the following chapters, the common thread is the element of critical thinking. These examples provide a great foundation for new and experienced educators alike.

Teaching thinking strategies requires a careful and deliberate plan of instruction. Educators must determine which thinking skills students have already mastered and which they have yet to learn. Educators must measure thinking skills regularly and should include thinking-skill development exercises and strategies throughout the course. Measuring student achievement is a challenge when the goal is simply measuring recall of information or psychomotor skill performance, but the process becomes even more complex when one adds to it measuring a student's ability to use information to think critically and to problem-solve. This problem is not unique to EMS education. A study on the evaluation of thousands of test items from K-12 education reveals that nearly three-quarters of these items tested the recall of information (i.e., a low-level cognitive skill), and very few tested the application of **higher-order thinking** skills.[2] Numerous studies in adult and elementary education have had similar findings.

Keys for Unlocking Higher-Order Thinking Skills

1. Instruction and assessment strategies that promote thinking skills
2. Practice with various methods of thinking that incorporate many strategies
3. Constant and consistent role-modeling of the process for students

Bloom's Taxonomy: Cognitive Domain

Level 1: Knowledge

Level 2: Comprehension

Level 3: Application

Level 4: Analysis

Level 5: Synthesis

CASE IN POINT

For example, after a session in which students learned and demonstrated the ability to ventilate a manikin using a pocket mask, the instructor asked these questions:

- How will you know if your breaths are getting into the patient?
- What does it mean if you do not see good chest rise and fall?

Some students immediately shouted the first answer that came to mind without giving it much thought at all. For instance, in response to the first question, one student said, "Because I know I gave a good breath." In response to the second question, a second student said, "The patient has something stuck in his throat." These answers may or may not have been correct; however, other conclusions had to be tested before these responses could be evaluated for correctness. To stimulate higher levels of learning, the instructor demonstrated excellent **facilitation** skills by asking follow-up questions, such as, "How can you be sure that the breath you gave is really adequate for the patient?" and "Is a foreign object the only thing that can obstruct an airway?" By offering additional probing questions, the instructor slowed the class down and encouraged students to process information carefully and thoroughly before responding.

Three key processes have been identified that enhance an educator's ability to assist students in the development of higher-order thinking skills. Key Process 1 involves the implementation by the instructor of various instructional and assessment strategies that teach thinking skills to students. To do this, educators must have a fundamental understanding of the thinking process and must possess the appropriate tools and techniques to assist students in acquiring the same. Key Process 2 requires that students be given ample opportunity to practice these methods. Educators should ensure that they schedule and provide opportunities for students to explore various learning styles and preference. In Key Process 3, the educator serves as a role model for critical thinking and problem solving to be emulated by students.

Teaching Tip >> *Instructors should provide critical thinking opportunities that appeal to a variety of student learning styles and preferences.*

Several valid strategies for grouping and classifying thinking skills have been developed. For example, Costa and associates organized thinking skills into the six R's of thinking: Remembering, Repeating, Reasoning, Reorganizing, Relating, and Reflecting.[3] This model is common to nursing education and is the framework for several of its strategies for the development of critical-thinking skills.

Barry Beyer, working with an inventory of operations common to curriculum developers and educators, classified thinking processes into three distinct groups: thinking strategies, critical-thinking skills, and micro-thinking skills.[4]

Techniques for Teaching Critical-Thinking Skills: The T.H.I.N.K. Model

A common nursing model classifies critical-thinking skills into five modes of thinking: total recall, habits, inquiry, new ideas and creativity, and knowing how you think. It uses the mnemonic T.H.I.N.K. and the processes proceed in the order of the spelling of that word.[5] The first two sections of the THINK model are not actually critical-thinking skills, but rather lay the foundation for critical thinking to come. These first two steps, Total recall and Habit, establish the reserve from which one will draw.

Total Recall

Total recall is the memorization of facts or remembering where to look for them. As a student practices total recall, it is important to distinguish which information should be recalled instantaneously and which can be looked up. Because patient safety is of the highest priority, it is becoming increasingly more acceptable in health care to use a job aid or reference material to avoid error. Many electronic references are available to providers to search for information such as drug dosages or poison control information at the bedside. Instructors should make clear to students which references may be used in practice and testing and which information is expected to be memorized.

Using patterns, or **mnemonics**, is helpful in improving recall. An example of recall occurs when a person remembers the following numbers in order: 5553561809. It looks daunting until they are organized like this: (555) 356-1809. Now, it resembles a phone number and is easier to remember. A common EMS mnemonic is PQRST (Provokes or Palliates, Quality, Region and Radiation, Severity, and Time) used to obtain the present and past medical histories in patients with pain.

Another example of recall might be asking the learner to look at a list of common words and to try to remember them: apple, car, yellow, pear, bicycle, blue, grapefruit, plane, and green. If the learner sorts the list according to the following patterns, called "grouping or chunking," it is easier to recall:

- Colors: yellow, blue, green
- Fruits: apple, grapefruit, pear
- Transportation: car, plane, bicycle

Another method of recall involves the association of facts with an experience. A person may quickly and easily remember a fact because it is associated with a strong emotion or a funny story. For example, few will ever forget where they were and what they were doing when they learned that commercial aircraft were being flown into buildings in America on September 11, 2001.

Habit

Habit, the second process of critical thinking, is any accepted way that works, saves time, or is necessary for the critical-thinking process to take place. Habits are thinking approaches that become second nature. Within the psychomotor domain, this level of **mastery** is called **naturalization**. Driving a car to school illustrates this principle for someone who has arrived at class without remembering the journey. Habits in the work environment can make performing a job a lot easier and free the mind to use your conscious thought for critical thinking. However, it is important that a person periodically reevaluate performance to ensure that he or she is not taking inappropriate short cuts. For example, students should consider whether or not they *always* cleanse the top of a medication vial with alcohol before withdrawing any medication from the vial.

Inquiry

Inquiry occurs as the student examines issues in depth and detail and questions what may seem immediately obvious. Although this single process of inquiry is often called critical thinking, the nursing model of thinking requires the action of all five modes of the T.H.I.N.K. model for critical thinking to take place. Inquiry is the primary kind of thinking used to reach conclusions, and conclusions are more accurate if inquiry is used.[5]

Inquiry requires the following six steps:

1. Receive information
2. Come to a conclusion, but collect additional information to rule in or out the immediate conclusion
3. Compare the new information with what is already known from past experience
4. Question biases
5. Consider one or more alternative conclusions
6. Validate the original or alternative conclusion

Perhaps determining a differential diagnosis is the most common use of the Inquiry step in health care, performed daily by practitioners everywhere. Of course, students will have to have recall of facts related to anatomy, physiology, pathophysiology, signs and symptoms, treatment protocols, and drug dosages as they approach any patient. Next, some of the student's thinking processes will be habit and require little or no conscious thought such as taking a radial pulse or noting skin signs, freeing the mind for the critical-thinking task ahead. This brings us to the steps of Inquiry where the provider will first receive information (from a patient, for example). After listening to, and confirming, the chief complaint and related symptoms the patient is experiencing, the provider will have a short list of possible diagnoses. Using step 2 of Inquiry, he or she will then gather additional information, say from diagnostic tests such as an ECG or labwork, to rule in or rule out the possible diagnosis from his or her short list. The provider will then compare these findings with what he or she knows from past experience, often needing to consider other possible causes for the patient's complaint.

After gathering this new information, the provider will determine a diagnosis and establish a treatment plan for the patient.

As one looks ahead to the last two processes in the THINK system, creativity and **metacognition** are upcoming. In this example of our patient diagnosis, creativity could be used if there is not an established treatment protocol for this differential diagnosis, or if the patient was refusing some suggested treatments. Metacognition would perhaps be implemented after the shift when exploring whether or not the treatment for this patient was proper, or while exploring how one arrived at the diagnosis in a journaling assignment about the shift required by the professor.

New Ideas and Creativity

New ideas and creativity is the polar opposite of the habit mode of thinking. Creativity allows the thinker to explore different pathways or alternatives for problem solving. A common phrase attached to this process is "to think outside the box." Creative thinking often leads to mistakes or ideas which will not be carried out but which can provide additional learning opportunities. Creative thinking allows practitioners of health care to individualize care and often to discover new solutions or improved processes. When performed at its highest level, the creative-thinking process allows for individual choices within the framework of medically acceptable behaviors.

Knowing How One Thinks

Metacognition is the highest of the thinking skills in the T.H.I.N.K. model. "Meta-" means "among" or "in the midst of," and cognition is the process of knowing. A student who attains this level can critically analyze his or her thinking process and make adjustments as needed.

Three major operations occur during the metacognitive process: planning, monitoring, and assessing.[6] Each process has several subprocesses. Planning is considered the most important facet of metacognition. It includes the following parts: stating a goal, selecting operations to perform, sequencing operations, identifying potential obstacles/errors, identifying ways to recover from obstacles/errors, and predicting desired and/or anticipated results.

Monitoring is the second process in metacognition. It includes steps for keeping sequencing in order by keeping the goal in mind, keeping one's place in the sequence, knowing when a subgoal has been achieved, and deciding when to progress to the next operation. Monitoring also involves spotting errors and obstacles and knowing how to recover from errors and obstacles.

The final step is the assessment of goal achievement. It comprises judging accuracy and adequacy of results, appropriateness of procedures, handling of obstacles and errors, and the efficiency of the plan and its execution.[4,6] Just as many learners never reach the naturalization level of psychomotor skill development or the evaluation level of the cognitive domain, many learners and professionals alike do not spend much time on metacognition or thinking about what they know and believe.

Teaching People Skills

It is the affective domain of learning that addresses not what we know about or do to patients, but how we go about it. The affective domain is about how we treat patients while we are treating them. Developing a generation of caring, compassionate providers who are self-motivated to do well and continue learning throughout their careers begins with a classroom environment which respects the learner as an individual who come to us with attitudes, beliefs, emotions, and experiences that are of value to the class. Affective skills impact any behavior or decision that one makes since all behavior includes an emotional component.

Educators have long known that the power of emotion can be harnessed to create a powerful learning environment. By tapping into emotion, instructors can build a vibrant classroom that takes students on an exploration of their profession and of themselves. Additionally, it has been shown repeatedly that students learn and remember more and at higher levels

Distinguishing Between Passive and Active Behaviors

Passive	Active
Quiet classrooms of note takers	Active classrooms of interactive learners
All work done alone	Work done in cooperative small groups
Rare participation in class	Regular participation to some degree
Classroom-guided materials	Creation of new and challenging assignments
Teacher-controlled lesson	Student- and teacher-controlled lessons
All tasks carried by the teacher	Classroom responsibilities shared by students

of cognition when the lesson was active and involved emotion or the senses. In the end, this student-centered, active-learning atmosphere brings about greater understanding and a more complete student and learning experience. This is why it is critical to begin to change classrooms from passive places of learning to active and engaging ones.

Educators are role models and are teaching values, whether they realize it or not. Every time an instructor relates a personal experience about how she or he was empathetic to a troubled patient or family member, communicates verbal and nonverbal reactions to student questions or performance, chooses subjects to be tested, and even emphasizes given topics in a lecture or presentation, the instructor is imposing values. The real issue for the instructor, then, is how to cultivate the ethics and values of our profession while setting aside his or her own personal prejudices, beliefs, and emotions. Educators have a much stronger influence on students than they may ever know or appreciate. Students learn from the behaviors that their educators model, including those instructor behaviors that they observe outside the classroom **(Figure 12.1)**.

Dr. Pat Croskerry, a physician and medical educator who studies and writes about how caregiver attitudes affect judgment and the quality of patient care, says "Our historical and continuing failure to acknowledge the impact of our feelings on the ways in which we interact with patients ultimately precludes optimal clinical reasoning and decision making."[7] Creating an environment in which students are engaged in activities to explore their emotions and also make critical decisions while under stress and in situations involving strong emotion, such as child abuse or a line of duty death, is the responsibility of the educator in the development of a more aware, accurate, affective, and ultimately effective medical workforce.

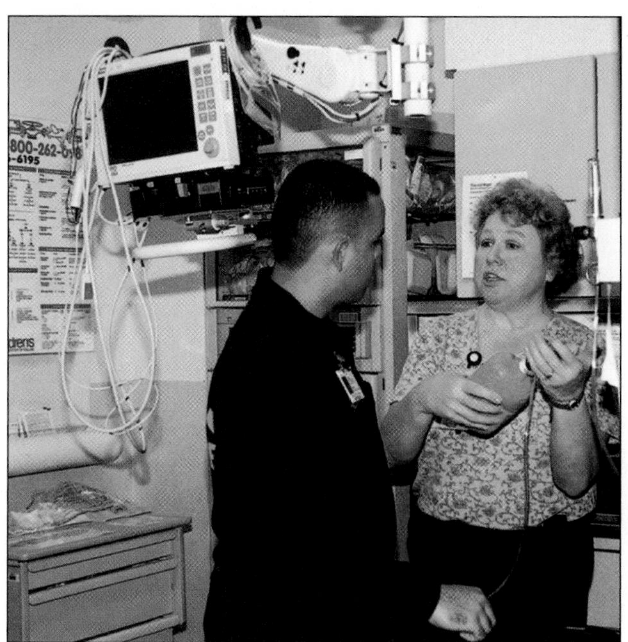

Figure 12.1

Educator model values and behaviors by everything they say and do within and outside of the classroom.

Teaching Tip >> *"If we don't model what we teach then we are teaching something else".*

Author Unknown

To appropriately affect a student's progress within the affective domain, an instructor must be consciously aware of the values, judgments, and beliefs that are inherent in the instructor's teaching but that may not be overtly apparent; then, the instructor must monitor changes in students to detect behaviors that indicate that they are adopting desired values and judgments. For example, in order for patients to feel cared for and respected, it is important to treat patients as human beings, not objectify them as their diseases or symptoms. Educators must be careful not to say things like "we responded on a chest pain last night," but rather to say, "we took care of an elderly patient with chest pain last night." Not only should instructors use the proper form of address and instruction, they must correct students who do not notice themselves treating patients with a lack of respect. This is just one example of how an instructor can model values and affect, but the opportunities to do so are endless—from learning and using patients' and students' names, to covering patients with a sheet or blanket to protect modesty, to wearing a clean uniform or dressing professionally when teaching. Each of these behaviors demonstrates to students the values of the profession of medicine.

Levels of the Affective Domain

As has been discussed in Chapter 7: Domains of Learning, Bloom identified five levels in the affective domain. Facilitation is the teaching technique that can be applied at all levels of the affective domain as well as to the cognitive and psychomotor domains. *Facilitation* is the process of assisting a learner in discovering information or abilities for him or herself. It is a technique distinctly different from lecture or demonstration in that the educator does not give answers, but rather questions or guides the learner in a way that promotes self-discovery.

Bloom's Taxonomy: Affective Domain

Level 1: Receiving

Level 2: Responding

Level 3: Valuing

Level 4: Organizing

Level 5: Characterizing

The next section discusses the steps in each level of the affective domain. Typically, students are expected to move through each step in each level; behavioral or performance problems can develop if one skips steps.

Level I: Receiving

Receiving is where the affective domain begins. It requires no more of the student than that he or she be aware of a given piece of information. This is usually cognitive in origin. The student has heard it, seen it, or read it. Receiving is made up of three successive steps. When a student demonstrates any of the actions described by these steps, he or she is operating at the receiving level.

These steps include the following:

1. *Awareness*: This step requires only that the student be conscious of the existence of a given piece of information or equipment. For example, the student sees the Hare traction splint in the classroom but does not display any interest in it. Another example might be that the student stays awake during the fracture management lecture. Of course, it may be very difficult to tell if the student was listening or not.
2. *Willingness to receive*: At this step, the student becomes curious enough about the piece of information or object that he or she is willing to devote some, but not all, of his attention to it. For example, the student begins to stop and look at the traction splint before sitting down in the classroom, or the student asks questions during the lecture on fracture management.
3. *Controlled or selected attention*: At this point, the student is so interested in the piece of information or object that it momentarily has top priority, despite the fact that other things are of interest at the same time. For example, the student would rather practice with the traction splint than discuss last night's events, or is so engrossed in reading the assignment that the student does not respond to his or her name when called.

   Exactly why the piece of information or object does or does not have top priority is up for interpretation and may be a function of what goes on in the classroom.

Assumptions of willingness to receive and of selected attention are precarious until the next level, Responding, is demonstrated. The Receiving level, however, forms the basis for all other levels. One must take care not to confuse verbalizations that show understanding of communicated stimuli with responding behaviors. Responding behaviors are demonstrated when "students act out behaviors consistent with . . . a particular value."[8]

Classroom Implications An instructor can promote Receiving by letting students know what is expected of them. This could be accomplished first by communicating the course objectives. Many times, it is not enough to just hand out the objectives. The instructor may need to explain what they are and how they can be used to the student's benefit.

Making lectures relevant to the student also enhances the Receiving level. The relevancy of the objectives and of what is being taught may need to be explained. Resources such as equipment, professional magazines and publications, manikins, posters, anatomy charts, and copies of lecture outlines and notes are also invaluable at this level of learning.

Perhaps one of the most important instructor techniques for enhancing the Receiving level can be accomplished by placing the emphasis on course matter where it belongs, and not where the instructor has a personal preference. Students will emulate what the instructor does without realizing that they are doing it, but they will also disregard what they are supposed to be learning if they perceive no clear reason or rationale for what is being taught. Therefore, when emphasis is placed on a subject, it is helpful for the instructor to explain why the emphasis belongs there. Likewise, instructors must be very wary of saying things such as "you don't really need to know that" or "I never do it like that" because in the position of authority and role model that is inherent to the teacher, the student may immediately disregard the information and choose not to learn it or have bias against it.

Level II: Responding

At this level, the student responds to some degree because of an outside influence. This is the point at which an observable change in behavior can first be seen and is often a response to instructor directives, course requirements, or job responsibilities. The student has not yet absorbed the value presented but is merely Responding to it. Like Receiving, Responding comprises the following three steps, the sequence of which describes the student's process of value acquisition within this level:

1. *Command response:* This step deals with appropriate responses that the student might not understand or accept the rationale for, and might not perform if certain requirements were not made. For example, the instructor states, "The traction splint must be applied correctly, according to your skills guide, at least once. By the way, you can't leave until you do." The student may call this bribery; the instructor calls this a necessary requirement. Another example of command response would be that the student is required to sign the EMT Oath & Code of Ethics before being allowed to participate in class.
2. *Willing response:* This step differs from the first in that the student responds, when asked, without the requirement making it necessary to do so. In other words, he or she will respond, when asked, without bribery. The exact motive is not known, but what is important is that the desired response was given. For example, the student will apply correctly the traction splint, according to the skills guide, when asked by the instructor. Or the student actually does sign the EMT Oath & Code of Ethics. The motive for the action comes from outside the person (i.e., the instructor), and the response is made because the student chooses to accept the instructor's request. Note that the reason behind that acceptance is not known, but what is important is that the action was done.
3. *Satisfaction response:* At this step, the voluntary response to sign the Oath or apply the traction splint is accompanied by a feeling of satisfaction or some other type of emotional response. For example, the instructor may want to relate this feeling to the one felt when the application of the traction splint was satisfactorily mastered, or the student is recognized for ethical behavior. It also could be compared with the student who frequently applies the traction splint because of feeling a sense of satisfaction when performing this skill. This step is directly affected by the response of the instructor, and it has a secondary effect on the student's self-esteem. This effect on self-esteem may be positive or negative depending on performance.

This brings up an important point. The emotional element is present at the Responding level in all levels of the affective domain, to different degrees, for the following three reasons: (1) This is the level at which the emotional element most often begins to occur, (2) this is the point where the emotional element becomes part of the motivation (The satisfaction or dissatisfaction gained during the response serves as its own reinforcement. How great a reinforcement is depends on both internal and external factors), and (3) the emotional element affects the student's overall perception of self.

Responding (Level II) is directly dependent on successful Receiving (Level I). This means that as Responding is observed, it may be concluded that Level I was attained. The degree to which it was attained may not be readily apparent. The reverse is also true—if Responding is not observed in a particular student, the Receiving level was probably not acquired or was not completed.

Classroom Implications Because this is the level at which the emotional element most often begins to occur, it has a direct effect on motivation and self-esteem, as has been stated earlier. Techniques directed toward this level include those that enhance motivation and self-esteem. Perhaps none is as important as ensuring a **safe classroom**. A "safe" classroom refers to an emotionally safe environment where a student will not be ridiculed for asking a question, experimenting with equipment, or failing an evaluation **(Figure 12.2)**. A great deal of learning can occur from a "failed" attempt. However, adults do not like to fail and often associate a failed attempt with "being a failure" or incompetence.[9]

Another technique for helping students move through the Responding level includes leaving equipment out and permitting students to practice in an open-lab environment, instead of having every encounter be instructor-led. The freedom to take

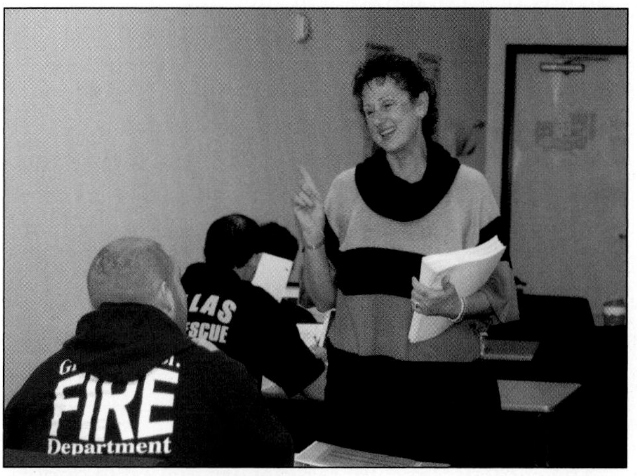

Figure 12.2

An emotionally safe classroom where students are freely allowed to ask questions and reveal their failings is conducive to a positive educational experience and promotes the Responding level of the affective domain.

equipment apart and put it back together, practice independently and in small groups, and challenge oneself to get faster, more accurate, or perform with more finesse is invaluable at this level.

Perhaps no other quality of an EMS instructor at this level is greater than respect for students themselves. This attitude of respect will guide and support the instructor's choices and, even when not spoken, will be perceived and communicated by students throughout the entire course.

Level III: Valuing

The third level of the affective domain, Valuing, refers to the point at which the student attaches importance and impact to a subject or phenomenon. In this way, a person's values begin to affect their judgment. These values are internalized slowly, a process that occurs through the entire student experience, which includes previous experiences before the course and interaction with peers, society, and significant others (e.g., instructors, partners, hospital staff, and spouses). The following three steps are involved in incorporation of the Valuing process:

1. *Acceptance (of a particular value)*: This step is similar to the awareness step of receiving, in that the student has become conscious that a particular action, subject, or phenomenon has worth. The instructor can assess whether this step has been reached by observing a student who makes the same or a similar response concerning the value in question, when confronted with a number of different stimuli. For example, if the student valued patient advocacy, the instructor would consistently observe the student choosing to do the right thing for the patient whether or not a supervisor were present or the patient was able to state his or her wishes. Whether anyone would "catch the student doing the right thing" is not the motivator of behavior when the student has reached the valuing level of the affective domain. The motivator is the value itself—in this case, being a patient advocate.
2. *Preference (for a particular value)*: In this step, the student not only has passively accepted the value but chooses to actively pursue it. In other words, when given a choice, the student will choose this value over other values that he or she may hold. The student typically takes every available opportunity to find out more about this value and those things related to it. Using our patient advocacy example, the student would choose to do the right thing for the patient even if it were inconvenient or uncomfortable personally, such as transporting the patient to the hospital even if it meant dinner would get cold or he or she might miss a potentially more exciting call that was just coming in to dispatch.
3. *Commitment (to a value)*: Here, the student is committed to his or her belief and may be seen trying to persuade or convince others to accept the value. It is at this point that the student has accepted the value without reservation. In the example of patient advocacy, a student might be observed convincing a fellow classmate to obtain a 12-lead ECG when indicated but not necessarily required, explaining how it may benefit this patient and protect the patient from harm. Or a student persists in obtaining an order for pain management when his or her partner does not want to bother with the pain issue since they are close to the hospital.

Simply put, this level is characterized by two things: a choice and, at its best, consistency between choices. At the lowest step in this level, the student is still open to reevaluating his or her position, so behavior is still tentative. At the highest step, the student is committed to this value and may be trying to further his or her knowledge of that value.

As with the previous two levels, this level is dependent on the attainment of Responding (Level II) and Receiving (Level I). It would be nearly impossible to have a student defend his or her position for providing pain management to a patient if the student did not first understand the negative effect on the patient both physiologically and psychologically (receiving) and that he or she possessed the skill, ability, and desire to relieve that pain (responding). It is important for educators to be aware that both the student and the instructor can get "stuck" at this level. If an internal valuing process has not developed, students will not progress beyond this level but will appear to do everything that the instructor tells them to do. They will do it the way they are expected to, every time they are observed (i.e., when the instructor is around). What happens when they are not observed or the instructor is not there is another thing.

If the student has adopted the values of a significant other, such as a partner or another instructor or mentor, without examining or testing these values for himself or herself, the values in question tend to be rigid and fixed. This tendency can be observed in the student or in the instructor. In the case of a student, the value may have been developed to gain approval from a rigid instructor, or the student may have lacked the confidence to take a risk. In the case of an instructor, the value may have developed because of lack of recent patient care experience, or the instructor may have perceived a questioning student as a threat. In either case, values tend to be fixed concepts, rarely examined or tested; as a result, certain values become so rigid that the student or instructor refuses to further his or her knowledge, even when presented with information that is contradictory. Such individuals tend to feel threatened when their value system is questioned. Student comments that suggest that the student or instructor has gotten "stuck" include the following:

"That instructor doesn't know what he's talking about!"

"I've worked in the field for 20 years and I'm not going to change now!"

"It doesn't say that in the book!"

Instructor comments or nonverbal clues include:

"Do it this way because I say to do it this way!"

"Who are you to question me?!"

The field of medicine changes rapidly, and keeping up with these changes requires that practitioners go to continuing educational events and subscribe to professional journals. Keeping an open mind,

CASE IN POINT

It was that dreaded time of year when the "last minute crowd" all register for the required refresher courses. The EMS educator always dreaded these refreshers because they are heavily populated with the most experienced and "hardened" EMTs and paramedics, who have waited until the last possible minute to register for their continuing education and refresher courses. To make matters worse, these experienced field providers view instructors as white tower "has been(s)" who do not do the job anymore and do not even remember what it was like being in the field. To cap it all off, the director made improvement of evaluations of the refresher courses one of the EMS educator's performance goals for the year. She was losing sleep over what to do, so she decided to stay up and read the EMS educator's textbook, where she found a few ideas that she thought might help her manage the situation.

As a first step, she set aside five days over two weeks to get out into the field and ride along with the crews. Second, she made a conscious decision to show respect for the EMS providers and their issues. She took the huge step of seeing situations from their perspective. After all, they are doing the job competently on a full-time basis all year; then they have to go into a classroom and practical labs to listen to a rehash of stuff that they believe they already know. Then they have to pretend to run codes and perform routine skills on plastic manikins. How boring it has to be, she realized. This led her to a breakthrough concept. She decided to go out on a limb and redesign the presentation format. She kept the same course objectives, the same content, and the same presentation and reference resources, but she changed the way everything would be presented.

On the first day of class, she mingled with the participants over coffee, chatting about the calls that she had been on over the previous two weeks. Next, she handed out the course materials and went over the objectives and schedule, but then made an announcement: "I'm not going to do any lecturing for this refresher. Because this is a *refresher* course, you are all very familiar with the content and how to do all the procedures. I'm going to ask you to 'discuss' the topics based on your experiences on calls. The only requirement will be that we all need to discuss every required topic in full. The way we do this will be up to you."

Everyone looked around uncomfortably. Most thought that it was going to be a complete disaster. To everyone's surprise, however, the group became animated, and a lively discussion began. Some participants tried to hijack the course and turn it into a social jam session, and others tried to become invisible, but most got on track and drove it in the right direction.

The result was a successful course that covered all course objectives and had a 100 percent pass rate on the final performance testing. The instructor, of course, was a nervous wreck after it was over, but the excellent course evaluations made it all worthwhile.

In this case, the EMS instructor took some very real risks and allowed herself to be vulnerable. First, she spent very rare and precious time in the field with crews, which helped to dispel the "ivory tower" stigma. Second, she decided that she would respect the responders and trust them. When she communicated this sincerely, they picked up on it and respected her and the process in return. Finally, she gave up the "security blanket" of presenting topics through traditional lectures in favor of letting participants form discussion groups and present their knowledge to each other. She realized that this approach might not work for every group or in every system, but she also suspected that opportunities for nontraditional approaches that incorporated trust and empowerment could probably be found in nearly every course, once she decided to look for them.

experimenting with students, and helping students to develop their reasoning skills all work to keep both the instructor and the student "unstuck." By extending one's own personal experiences to students, the educator can ensure that the values she or he holds are continually being reinforced or modified and kept up to date.

Classroom Implications Elizabeth King maintains "the learning of an attitude occurs when a respected role model makes a verbal communication to the learner regarding desirable choices of action or displays these actions directly."[10] The implications of this are clear. We must think about what we, as educators, say and do at all times. We must display an interest in our students and accept, guide, and encourage them while we give them the tools they need to support their own conclusions. If a safe classroom environment has been maintained, students will find the freedom to fail, and in that failing, they will explore the values and choices the instructor has shown them in the classroom. Students need the chance to analyze and synthesize for themselves, so they can claim values as their own. Students can be helped in this process by an instructor who supplies them with a good background in general knowledge, then forces them to explore new concepts and ideas, to analyze what they are learning, and to synthesize new ideas and concepts on "their own." An instructor may teach the definition of substance abuse and associated signs and symptoms. But in order for all students to make decisions about their values associated with this population of patients, instructors will need to allow students to explore this topic further. For example, the teacher may ask students to create their own definition of "a substance abuser" or give scenarios where the student must judge the description of behavior in the scenario against the definitions created, possibly forcing students to explore (with instructor facilitation) the emotional issues around identification and care of substance abuse patients. All of this forms the basis for the next level.

It has been said that good judgment comes from experience, and experience comes from bad judgment. Is it not best to start the student's experience from bad judgment in the classroom so they can develop good judgment in the field? One way to start this process is to present challenging, realistic simulations in the classroom, where it is safe for students to fail. After all, the patients are actors or plastic manikins and their emergencies are not real. For simulations to be effective in helping students move through the valuing level of the affective domain, the choices that they will face in the field must be made available in the classroom. Careful planning and coordination are necessary if students are to make the most of simulations in the classroom that will have real-world applicability in the field, clinic, or hospital.

Students who are "stuck" at this level are often found in continuing education classes. They are the ones who already have a strong value and belief system that they have formed over years of experience and other training. To "get through" to these students and really offer them a worthwhile educational experience, the educator must appreciate their educational experiences from the students' perspective. First, such students not only have ideas and concepts that are already deeply rooted and that work for them, they also frequently are fearful, and fear of failure is very strong for adults.[11] Their fear does not need to be realistic or rational from the perspective of the educator to be very real to the adult student learner. This fear need involve only a perceived threat. The most likely threat is that to the student's esteem and his or her self-perception of competence, as failure is associated with incompetence. Therefore, the ideal strategy for the educator is to calm the fears of these students by making the classroom and laboratory a safe place to make and learn from their mistakes. This means that not only will instructors respect students, but shall insist that students respect each other as well. No horseplay, teasing, or ridicule should be tolerated if a student's performance is sub-par.

To achieve a change at this level when students are "stuck," the educator can go back to the Receiving level and use techniques that have already been suggested, such as making the information or change relevant by conveying to students why the training is necessary. The educator can then move to Responding by showing examples and asking for student responses to specific situations, then creating activities that require a response. The educator can then move to Valuing, where learners will have a chance to tear the subject matter apart and put it all together again (analysis and synthesis of the value in question). These activities generally are best accomplished through the use of challenging and realistic scenarios, case studies, or problem-based learning activities.

Level IV: Organization

During the formation of values and attitudes, students begin to recognize several values that apply to the same situation. Students begin to categorize these by how much worth the new value has in relationship to the other things they value that apply to this situation. By doing this, students establish an order of values that they can defend and justify. When this is done, the student is operating at Level IV, Organization. Two steps are required for a student to acquire this level:

1. **Conceptualization (of the value)**: The student identifies the basic concepts of the new value as characteristics that are common to any one value already held. He or she then interprets these common characteristics into a subject or "heading" that can easily be recognized for reference purposes. An example is a student who chooses from a group of publications all those with articles that discuss EMS topics.
2. **Categorization (of the value)**: At this step, the student organizes his or her own values that have characteristics in common into a relationship or hierarchy based on what has been learned in class, through skill demonstrations, and during personal experiences, as well as through the influence of those the student holds in esteem. This allows the student to defend and justify his or her actions. If Level III has been fully integrated and the instructor has allowed creativity and has supported lectures and demonstrations with adequate and sound medical reasoning, the student will more easily attain this level. The more concretely the student can justify and defend his or her actions, the more confident the student becomes, and the more secure his or her value system will be. Ideally, this hierarchy of values, or value system, should be harmonious and consistent.

To reach this point, the student generally needs to have completely integrated Levels I, II, and III into personal thought processes.

Classroom Implications The foundation of this level is set in the quality of supporting information (e.g., anatomy, physiology, pathophysiology, pharmacology) that the student has acquired. The implications for instructors are strong. Instructors must themselves have a good background in basic medical science if they are to help students. The need for the instructor to keep up with information and continue to expand personal horizons cannot be overemphasized. However, it is equally important for instructors to recognize that they cannot know everything. Therefore, making sure that instructors have access to a good library and reliable resources is a must, as is making good use of those resources on a regular basis. Instructors must look up things that they do not know. It is critically important for instructors to remember at all times that they are the students' primary resource, their mentor, and the model that they will be emulating. This is an onerous responsibility for all educators.

Information that instructors provide should allow students to begin to reason out the "whys." Instructors should start the reasoning in the classroom by monitoring and correcting student actions when necessary. For example, the instructor may ask students to compare patient situations, given two patients, both of whom are complaining of abdominal pain; one is a 25-year-old female, and the other is a 65-year-old female. Students can then be asked to discuss the keys of assessment (physical examination and history), explore the differential diagnosis, and compare treatment options. Then, the instructor can make the 65-year-old a patient with diabetes and ask students to explain how this changes their answers and treatment choices.

Teaching Tip >> *Exercises that force the student to compare two patients with similar complaints demonstrate to the student how values may apply to similar situations, and how values may differ from one situation to another.*

Use of scenarios to force students to examine two values facilitates organization of values according to sound medical reasoning. The reader can consider this example: A patient falls and twists her neck. Upon assessment, she is not breathing adequately. Clearing her airway does not improve her ventilations. The student is faced with immobilizing the patient where she lies, or gently moving her head and neck into alignment. What should the student choose and why? Have students justify their answers. Have discussions involving two value systems, exceptions to the rule, and immediate life threats. These all help students to organize their values.

Use of scenarios is especially helpful at this level. Discussions of why certain signs and symptoms appear, what (if appropriate) expected signs/symptoms are *not* apparent and why that may be, and which treatment should be selected and why, all go toward helping students justify their actions with the use of sound medical reasoning. "Because it says so in the protocol" is a weak answer from a student at any learning level.

Level V: Characterization

At this level, the value system is so ingrained in students' behavior patterns that it becomes part of their lifestyle, and students' values become integrated into a total philosophy of care. Experience is required to attain this level. Therefore, this level is not usually observed in the classroom unless continuing education is being taught to a group of seasoned providers.

The two steps that constitute this level help describe a person who has attained it:

1. *Consistency*: This means that when the student is confronted with a number of situations that involve a reaction based on the same value system or characteristics, the student's reactions are automatic and predictable. The key here is consistency. When confronted by a situation that demands a choice between values, the student is consistent in his or her choice and is able to consistently defend that choice with sound medical knowledge and judgment based on balancing of values, "book learning," skills, and experience. The instructor is able to predict how the student will act in a given situation. For example, a student who believes in treating all patients with dignity will consistently complete a full assessment and care plan for the intoxicated homeless patient regardless of how many times that same patient has called EMS. The instructor, or later, coworkers and supervisors, will be able to accurately predict that this provider will not take short cuts or dismiss the patient simply because he or she has cared for the patient many times before.
2. *Characterization*: Now, the student is so closely associated with the value or characteristic in question that people use the characteristic to describe him or her, like ALS Amy who tends to err on the side of caution and ride in with advanced life support measure in place on nearly every patient, or Safety Sam who always wears gloves and eye protection no matter how clean the patient appears. The student has integrated attitudes, values, and ideas into a total philosophy. Typically, this level is associated with a high level of student pride in accomplishments, as well as a high degree of satisfaction in work performed.

It is important for the instructor to recognize that students' experiences may greatly contribute to their attaining this level in one area and not in all. For instance, students may attain the level of Characterization with behavioral patients, but they may attain only the first steps of the Valuing level with pediatric patients. This may be so because of the population groups they serve, or it may be a result of where their interest lies. The interest and comfort levels of students dictate choices, such as always caring for behavioral patients while preferring their partner to care for all of the pediatric patients.

Peers, especially partners, receiving hospital staff, administrators, and life events may directly affect attainment of this level. A provider may demonstrate characteristics of this level but then vacillate between levels, depending on what is going on in his or her life. For instance, a provider may be on his way to acquiring Characterization when suddenly faced with the death of a coworker, a divorce, administrative decisions that negatively affect his or her ability to deliver patient care, or a receiving hospital staff whose attitudes are demeaning. If so much stress is introduced that basic value systems are called into question, an individual may revert back to Receiving or Responding. Personal stressors may become powerful inhibitors to acquiring or maintaining this level.

Classroom Implications The most important action instructors can take is to model this level. Participating in continuing education as students, belonging to professional organizations, reading professional journals and discussing articles with students, extending their knowledge base to other disciplines, ensuring that classroom topics are relevant and applicable to the field, and being sensitive to what happens to students when they leave the classroom, all help to contribute to the acquisition of this level by instructors—not only for themselves, but also for students.

Teaching Psychomotor Skills

The learning, mastery, and performance of skills are, and will remain, an important part of the medical field from the medical assistant who takes vital signs to the surgeon performing a delicate operation. Therefore, it is imperative that medical educators be proficient in the teaching and evaluation of skill performance.

Psychomotor skill development is crucial to good patient care. All the effort put forth at the scene of an EMS incident is dependent on the provider's ability to select the right skill, at the right time, and to carry it out in the right manner. In addition, many of the skills routinely performed at an EMS call are critical to patient survival and leave little or no margin for error. As an example, correct placement of an intraosseous infusion is vital to securing and maintaining a route for fluids and medications in an infant. However, this procedure allows no margin for error. The device must be placed in the correct location or the patient will not get needed medications. Thus, teaching paramedics to place intraosseous infusions must be done correctly, efficiently, and in a manner that ensures learner success. This can be accomplished only when the instructor has a solid understanding of psychomotor skill training, mastery, and performance.

Understanding the Psychomotor Domain

The psychomotor domain comprises the skill, action, muscle movement, and manual **manipulation** related to performing a physical action. Similar to all domains, the physical activities addressed in the psychomotor domain also have affective and cognitive dimensions. A learner who is being taught to start an intravenous line (IV) needs not only to learn the physical movements and manipulations needed to insert an IV catheter, he or she must appreciate the discomfort the procedure causes, which are elements of the affective domain, as well as the why and when associated with starting an IV, which is the "psycho" or cognitive part of the psychomotor domain, or in some cases, elements of the cognitive domain applied here. In addition, the context or environment in which the skill will be performed is important. Many medical procedures are carried out in a field environment that is very different from that of a hospital or classroom. As one of the basic parts of a behavioral objective, as discussed in Chapter 8: Goals and Objectives, a condition is specified under which the desired behavior is to occur. When psychomotor skills are taught, it is imperative that the instructor stress, and if possible simulate, various conditions in the classroom in order to prepare the student to perform those skills in real-world settings such as with the patient seated in a lab chair, lying in a hospital bed, or ambulatory at the scene of a motor vehicle crash. It would be unfair for a learner to master a technique while not wearing personal protective equipment (PPE), then suddenly find that he or she is unable to do, or feels awkward doing, the same skill in a field setting wearing PPE. And, as with all learning experiences, modeling plays an important part in the learning experience. It is imperative, therefore, that the instructor and all other instructional personnel carry out skills and procedures in a manner consistent with that expected of the learner. In this example of PPE, the instructors, then, should be wearing gloves and goggles while demonstrating the skill.

When teaching psychomotor skills, the instructor must consider learner "prerequisites" needed if the student is to learn the cognitive material. The ability of the learner to actually perform a skill is dependent on a number of parameters. The instructor should consider the following:

- *Physical strength of the learner.* Can the learner, for instance, lift a stretcher containing a 150-pound patient? Can he or she carry equipment and equipment containers up a flight of stairs?
- *Physical endurance.* Can the learner do cardiopulmonary resuscitation (CPR) at the proper rate and depth for several minutes at a time?
- *Coordination.* Does the learner possess significant coordination and fine motor control, or is he or she "all thumbs"?
- *Sensory acuity.* Can the learner see fine detail? Exhibit sufficient depth perception? Does he or she wear bifocal glasses that make intubation difficult? Can he or she hear well enough to note different heart tones or breath sounds?
- *Composure.* How does the learner perform under stress? Does he or she develop tremors that interfere with delicate procedures? Does the learner become impatient, and thus tend to perform skills brusquely or without proper attention to detail? Conversely, if the skill produces discomfort for the patient, does the student freeze and fail to complete the skill?[12]

The instructor is cautioned that when these parameters are evaluated, measures appropriate to the actual job description of the provider should be followed, as should the requirements of the Americans with Disabilities Act. (For more information on the Americans with Disabilities Act, see Chapter 10: Legal Issues for the Educator.)

Teaching a skill involves more than just correct demonstration of the skill. The instructor must analyze the skill and must recognize that every skill consists of a series of subcomponents. The actual terminology and number of components vary in the literature, but the essential actions include gross muscle movement, fine muscle movement, and **spatial awareness**. To understand these relationships, one can consider the skill of intramuscular injection. Providers engage in gross muscle movement as they move their arms up and forward toward the injection site. As the needle enters the patient, fine muscle movement adjusts to **tactile stimulation** to steady the path of the needle and handle gauge resistance. Spatial awareness tells providers where their extremities are in relation to their bodies and the environment. This information allows providers to "aim" the needle and determine when to stop advancement. Because awareness of the environment is so important, sensory acuity and perception are also important aspects of skill mastery. In this example, if the patient had moved, the provider would have to sense this and adjust his or her movement accordingly. Thus, when teaching skills, the instructor must understand not only the steps and sequence involved, but the kinematics of the procedure as well.

Levels of Psychomotor Skill Development

It would be convenient if learners could see a skill demonstrated once, then be able to exactly reproduce the skill immediately and permanently. However, this is not the case. Learning a skill and assimilating it into a rote response involves a number of developmental steps. As with the other domains of learning, a taxonomy of psychomotor skill development has been devised. However, unlike with the cognitive domain, for which most educators use Bloom, different taxonomies are reported in the educational literature for psychomotor skill development. For the purposes of this textbook, we will use Bloom's taxonomy of psychomotor skills development.

> **Bloom's Taxonomy: Psychomotor Domain**
>
> Level 1: **Imitation**
>
> Level 2: **Manipulation**
>
> Level 3: **Precision**
>
> Level 4: **Articulation**
>
> Level 5: **Naturalization**

Imitation

The most basic psychomotor skill is repeating or modeling a skill that is demonstrated to the learner by an expert. In this "see one, do one" approach, the instructor demonstrates the skill, then asks learners to repeat it. Usually, the instructor talks or guides the learner through the steps of the skill. This method works best for skills that are simple and can be understood easily through observation. For more complex skills, the instructor begins the learning process at the imitation stage by breaking down the complex skill into simpler, more easily learned skills that can be modeled by the beginner. Because learners are receptive to modeling the behavior of the instructor or another expert, it is important that the instructor avoid modeling incorrectly. This can be difficult in that the instructor has progressed to the naturalization level and may not even be cognizant of how he or she is performing the skill. However, should a skill be modeled incorrectly, it will take many more practice attempts to "untrain" the incorrect behavior than it would have taken to teach the behavior to mastery level in the first place.

Manipulation

The second phase of skill mastery is manipulation. During this stage, learners move away from simple modeling to performing the skill according to guidelines, such as skill sheets. They "manipulate" the various parts of the skill in such a way as to develop their own basis or foundation for doing the skill. Because learners are still exploring the skill, mistakes are common and are to be expected. However, mistakes help learners to better understand the skill through the corrective actions needed. It is important for the instructor to closely monitor learners as they practice skills to ensure that no incorrect actions or "bad habits" are learned as part of the skill. Because each learner is different, some variation in performance may occur, but by and large, the learner must perform the skill as modeled by the instructor or according to the skill sheet or established standard. It is also important at this stage for the instructor to explain to learners why a particular action or technique is used. This is especially important if skills taught later in the program will require this action. For example, proper placement of limb leads in obtaining an electrocardiogram (ECG) may not be critical for a 3-lead ECG, but it becomes more important when a 12-lead ECG is obtained.

This is also the period during which the learner begins independent practice of the skill. It is important that skill sheets or procedures be explained clearly and in sufficient detail. Practice sessions should be observed closely, and any incorrect behaviors should be immediately identified and corrected. Because the learner is discovering the new skill, group practice may provide a supportive environment and can allow learners to explore the new skill together.

Precision

At the precision stage, the learner can perform the basic skill without coaching or the skill sheet and with few, if any, mistakes. However, the learner still has not developed the expertise to perform the skill in various contexts. For example, the learner may be able to splint a fractured arm on a simulated patient who is sitting up without angulation. However, any variation of the patient position or severity of injury, such as the patient lying down, will reduce the learner's precision. Precision is often the level students are at when they are tested on a psychomotor skill. They can perform the skill correctly without the skill sheet, but often only in a controlled environment without distraction or variation.

Articulation

This stage blends psychomotor skill development with the cognitive and affective dimensions of a skill or procedure. The learner understands why the skill is done in a particular way and knows when the skill is indicated. The learner can now evaluate the context in which the skill is performed and can adjust his performance to the situation. In the previous example, the learner would now be able to splint an arm, regardless of patient position or other conditions. The learner is now performing the skill without mistakes and without the assistance of props such as skill sheets or instructor prompting. This is the level of psychomotor skill performance that is expected of an entry level provider. However, students are often never tested at this level. Given constraints on classroom and lab time, students may not get past the Precision level in class. Often, clinical time, internship, or even on-the-job-training is required to reach articulation level. Instructors should be aware that potential employers may be expecting a higher level of performance than can be delivered by a new graduate of their medical educational program.

Naturalization

At this stage, the learner can perform the skill flawlessly and without much conscious effort. In a scenario, simulation, or actual patient care situation, the learner will be able to perform the skill while continuing to monitor the context and environment. The learner will be able to multitask effectively **(Figure 12.3)**. The learner has achieved what is known as "muscle memory," that is, the skill has become rote and can be initiated and performed with minimal sensory awareness. A common example of this level of mastery is the provider who is seen performing a manual skill, such as a pulse or neuro-check, while obtaining an oral history from the patient. This level is rarely seen in the classroom learner or entry level provider. It develops later as the provider gains experience on the job.

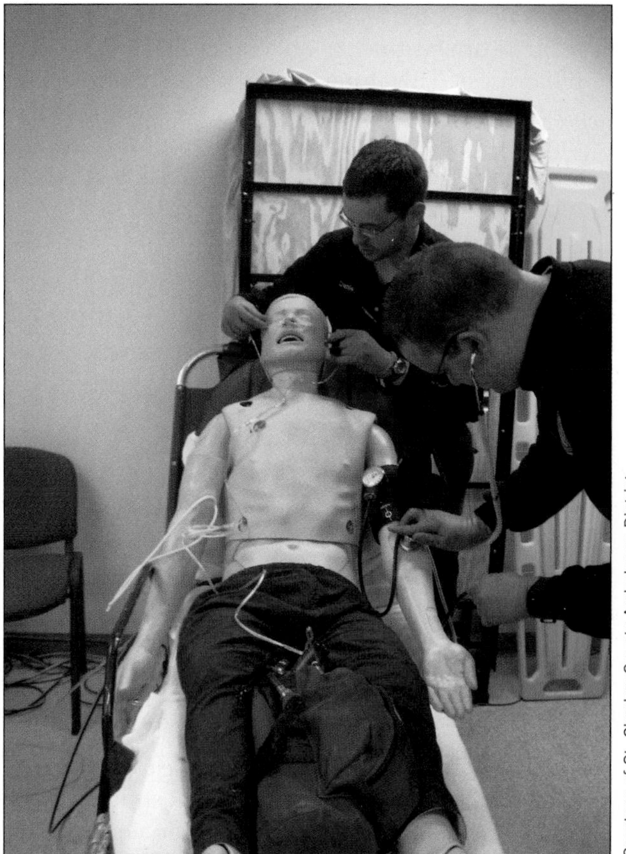

Courtesy of St. Charles County Ambulance District

Figure 12.3

Naturalization of a psychomotor skill is achieved when the student is able to multitask effectively.

Teaching Psychomotor Skills

Effective teaching of psychomotor skills involves more than just demonstrating a skill and having learners practice. As with any instructional activity, preparation and teaching technique are important aspects of the overall experience. This is especially true in the psychomotor domain because of the complexity of many EMS skills.

Because EMS skills almost always involve equipment and, to be effectively demonstrated, usually require special teaching aids or manikins, preparation is important. To begin, the instructor must review the lesson goal, objectives, and lesson plan to ensure that he or she is familiar with the lesson. Necessary equipment, supplies, and teaching aids should be identified and secured. The instructor is cautioned not to assume that equipment and materials will be available in the classroom. This is especially true in multiple-use facilities, where different instructors and different classes may meet in the same facility. If the instructor arranges for an in-service unit to provide lesson props, a backup plan should be in place in the event the unit suddenly becomes unavailable. The same applies to lessons planned for outdoors that may be canceled or modified because of weather.

When setting up the classroom or drill ground, the instructor should consider the following:

- *Safety.* The instructor should consider safety, not only in terms of practice by the learners, but as it relates to any inherent danger associated with demonstrating the skill. For example, caution is needed when one is demonstrating auto extrication skills. Vehicles and equipment can shift, or parts may fly off, during certain activities. The instructor should clearly define and mark safe zones. Other safety considerations include sharps, medical waste, restraining of simulated patients on hard surfaces, and lifting and moving exercises.

- *Visibility.* For the learner to model and imitate a skill, he or she must be able to see all aspects of the process. Therefore, it is important that the instructor provide visibility. This may involve moving learners, breaking into small groups, using video demonstrations, or using special, large-scale models or cameras and video projectors.
- *Rehearsal.* Regardless of how many times an instructor has performed a skill, or how well he or she can do it, it is always prudent to practice the skill before class. This is especially true when one is using special models or equipment that is different from that routinely used. Nothing kills an instructor's credibility more effectively than an inability to use the equipment that he or she is teaching about. If something is to go wrong, it will surely happen during the class session.
- *Classroom preparation.* The instructor should arrange the classroom to ensure visibility and to accommodate the equipment and instructional props. The instructor should check in advance for electrical or oxygen connections, venting, and so forth.
- *Practice space.* If learners will practice a particular skill, the instructor must ensure that sufficient space is provided, as well as appropriate equipment, at each skill practice area. If learners will rearrange a classroom before they begin practice, the instructor must ensure that this can be done and will not be disruptive to the learning process.
- *Group size.* Most physical or psychomotor educational programs recommend no more than a 10:1 student to instructor ratio to ensure students are properly supervised, can see all demonstrations, and will receive adequate practice time and feedback from the instructor. However, many programs find that 6:1 is a more realistic ratio, and that regardless of group size, students will rarely get enough practice to reach precision, articulation, or naturalization levels during class time. A "skills disclaimer" or statement in the course policy manual alerting students to the fact that they will need to practice outside of scheduled classroom and laboratory hours will help set this expectation.

Whole-Part-Whole Instruction

The standard technique used for teaching EMS skills is the **whole-part-whole method**. To use this technique, the instructor demonstrates the skill three times:

1. *Whole.* The instructor demonstrates the entire skill from beginning to end, while briefly naming each action or step. If possible, the skill should be performed under the conditions specified in the psychomotor behavioral objective such as "The paramedic student will successfully demonstrate initiating an IV line on a patient in the emergency department with no critical errors." Because it is so important that the initial imprint is a perfect demonstration, many instructors choose to use a video of the skill for the first "whole" demonstration. As video can be edited, the instructor can be positive that the demonstration is a match for the established technique or standard.
2. *Part.* The instructor demonstrates the skill again, step-by-step, explaining each part in detail. It is important that the instructor select proper size "bites" of the skill. If the information is too specific, the learner can be overloaded with detail; too broad, and the learner may not be able to make the connection from step to step
3. *Whole.* The instructor demonstrates the entire skill from beginning to end, without interruption, and usually without commentary

This technique provides repeated, accurate examples of how the skill is done. If a learner was not completely focused on the skill demonstration the first time, two other opportunities for observation are provided. This approach also provides a rationale for how the skill has been performed. During the "part" presentation, the instructor can integrate affective and cognitive objectives and encourage student interaction and questions. Finally, it has been proved that the technique works well for both analytic and global learners. Analytic learners appreciate the step-by-step instruction, and global learners get the chance to see the skill performed in context.

Progression Through The Psychomotor Domain Levels of Skill Acquisition

As has been discussed, the learner moves through a progression of increasing proficiency, eventually reaching the mastery level. When teaching psychomotor skills, the instructor must provide an environment that fosters this development.

The instructor should first work with learners to move from novice to expert, that is, being able to perform the skill at the precision level. When moving learners in this direction, the instructor should keep the following in mind:

- Learners should be allowed to progress at their own pace. If learners are moved too quickly, they may not understand what they are doing and will not acquire good thinking skills.
- Although the demonstration may provide information on the performance of the entire skill from start to finish, learners should be allowed to learn the individual parts of the skill before pulling it all together and demonstrating the whole skill. For example, learners may need to learn how to hold or operate a piece of equipment before they can be taught the sequence of applying or using the device.
- Learners should master individual skills before placing them in the context of a scenario or simulation.
- Learners should be allowed ample time to practice a skill before they are tested.
- The need for constant direct supervision should diminish as practice time increases and skill level improves.

Taking this into consideration, the instructor should plan skill learning to follow a sequence similar to the following:

1. The instructor demonstrates the skill to learners three times using the whole-part-whole method.
2. Learners attempt the skill under direct supervision of the instructor who can correct sequencing or technique mistakes before or as they happen.
3. Learners practice using a skills check sheet.
4. Learners memorize the steps of the skill until they can verbalize the sequence without error.
5. Learners perform the skill, stating each step as they perform it.
6. Learners perform the skill while answering questions about their performance.
7. Learners perform the skill in the context of a scenario or an actual patient situation **(Figure 12.4)**.

Honest feedback about the learner's performance should be provided regularly. The instructor should not hesitate to correct improper performance, but whenever possible, should include positive feedback as well to ensure that the learner continues the correct behaviors while modifying the actions that were not quite right. This is especially critical during the early stages of skill development. If incorrect behaviors are not effectively corrected, mastery or muscle memory of the wrong technique will occur, and correcting this later on will be more difficult. The instructor may allow advanced learners to identify and correct their own errors under limited supervision. To reinforce correct behaviors, the instructor could end practice sessions with a demonstration of correct performance.

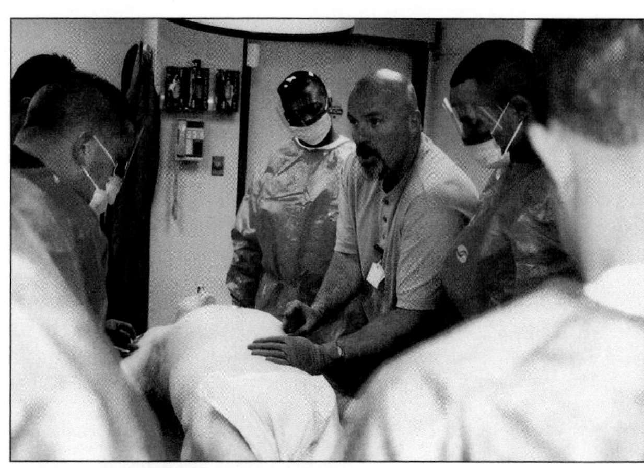

Figure 12.4

Learners should move through a progression of increasing proficiency and achieve mastery before using skills on real patients. Shown is a cadaver lab that is used to assist students in achieving mastery.

As a learner masters a skill, it is important for the instructor to appreciate the level of mastery required of the learner. Too often, instructors and practical test evaluators expect a learner to perform a skill at a level beyond that attainable by an entry level provider. Some instructors and evaluators expect performance that matches their own level of mastery. This is not only an unrealistic expectation, it is unfair to the learner as well. It is important for instructors and evaluators to accept that many skills may be performed in a number of different but medically acceptable ways. Just because a learner performs a skill in a way that differs from the instructor's performance does not mean that the learner's performance is wrong, unless it is medically incorrect or may harm the patient.

Skill Sheets

When new skills are taught, it is important for the learner to know clearly what is involved in the skill, in terms of both actions and sequence. Although the instructor demonstrates the skill, the use of a detailed skill sheet or task analysis enhances the learner's comprehension. The skill sheet also serves as a review for skill performance. For visual and concrete learners, it provides the needed framework on which mastery of the skill can be built.

When preparing a skill sheet, it is important for the instructor to clearly list the various steps of the skill at a level consistent with that used in the teaching demonstration. In other words, if six steps are demonstrated in completing a skill, the skill sheet should list six steps. The skill sheet should not be used to break the skill down to a level that is more finite than the one taught, or conversely, to compress actions into fewer steps. It is also important for the instructor to design the skill sheet with emphasis on areas that are critical to proper skill performance and subsequent skill evaluation. If process is important, it should be included. Likewise, if sequence is important, sequencing should be delineated on the skill sheet, and it should be clearly communicated to the learner that it is important.

A common practice is for instructors to provide students with the practical evaluation skill sheets of the National Registry of Emergency Medical Technicians (NREMT) for use during practice. While it is appropriate for students to have and use the National Registry skills sheets, it should be remembered that these were intended as evaluation tools, not teaching tools, and they lack sufficient step by step detail for the student new to the skill to understand how and why each step is executed. A skills video, skills manual, or skills textbook may be necessary in addition to the skills sheets.

Improving Psychomotor Skill Development During a Skills Session

Skill sessions provide valuable time for the learner to practice and master skills. However, for full support of skill mastery, it is important that the skill session be used to maximum advantage. To accomplish this, the instructor should keep the following in mind:

- Have all necessary equipment setup before the session begins. However, if the setup is complicated or the class is large, the instructor may have the learners retrieve equipment from a storage area and set up the practice stations. In a similar manner, learners can be asked to put away the equipment.
- Use realistic and current equipment that is in proper working order. Do not expect learners to master a skill if they do not have the right equipment to use.
- Use standardized teaching tools such as skills videos and skills sheets.
- Allow ample practice time in class, at breaks, and during other times. However, ensure that all practice sessions are conducted safely and with proper supervision as needed.
- Always model correct psychomotor skill behavior.
- Keep learners active and involved. This can be difficult, especially as learners become more proficient; they may not wish to engage in repeated practice of a skill. Consider adding context to practice, such as placing the manikin on the floor, or in a chair, or under a table to simulate different positions in which patients may be found.
- Insist that learners respect equipment and skills.
- Ensure competence in individual skills before using scenarios. Scenarios should be designed to tie together basic skills, once they have been mastered.
- Consider videotaping a skill and allow students to review their performance.
- Add realism. It is important for the instructor to place skills in the context of on-the-job situations. When using scenarios, do the following:
  - Limit the objective of the scenario to three learning points.
  - As learners become more sophisticated with the use of critical-thinking skills, add dimensions to the scenario.
  - Make the scenario realistic, especially in terms of the performance objective and the safety requirements, such as wearing protective equipment.
  - Use actual equipment.
  - Consider the use of moulage, props, background noises, and so forth.

Managing the Skill Session

Skill practice time is an essential component for skill mastery to occur, especially in certification courses like Emergency Medical Technician. It is imperative that the instructor plan practice time to provide maximum opportunity for the learner to master skills. This is best achieved when some degree of structure is provided during the session. Simply providing a room full of equipment and instructing learners to practice skills will usually result in chaos and little active practice by the learners. This is especially true when skills are being reviewed that the learner believes he or she has mastered. Instructors teaching refresher or renewal courses are often faced with the challenge of motivating learners to perform skills they believe they already know. To ensure maximum use of practice time, the instructor should plan activities to keep the whole class engaged for the entire length of the practice session. This is especially important if only one or two instructors are managing a large class.[13] After appropriate introductory material, and with adequate resources such as skill check lists, some student groups can be independently assigned for peer evaluation.

A few issues about the use of assistant instructors must be mentioned. Assistants can be a great help to an instructor, and they may provide direct assistance and feedback to learners. However, it is important that the lead instructor and assistant instructors teach the same skill in the same manner. Instructor development meetings where the teaching tools, skills sheets, equipment, and evaluation tools can be reviewed together can go a long way in helping assistant instructors remain consistent with program goals. **Inter-rater reliability** (IRR) exercises should be conducted for all evaluators. IRR is the process of calibrating instructors to the evaluation tool so that each instructor is grading exactly the same way. Often, a video of a medical skill is played, then the student in the video is rated by all instructors present. Scores for the student are shared, and often, are wildly different. A lead instructor or program director then reviews the skill, the standard, and the evaluation tool with the instructors. They then watch the same video again, grading according to the instruction they just received. Usually, the scores among all instructors are much closer together. If necessary, the process can be repeated several times until all evaluators understand which behaviors should and should not be counted as correct.

Maximizing Skill Session Time

To ensure that practice time is used as efficiently as possible, instructors should plan activities to fill the entire instruction time. Instructors should consider assigning roles to learners during skill practice. In this way, learners will have the chance to practice different skills and rotate through different roles during the skill practice. This approach works well to occupy learners who otherwise would be waiting to practice a skill or to move on to the next skill. Detailed skill sheets allow students to self- and peer-evaluate during the skill sessions.

Learners can be assigned to the following roles, depending on the size of the practice group:

- *Evaluator.* Uses a skill sheet or records steps as they are performed. This allows learners to appreciate the challenge of evaluating a skill and reinforces learning through observation of the skill that is being performed.
- *Information provider.* Facilitator uses a script and provides information as it is requested; for instance, vital signs when they are taken.
- *Team leader.* Is primary patient care provider and leader of the team performing the skill(s).
- *Partner or assistant.* Assists the team leader and performs care as directed by the team leader; depending on practice parameters, may be silent or may be able to suggest and interact with the team leader. More than one team member or partner may be needed for safety such as during spinal immobilization or patient restraint.
- *Patient.* Faithfully portrays signs and symptoms according to scenario; may be moulaged for realism. This role also familiarizes the learner with the experiences of the patient and promotes empathy.
- *Bystander(s).* Additional practice team members can assume the role of bystanders and can act as distracters or helpers. It is important for the instructor to monitor learners in this role to ensure that they do not get too carried away with their role-playing, thereby disrupting the actual practice of the skill in a realistic setting.
- Additional roles, if groups are large, might include first responders, members of the fire department or law enforcement, or a hospital charge nurse to whom the report will be given.

When designing a practice session, the instructor should distribute a written scenario to practice groups. The scenario should be realistic for the learner's level of expertise and local operational capability. It should also match the performance objective that is being reviewed. Sources of scenarios include actual calls, medical scenario books, EMS textbooks, instructor toolkits, and professional organization websites.

To begin the practice session, the instructor should have the information provider read the dispatch information. Whenever possible, learners should be allowed to complete the scenario without interruption. At this point, the learner should have mastered individual skills, so stopping for correction should not be necessary. Once the scenario has been completed, the group as a whole should evaluate skill performance, beginning with the team leader. By allowing the team leader to identify his or her own mistakes, the instructor is able to determine the degree of self-awareness possessed by the team leader. Additionally, the instructor can compare the learner's assessment of his or her performance to his own assessment of the same, helping to calibrate the learner to the standard of professional performance.

The various role players should next be called upon to critique the performance. It must be remembered that learners are often their own greatest critics. They should be encouraged to look for the positive aspects of their performance. Otherwise, they may focus on what they perceive as poor performance. The assistants, patient, and bystanders all should take turns providing feedback. Finally, the evaluator should comment on timing, sequencing, prioritization, and skill performance.

Regardless of how an evaluator is issuing the critique, it should be a positive learning experience—not a learner bashing. To provide a positive experience, a positive-negative-positive format is often used, but has come under scrutiny in recent years. It has been suggested that the positive-negative-positive approach, or "feedback sandwich" as it has been called, is manipulative and minimizes the value of anything positive said because the listener already knows something negative is coming and is now able to focus only on the negative.[14] To make sure this does not happen, the positive feedback should be specific and personal, focused on a single behavior in a single discussion. The instructor should next move to constructive feedback and areas for improvement, citing specific actions or decisions of concern. Comments must be consistent with what learners have been taught, and they must follow the skill sheet. The instructor should end the review with a positive comment such as, "I was especially impressed by how you applied the traction splint, given the location of the fracture."

Once the scenario has been critiqued, learners should change roles. Sufficient scenarios and time should be provided for all learners to have at least one chance to play each role. However, time constraints may not permit this, so it may be helpful for students to develop a rotation in their group where the roles are rotated not just during one skill lab, but each time the students are practicing skills. Additionally, instructors may want to script the scenarios to ensure that by the end of the course each group has participated in a sufficient variety of patient care situations.

CASE IN POINT

The EMS instructor was conducting the cardiac arrest skill session for six EMT students. He began by asking, "Who wants to be the team leader first?" A lively, bright, and aggressive student jumped up to the head of the manikin and said, "I'll do it." The information provider presented the case of a witnessed arrest with bystander CPR and no automatic external defibrillator (AED) when the crew arrives.

"The first thing I'm going to do is BSI and scene safety, and I'll determine whether I need any help. Are there any other patients? Any hazards, like downed electrical lines? He didn't get electrocuted, did he?" He immediately gave out team assignments to check for unresponsiveness and signs of breathing, put on the AED, assess for circulation, and begin cardiopulmonary resuscitation (CPR) beginning with chest compressions. After determining there was no pulse, the AED indicated a need for shock, and everyone stood "clear" while it delivered a shock. Chest compressions were started and the other team member alternated with bag-mask ventilation until the next shock was indicated. The instructor then conducted a brief critique of the session, allowing the patient care provider to go first, then allowing others in the group to provide input.

Addressing the team leader, he said, "Your initial steps and team management were very well organized and effective. Well done." To the team member who managed the airway, he said, "Your assessment and ventilations were fine, but you didn't use an oropharyngeal airway. I was wondering why not?" After the team member shrugged and looked around for support, the instructor said, "I understand you may have overlooked it, but realize that the oropharyngeal airway is the most neglected adjunct in the basic life support tool kit. Everybody should keep it in mind. Can you think of why?" The discussion went on with the instructor providing constructive nonjudgmental feedback in a positive learning environment.

This was a typical cardiovascular skill assessment session in which realistic manikins, an AED, and airway and ventilation devices were provided. The instructor's feedback to participants was nonjudgmental, honest, and helpful. The organized setup, combined with a qualified and prepared instructor, provided the next best learning environment that we have after actual clinical settings.

Summary

Comprehensive EMS education involves teaching in every domain and at all levels. Educators must be conscious of the three domains of learning and must apply appropriate teaching methods for the purpose of developing competent, compassionate care providers. In addition to giving attention to each domain, the educator must be aware of the multiple levels of learning that students go through in becoming fully competent. Each level requires that the instructor (1) be aware of the signs of progress and (2) know the teaching methods that help move students toward higher levels of learning and critical thinking.

Glossary

active behavior The student is actively thinking or doing something to learn.

articulation The fourth stage of psychomotor skill development is to blend the skill with the cognitive and affective dimensions of a skill or procedure so that the learner understands the "whys" and "whens."

categorization of the value The student organizes his or her own values that have characteristics in common into a relationship or hierarchy that has characteristics common to based on what has been learned in class, through skill demonstrations, and during personal experiences, as well as through the influence of those the student holds in esteem.

command response A requirement of the student.

composure Has to do with how the learner reacts; maintaining a sense of calm under stress.

conceptualization of the value The student identifies the basic concepts of the new value as characteristics that are common to any one value already held.

critical thinking: As described by John Dewey: ". . . the active, persistent, and careful consideration of a belief or supposed form of knowledge in light of the grounds which support it and the further conclusions to which it tends." Higher level cognitive skills, or problem solving skills.

facilitation Assisting a learner in discovering information or abilities for him or herself.

higher order thinking Has to do with Bloom's higher cognitive levels to include analysis, synthesis, and evaluation; critical thinking, problem solving.

imitation The first phase of psychomotor skill development is the ability to repeat a skills demonstrated by an expert.

inter-rater reliability Consistency among evaluators or evaluation methods.

manipulation The second phase of psychomotor skill development is the ability to perform the skill by developing the student's own method of skill manipulation.

mastery Possession of a skill.

metacognition simply put, thinking about thinking; literally, "in the midst of knowing"; an awareness and control of one's thinking.

mnemonics Using patterns to assist in recall.

naturalization The fifth stage of psychomotor skill development is where the skill becomes a habit and is performed flawlessly and without much conscious effort.

passive behavior The student is not engaged or active but only receives information or ideas.

precision The third phase of psychomotor skill development is to perform the skill precisely in a controlled environment without distraction or variation.

safe classroom An environment in which the student feels little risk of emotional harm while actively participating in learning activities.

satisfaction response A voluntary response that brings on a sense of self-esteem.

sensory acuity Ability to perceive fine detail.

spatial awareness Awareness of the location of one's extremities in relation to their body and the environment.

T.H.I.N.K. A model or system; a mnemonic used for a model to teach critical thinking skills which stands for "T" - total recall, "H"- habits, "I" - inquiry, "N" - new ideas and creativity, and "K" - knowing how you think.

tactile stimulation Activation of the sensation of touch, texture, temperature, and other touch sensations.

whole-part-whole instruction A teaching technique that first provides the big picture, then breaks it into separate parts and steps, then completes the technique with another overview of the big picture.

willing response The student agrees to respond from something inside the student.

References

1. Dewey, J. (1963). *Experience and education.* New York, NY: Collier.
2. Stiggins, R. J., Rubel, E., & Quellmakz, E. (1986). *Measuring thinking skills in the classroom.* Washington, DC: National Education Association.
3. Costa, A. L., Hanson, R., Silver, H. F., & Strong, R. W. (1985). Building a repertoire of strategies. In A. L. Costa (Ed.), *Developing minds: A resource book for teaching thinking.* Alexandria, VA: Association for Supervision and Curriculum Development, 141–143.
4. Beyer, B. K. (1987). *Practical strategies for the teaching of thinking.* Boston, MA: Allyn and Bacon.
5. Rubenfeld, M. G., & Scheffer, B. K. (1995). *Critical thinking in nursing: An interactive approach.* Philadelphia, PA: J. B. Lippincott.
6. Beyer, B. K. (1988). *Developing a thinking skills program.* Boston, MA: Allyn and Bacon.
7. Croskerry, P. (2007, February). The affective imperative: Coming to terms with our emotions. *Society for Academic Emergency Medicine, 14*(2), 184–186.
8. Lorber, M. A., & Pierce, W. D. (1983). *Objectives, methods, and evaluation for secondary teaching* (2nd ed.). Englewood Cliffs, NJ: Prentice Hall.
9. Norman, G. R. (2000, March). The adult learner: A mythical species. *Academic Medicine, 75*(3), 217–218.
10. King, E. C. (1984). *Affective education in nursing: A guide to teaching and assessment.* Rockville, MD: Aspen System.
11. Wlodkowski, R. J. (1999). *Enhancing adult motivation to learn.* San Francisco, CA: Jossey-Bass.
12. Sage, G. H. (1984). *Motor learning and control: A neuropsychological approach.* Dubuque, IA: W.C. Brown.
13. Zipp, G. P., & Gentile, A. M. (2010, February). Practice schedule and the learning of motor skills. *Journal of College Teaching and Learning,* No. 2, 35–42.
14. Johnson, S., & Johnson, C. (1986). *The one minute teacher: How to teach others to teach themselves.* New York, NY: William Morrow.

Additional Resources

Amato, T. (2007). Respecting the power of denial. *Academic Emergency Medicine,* No. 2, 184.

Croskerry, P. (2002). Achieving quality in clinical decision making: Cognitive strategies and detection of bias. *Academic Emergency Medicine.* No. 9, 1184–1204.

Croskerry, P. (2005). Diagnostic failure: A cognitive and affective approach. In *Advances in patient safety: From research to implementation.* AHRQ publication No. 050021, Vol. 2. Rockville, MD: Agency for Health Care, Research and Quality, 241–54.

Croskerry, P. (2005). The theory and practice of clinical decision making. *Canadian Journal of Anaesthesiology, 52*: R1–8.

Damasio, A. R. (1994). *Descartes' error: Emotion, reason and the human brain.* New York, NY: Grosset/Putnam.

Docheff, D. M. (1990, Nov/Dec). The feedback sandwich. *Journal of Physical Education, Recreation and Dance.* Vol. 61, 17–18.

Kassirer, J. P., Kopelman, R. I. (2002). *Learning clinical reasoning.* Baltimore, MD: Williams and Wilkins.

Krathwohl, D. A., Massie, B. B., Bloom, B. S., *et al.* (1964). *Taxonomy of educational objectives handbook.* II: *Affective domain.* New York, NY: David McKay.

McCombs, B. L., McNeely, S., (Eds.), (1996). *Psychology in the classroom: A series on applied educational psychology. Teaching for thinking.* Hyattsville, MD: American Psychological Association.

Musinski, B. (1999, Jan–Mar). The educator as facilitator: A new kind of leadership. *Nursing Forum, 34*(1), 23–29.

Regehr, G. (2004). Self-reflection on the quality of decisions in health care. *Medical Education,* No. 38, 1024–1027.

Sternberg, R. J. (1985). *Beyond IQ: A triarchic theory of human intelligence.* New York, NY: Cambridge University Press.

Wlodkowski, R. J. (2008). *Enhancing adult motivation to learn: A comprehensive guide for teaching all adults* (3rd ed.). San Francisco, CA: Jossey-Bass.

13

Tools for Individual Learning

You cannot teach a man anything; you can only help him find it within himself. — GALILEO GALILEI

As has been discussed in earlier chapters, adult learners respond best in an environment that offers a variety of learning methods. Adult learners frequently have a motivation for learning that is not present in younger learners. They have consciously made the choice to acquire new knowledge and often seek out ways on their own to broaden and apply their new-found knowledge. This chapter introduces a variety of methods best suited for individual or self-directed learning.

Individual learning can involve one-on-one learning with an educator or with another student. It can refer to self-directed learning that is indirectly facilitated by an educator, or it may be used in describing an individual who is working on his or her own to further knowledge on a given subject. Additionally, this chapter explores techniques used inside and outside the classroom that encourage self-directed learning.

CHAPTER GOAL: This chapter introduces a variety of methods best suited for individual or self-directed learning.

Reading Assignments

Most EMS instructors assign textbook reading and journal assignments to supplement content presented during the class, or to prepare students for classroom activities that enhance understanding of the subject. These assignments can reap benefits for both faculty and the learners. Students who value and complete reading assignments have better exam scores, increased class participation, and increased understanding.[1] Despite these benefits, in many classrooms a substantial number of students fail to complete the required reading. Some researchers determined that less than 30 percent of the college students they studied completed assigned reading.[2, 3]

Students' failure to read may be associated with the following:

1. Low self-confidence.
2. Lack of interest in the topic.
3. Failure to realize the importance of the reading assignment.[1]

On the other hand, faculty may not take measures to ensure reading is done because of their perceptions on how it will make students feel about them, their belief that it will lead to poor evaluations or a general lack of motivation of some instructors.[1]

There are several possible solutions to increase reading. Some "value" should be assigned to assignments designed to assess reading compliance. Graded exercises such as quizzes, summary statements, or worksheets can be used. Some instructors allow students to prepare a handwritten index card based on the reading that can be taken into the test or quiz as a motivator to read. If instructors do not monitor reading, it can quickly become the class norm to not do it.

In some cases, students do read the material, but fail to understand it. In many instances, these students have not learned how to read effectively before they enter the EMS classroom. It may be helpful to offer the student some alternative reading strategies. This may include having the student outline content or pause after reading a section of text and do the following:

1. Consider whether they fully understand what it means or if they need to clarify it further.
2. Reflect on how this fits what they already know about the subject.
3. Infer how this new content might "look" in a patient or how it might affect their response to a 9-1-1 call.
4. Decide the most important points in the section.

These strategies, when used appropriately can increase the students' ability to read for meaning and to incorporate the new material within their schema of knowledge related to that topic.[4] If possible, refer students who are struggling for reading assistance to the school resource center.

Textbooks as Tools

Although the usefulness of textbooks in education is often debated in the literature, a textbook can be an important tool for individual learning if it is used appropriately. Before the educator can begin to maximize the potential of a textbook, however, an understanding of the book and its elements should be reached. Educators should view a textbook as a tool and should study its structure and function, as one would study an anatomy lesson. In keeping with the earlier discussion of a purely lecture instructional format, the textbook should not be used as the sole source of information. Instead, it should provide a foundation of knowledge from which an educator can expand and enhance the student learning experience, and as a tool for answering questions and providing feedback.[5–7]

Know the Textbook

The educator can begin by taking a critical look at the textbooks that are currently used for the course. He or she can review the table of contents and take note of the order in which the topics are presented. Does this order follow what happens in the classroom, or not? The educator should become familiar with the content covered within each chapter and should note those topics that might be considered enrichment—that is, material that goes above and beyond the required curriculum.

The front matter of most current texts provides a description of "features" or tools included within the book to enhance learning and provide structure to the content. These features are generally highlighted and explained as part of the introduction to students and instructors. Studying each of the features and beginning to plan and strategize how they might be used in the classroom is a good approach. For example, the instructor may want to provide examples and suggestions for students as the class progresses through the book. The text box on this page outlines strategies by which learners can benefit most from their textbooks.

Strategies for Getting the Most from the Textbook[6]

1. **Preview-Connect-Predict**

   Preview with the students the content in textbook chapters by having them work in small teams and look at headings, pedagogical elements, and so forth. Explain to the students the importance of the goals or learning objectives listed in the textbook. Explain to the students how to use the objectives when reviewing for exams. While previewing, have students discuss connections to their individual life experiences and knowledge. Finally, have students predict what they will learn in the chapter.

2. **Think-Pair-Share**

   Have students work with a partner. Pose an application question related to a section of the text and ask each student to reflect on the answer alone for a minute. After the silent reflection, the pair takes a minute or two to discuss their individual thoughts. Finally, the instructor asks each pair to share their response with the class. Describing their answer in their own words demands greater comprehension of the material.

3. **Admit-Exit Tickets**

   Have students enter the classroom with a written-down "fact" that they learned from the assigned reading. This fact "admits them" to the discussion for the day. After the discussion has ended, students reevaluate what they have learned and list new concepts and thoughts as their "Exit" card. The exit card is their ticket out of the classroom.

Modeling Use of the Textbook

One of the best ways to encourage students to open their textbooks and begin using them is to model the behavior as an educator. Although teaching straight from the textbook is inappropriate, the instructor can have a positive impact on appropriate student use of the text. How is the textbook that has been assigned to the class used by the instructor in the classroom as he or she teaches? Is the textbook merely used as a means to get students to read outside the classroom? Does the instructor make the class text a living, breathing part of every class session? Or, does he or she refer to it only when providing the next reading assignment? The educator should assign the textbook a role in the overall learning experience, using it as a baseline for knowledge and a reference for questions or clarifications.[7,8]

Teaching Tip >> *When students make the inevitable "but that is not in the book" comment, take the opportunity to get students to research the missing or controversial topic, then present to the class the reasons why they think the information in the text is missing or presented in the way that it is. Additionally, textbooks are usually written to a national standard, and information in the text may be inconsistent with local protocols. The instructor should use this opportunity to have students research and discuss differences.*

Pedagogical Features

Many textbooks have specific elements designed to enhance student learning and retention. Some studies have shown that it is these various elements that are read most frequently by students.[7] Elements such as learning objectives, case scenarios, review questions, and enrichment information all offer opportunities to enhance individual learning. Following are examples of how each learning feature can be used.

Learning Objectives

Objectives developed based on the National EMS Education Standards[9] drive Emergency Medical Services (EMS) educational programs. They determine what is taught and describe desired outcomes (see Chapter 8: Goals and Objectives). Knowing where they are placed in the textbook, how they integrate with the three learning domains (cognitive, psychomotor, and affective), and what their purpose is will be helpful to many students. The instructor should take the time to explain these resources at the beginning of a program and should describe how all three learning domains will be incorporated into the course.

Students should be encouraged to review the objectives before they read the content. They should refer back to the objectives as they read the text content to ensure that they are identifying the most important information.

When using objectives for individual learning, the instructor should encourage students to review them before taking a cognitive or skills exam. Students should be urged to shape each objective into a question and should confirm that they can confidently answer each of these questions. For objective questions that they cannot answer, students must return to the content of the text or seek answers from other students or the educator.

CASE IN POINT

This technique can be modeled in class either before or after a lesson is presented. Specific objectives are selected and are reworded as questions. Students are instructed to hold their answers until chosen, then to state the question out loud. Students wait several seconds (20–30) before they select another student, who must give the answer. Students should be encouraged to do the same for themselves as they review the material before an exam. If they cannot confidently answer the objective, they can return to the content to reread the information that was missed the first time around. This may also encourage students to use review of objectives as a reading strategy before they come to class; this promotes individual learning.

Case Scenarios

Case scenarios are another common element of many textbooks. For example, some texts begin each chapter with a scenario in an effort to put what is about to be read into a meaningful context for the student. The case study also serves as a motivational tool to help the learner identify why the topic is important. Scenarios can be excellent tools for students as they learn to think critically and improve their problem-solving skills. When course material is put into the context of a patient scenario, it frequently becomes more real for the learner and thus more easily understandable.

CASE IN POINT

The instructor begins the renal failure lesson using a scenario about a 9-1-1 call for an unresponsive patient at a dialysis center. It is presented at the beginning of a lecture, and the instructor asks students to write down a response to questions such as: What hazards should you anticipate on this scene? What conditions might cause this chief complaint? The instructor should allow students just three to four minutes to jot down some thoughts before asking them to share their comments with the student sitting next to them. Comparing answers is a great way for students to see through someone else's eyes; it opens them up to other possibilities.

In the same manner, the instructor may choose to end a class session by reading or assigning a scenario from the next chapter. Students should be encouraged to think about the scenario and should come to the next class meeting prepared to discuss it.

Students can also develop their own scenarios from events they have experienced. Ask them to develop some key questions for their classmates based on their scenario. Names and dates should be changed or withheld to ensure privacy for patients.

Review Questions

Many textbooks also offer some form of content review at the end of each chapter or section. Chapter review questions are often used to test or validate that the student has learned or gained some new knowledge from the reading. These questions can become a valuable tool for the student, especially if the educator models their use and incorporates them into classroom discussion or quizzes.[10]

Learners can use review questions as a self-evaluation tool to prepare for exams or to gauge their understanding and progress as they move through the content.

Students can develop exam or review questions to share with other students. A "student-developed" question bank can be used to promote discussion. Student questions can be placed on index cards and drawn from a "question deck" or placed in a fish bowl and used as a review when the class needs a break or a change of pace.

CASE IN POINT

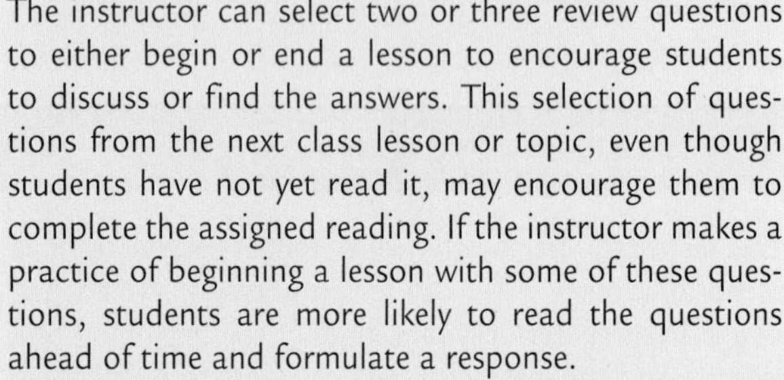

The instructor can select two or three review questions to either begin or end a lesson to encourage students to discuss or find the answers. This selection of questions from the next class lesson or topic, even though students have not yet read it, may encourage them to complete the assigned reading. If the instructor makes a practice of beginning a lesson with some of these questions, students are more likely to read the questions ahead of time and formulate a response.

Enrichment

Enrichment content refers to information presented in a textbook that goes beyond the required curriculum. Enrichment information often presents topics that are closely related to, but not directly contained within, a respective curriculum, and they can be used as a valuable tool for individual learning if this is modeled by the instructor.

Enrichment content can be a great place for a student to begin looking for topics for research papers or extra credit assignments; it can be used to motivate students to think beyond what is "required" of them.

Addition of enrichment information can be detrimental if it is added to an already heavy, required learning load. Educators should choose this material carefully so they do not burden students with information of little value, or will not directly affect how they may care for a patient. For instance, if presented well, the basic pathophysiology of congestive heart failure can help students identify afflicted patients sooner. On the other hand, presenting extensive details about jellyfish stings to a class of emergency medical technicians (EMTs) in Nebraska may not be the best use of class time.

Key Terms and Glossary

Terminology and definitions are paramount for student comprehension. Key terms are often listed at the beginning of the chapter and called out in bold text the first time they appear during the chapter. The glossary is typically located at the end of the text and includes all key terms. Students can use the key terms and glossary as review tools. Students highlight the terms they know and place terms they do not know on flash cards or index cards for quick and mobile review tools. Periodic review of the glossary should lead to an increase of highlighted terms. As a final review, all terms should be highlighted demonstrating a mastery of the important terms in the textbook.

Appendix

Important reference materials such as drug descriptions, forms, tables, or enhanced content may be placed in the appendices. On occasion, other reference materials or practice exercises, such as ECG strips, are included in an appendix.

Textbook Ancillaries

Not so long ago textbooks were the one and only tool used to support classroom learning and individual study. Today, the choices of instructional tools are many. Textbook support materials may include items such as workbooks, companion CD-ROMs, companion websites, pocket guides, and exam review manuals. All these instructional formats are potentially valuable tools for self-directed learning in initial and refresher training. However, as with textbook use, it is incumbent upon the educator to reinforce the use and importance of these ancillary materials.[11]

Student Workbooks

Print workbooks that accompany textbooks typically consist of questions and written exercises that are specific to each chapter. They are ideally suited for individual learning because the workbook material is self-paced, generally follows the format and content flow of the textbook, and promotes active learning through content reinforcement exercises.[11] For example, students can use workbooks for exam preparation, remediation, and reinforcement of concepts **(Figure 13.1)**. Educators can use them for homework assignments and for assessment of student understanding and growth. The disadvantage of the workbook is that it requires an additional cost to the learner, and it can be time-consuming and subjective for educators to grade.[11] At the very least, however, educators should make students aware of such resources and should encourage their use. An example of encouragement may be to offer extra credit for completed workbook assignments, or the instructor can present workbook activities during class time.

Electronic workbooks have also become available. These workbooks are generally available online (not in print format), and they include interactive activities that provide immediate feedback. Again, these are ideally suited for individual learning, and the online feature of immediate feedback can make grading easier for the educator. One study that compared the use of print workbooks and electronic workbooks found that, although learner satisfaction was greater with the electronic product because of ease of use and time savings, no significant difference was noted in post-test performance.[11]

Companion CD-ROMs or DVDs

A companion CD-ROM or DVD is packaged with a textbook. Such media use technology to extend the functionality of the textbook by offering such items as review questions, images, animations, skills videos, video cases, interactive media, audio glossaries, case studies, and an assortment of games—all designed to encourage independent learning and enhance the content of the textbook. In the future, many of these ancillaries will be published on the website or within the learning management system. Educators should model the use of these tools in the classroom so that students become aware of their existence and purpose as learning tools.

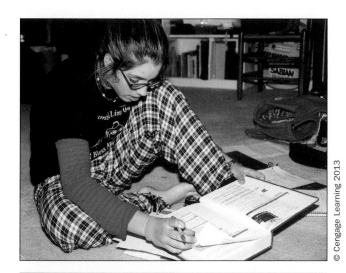

Figure 13.1

Workbooks can be a valuable tool for examination preparation and content reinforcement, especially if the content is applied to case scenarios.

Teaching Tip >> *If technological resources are available in the classroom, once a week or so the educator can select a feature or topic of the companion DVD or CD-ROM or website to highlight and demonstrate for the whole class. Alternatively, a student can be asked to demonstrate the use of the tool and to begin a discussion on the topic. If technology to demonstrate these resources is not available in the classroom, the educator should make a point of creating an assignment that encourages learners to access them on their own.*

Not all learners have convenient access to a computer to use the electronic content in companion media, but with a little brainstorming, some simple solutions can be offered. For example, these activities can be printed out by a fellow student or the instructor and can be provided as a handout. In other cases, learners may have to use a friend's computer or one at the local library or college computer lab. With enough forethought and planning, most barriers to computer access can be overcome in a reasonable manner.

Companion Websites

Many publishers have created online tools that are ideally suited for individual learning and exploration. These tools typically are contained on a website that has been developed and is owned by the publisher for a specific book, hence the name "Companion Website" **(Figure 13.2)**. These sites generally contain information such as learning objectives and various activities that reinforce content from the text. Instructor tools are also available, including instructor manuals, lesson plans, and test banks.

In many instances, companion website activities are similar to those found in the electronic workbook, described earlier. They can take the form of simple labeling exercises that are provided along with a variety of quizzes. Additional resources that can extend the capability of the book include audio glossaries that

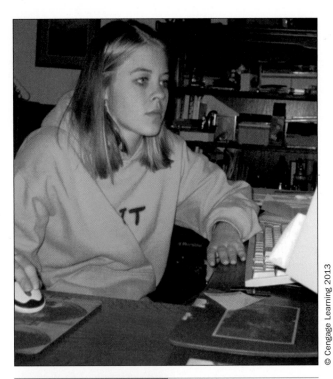

Figure 13.2

Studying on a companion website may suit the needs of younger students because of the advantages of audio and visual movement.

allow students to actually listen to a medical term being pronounced, and links to pertinent websites that include more information on the specific topic. Most of the tools offered on companion websites require very little bandwidth. However, as more interactive elements and streaming video become available, bandwidth may become an issue. This can be an important consideration for the educator who assigns some of these more complex activities.

Most EMS companion Web resources are found within a learning-management system that offers many course-management activities at no charge. When instructors use the learning-management features in these sites, the student can check grade and attendance records on line, take quizzes, and find many course resources. More information on companion websites and learning-management systems can be found in Chapter 17: Tools for Distance Learning.

Electronic Textbooks

Many EMS textbooks are available in electronic format. The electronic textbook contains all content as in the hard-copy version. In addition, most electronic texts allow the student to highlight, make notes within the text, and copy small sections of key text. The search features in electronic textbooks are very helpful to students who are struggling to understand a term or concept. When the student enters a search term such as "shock", every occurrence of that term appears in a navigation frame where the student can simply click to be taken to that section of the textbook.

Research and Professional Journals

Most textbooks provide an overview of content within a specific area. While this is important for student's big-picture understanding of a topic, the content in the text may lag behind current research or lack sufficient detail. Assigning reading from professional journals can assure that the students are familiarized with the most up-to-date research about a topic. Reading assignments can also provide the basis for discussion about controversies in emergency care and allow students to explore evidence for and against some emergency care practices. It will also prepare them to find relevant information after they graduate, paving the way for independent lifelong learning.

Teaching Tip >> *Assign a project where students must examine the case for and against an issue related to prehospital emergency care. Require them to find relevant articles to support and refute their position. Topics could include emergency care issues such as endotracheal intubation, benefits of advanced life support medications in cardiac arrest, or use of lights and sirens during emergency response.*

Independent Study

Sometimes the best way to teach is to be seemingly absent from the learning process. In this type of teaching, the educator's role is more that of a facilitator. The educator can assist the learner in setting his or her own educational goals, then can help the learner create a strategy for attaining these goals outside the traditional classroom. In general, an educator's role in facilitating self-study is to assist the learner in discovering helpful resources and supportive experiences that can serve as source material. Once the learner is in touch with the source material, the educator can assist with identification of key learning elements and can help put the newly acquired knowledge into context.[12] Self-study helps the student to become more independent and to develop skills that will lead to internal motivation to seek out knowledge throughout his or her career.[13,14]

In a more directed or programmed approach, an educator might construct predetermined goals and clear exercises through which a learner can reach these goals. In the context of EMS education, this type of directed, independent study assignment can be a helpful adjunct to learning. It is often a challenge for the instructor to cover the entire curriculum prescribed in EMS courses. Independent study offers options for learning to take place outside a traditional classroom setting.[15]

Adult learners in particular can be well suited to independent learning. Many are mature enough, are internally motivated, and have strong study habits that will allow them to succeed. It should be noted that younger students may misinterpret the customization and flexibility of independent study as an "easy" way to acquire knowledge. Self-directed learning, however, can be difficult. The learner must be self-motivated and, when expert consultation is not immediately available, must have the curiosity and discipline needed to search for a correct answer. Understanding a complex subject without the explanation provided by an instructor in the classroom might be more difficult than some students originally predict.

The proliferation and widespread availability of televisions, DVD players, computers, tablets, smartphones, and the Internet have given a new look to self-directed learning. It is important to note that although the latest methods for self-study have focused on electronic and audiovisual media, this kind of learning does not have to be driven electronically. Research has proved that reading printed materials, reflecting on the meaning of their content, and writing a summary of what has been learned is an effective educational method.

CASE IN POINT

Certification courses such as National Incident Management System (NIMS), Hazardous Materials Awareness, and Medical Terminology can be assigned for students to complete independently online. These courses are offered at no cost and can free valuable classroom time.

Examples of Independent Study Assignments

- Workbooks
- Self-assessment quizzes, puzzles, and games
- Step-by-step tutorials
- Computer-aided instruction
- Library research
- Additional reading
- Guided exercises for reviewing and organizing notes
- Interviews or discussion with experts or other individual persons or groups such as stroke survivors
- Listening to a podcast or other recorded information
- Web searches

Note Taking and Reviewing

One way to enhance individual student learning is to encourage note taking during lectures and reading assignments, and while the student is completing other assignments. Taking notes is a cognitive activity that helps many students process information and capture key concepts for later review. Students can write or draw notes. Research suggests that the activity of transferring cognitive thought onto paper alone enhances student learning. Future review of these notes and further reading have been shown to further enhance retention.[15–17]

Note taking that requires that the learner listen, sort out the more important information, capture something that will stimulate his or her memory and understanding, and summarizes or answers questions in their own words improves comprehension and retention.[18] The more the notes incorporate previous knowledge, and the more often the student translates the information into his or her own words, the greater is the likelihood that the student's learning will be enhanced by note taking.

Educators can facilitate and guide effective use of notes by pacing the delivery of lectures and emphasizing key points. They can also prompt students to write down and remember elements that might be critical to an understanding of future concepts or information that will be tested. New technology allows students to takes notes within the electronic textbook on their laptop or pad device.

Some experts suggest the use of a structured lecture process called the "guided lecture procedure" (GLP). This allows for a formal 5- to 10-minute pause during which students try to encapsulate what they have just heard, followed by 10- to 15-minute small group discussion during which students can compare notes and discuss lessons learned.[17,19] Chapter 15: Tools for Large Group Learning discusses guided lecture in greater detail.

A handout or organizer with the general outline of the lecture topic or assignment can also encourage note taking and can provide organization and structure to the lesson. When electronic presentation tools (such as PowerPoint) are used, it is possible for the instructor to provide to students a complete lecture summary. It is probably best for the instructor to hand out general outlines and to avoid giving out full slide summaries before the lecture. Studies have shown that review of instructor-provided lecture summaries is effective for short-term recall, but that retention is significantly enhanced when the learner has taken his or her own notes. The combination of taking one's own notes and reviewing these notes between lectures is most effective.[20]

In all cases, educators should encourage active learning techniques to prompt students to review materials. Passive listening is one of the least effective methods of learning.[21]

Independent Assignments

Educators can facilitate independent learning and studying through the use of independent assignments. Examples of individual learning strategies that could be distributed to students are listed here. This section highlights the use of flashcards, research, journaling, and portfolios. The text box on this page can help students maximize their learning experiences by adopting the evidence-based strategies.

Flashcards

The literature on flashcards typically describes their use in teaching children how to read. Although some critics claim that flashcards promote only rote learning and not comprehension, their usefulness has more recently been explored; research shows that flashcards can improve the speed of reading, which then improves comprehension of the subject matter.[24] Accordingly, flashcard use in EMS education may be most appropriate for subject areas that require memorization and learning of another language, such as medical terminology or pharmacology.

Making the Most of Learning for Students[22,23]

1. Study information in "chunks" that contain no more than seven key concepts.
2. When reading, summarize each paragraph in one sentence using your own words.
3. Organize key concepts into sequences, pictures, models, or algorithms as you study them.
4. When reading new material, consciously relate it to something you already know.
5. Your motivation to succeed and your belief that you can are essential elements to your success in learning. Focus on your end goal so you will put in the work needed to learn the material. Break content into small pieces so it is manageable to learn.
6. Think about how you learn most effectively and try to use those strategies. When given an assignment, consider what will be involved and what parts of it you might find difficult. Then identify the steps needed to complete it successfully.
7. Meaningful learning does not occur if you play the passive role of a chick waiting for the mother bird to drop a worm into your mouth. To really learn something, you must actively participate in the learning process. Your teacher guides the instruction, but you must work to understand new knowledge and to see how it fits in with what you already know.
8. Apply what you are learning to a situation you might see on the ambulance and predict how the scenario would progress. Ask yourself, What would this patient look like? What would her vital signs be? How might her condition change as time passes if no interventions are performed? How would I manage the situation?
9. When learning a new concept or fact, know the "why" associated with it. For example, a patient with a heart rate of 30 is likely to have signs of shock. Ask yourself "why" that is.
10. Practice the new concepts and skills you have learned often and in as many different situations as possible.
11. Monitor your progress. If you are struggling with specific knowledge or skills, change your learning strategy to be more successful. Seek help from class peers or instructors.
12. Learning new complex material takes time and repetition—plan for both.

The use of electronic media to produce image-enhanced flashcards can also help learners (particularly visual learners) retain information.[25] Commercial products are often available, or the educator or learner can make cards using blank index cards or programs such as PowerPoint. Free internet-based flashcard programs and apps are also available and may be more desirable for some learners.

Teaching Tip >> *Flashcards can easily be incorporated into lectures by the use of features in presentation software such as PowerPoint. A word, phrase, or image can be placed on a single slide, and features such as build and dissolve can be used to place the "answer" on the bottom of the slide or on the next slide.*[25]

Research Projects

Research is an important component of individual learning, both as a resource for finding information and in the discovery or validation of information. Conducting research may be required in some educational programs; however, this section focuses on individual research assignments.

Educators should always encourage students to expand their knowledge. One of the best ways for them to do this is through research. With the availability of the Internet and all that it has to offer, students are more eager than ever to do a little "surfing" and expand their knowledge. Research projects can be both fun and informative and should include a variety of formats and styles. In addition to an Internet or library search of the current literature on a topic, research may involve such things as student-led comparisons of products and equipment, or a study of the trend of class blood pressure measurements over the semester to see if readings run higher on testing days. For many students, the difficult part of the research project is not the research itself but the selection of a topic; therefore, it is a good idea for the instructor to provide a list of suggested topics that can be offered to students who wish to complete a research assignment.

Research projects can be given as a mandatory assignment that all students must complete, or they may be used as an optional assignment that offers students the opportunity to earn extra credit. Whichever the case, the instructor must provide clear direction and must outline expectations for the project in as much detail as possible. Details such as the nature and scope of the topic, the length of the final paper, the due date, how much class credit it is worth, and acceptable format for submission should all be spelled out before any research is begun.

Teaching Tip >> *Without some guidance and direction from the instructor, students may select topics that are too broad in scope or that do not relate to EMS at all. The instructor should have each student select a topic and submit it for approval before he or she begins the research. Students may choose topics that are very familiar to them or they feel comfortable with. Instructor input into the choice may encourage students to research current topics and expand their vision.*

A student may wish to do research on the pay rates of EMTs. If the student's goal is to find a job as an EMT in a local department or agency, it may not benefit the student or the class if he or she begins researching EMT pay scales across the United States. One instructor suggestion might be to focus on EMT jobs within a 100-mile radius of home, thus providing more useful information not only for the student who is conducting the research but for the rest of the class as well.

Another tool that the instructor may use, especially if the research project is optional, is a list of preselected topics that can be assigned as students express an interest in doing a project. Ideas for topics can be gathered from news and magazine articles or from current events. The instructor should keep a running list of ideas that can be used when students come up empty-handed. "Enrichment" topics included in some textbooks may be helpful as well. These topics typically go beyond the curriculum and are of interest to many students.

Teaching Tip >> *It is important that instructors spell out what they expect from completed research projects. Develop a grading rubric (outline) that specifies how points will be awarded relative to style, content, and organization. Specify the minimum number and type of appropriate references (Internet sources, journal articles, personal interviews). It may be necessary to further specify which journals or Internet sites are considered acceptable. Minimum word count requirements will also indicate to the student what is expected. The more direction the instructor provides, the more successful students will be with their projects.*

Journaling

Encouraging learners to write about their experiences during a training program can be enlightening for both the learner and the educator. Journal writing (journaling) is an effective method of allowing learners to reflect on what they have been learning and to put it into words that can be read by or shared with others as appropriate **(Figure 13.3)**. Journaling also provides an opportunity for students to explore feelings about experiences—a task that taps into the affective domain.

Journaling can take many forms, ranging from a formal composition notebook that is submitted for a grade to less formal online discussion boards or private blogs. Before assigning the journal, the instructor should consider the specific objectives it is designed to achieve. Topics can range from a general class experience to specific experiences in clinical and field settings. One example of a journaling assignment is to ask students to track all medications encountered during clinical or field internships. Students must research each medication encountered and must list the most common indications, contraindications, and adverse effects. Another journaling technique is to ask students to document any questions that may arise as they read the text. Students must then seek out the answers to these questions from fellow students. Because the actual task of journaling is conducted throughout an extended class, such as an EMT or paramedic program, students can use the journal as a reflective tool through which they can observe changes in their knowledge base and can assess how acquired knowledge has affected the way they treat patients. Journals can also serve as a great study tool for major division exams and finals.

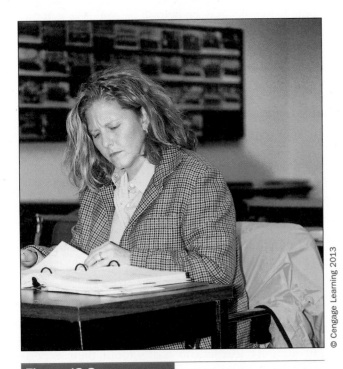

Figure 13.3

Journaling allows students the opportunity to reflect on their experiences and explore their feelings.

As with any appropriate assignment, expectations should be clearly defined at the beginning. What form will the journal take, and what will it contain? Will the instructor accept handwritten journals? Or, must they be typewritten before submission? When will the journal be due, and what point value, if any, has been assigned? These are all questions that must be addressed so that students can begin with a clear understanding. A grading rubric should be made available to the students with the details of the assignment. Even with the most explicit of instructions, students may interpret things differently than the instructor intends. For this reason, it is appropriate for the instructor to inform students that he or she will be sampling their journals on a random basis throughout the program and will offer informal feedback along the way. This helps the instructor to identify students who are not doing the assignment at all, or who may be headed in the wrong direction. Anonymous examples of journals from previous classes also help students to understand what is expected.

Educators can also use journaling as a way to individually explore their own teaching methods and effectiveness.[26]

Case-Study Projects

Most allied health professions and fire service standards are expressed in terms of what the provider will do or be able to perform once on the job. The standards or objectives are expressed using verbs. These verbs determine the level of performance and therefore determine the teaching and evaluation levels. For verbs such as "identify" or "label", a lower level of learning is occurring. When verbs such as "assess", "evaluate", "manage", "develop", or "create" are driving the end learning outcome, teaching and evaluation must occur at higher levels. Complex case-study projects create a learning environment where students can create or develop thinking and performance skills at the higher levels of Bloom's taxonomy.

For this type of assignment, students are given a scenario, data (examples include response times, payroll, population demographics), and specific information that challenges the learner to solve a series of problems, develop policies and procedures, or "invent" a solution. This is different from research projects where students research a given or selected topic that has a goal of developing "new" cognitive knowledge. In this type of case-based assignment, students are required to use their current knowledge and experiences to solve problems presented by the data given. The goal is to create and develop critical thinking and decision-making skills. Instructors provide an enriching learning activity by creating hidden problems and challenges that evaluate both cognitive and affective learning domains. Projects are used to test knowledge at higher-level thought processes. Projects provide an opportunity for multiple "correct" responses from individual students. Presenting project results can lead to meaningful discussions in the classroom.

Portfolios

A *portfolio* is a collection of student work that demonstrates progress and attainment of educational goals.[12, 27, 28] Portfolios are not a new idea. The concept is borrowed from the arts, wherein the portfolio is a collection of work used to demonstrate an artist's talent. Portfolios have also been used in other educational settings, including college business programs, high school technical programs, elementary schools, and fire service certification courses. Portfolios can be used in many ways, depending on their purpose and intended audience:

- *Working portfolios* act as containers through which the student and the instructor interact on progress made through assignments and tasks.
- *Showcase portfolios* represent the student's best work.
- *Assessment portfolios* document student learning and demonstrate mastery of concepts; they are graded by the instructor.

The key characteristic of a successful portfolio is that it is carefully planned and purposeful.

Topic assignment is an important first step in the creation of a portfolio. The instructor should approve the topic and the forms of expression used. The instructor can provide a list that includes a variety of options, such as oral presentations, debates, original games, visual presentations, flow charts, time lines, demonstrations, role playings, musical/rhythmic presentations, skits, journals, creative visualizations, poster presentations, and Web pages. This list can guide students as they plan their collections of tasks or projects.

The instructor should monitor the developmental stages of the portfolio. One method of monitoring student progress is requiring the student to submit intermediary steps for consideration and possible impact on the course grade. For instance, the instructor may require a check-in for the following steps: (1) Overall plan with areas of interest or broad topics to be covered; (2) tasks to be completed under each area; (3) major points or objectives to be completed with each of the tasks; (4) specific formats for demonstrating or documenting objectives (needs list that may contain photographs, brochures, posters, written reports, surveys, records, policies, procedures, budgets, drug cards, skill sheet check-offs, clinical records, interviews, journals, video clips, website links, etc.—check lists with timelines should be developed); (5) method or methods for presenting the completed portfolio. Check-ins should occur on a regular basis and be applied to all forms that the student plans to use, whether they involve a written presentation or another style of presentation.

Assembling the portfolio is an active-learning and self-reflection process. The student and instructor can select elements that best represent the student's progress. The student then reflects critically on his or her work and the types of elements that will best represent achievements. This activity encourages students to pay closer attention to their own performance and prompts students to work on areas where performance has been weak.[27]

Portfolios can be used to enhance self-reflection and ownership of learning. Assembling the portfolio encourages students to reflect on their own progress and performance as they select the most positive aspects of that performance. Students take responsibility for their accomplishments, and they take on ownership of their learning.

Billings and Halsted[12] warn that this method of instruction may require new ways of thinking on the part of educators. It is important for instructors to teach students how to take advantage of this learning process. Students must see the clear objective and benefit of the portfolio, or it might be viewed as "busy work." Billings and Halsted also suggest specific inclusion criteria for the portfolio so that it does not become too bulky. If the portfolio is being used to

Characteristics of a Carefully Planned Portfolio

- The portfolio should contain a definition of its goals.[6] Objectives are determined jointly by the student and the instructor.
- The focus is on successfully completed student accomplishments, tasks, or a collection of projects.
- Evidence of progress is documented.
- Student strengths are emphasized instead of mistakes.
- Students help decide what will be included.
- Students have access to their portfolios.
- Evaluations with clear grading criteria are reviewed by the student, instructor or team of evaluators, and peer reviewers.

CASE IN POINT

Sample materials to include in a portfolio for an EMS student:

- Summaries of attendance and course completion(s)
- Successfully completed skill station check sheets
- Summaries of clinical hours, locations, contacts, skills, and preceptor evaluations
- Summaries of major exam scores
- Personal mission, oath, or career goals
- Essays, research papers, or review articles

assess student performance, grading criteria and expectations should also be clearly identified. Students should be required to continually evaluate their own products, and educators should schedule conferences with students during which they can provide feedback and guidance.[17]

For information on evaluation of portfolios, see Chapter 22: Other Evaluation Tools.

Independent Learning Labs

Independent learning labs, known as the "learning resource center" (LRC), provide a variety of learning activities that stimulate students' senses of sight, sound, and touch. Although the LRC originally focused on psychomotor skills, the LRC of today has a wide array of technology and various resources that are made available to students to help them acquire cognitive, affective, and psychomotor skills. Through the LRC, students are encouraged to learn, make decisions, and think critically in a low-stress environment.

Some students do well independently in the LRC. Some institutions have developed various types of modular learning approaches for teaching and evaluating skills. These generally are specific instructional units with pretests, post-tests, objectives, structured activities, resources, and evaluation tools. Such learning approaches may be computerized, or they may use multimedia along with models or hands-on materials. One medical school, for example, used problem-based assignments, case studies, and computer-based simulations and exercises to direct individual learning.[29] The LRC approach is self-paced, and assignments can be completed whenever the student is available, as long as the LRC is open. The environment is a nonthreatening one, and the student can linger on a particular topic as long as he or she desires.[12]

Targeted Internships

A **targeted internship experience** is a focused area of clinical experience (hospital or field) through which learning is enhanced or remediated. Students who report back on their experiences can enlighten fellow students about a particular specialty area. Such experiences require objectives for the rotation, learning activities, and means of measuring achievement of the objectives. A student who becomes intrigued by behavioral disorders may choose to spend some time in the in-patient psychiatry area to observe how patient behavior changes after an acute episode. A student who is struggling with electrocardiogram (ECG) interpretation may benefit from clinical experience in a cardiac stepdown unit, where he or she can observe many ECGs over time. A student who is interested in rural EMS may be interested in spending focused time with a rural EMS unit.

Peer Teaching

"See it, Do it, Teach it" has long been a goal for some instructional entities. Students can learn by teaching. Students develop their own teaching outline and PowerPoint on a selected topic and then present it to the class. Like a research paper, the topic should probably be preapproved and relatively narrow so that the student is able to present in a 5- to 8-minute time frame, depending on how much class time is available. Quizzes, puzzles, or a worksheet can be developed by the student to evaluate comprehension.

Learning Contracts

Learning contracts serve as a medium through which an adult's experience can be combined with new learning. Contracts can take a variety of forms (e.g., paper-based, audio, descriptive statements) that can be as individual as the learner. Similar to personal development plans used in the work environment, learning contracts provide a pathway through which learners can personalize their learning and apply it to immediate and future situations and goals.

When a learning contract is arranged, learning objectives are not set by the educator or presented

Student Guide to Creating a Learning Contract[30]

1. Specify your learning objectives.
2. Specify learning resources and strategies.
3. Identify target dates for completion.
4. Specify evidence that objective is met.
5. Describe how the learning will be validated.
6. Review your contract with faculty.
7. Implement the contract.
8. Discuss the results with faculty.

in a textbook; instead, the learning contract provides an avenue by which learners can assess their personal learning needs and set their own goals and objectives. The keys to successful learning contracts include (1) setting measurable, achievable objectives and goals and (2) changing the contract as time and needs progress and change. Educators can introduce this tool[30] to learners and can help them define their own individual learning goals and framework.

Summary

Students enrolled in EMS programs generally are highly motivated and have a sincere interest in what they are learning, especially those who have chosen the path on their own. The instructor must recognize and exploit this motivation for the benefit of the learner. As has been discussed in this chapter, an instructor can use many methods to maximize the benefit of this motivation by providing a wide variety of individual learning opportunities for the student.

The educator should become intimately familiar with the many tools available for individual learning to push students to expand their learning beyond the classroom. In addition, individual learning aids can assist struggling students. Individual learning aids can be tailored to each student's needs. The keys to success for the individual student who uses any of these tools are (1) to establish clearly defined expectations to guide the student through the assignment, (2) to model the use of learning aids in the classroom, and (3) to integrate their use into the curriculum.

Instructors must remember that not all learning occurs within the four walls of the classroom. EMS students often are eager to extend their learning beyond the classroom and to develop critical thinking-skills that will remain useful throughout a lifetime.

Glossary

independent learning labs (learning resource center) An area with technology and various resources available to students to help them acquire cognitive, affective, and psychomotor skills.

pedagogical features Features of a book designed to enhance student understanding.

targeted internship experience A focused area of clinical experience (hospital or field) through which learning is enhanced or remediated.

References

1. Lei, S. A., Bartlett, K., Gorney, S., & Herschach, T. (2010). Resistance to reading compliance among college students. *College Student Journal, 44*(2), 219–229.
2. Sappington, J., Kinsey, K., & Munsayac, K. (2002). Two studies of reading compliance among college students. *Teaching of Psychology, 29*(4), 272–274.
3. Burchfield, C. M., & Sappington, J. (2000). Compliance with reading assignments. *Teaching of Psychology, 27*(1), 58–60.
4. Nash-Ditzel, S. (2010). Metacognitive reading strategies can improve self-regulation. *Journal of College Reading and Learning, 40*(2), 45–63.
5. Lidstone, J. (1995). Teaching with textbooks in undergraduate geography courses. *Journal of Geography in Higher Education, 19*, 335.
6. Robb, L. (2003). Strategies for getting the most from textbooks. *Instructor, 112*, 5.

7. Van Boxtel, C., van der Linden, J., & Kanselaar, G. (2000). The use of textbooks as a tool during collaborative physics learning. *Journal of Experimental Education, 69,* 57.
8. Holmes, J. (1995). Are textbooks inevitable?*Journal of Geography in Higher Education, 19,* 339.
9. National Highway Traffic Safety Administration (2009). *National EMS Education Standards.* (DOT HS 811 077A). Washington, DC: Department of Transportation.
10. Kellum, K. K., Carr, J. E., & Dozier, C. L. (2001). Response-card instruction and student learning in a college classroom. *Teaching of Psychology, 28,* 101–104.
11. Gutierrez, C., & Wang, J. (2001). A comparison of an electronic vs. print workbook for information literacy instruction. *Journal of Academic Librarianship, 27,* 208.
12. Billings, D., M., & Halstead, J. A. (1998). *Teaching in nursing: A guide for faculty.* Philadelphia, PA: W. B. Saunders, 334.
13. Brookfield, S. (1986). *Understanding and facilitating adult learning.* San Francisco, CA: Jossey-Bass, 41–75.
14. Yeazel, M. (2004). Demonstration of the effectiveness and acceptability of self-study module use in residency education. *Medical Teacher, 26,* 57–63.
15. Davis, B. G. (2001). *Tools for teaching.* San Francisco, CA: Jossey-Bass.
16. Morrison, E., McLaughlin, C., & Rucker, L. (2002). Medical students' note-taking in a medical biochemistry course: An initial exploration. *Medical Education, 36,* 384–386.
17. Toole, R. J. (2002). An additional step in the guided lecture procedure. *Journal of Adolescent and Adult Literacy, 44,* 166–169.
18. King, A. (1992). Comparison of self-questioning, summarizing, and notetaking—Review as strategies for learning from lectures. *American Educational Research Journal, 29*(2), 303–323.
19. Kelly, B., & Holmes, J. (1979). The guided lecture procedure. *Journal of Reading, 22,* 602–604.
20. Thomas, G. (1978). Use of student notes and lecture summaries as study guides for recall. *Journal of Educational Research, 71,* 6.
21. Erlendsson, J. (n.d.). Learning retention rates. Available at: http://www.hi.is/~joner/eaps/cs_reten.htm. Accessed August 11, 2003.
22. Mayer, R. E. (2011). *Applying the science of learning.* Boston, MA: Pearson.
23. Ambrose, S. A., Bridges, M. W., Lovett, M. C., DiPietro, M., & Norman, M. K. (2010). *How learning works: Seven research-based principles for smart teaching.* San Francisco, CA: Jossey-Bass.
24. Nicholson, T. (1998). The flashcard strikes back. *Reading Teacher, 52,* 2.
25. Burmark, L. (2004). Visual presentations that prompt, flash, and transform. *Media & Methods, 40,* 6.
26. Dicker, M. (1990). Using action research to navigate an unfamiliar teaching assignment. *Theory into Practice, 29,* 203–208.
27. Lyons, R. E., McIntosh, M., & Kysilka, M. L. (2003). *Teaching college in the age of accountability.* Boston, MA: Allyn & Bacon. 217–220.
28. Orlich, D. C., Harder, R. M., Callahan, R. C., & Gison, H. W. (2001). *Teaching strategies: A guide to better instruction* (6th ed.). Boston, MA: Houghton Mifflin. 369.
29. Whitaker, E. M. (1994). How we teach physiology. *Medical Teacher, 16,* 213.
30. Berger, N. O., Caffarella, R. S., & O'Donnell, J. M. (2004). Learning contracts. In M. W. Galbraith (Ed.), *Adult learning methods: A guide for effective instruction* (3rd ed.). Malabar, FL: Krieger Publishing.

14

Tools for Small Group Learning

The dilemma for the humanistic educator was to devise alternative ways of working within an education system characterized by a prescribed curriculum, similar assignments for all students, lecturing as the only mode of instruction, standards by which all students are externally evaluated, and instructor chosen grades as the measure of learning, all of which precluded meaningful learning. — Carl Rogers

Small group teaching is well recognized as an important means of facilitating learning. A small group format encourages learners to express their comprehension and compare their ideas with others, thereby improving their understanding of the subject. The basic tenet of small group teaching focuses on teamwork and cooperation; educators and learners work together to solve problems and develop critical and higher-order thinking skills. Educators should facilitate learning within small groups and provide the opportunity for learners to monitor their progress and become more self-directed.[1]

A group can consist of two or more students working together.[2] However, the size of the small group is relative to the educational environment. If an educator is used to teaching groups of 100 to 200 or more learners, a small group may consist of 40 to 50 students. Alternatively, if a large group consists of 35 to 40, the small group may comprise fewer than 10 learners. For the purposes of this book, a small group is defined as consisting of 4 to 10 learners.

Small group learning has many characteristics that set it apart from other models of teaching and learning in both approach and delivery method. This chapter explores the concepts of facilitation in small groups and provides examples of different strategies that educators can use in teaching small groups.

CHAPTER GOAL: This chapter explores the concepts of facilitation in small groups and provides examples of strategies educators can use in teaching small groups.

Advantages of Small Group Learning

Small group learning offers many advantages. It allows learners to bring their own experiences to the learning process and increases active learning. It encourages creativity, stimulates discussion, and has been shown to improve confidence and performance.[3] In addition, small groups encourage and assist students in developing such transferable skills as teamwork, communication, collaboration, and leadership. This is particularly true in the field of health care, where small groups are used outside the classroom in continuing education environments such as journal clubs and case reviews.[4]

Working in small groups allows students to learn from others—from the examples they offer and their insights, opinions, and mistakes. The educator facilitates the learning objective. For example, one learner may learn a task more quickly than the others, then may offer to demonstrate to others how the skill was mastered.

Although some schools of thought claim that small group learning requires more instructor time and preparation, others claim that it actually decreases lecture load and overall workload.[2, 3, 5]

The primary purpose of teaching and learning in small groups is to develop learners' knowledge, skills, and attitudes so that they can meet desired educational outcomes. This is done in association with the learning outcomes that are described in the curriculum. Because of the intensive nature of the instruction provided with a ratio of one instructor to a small number of students, small groups afford the student the opportunity to learn the finer details of the profession.[6]

Disadvantages of Small Group Learning

Disadvantages of small group learning seem to center on the time it takes to plan appropriate activities and to initiate a "learning change" with learners. Developing a small group learning environment can take time and requires a change from typical educator-centered lectures to learner-centered activities.[3] Learners may resist, and educators may find themselves wanting to give lectures rather than facilitate discussion. Management of group dynamics can become an issue, and workloads within groups may not be equally distributed (see Chapter 11: Introduction to Teaching Strategies). The small group learning format requires that more time be spent on a lesson, and educators may not be able to cover all subject matter in the curriculum.[5] Some believe that teaching small groups can be very demanding in terms of preparation in that individual student learning styles must be identified, and the instructor must respond to those learning styles by adopting teaching methods that meet individual needs. Facilitation may be complex because of the diverse range of learning styles, as well as variation in abilities, personalities, age differences, and different cultural backgrounds, and because students may be unmotivated or passive learners.[6]

Most of the cited disadvantages, however, can be overcome with effective planning and time management. The following text box lists some techniques for successful small group learning.

Creating Successful Small Groups[2,5]

- Design challenging exercises to be done in a limited time frame.
- Ensure that work assignments are clearly defined.
- Assess both individual and group work.
- Use both peer evaluation and self-assessment.
- Monitor and facilitate small group work (remain visible).
- Ensure that the learning environment is suitable to the task.

Types of Groups

Small groups can be formal or informal. Formal groups typically have a planned purpose, require a formal selection process, and assign roles to each group member **(Figure 14.1)**. A formal small group, for example, may be used for problem-based learning, case discussions, or simulations. Informal groups can work over a much shorter duration without assigned roles **(Figure 14.2)**. For example, breaking up a large class by having learners turn to their neighbors to discuss a concept or problem is one example of an informal small group approach.[5] Having students move between different lab stations to learn isolated skills is another example.

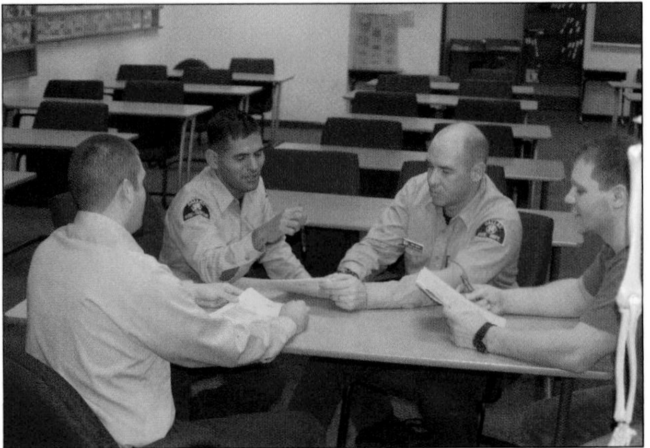

Figure 14.1

Small groups can be formal with a planned purpose and roles, as in problem-based learning.

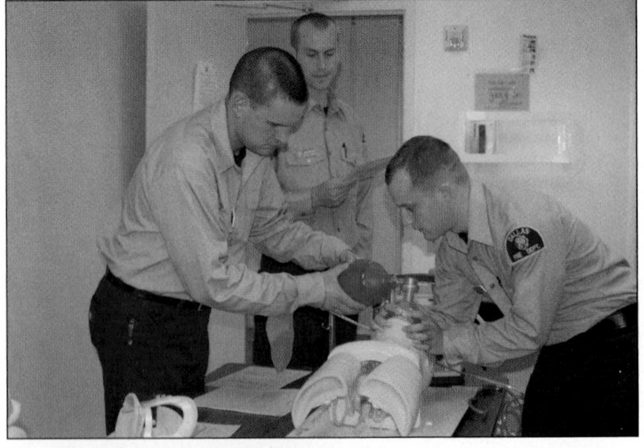

Figure 14.2

Groups can be informal, as in a skills practice laboratory. Both formal and informal groups can promote effective learning.

Many educators deliver lectures to larger groups, then subdivide students into smaller tutorial groups to create a manageable environment, particularly when the goal is psychomotor development within practical skills laboratories. Ideally, these smaller groups comprise a mix of different types of students (e.g., age, cultural background, personality) and skill; the diversity of students adds a dimension of richness to the group.

Cooperative and Collaborative Learning

Cooperative learning and collaborative learning represent two key models of small group teaching and learning. In these types of settings, the educator poses the learning theme, and students work together to find associated details. Cooperative and collaborative learning methods differ from traditional teaching approaches in that students work together instead of competing with each other. Although these two approaches have similarities, they are characterized by significant teaching differences.

Features of Cooperative Learning[8]

- *Intentional group formation*—Group members are selected according to predetermined criteria. For example, recent high school graduates mix with older students.
- *Continuity of group interaction*—Members have regular group meetings to deal with the assignment and, in turn, a social network develops. For example, the group may elect to meet in the cafeteria, where, over coffee, they can divide out the work.
- *Interdependence among group members*—Groups work toward a common goal; each member is assigned a specific role associated with the learning process.
- *Individual accountability*—Students are graded individually to reduce "social loafing." Each student makes an independent contribution to the learning; therefore, each assignment is graded on an individual basis.
- *Instructor as facilitator*—The instructor circulates in the group to clarify the task and to offer encouragement.

Cooperative Learning

Cooperative learning is defined as a division of labor undertaken to solve a problem.[7] For any given task, students divide up the work, then come together to present findings. Each student makes an individual contribution.

Collaborative Learning

There have been recent demands from employers for students who graduate from their courses to be flexible, to be team-players, and to have good interpersonal skills. **Collaborative learning** experiences encourage students to think for themselves, compare their thinking with others, and to engage in higher-order thinking processes.

Collaborative learning involves the following:

- Discussion
- Negotiation

CASE IN POINT

A 28-year-old female patient with severe abdominal pain calls 9-1-1. The patient is planning to start a family, so she might be pregnant.

To provide appropriate patient care, students must learn about abdominal pain associated with ectopic pregnancy.

If five students constitute the group, a specific learning task should be allocated to each student, such as:

- Normal anatomy and physiology of the female reproductive system
- Pathophysiology of ectopic pregnancy
- Clinical presentation of ectopic pregnancy
- Clinical problems and complications that may be anticipated
- Patient care required before time of arrival at the hospital

In turn, each student presents his or her findings to the whole group. If additional students are available, the educator has the option to subdivide tasks (e.g., one student is allocated the anatomy of the reproductive system, and another is asked to find out about the physiology). Alternatively, two students could be allocated to work on a task together.

- Problem solving
- Clarification
- Interpreting

Collaborative learning, in contrast to cooperative learning, focuses on learners working together and being jointly responsible for successful learning outcomes. It encourages active student participation in the learning process by requiring that individual students do an assigned task and think about the approach they must take. Each student must participate in discussion and justify his or her position. Collaborative learning is one way that students can learn from each other—it is a powerful learning tool in that an element of subliminal peer pressure develops between students when one student is seen to be more knowledgeable than the others. Each member of the group researches a section of the task to find information that assists other members of the group.

Small Group Student Dynamics

As individuals, human beings are all different; they have different needs, wants, perspectives, beliefs, and values. Similarly, students differ from each other. Within small group teaching and learning environments, the effective educator will notice the way in which the group interacts. Some students might not readily verbalize their ideas in class and might appear withdrawn and passive. Alternatively, other students might dominate discussions about their experiences and opinions. This may result in negative arguments, group dissension, and personality difficulties that can cause ineffective group productivity.

At times, the instructor will need to employ skillful group-management actions to arbitrate the potential challenges they might experience in association with dysfunctional collaborative learning groups. Some students might complain that others in their assigned group have not contributed equally to the learning exercise. Other students might express their dissatisfaction when their grade is less than what they anticipated due to another student's weaker submission. Therefore, it is essential that clear guidelines are given to students to ensure each knows what is expected from them and the criteria for grade parameters.

To encourage a productive collaborative learning environment, the successful educator will do the following:

- Ask each student a given number of questions.
- Ask open-ended questions as a strategy to engage quieter students.
- Seek clarification or ask probing questions so that students can expand their thoughts.
- Moderate the amount of time and frequency that eager students proffer their discussion, that is, "Shared Air Time."
- Promote students to work towards a common goal: The success of their learning.

CASE IN POINT

The instructor poses the scenario to which students are to respond.

"Matthew is wheezing really badly—he's an asthmatic and is having trouble breathing!"

As a group, students research information that explains the following content:

- Anatomy and physiology of the respiratory system
- Causes of asthma—what triggers an asthma attack, how asthma develops
- Home management to maintain healthy lifestyle—"reliever and preventer" inhalers
- Pharmacology to relieve the impact of asthma—how these medications work on the body
- Medical intervention in asthma crisis/respiratory arrest—oxygenation, intubation, medication, injection
- Hospital treatment of acute asthma
- Patient education to manage asthma

Preparing for Small Group Teaching

Within any classroom, the role of the educator is to engage students in learning. Because of the intimacy of small groups, the educator may take on various roles as needed, such as instructional guide, content expert, examiner, facilitator, teacher, learner, and advocate. Each role is determined by the dynamics of the group and the topic that is being presented. On one hand, a firm or semiauthoritative approach may be needed when student requirements for successful completion of the course are outlined; on the other hand, a relaxed, friendly, and casual approach may be used to create a comfortable learning environment when that is the goal.

Planning the Class Session

With any teaching assignment, the instructor must first consider what learners need to achieve so that learning objectives can be identified. Each step of the learning process must include clear tasks so that students can build on existing knowledge and relate new information to previous learning. Each step must be delivered at a level that learners understand, and learners must comprehend relationships at each point.

Chapter 9: Lesson Plans provides details on how the instructor should develop lesson plans for a standard class session. Methods of delivering instruction to small groups are consistent with the basic techniques used for a group of any size. The instructional session should begin with an introduction that sets the scene and provides a focus for the learning that is to come. The introduction should include a statement that illustrates the significance of what is to be learned and explains why it is important for students to develop knowledge and skills associated with the learning objectives of the session.

The body of the instruction is set out in logical and sequential manner. The instructor is challenged to design the instruction in such a way that new knowledge is constructed by building on existing knowledge. Various activities that involve students are incorporated into the lesson. Examples of such activities include student identification of cases for discussion, simulations, and role-playing.

The conclusion of the lesson brings together its significant features. The conclusion provides an opportunity for the instructor to restate the main components. This statement reminds students of the important things they need to study to consolidate their learning. At the end of the session, it is a good move for the instructor to describe the students' original knowledge base and point out the new knowledge that they have acquired since the lesson began.

Selecting Groups

Assigning students to specific groups is more effective when dealt with ahead of time. If this is not possible, it should be quickly attended to at the commencement of class so as not to waste time.

Teaching Tip >> *It must be remembered that EMS personnel will not always work with the same partner or crew. Variation in the memberships of groups, as well as in their skill levels, can enhance the overall performance of individual members and of the team.*

The instructor can use several methods to assemble groups. Randomization techniques such as counting off or drawing numbers allow learners to maintain minimal control in the random-sorting process. The educator can control the selection before class time based on knowledge of the group, keeping in mind individual strengths and limitations. The educator might assign groups according to students' age, sex, relative ability, or study major. Student control of selection allows individual or collective formation of groups based on the wishes of group members. However student self-selection is generally not recommended as students might not consider the demands of the study task when choosing fellow group members. This option may prove to be less effective because the student strength might not match the task at hand.[9]

Common Small Group Strategies

Various types of small groups can participate in diverse learning activities. Included in this chapter is a discussion of tutorials and seminars, case discussions, role plays, and problem-based learning. Some strategies for small group learning are outlined here, as well as elements of a small group strategy known as "Team-Based Learning."

Tutorials and Seminars

Lectures presented to large groups of students are usually planned to work hand-in-hand with tutorials and seminars. The lecture provides the formal academic point of view, whereas the purpose of tutorials and seminars is to transfer theory into applications for

Additional Small Group Applications[5]

- Begin class discussion with small groups to motivate learners and set the stage for learning.
- Break up a lecture with small groups to deepen and assess understanding.
- End class discussion with small groups to summarize the learning tasks of the day.
- Use small class format for exam review.
- Work in small groups for exam debriefing.
- Use small group activities as an adjunct to audiovisual presentations.

Team-Based Learning[10]

Team-based learning is another method of group learning. In this process, the instructor divides the class into permanent teams. Team readiness for activities is assured using the following:

1. Preassigned reading
2. Individual multiple choice assessment
3. Multiple choice assessment repeated with group
   - Assessment self-graded by group using a progressive disclosure method until all correct answers are known
4. Teams may appeal answers with instructor
5. Mini-lecture by instructor based on material learners are struggling with

Each team is assigned an in-class activity (4 S's):

1. *Significant* problem to solve collaboratively
2. *Same* problem is assigned to each group
3. *Specific* choice (answer) is developed by each group
4. *Simultaneous* report-out is conducted
   a. Each group defends its choice using evidence.
   b. Describe how they came to their conclusion

Summative peer evaluation is conducted several times throughout the semester.

clinical practice. It is common for tutorials and seminars to be included within the format of a class.

The tutorial is achieved primarily through discussion. The educator usually leads the tutorial, and learners are expected to provide input. The tutorial provides a wealth of opportunities through which students can learn. It is in this class that the relevance and meaning of what students are doing become apparent. Effective tutorials require clear guidelines that enable learners to achieve expected learning outcomes, along with expectations that everyone will participate in the learning process and that decisions will be made by group consensus.

In situations in which questions and statements for discussion are drawn from the lecture content, the educator should have an outline prepared in advance. This outline is the road map that guides the learning process. Development of questions for the tutorial requires thorough attention to the preceding lecture content. If another faculty member has delivered the lecture, it is useful for the instructor to liaise with him or her to ensure that the outcome is in accordance with overall curriculum requirements.

Teaching Tip >> *The main task that the educator faces is getting the discussion going; this can be a challenge for the new instructor. As with most other teaching methods, getting students involved creates a functional learning environment. One of the most disappointing situations that the instructor can experience is a silent group. If no one offers to start a discussion, the instructor must take the lead. The instructor should ask students for their opinions and have students share experiences with the group. Students do not always recognize what they do not know. The tutorial provides a means by which students can identify shortcomings, so they can review and work on those areas. For this purpose, the wise instructor pays attention to the tutorial preparation.*

Seminars are typically led by students while the instructor facilitates the learning theme. Seminars, like tutorials, are usually associated with a parallel lecture; a seminar provides a forum in which learners can raise learning issues by working through allocated tasks. During seminars, learners and educators discuss a topic that is part of the course content in an environment that does not demand the rigor of academia.

At the commencement of the course, seminar tasks are usually allocated to learners who are required to prepare a theme for discussion. For example, if the focus of the lecture is myocardial infarction, the seminar could address such topics as physical exercise and nutrition for a healthy heart, or associated physiology of time-related activity of cardiac markers after an infarction.

Handouts distributed at seminars and tutorials provide insights into the content discussed. Handouts help the student recall the topic as discussed in class; a reference list of available texts and resources for independent study can be provided as part of the handout. Students are encouraged in this way to read more about the topic than is provided in the handout.

Case Discussion

The relevance of bringing together theory and practice has impact when each learner is asked to describe a particular case that he or she has experienced as part of field internship. The case can be dissected into specific sections for analysis.

A diabetic crisis is used to illustrate how each section can be analyzed. For example:

- *The situation in which the victim was found*—What clues provide information that could assist EMS personnel to determine the cause of the incident?
- *The clinical features of the patient*—What were the clinical features, and how do they relate to the underlying pathophysiology?
- *Associated medical conditions of the patient*—Some medical conditions such as diabetes may be accompanied by retinopathy, a vision problem. How and why does this develop?
- *Prehospital care*—What care was provided? Why was this done? What could or should have been included when this care was provided?
- *Patient education*—What does the patient need to learn to manage his or her diabetes at home?

Because each learner has a personal interest in the case, the student group and the instructor provide detailed discussion that creates a great learning opportunity. Additionally, case studies can provide a great opportunity for the program medical director to become involved in the learning process.

Role Plays

Role-playing is a group-oriented process that involves at least two participants in a classroom dramatization. Role plays can involve as many as seven to ten characters but are usually limited in duration and scope. This type of classroom drama can be used to investigate and bring alive almost any topic. The technique is meant to create a situation in which each participant adopts a realistic character, or type of patient, and interacts with others in the role play according to how the character would act in real life.

Adequate preparation and facilitation skills are essential for the successful use of a role play. In general, the extent to which the acting performance is realistic determines the degree of learning that will occur. Instructors should set the stage so that students take the exercise seriously. Giggling, joking, and outbursts of laughter are often related to discomfort on the part of the role players, or students. These outbursts tend to diffuse needed tension and can break the concentration of players, minimizing the importance of the event. It is important for the instructor to remind students that they may face this very situation in an actual patient care environment. Debriefing and discussion are key elements in reinforcing important learning points and integrating the performance into the lesson plan. Acknowledgment of the stress involved in the performance and appropriate use of humor can be encouraged once the goals of the role play have been achieved.

Essential Elements of Role-Playing[11]

- *Briefing students*—Explain the subject, goals, and key elements of the situation. If particular physical behaviors are needed, such as facial expressions or body position, the instructor should coach the role players on a realistic way to reenact actual patient presentation.
- *Conducting the drama*—Act, or set the stage and environment so others can act.
- *Debriefing*—Identify key concepts that have been learned, and facilitate a constructive conversation about the performance of the players.

Care should be taken to respectfully diffuse the anxiety of participants so that a safe learning environment is created. Students may try to psychoanalyze the players based on their roles; it is important for everyone to be reminded that these are only dramatizations and improvisations—not necessarily the real feelings or actions of the participants. Inviting guests such as past patients, acting students, local crisis team workers, Community Emergency Response Team (CERT) members, or EMS program graduates to play a role can often lead to a higher level of intensity and learning. Videotaping can enhance this activity, allowing for retrospective group or individual performance review and evaluation.

Role plays differ from scenarios in that very little medical equipment is used. Role plays focus on human interaction, case presentation, symptomatology, interview approaches, de-escalation, and communication skills. Crisis intervention, therapeutic communication, and courtroom-testifying skills are particularly well suited to this type of group process.

Some types of role-playing include the following:

- *Student–student scripted role play*—A group of two to ten students dramatizes a patient encounter, taking on the roles that would be involved—from patient(s), family members, and bystanders, to first responders, and EMS crew members.
- *Student-directed improvisational role play*—A group of students creates a situation to which another student (or team of students) must respond. Students prepare the dramatization in advance, researching the signs, symptoms, and possible actions or reactions that might occur during such an

event. Students who prepare the role play might anticipate what occurs when a patient is treated inappropriately or is not treated at all.

- *Instructor–student role play*—The instructor pretends to be a patient and interacts with two or more students as they try to interview and take care of him or her.
- *Guest role play*—A person unknown to the class is invited to dramatize a case. Students are placed in the role of EMS responders who try to take care of the guest.

Problem-Based Learning

Problem-based learning (PBL) is an instructional method by which the instructor creates a complex, well-structured problem that a group of students tries to solve. Although the term "problem-based learning" is used loosely as an educational tool for any real-life patient problem or situation, the true form of PBL is well defined and structured. The problem presented is realistic and serves as the catalyst for learning. Students first work to uncover the facts and basic science behind the problem. In subsequent steps, students create possible explanations (hypotheses) about the problem and propose ways to solve some of the issues presented.[12,13]

PBL is not a new concept in education. Socrates and Plato pushed their students to think and search for answers and debate their hypotheses in an educational environment. In 1968, PBL was more formally established by Barrows and his colleagues at McMaster University in Ontario, Canada, as a way of helping students apply basic scientific methods to clinical problems.[13, 14]

The educator in PBL serves as a coach (also referred to as a "facilitator," "guide" or "tutor") and helps balance and guide the direction of student inquiry. As a facilitator, the educator sets the tone for a positive and respectful exchange and for critical discussion of ideas. Feedback is essential to this facilitation.[14,15] The belief behind this method is that by discovering the issues and processes that characterize a problem, students acquire basic knowledge and immediately apply that knowledge to solve the problem.

Research evidence has been steadily mounting to show that PBL improves clinical reasoning skills and helps students better organize and apply clinical knowledge. This type of group learning fosters cooperative working and improves assessment skills.[16–19] Some studies have shown that PBL reduces the stress of intense medical education.[16]

Advantages of PBL include the development of interpersonal skills, research approaches, communication techniques, prioritization of time and resources, teamwork, and potentially, learner confidence. Additionally, students are motivated by working on a relevant, real-life problem, and they are given the opportunity to be self-directed to some extent. Some disadvantages of PBL include the difficulty of stepping back from a traditional information-delivery model, the time and resources needed for setup, and the ongoing need for facilitation.[17] Also, protected time for independent research and study is essential and may not be available because of the requirements of the curriculum.

Sample Class Sessions with Problem-Based Learning Technique

CLASS 1

Morning: Group meeting to (a) review case, (b) review terminology, (c) identify critical data, (d) discuss possible explanations, (e) discuss group action plan, and (f) identify learning issues for group and individual persons

Afternoon: Lecture or lab to support problem

CLASS 2

Morning: Independent research to support problem: reading on core issues, writing down individual issues

Afternoon: Lecture or lab to support problem

CLASS 3

Clinical experience to support problem

CLASS 4

Morning: Independent research to support problem

Afternoon: Lecture or lab to support problem

CLASS 5

Morning: Group meeting to discuss how new learning applies to the analysis and resolution of the case

Parameters for PBL

Although problem-based learning units can be presented in various formats, the following principles remain consistent:

- In a PBL unit, the ill-structured problem, as described below, is presented first and serves as the organizing center and context for learning.
- The problem on which learning centers:
  - Is ill structured;

- Is presented as a "messy" situation;
- Often changes with the addition of new information;
- Is not solved easily or formulaically;
- Does not always have a "right" answer.

- In PBL classrooms, students assume the role of problem solver; teachers assume the roles of tutor and coach.
- In the teaching and learning process, information is shared, but knowledge is a personal construction of the learner. Thinking is fully articulated and is held to strict benchmarks.
- Assessment is an authentic companion to the problem and the process.
- The PBL unit is not necessarily interdisciplinary in nature but is always integrative.

Teaching Psychomotor Skills

Teaching psychomotor skills provides an excellent opportunity for the instructor to teach in small groups. Psychomotor skill development is crucial to good patient care. All the effort put forth at the scene of an EMS incident depends on the provider's ability to select the right skill at the right time, and to carry it out in the right manner. Many of the skills routinely performed at an EMS incident are critical to patient survival and leave little or no margin for error. Details of teaching psychomotor skills can be found in Chapter 12: Teaching in All Domains.

Simulations

Simulation exercises provide an excellent opportunity for students to incorporate cognitive, psychomotor, and affective skills while working in groups

CASE IN POINT

EXAMPLE OF A PROBLEM FOR PBL

Scene

EMS is dispatched on a Saturday evening to an affluent shopping mall for a "girl who is acting strangely and talking out of her head." The dispatcher says that mall security initiated the call, and that the patient is somewhat verbally aggressive. When the crew arrives, they meet a provocatively dressed young woman who is smoking a cigarette and says she is 20 years old and was just pushed by a man she met inside the bar. She says she is "fine" and would be "better if the ? @** police would stay out of her life and leave her alone." Mall security indicates they smell alcohol on the patient's breath. The police officer on the scene states that this could be her cologne, and that she appears to be constantly staring at the floor.

Assessment

The patient admits to occasional drug abuse but says she has not taken anything recently. EMS notes that she has an abrasion on her knee and a medic alert bracelet on her wrist, indicating allergy to haloperidol and benzodiazepines. The police have searched the patient for weapons and have given EMS empty bottles of rifampin, metformin hydrochloride, and valproic acid. The patient is refusing to be treated and states that she is being "set up" for another hospital bill because the "police said the detox unit is full." She just wants to go home. Her blood pressure is 160/90; pulse is 124; respirations are 20 per minute, and SpO_2 is 80 percent on room air.

In their own defense, the police privately admit that the county detoxification unit is full, but they are willing to arrest her for disorderly conduct if the EMS crew medically clears the patient.

Questions for the First Group Meeting

1. What key elements are included and/or missing in the patient assessment?
2. What physiologic mechanisms might be responsible for the symptoms present?
3. What field impressions should the EMS crew consider?
4. What legal principles are at play? What psychosocial issues are implicated between each of the agencies responding to the call (Mall Security, Police, and EMS)? How would each of those be managed?
5. What is the patient's possible medical history based on the assessment findings?

Complications to Be Discovered After the First Discussion Is Completed

Case Continuation: As the crew questions the patient, she has a tonic seizure (arms only) and then is unresponsive to any stimuli.

- How should EMS manage this patient?
- Should the patient awaken and become violent, what type of physical and alternative restraint systems might be used?

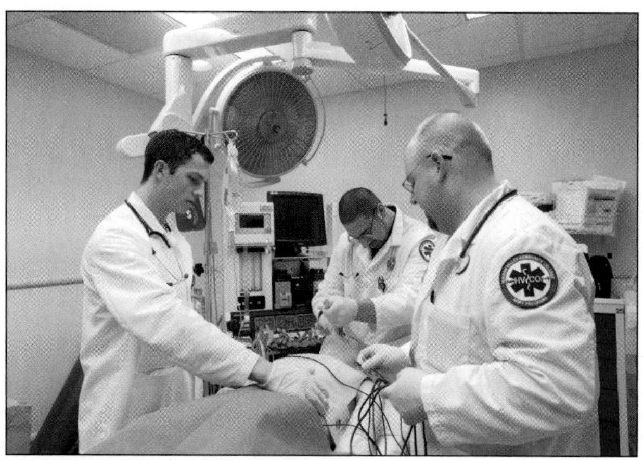

Figure 14.3

Simulation exercises are typically popular with students because they give students the chance to practice what they have learned and to self-evaluate.

(Figure 14.3). The purpose of simulation is to create problem-solving situations that students can expect to deal with during their careers. It is useful to base the problem around student's current learning and clinical experiences to ensure that the scenario is within reach of each student's level of training and degree of expected competence.

Similar to role plays, simulations require a patient actor or high-fidelity manikin, a responding crew, bystanders, and a facilitator. Using moulage to simulate illness or injury can enhance the realism of this experience. Simulations can be used to open a class by stimulating discussion, or to close a class by evaluating student understanding of the covered material. Simulations can be done as remediation during clinical or field rotations when similar cases have been seen. Finally, they can be done during lab time as a "put it all together" activity for students. Simulation is discussed more fully in Chapter 18: Tools for Simulation.

CASE IN POINT

Vehicle extrication is one example of a simulation exercise. Although it might be difficult to acquire or use actual car wrecks, the simulation is effective when an actual vehicle is used. With relevant training equipment, each student takes the role of the victim to be extricated from the vehicle. If different types of vehicles are available, it is beneficial to repeat the exercise in different vehicles to enhance students' awareness of the problems to be encountered in various real-life situations.

Different scenarios can be created to dramatize problems of advanced complexity that must be solved—extrication of the patient who has spinal injuries, or a potential leg fracture, or a major hemorrhage and crushed chest. Each scenario will require actions and practices that demonstrate standard competencies of prehospital care.

Teaching Tip >> *To make simulations more realistic, move students to a different location such as outdoors, in the hall, or in the bathroom. Use moulage, background noise, and props such as medical supplies, medication vials and bottles, or other products; have simulated patients follow a scripted storyline.*

Simulation exercises offer many benefits. Each scenario can be stopped at any time to draw attention to certain aspects to which the participant must give due attention. Because the demands associated with real-life events are not a part of the exercise, each part of the scenario can be discussed at the point of activity, and each can be supportively critiqued at the conclusion.

Summary

For EMS educators, working with small groups is both challenging and rewarding. Not only does the use of small groups help to promote a higher level of thinking and understanding in the classroom, it also fosters "life after class" skills of leadership, teamwork, communication, and accountability. Whether the entire curriculum is designed around small groups, or they are simply used to break up lectures or to teach psychomotor skills, small group instruction can be an extremely effective educational strategy.

Glossary

collaborative learning A group learning activity in which the educator poses the learning to them and the students divide the labor to find associated details.

cooperative learning A group learning activity in which the educator poses the learning to them and the students work together and are jointly responsible for learning outcomes.

problem-based learning (PBL) An instructional method by which the instructor creates a complex, well-structured problem that a group of students tries to solve.

role-playing A group process that involves students in a dramatization.

References

1. Jaques, D. (2000). Learning in groups. In *Handbook for improving group learning* (3rd ed.). London, UK: Kogan Page.
2. Healey, M., & Matthews, H. (1996). Learning in small groups in university geography courses: Designing a core module around group projects. *Journal of Geography in Higher Education, 20,* 167–181.
3. Sobral, D. T. (1998). Productive small groups in medical studies: Training for cooperative learning. *Medical Teacher, 20,* 118–121.
4. Jaques, D. (2003). Teaching small groups. *British Medical Journal, 326,* 492–494.
5. Cooper, J. L., & Robinson, P. (2000, Spring). Getting started: Informal small-group strategies in large classes. *New Directions for Teaching and Learning. 81,* 17–24.
6. Cooper, L., Lawson, M., & Orrell, J. (1997). *Raising issues about teaching: Views of academic staff at Flinders University.* Adelaide, Australia: Flinders Press.
7. Roschelle, J., & Teasley, S. (1995). The construction of shared knowledge in collaborative problem solving. In C. E. O'Malley (Ed.), *Computer-supported collaborative learning.* Heidelberg, Germany: Springer-Verlag.
8. Maughan, C., & Webb, J. (2001, November). Small group learning and assessment. UKCLE Seminar, "From Little acorns . . ." Available at: http://www.ukcle.ac.uk
9. Cross, K. P., & Steadman, M. H. (1996). *Classroom research: implementing the scholarship of teaching.* San Francisco, CA: Jossey-Bass.
10. Sibley, J., & Spirdonoff, S. (2011). *What is TBL? Getting started with TBL* Retrieved 1/09/12, from http://tblcollaborative.org/starting
11. Orlich, D. C., Harder, R. J., Callahan, R. C., & Gibson, H. W. (2001). *Teaching strategies: A guide to better instruction.* Boston, MA: Houghton Mifflin. 296–297.
12. Center for Problem-Based Learning, Illinois Mathematics and Science Academy. Available at: http://www2.imsa.edu/programs/pbl/whatis/whatis/slide12.html. Accessed October 12, 2004.
13. Wang, H., Cos, A., Thompson, P., & Shuler, C. Problem-based learning—PBL quick facts. USC California Science Project Leadership Cohort. Available at: http://www.usc.edu/hsc/dental/ccmb/usc-csp/Quikfacts.htm. Accessed October 12, 2004.
14. Barrows, H. S. (1996). Problem-based learning in medicine and beyond: A brief overview. In L. Wilkerson & W. H. Gijselaers (Eds.), *Bringing problem-based learning to higher education: Theory and practice,* Vol. 68. San Francisco, CA: Jossey-Bass.
15. Wilkerson, (2004, September). An introduction to problem-based learning. Presented at: 2004 National Association of EMS Education Symposium; Los Angeles, CA.
16. Mensink, D., Kaufman, D., & Day, V. (1998). Stressors in medical school: Relation to curriculum format and year of study. *Teaching & Learning in Medicine, 10,* 138.
17. Whitfield, C., Mauger, E., & Zwicker, J. (2002). Differences between students in problem-based and lecture-based curricula measured by clerkship performance ratings at the beginning of the third year. *Teaching & Learning in Medicine, 14,* 211.
18. Walters, J., Croen, L., Weissman, Z., & Reichgott, M. (1999). A small group, problem-based learning approach to preparing students to retake step 1 of the United States Medical Licensing Examination. *Teaching & Learning in Medicine, 11,* 85.
19. Kilroy, D. (2004, July). Problem-based learning. *Emergency Medicine Journal, 4,* 411.

Additional Resources

Aaron, S., Crocket, J., Morrish, D., Basulado, C., & Kovithavongs, T. (1998). Assessment of exam performance after change to problem-based learning: Differential effects by question type. *Teaching & Learning in Medicine, 10,* 86.

Bertola, P., & Murphy, E. (1994). *Tutoring at university: A beginner's practical guide.* Curtin University of Technology: Paradigm Books.

Billings, D. M., & Halstead, J. A. (1998). *Teaching in nursing: A guide for faculty.* Philadelphia, PA: W. B. Saunders. 415–416.

Blackman, I. *Rasch scaling—Blood pressure.* School of Nursing, Flinders University, South Australia.

Cooper, J. L., MacGregor, J., Smith, K. A., & Robinson, P. (2000, Spring). Implementing small-group instruction: Insights from successful practitioners. *New Directions for Teaching and Learning.* 81.

Deeny, P., Johnson, A., Boore, J., Leyden, C., & McCaughan, E. (2001). Drama as an experiential technique in learning how to cope with dying patients and their families. *Teaching in Higher Education, 6,* 99–112.

15

Tools for Large Group Learning

My play was a complete success. The audience was a failure. — Ashleigh Brilliant

Teaching a large group requires a different approach than is used to teach a small group, but the principles of teaching methods are retained. This chapter offers teaching strategies for instructors to use when they face the challenge of teaching large numbers of students.

What constitutes a "large group" cannot be firmly defined because this is relative to the educational setting and the circumstances of the instructional event. In some situations, a "large group" may constitute 40 or 50 students; in others, more than 100 students may be included. At a regional or national conference, it is not uncommon for a class to be filled with 200 to 400 or more students. Therefore, the concept of "large group" is subject to interpretation. For the purposes of this text, a large group is defined as a greater number than can be easily handled for small group activities (i.e., more than approximately 40 students).

The advantage of teaching a large group is that content can be presented to many individuals at the same time. This saves instructor time, thus reducing costs. One instructor who teaches 45 students is more cost-effective than one who is teaching 15 students over three sessions. On the other hand, teaching a large group requires teacher-centered learning techniques such as lecture, rather than a learner-centered classroom.

Lecturing is the strategy most often used for teaching large groups. Variations of the lecture format and diverse techniques can promote learning and interactivity. Other large group teaching techniques include debate and student presentations. Although a large class can be a challenge for an instructor, effective methods can be identified and applied with careful planning.

CHAPTER GOAL: This chapter offers teaching strategies for instructors to use when they face the challenge of teaching large numbers of students.

Lecture

Despite the interest of educators in more student-centered techniques, the lecture remains the most widely used teaching method in medical education.[1] **Lecture** is a teaching session in which the instructor is the principal teacher. Lectures allow the educator to disseminate large amounts of information to learners in a very direct and cost-effective manner. The lecture format has been well described as effective in the literature.[2–4] This method allows the focus to remain on the educator and the educator to be the center of control for the flow of information.

Educators teach as they themselves have always been taught. The model has been the same for as long as anyone can remember. Teaching this way is comfortable for both educator and learner. Lecturing is a traditional strategy to which every student can relate, and it certainly has its place in the educational process.

Advantages and Disadvantages

When used effectively, a lecture can facilitate new learning and clarify complex or confusing concepts that may need special explanation. Lecture can also be used to organize thinking, promote problem solving, and challenge attitudes.[5,6] It may be used as a change of pace from other teaching strategies, or for delivery of material that is not otherwise available to students.[4] The lecture can also stimulate student thought and questions that can then be used with smaller group teaching strategies.[7]

Cooper and colleagues[8] note the consensus among university faculty members that transmission of knowledge through lecture is an important educational strategy, and that there is an interdependent relationship between lectures and other modes of teaching. Most instructors would agree that lectures are significantly

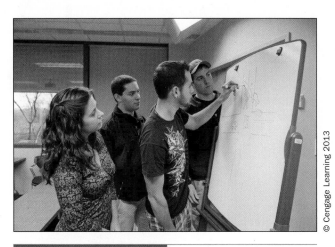

Figure 15.1

Techniques can be used to enhance the lecture format and contribute to student learning.

more valuable when complemented by tutorials and student-to-student interaction **(Figure 15.1)**.

Many have questioned the role of the lecture in teaching. Some educators believe that lecturing is a poor method for developing thinking skills or attitudes because students are passive, unengaged learners.[4] Certainly, decreased student involvement is a disadvantage. Lecture alone without the use of visual aids favors auditory learners and may easily result in the lost attention of visual and kinesthetic learners.

Clearly, the lecture method entails both advantages and disadvantages. However, thorough preparation and knowledge of methods of enhancing the lecture can make it an effective learning experience. Students have identified features that enhance lecture delivery which include the following:

- Educators use of variety of teaching and communication processes
- Educators should be organized so learners can follow the train of thought
- Educators model behaviors they expect students to demonstrate [9]

Basics of Lecture Preparation

Once the learning objectives of the lecture have been identified, preparation is focused on developing the lesson plan to ensure that the lecture content meets those objectives. Previously used lectures should be updated periodically to reflect current protocols and procedures. Educators can take the following steps to enhance lecture preparation:

- Conduct research to find the most recent information, statistical data, and clinical practices that relate to the lecture content or objectives.
- Identify the most important points that students must understand and retain. Key points are intended to encourage higher levels of thinking.
- Distinguish between knowledge and concepts that are essential and those that are not part of the core message. The aim is to focus on the most important aspects of the topic, rather than to synthesize a large amount of material. If the topic is not part of the core learning objective, it can be included in the supplementary readings or identified to the students as "nice to know."
- Create lecture notes and/or an outline in an effective format so as to keep on track and deliver the content in a sequential and logical manner.
- Be prepared with more material than needed so as to be confident and have a sense of knowing the topic thoroughly; however, it is important not to *over* prepare or provide all the researched information to the students. The goal of the lecture is to teach students relevant information—not to prove how much the instructor knows.
- On the day of the lecture, educators should prepare for their best personal presentation and should prepare the environment itself.

Instructors must assess their own personal attributes to evaluate how they project themselves as teacher, role model, and professional. Due attention to dress and grooming allows the instructor's appearance before the audience to be seen as professional and to reflect a professional approach to work; at the same time, it enhances self-confidence. Stage fright is frequently related to insecurities about physical appearance. Modest, conservative clothing is always appropriate. For men, not wearing a tie when the men in the group will likely be wearing them can convey disrespect. Looking one's best helps one to be confident and comfortable in front of the class. Comfortable clothes and shoes are helpful. Hair should be styled in such a manner that it does not create distractions (such as flicking long hair out of one's face). Being clean and tidy works every time. Silently reciting positive affirmation statements can boost the instructor's self-confidence.

Some lecture classrooms have fixed seating; others are furnished with stackable chairs. If chairs require setup, the instructor should position them in an arrangement that offers the greatest possible degree of interaction. The heating and cooling controls should be checked and windows adjusted to promote airflow and comfort. Ensuring the physical comfort of students significantly aids their attention span.

Instructors should arrive early to set up equipment that will be used. Many institutions do not have technical personnel to attend to this requirement, so it becomes the instructor's responsibility. At the podium, materials should be organized so that the lesson plan and any other needed materials are readily accessible. On occasion, the instructor may be required to lecture off-site and at a location with which he or she might not be familiar. On such occasions, it is wise to request the necessary equipment and to confirm the availability of basic technology such as laptop, audiovisual projectors, and DVD players. Have back-up materials such as USB drives or CDs at hand in case the expected technology is not forthcoming.

Parts of a Lecture

After research and identification of key points to be delivered during the lecture, the instructor develops the three parts of the lecture: introduction, body, and conclusion. These parts are common to any instructional activity. Although most lecturers begin with the development of the body of the lecture, this discussion proceeds in presentation order and begins with the introduction.

Introduction

The purpose of the lecture introduction is to capture students' interest and attention. The lecture should be started with a thought-stimulating statement, an analogy, a thought-provoking challenge, a video or audio clip, a case study, or a question that arouses curiosity. This approach grabs students' attention and focuses their minds on the topic of the lecture. Some examples are as follows:

- "After cardiac arrest, very few patients walk out of the hospital neurologically intact . . ."
- "Patients who require long-term or ongoing institutional care are often the result of life-saving efforts by paramedics and emergency room personnel . . ."

The introduction should establish the intention and relevance of the topic and should identify how this piece of information fits into the "big picture," such as, "Strokes are a leading cause of death in America. Disability from strokes alone costs society millions of dollars. Early recognition and management of the patient with stroke can significantly decrease the devastating disability that results from strokes."

Another effective introduction is a case study, that is, information from a real emergency call. Some lecturers choose to use a portion of the case study as an introduction, then to complete the case study, perhaps with the patient outcome and diagnosis included, as the conclusion.

The introduction can provide the ground rules for the lecture. Students should be told whether it is appropriate to ask questions during the lecture, or if they should wait for a question-and-answer session at the end. Also, students should be told whether comments are allowed during the class session. The lecturer can identify an approximate time until the next break, which should occur approximately 45 to 50 minutes after the lecture begins.

> **Teaching Tip** >> *Students should be given index cards so they can write down questions that they may have during the lecture. These are handed in at the end of the session, and the instructor can discern themes or areas that need reinforcement or clarification. This allows a student to ask questions without having to interrupt, speak up in class, or fear being accused by fellow students of asking "dumb questions."*

Some presenters find it helpful to write out the complete introduction so that in the first few minutes of public speaking, they can rely on that as a crutch if necessary. This reassurance can assist the instructor in overcoming initial nervousness.

The introduction should not include an apology for the lack of time or the amount of information to be covered. These statements indicate poor teacher preparation.

Body

The body of the lecture must present key points to be discussed in achieving the learning objectives. Although the instructor has some freedom to select an approach for delivery of information, the lecture must follow a logical order and must be well organized. One example is as follows:

- Describe the cause of the medical condition; discuss incidence of the condition.
- Explain relevant medical terminology that is used.
- Identify the major clinical features of the illness.
- Discuss the pathophysiology.
- Explain the care that should be provided, and relate this to the pathophysiology.
- Provide an overview of follow-up care.
- Offer strategies related to health and safety issues (e.g., reducing risk of personal injury or contamination).

Although it may be necessary for the instructor to provide more detailed information during the lecture, it is important that the main principles and ideas are not lost. At regular intervals during the lecture, it is useful for the instructor to summarize the main points. Students do not retain every detail that is presented; therefore, repetition brings focus to the message and reminds students of what they have learned.

Teaching Tip >> *The lecturer should provide commercial breaks! Today's generation has grown up with television, with material routinely presented in a half-hour or hour-long format interrupted by commercials, sometimes as often as every eight minutes. So lecture material should be presented in segments, then a "commercial" should be added, such as a summary or illustrative point. This allows students to process information in chunks, and it gives students who are taking notes the chance to get caught up.*

Conclusion

The lecture requires some form of closure. This can be achieved in various ways, such as the following:

- Summarize the main points of the lecture by providing a new example that illustrates the main points of the material. This new example provides students with an opportunity to confirm their learning.
- Make a statement that identifies what the instructor expects the students to gain from the lecture.
- Ask a student to provide a summary of the main points.
- Relate the lecture to previous and future learning.
- Direct students' attention to additional learning resources related to the lecture.
- Hand out 3 × 5 cards on which each student can summarize key points before returning them to the instructor. Through this technique, the instructor receives important feedback on his or her effectiveness and identifies concerns that can be clarified in the next lecture.
- Conclude the lecture by asking for questions and answering them.
- Prepare the students for material to be covered in the next session.

When a student asks a question, it may be important for the lecturer to repeat the question so all students can hear it. After the question-and-answer session has concluded, a second powerful closure to the lecture can be used.

Another closing technique is to complete a case study that was begun as the lecture introduction. The actual patient diagnosis and outcome can serve as the ending of the lecture. Some teachers end the lecture with something memorable such as a motivational story or a challenge. The ending can strongly influence what information students take home.

Techniques for Enhancing Lectures

Because the lecture format has some disadvantages, instructors must develop methods by which to enhance the lecture to promote the acquisition of knowledge. Various techniques can be used, and instructors can explore which of these works best for their style and that of their students.

Humor

Humor can be an effective teaching tool when used correctly. The purpose of integrating humor into a lecture is not to have the lecturer receive high evaluations or to entertain the class. Laughter can be a valuable learning tool that reinforces the learning experience. It helps the lecturer connect with students and arouses interest. Laughter can help people relax and gain or keep attention. Humor can make information more memorable and can highlight an issue. Visual humor can facilitate learning and combat short attention spans. Students can look up at the picture or cartoon or prop and refocus on the lecture. The humor used should always be relevant to the topic under discussion.

CASE IN POINT

One method of using humor in a lecture is to make a point, illustrate the point with a short humorous illustration, then remake the point. An example is as follows:

> Clear communication with the patient and with his or her family is essential. It is like the EMT who responded to the scene of a shooting. Wanting to be able to quickly assess the injury, the EMT asked the patient where he was shot. The patient responded "over on Hatcher Street!"

Clear communication is an essential component of patient assessment.

Instructors must be careful about how they use humor in the classroom because it may be perceived in a very personal way. Attempts to emulate people from television or others who have a great sense of humor may not translate readily to an instructor's style. As a result, attempts at using humor may not be effective. Caution is encouraged when one uses humor in the classroom because one person's humor may be another person's insult. Instructors should be safe if they use gentle and quirky humor in the classroom setting.

Storytelling

Relevant stories relating to the specific objectives of the lecture can enhance lectures. Stories can effectively illustrate and elaborate points. "War stories," or personal stories of a real incident, can assist students in applying information to patient situations. Stories based on actual cases provide an element of realism that reinforces the notion that students will one day encounter the difficulties associated with similar patients with similar problems. Storytelling can be a powerful and effective teaching tool because it can be used (a) to analyze and problem-solve certain elements of the patient care that was provided and (b) to stimulate critical thinking about patient care decisions. Inconsequential details should be eliminated so the story is not too long and student interest is maintained. Stories should be spaced throughout the presentation to provide a change of pace and to reemphasize the message. Storytelling should not allow students to digress into nonpurposeful discussion. It is imperative that the storytelling not violate patient privacy. This is essential not only to comply with the law, but also to model the importance of protecting patient privacy for the learners.

Case Studies

A **case study** is an analysis of a real-life patient situation as a way of illustrating information. Case studies help students learn to apply information to patient care situations. Cases used in lecture should be well designed and should illustrate the important points of the class. Such cases, especially when used with interactive methods, can stimulate critical thinking and problem solving.

Handouts

Handouts can be an important learning aid. Handouts provide a summary of the key points of the lecture and supporting instruction, but they do so without exhaustive explanation. Handouts provide students the opportunity to reflect on the lecture topic and to expand their understanding. A handout allows many students to reflect on what the presenter is saying instead of worrying about taking notes. Careful listening allows students to think about the applications and implications of the lecture. In addition, the learner can review and reflect on the class at a later time to better integrate learning.

Although speakers typically say 120 to 180 words a minute, most audiences think at a rate that is 10 times faster. A handout can keep the learner focused on the spoken material rather than allowing time for the mind to wander. Handouts can also provide more in-depth information that is not included in the lecture, along with references through which students can enrich their learning.[10] In some cases, handouts can present material in an alternative format to the textbook that may promote student understanding. Student organizers are a type of handouts. These present the material in visual or tabular formats that assist learners to compare and contrast information or to put it into a schema that integrates it with their previous knowledge. Organizers should not be completely filled in. Rather, they should be structured so the learner must identify and fill in missing elements to complete them. Examples of organizers include concept maps, outlines, Venn diagrams, algorithms, tables, and diagrams.

In general, handouts should be provided to learners at the beginning of the lecture, so they can follow the sequence of the lecture. Although lecturers may state, "don't worry about taking notes—it's all in the handout," conscientious students may find themselves worried that it is not all there and may wish to write down information "just in case." If the handout is not an exact version of the presentation, the lecturer is more likely to keep student attention. However, in this case, the handout should be given out at the end of the lecture.[10]

Instructors should encourage students to study the lecture material beyond the content provided in the handout, because handouts usually are abbreviated to focus the theme of the required learning. Students will find handouts helpful if they include a list of reference materials for further reading.

In addition to outlining or listing key points, handouts may include: a glossary with definitions of unfamiliar terms; a list of steps such as a skill task analysis sheet, diagrams, or flow charts; and a reference list.[10]

Audiovisual Aids, Props, and Models

Audiovisual (AV) aids are instructional media such as audiotapes (e.g., from a 9-1-1 call center), video-related technologies (e.g., YouTube), and television footage (e.g., from news services). Incorporating AV material into lectures stimulates the students' senses of sight and hearing. Props and models are additional visuals that can be used during a lecture. These tools are used primarily to accompany a class presentation for the purpose of enhancing learning.

AV aids offer many benefits, especially when a combination of more than one medium (multimedia) is used. Multimedia presentations can be applied to a variety of learning styles and may facilitate learning. Use of multimedia can reduce the costs of teaching and learning and may improve learning effectiveness. This is accomplished through increased learner motivation, improved retention of learned material, and enhanced interactivity.[11] The instructor should ensure that all students can hear and see the AV aid, model, or prop. A document camera may be helpful in facilitating this. For more complete information on the use of audiovisual materials, see Chapter 16: Using Technology to Enhance Classroom Learning.

Guided Discussion and Questioning Techniques

Teacher-led discussions help students develop strong thinking skills and gain a sound understanding of the course material. In a large group, it is not always possible for the instructor to use a teaching tool that encourages students to discuss a particular learning point among themselves. However, teacher-led guided discussion allows students the opportunity to have their learning challenged. Guided discussion is designed to give students the chance to develop critical thinking and to increase student's comprehension by exploring an area of learning that is currently unfamiliar to them. The instructor poses a question to the whole class, and learners offer responses or additional questions to broaden the scope of the discussion **(Figure 15.2)**.

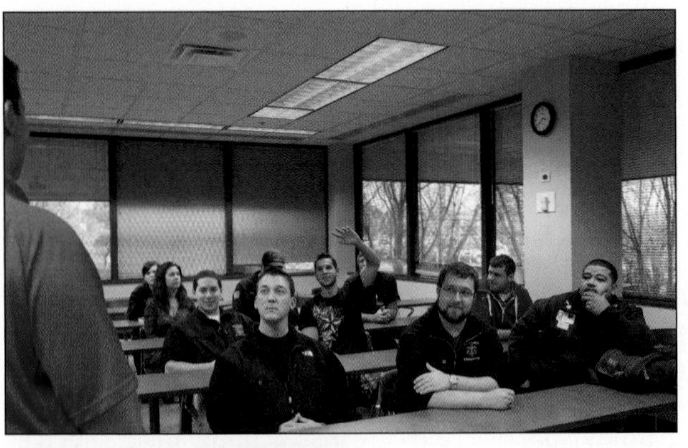

Figure 15.2

Effective questionning techniques can be used in a large group. However, the instructor must be prepared to manage the discussion.

Although questioning techniques can be used in a large group just as in any group, these techniques must be more carefully controlled in a large group setting. Discussions initiated within large groups can yield great results that assist students in learning; however, for a new instructor with limited experience in managing very large groups, this can readily turn to chaos. In some cases, two or three students may wish to dominate the discussion and argue their perspective as the model to be followed; they may even become argumentative. Members may not listen to each other, and each faction can become deferential toward the instructor. Discussion may tend to focus on one section of the group, and the rest may stop joining in. Additionally, when a student who is called on speaks, other students may begin talking among themselves, which can be very disruptive in a large classroom. Students should be instructed to remain silent until they are called on. Large group discussion must be undertaken with careful planning and caution.[7]

During a large group discussion, it is important for the instructor to make sure that the acoustics are adequate or that students use a microphone, because otherwise, only those in the immediate vicinity of the responding student may be able to hear. Presenters should come to the podium and use the microphone to present their findings. Additional information on questioning techniques can be found in Chapter 11: Introduction to Teaching Strategies.

Activities

Many instructors would be aghast at the idea of having large groups of students participate in activities during the lecture. Students in this situation become noisy, and the instructor must worry about whether students are actually undertaking the task at hand or are using the time for social chatter. Instructors may be concerned that time will be wasted if students are permitted to become involved in an activity. Despite these concerns, some simple activities have been designed that can readily be worked into a lecture.

Lecture content can be reinforced by an activity that is used to review material. By putting forth an application problem, the lecturer challenges students to find solutions to problems in ways that they must do so in the field—by actively participating with others in the group. Under the instructor's direction, learners may conduct a review or even play games that have been structured to allow students to apply the knowledge they have gained in ways that they may never have imagined. Movement from passive to active learning is what makes facilitation such an exceptional educational strategy.

Students can be given specific tasks to attend to during the lecture by assigning "listening teams".[12]

At the commencement of the lecture, the instructor assigns a section of student teams.

- *Clarification Team* identifies issues that need clarification within the lecture content.
- *Elaboration Team* suggests points that require further elaboration.
- *Rebuttal Team* finds points on which they disagree.
- *Application Team* identifies problems of practical application they request the instructor to identify.

At the end of the lecture each group is allocated time to present a summary of their findings.

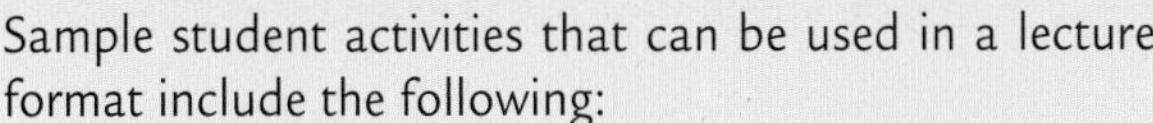

Sample student activities that can be used in a lecture format include the following:

- At a key point in the lecture, the presenter can summarize learning by posing some multiple-choice questions. Students must hold up a card or erasable white board with A, B, C, or D on it,[13] or four different-colored papers can be used to represent choices A through D. Obviously, the instructor must prepare the cards or paper before class time.
- A multiple-choice question can be presented on the screen so that all students can see and read it. The presenter can invite students to identify the correct answer, then can call for volunteers to justify why the other options are incorrect.

Work Sessions and Guided Lecture

Another way that the instructor can modify the lecture format is by pausing every 12 to 18 minutes for a short 2- to 3-minute student "work session." This session assists students in clarifying and assimilating material just presented. Activities may be varied and can include the following:

- Students or student groups of two or three write down everything they can recall from the material just presented with special attention to the main points.
- Students working with a partner or two write down everything they can recall from the class, then reconstruct and discuss the lecture (students may not take notes during the lecture).
- Students or student groups develop test questions and answers from the previously presented content.
- Buzz groups of two or three students can be designated as discussion groups for the lecture. The groups can be given specific, time-limited assignments during the lecture such as developing a list of questions they hope the instructor will answer during the lecture. Other open-ended questions can be posed to these groups to identify areas of understanding or confusion.[9]

During the work session, the instructor should be available to clarify any issue that may arise. These short "work sessions" can be followed by a brief student discussion and clarification of material as a large group.[14]

Interactive Lectures

Available technology now assists instructors in changing a passive lecture to one that is interactive. Public area display systems (PADSs) (also called "classroom feedback," "audience-response systems," "personal response systems," or "clickers") are remote-control units from which the audience is able to interact with lecture content through a computerized visual display. The instructor poses a question that has several potential answers, and from the remote-monitor-control unit provided for each participant, one response is selected. Data can then be manipulated to provide immediate feedback that reveals participants' responses. Displaying the anonymous response feedback permits both instructor and learners to identify whether concepts have been mastered or need further elaboration. This technology is a nonthreatening manner for everyone to actively participate in the lecture. This type of technology can also be used to facilitate television game programs in which the opinion of the audience is sought. This format is effective when discussing ethical issues that some students may be reluctant to discuss. There is evidence to suggest that use of PADS improves student participation, increases student-faculty contact, and enhances student learning outcomes.[15]

Considerable content within EMS educational programs can be enhanced through a "talk-show host" approach. The instructor poses a general question or statement, and student group members offer responses that describe how they would deal with the scenario. This approach works especially well in sociologic situations for which no answers are absolutely right or wrong.

The new instructor may feel anxious about using this method for the entire lecture period; however, it is advantageous to schedule a 5-minute section that incorporates this method into the lecture. It is a helpful technique to recap material and assess whether learners are ready to move on to the next topic.

This allows the instructor to develop experience in this teaching approach.

Teaching Tip >> *A low-tech audience-response system can be constructed by having the local hardware store cut 12 × 12 inch squares from the 8 × 4 ft white tileboard sheets they sell for about $20.00 to produce mini-white boards. Each student is given a whiteboard, a paper towel, and a dry erase marker. After asking them a question, the instructor has the entire class hold up their whiteboards at the same time. This involves the class in the lecture, and allows the instructor to determine whether the class is mastering key concepts. It also permits students the chance to show creativity as some answers can be drawn, rather than written.*

The text box on this page offers several tips for effective public speaking techniques that instructors can incorporate into lecture sessions.

Guest Lecturers

Many instructional organizations invite people who are knowledgeable about a particular topic to deliver a lecture. An invited guest lecturer must realize that preparation is crucial to the success of the lecture. Preparation is vital in ensuring that content stimulates student learning. The following focal points require significant attention to ensure that delivery meets the expectations of both the institution and the students:

- *Find out how the lecture topic fits with the standards and course curriculum.* It is important for the guest lecturer to find out as much about the context of

Essentials of Public Speaking

PREPARATION

When instructors know that they and their materials are well prepared, their self-confidence is boosted; this can help reduce the amount of anxiety that new lecturers experience. Although practice delivery of the lecture in private surroundings is encouraged, actual delivery on the day provides vital experiences for the new lecturer.

VOICE MODULATION

Lecturing requires the use of one's voice; lecturing to a large group requires additional attention to the speaking voice. Instructors who have not used a microphone before should practice using one. A natural speaking voice should be adopted, and enunciation should be clear. The pace and pitch of voice should be varied; this increases students' attention to the topic and reduces the likelihood that students may lose concentration through a hypnotic monotone. Timely pauses should be included to give students time to write notes.

ENTHUSIASM AND PERSONALIZATION

Instructors should keep in mind that they have already put a lot of work into developing the lecture. Conveying enthusiasm for the material through use of colorful language and dramatic adjectives enhances the core concept of the material. First- and second-person pronouns (I, we, you) should be used because these personalize the instruction and lend status to and emphasize the importance of the topic.

EYE CONTACT

Eye contact is key to effective communication and is an important aspect of lecturing and teaching. Even with a large group, students should sense that the teacher is looking directly at them at some time during the lecture. With fewer students, it is a worthy goal to look at each student during the course of the lecture. The speaker's eyes should be alert and should convey emotion, enthusiasm, and passion for the topic. As the speaker looks at students and into their eyes, he or she should observe clues from students' body language. Boredom, sleepiness, confusion, and frantic note taking can all speak to the teacher who listens. Alterations can then be made in the style or pace of the lecture, or a break in, or addition of, an activity may be needed.

GESTURES AND BODY LANGUAGE

Effective lecturers use gestures and body language to help convey their message. Nonverbal clues can speak much louder than spoken words can, so it is important that they match. A lecturer who says he is excited about the ability of EMS providers to positively affect the outcomes of patients with the use of new equipment is difficult to believe if his body language does not say the same thing. The key to using gestures is to use those that come naturally. Natural gestures come more easily when the lecturer is relaxed, comfortable with the topic, and prepared for the class. As the lecturer becomes more at ease with speaking, it also becomes more natural to move from behind the podium and change places in front of the class. Some lecturers change positions when they change subjects or emphasize points.

the lecture as possible, and to identify where it fits into the overall course program. The guest lecturer should meet with the course coordinator to clarify how the lecture should reflect course learning objectives. Topic learning outcomes should guide the guest lecturer in that these are the working documents that describe the topic content. The lecture is expected to address each outcome.

- *Find out a little about the students.* Knowing about the age range of students, as well as their educational levels and cultural backgrounds, will assist the lecturer in preparation and will allow the guest lecturer to use relevant examples.
- *Find out what knowledge the students have about the topic.* The course coordinator and teaching colleagues will be able to provide insight so that the appropriate **pitch of lecture delivery** can be achieved. In other words, the lecture language should be commensurate to the students' level of learning.
- *Find out how students will be assessed.* Knowledge of how students are to be assessed should affect lecture preparation. In contrast to assessment conducted through a major essay paper, assessment performed through multiple-choice questions or short-answer information-recall questions requires helpful study resources and handouts that specifically address examinable material; these should be made available to students at the beginning of the course.
- *Find out the scheduled duration of the lecture.* Although many institutions allocate lecture periods of a "50-minute hour," lecture length should be confirmed in advance with the course coordinator or program director.

At least a week before the lecture delivery date, the guest lecturer should check out the venue if possible. He or she must learn how to get there and must become familiar with the location of access and exit doors and the room's physical layout. Information should be obtained about technical equipment provided within the lecture hall, and each piece that will be used should be tested to ensure that it is in working order. The lecturer must determine which equipment must be ordered from another location.

Instructors and guest lecturers should make sure they know how to confidently use the technical equipment needed for their presentation. Arriving early to practice each function of the equipment before commencement of the class builds confidence, so instructors know that when the time comes for delivery of the lecture, the equipment can be used with no hitches. If microphones are available, the lecturer should test his or her voice against volume control, pitch, and clarity. The best advice: Be prepared in case the technology fails!

Debates

In the course of their work, EMS personnel encounter a variety of situations that differ from their own personal standards, beliefs, and social values. Another teaching strategy for large group settings is **debate**, or structured controversy. A *debate* is a structured contest of reason and logical arguments aimed at identifying truth. The session is bound by predetermined rules and can be used any time that the topic is open to opposing points of view. Debates are best used for higher-level cognitive thinking concepts. As a teaching strategy, the debate can foster critical-thinking skills and reveal complexities of health care issues. Often, in many of the sociologic situations that confront EMS providers, no definite right or wrong decision-making actions can be identified, as each case requires individual attention. Numerous factors may have an impact in compounding patient care decisions. Therefore, classroom debate on those issues encourages students to critically think about the consequences of their actions when they deal with patients in real-life situations. Debate can facilitate understanding of the points of view of others and can promote development of communication skills. The basic structure and format of a debate should be introduced far enough in advance that students can adequately prepare. Structure and techniques should not be the focus of the session, as relevant material may be lost in the process.[7]

The primary disadvantages of the debate approach are student anxiety and the need for adequate preparation time. Some students become anxious because of the public-speaking skills required and the confrontational nature of debate. Some students do well with this strategy. Debate generally requires that students engage in research.[7] Participants require clear guidelines about the topic that they are to debate, and these guidelines must reflect the learning objectives of the course. It is useful for students to meet with the instructor before the time of the event so that each team can incorporate key learning themes into the debate.

Debating teams require information to be used in developing and printing handouts for the student group, as well as other resource material that can be used within the debate presentation; they also do well when they use available AV technology to enhance their presentations.

Typically, a debate involves five to seven students: two to three to present the "pro" side, two to three to present the "con" side, and one who acts as a moderator.

Students must have knowledge of both sides of the issue if they are to argue intelligently. Generally, each side presents opening comments for a specified time, then each side presents its viewpoint, followed by a rebuttal from the other side. The debate ends with a summary from each side. Time limits are clearly defined, are equal for each side, and are strictly enforced by the moderator. At the conclusion of the debate, the class can vote for the best-presented argument.

CASE IN POINT

Some suggestions for debate—one side must argue "yes" and the other "no":

- Should paramedics be permitted to perform endotracheal intubation?
- Which model of EMS delivery is most effective?
- Should EMTs acquire and transmit 12-Lead ECGs?
- A paramedic's work is professional and the profession should work autonomously with minimal medical oversight.

Student Presentations

Collectively, students are incredibly creative. They usually enjoy the challenge of demonstrating their ingenuity. Student presentations offer an effective teaching method. In turn, and at allocated times, each student is required to present information to the group on a predetermined topic. This approach has advantages and disadvantages. The strength of this approach lies in the empowerment that it gives each student to research and learn about the theme to be presented. The weakness is that many students are distracted by concern for their own presentation and do not concentrate on material presented by other students. Establish clear rules related to civility and appropriateness of information. Develop an evaluation rubric so students know grading criteria clearly in advance. New instructors may need to liaise with the program director to determine the logistics involved with having a large number of students make individual presentations in a timely and effective manner.

CASE IN POINT

At some time before the event, a group of four or five students can be asked to collaborate in developing a short presentation that demonstrates a concept that complements the lecture topic. Three examples are given here:

1. Discuss methods to effectively communicate with hearing-impaired patients.
2. Discuss a chronic neurologic disease such as multiple sclerosis, and explain its prehospital care implications.
3. Illustrate polarization and repolarization of the cardiac conduction system.

Although each of these presentations need take only a few minutes, it is wise for the instructor to allow more time for the audience to reflect on the learning point and to regain composure before the instructor proceeds with the lesson. It is helpful to give the students in the audience an assignment before the presentation, such as "Identify the three most important things you learned from this presentation" to keep them focused on the message, rather than the presentation method. The instructor must listen carefully to correct any misstatements and to fill in essential content the presenters may have missed.

Summary

Teaching to large groups is an effective method of instruction when attention is given to the finer points of development, delivery, and management of the event. Mastery of the skill of lecturing takes considerable time and effort; with collegiate assistance, encouragement, and practice, the task becomes easier.

Effective teaching to large groups requires the attention of the instructor in learning how the lecture fits with the overall course curriculum. Armed with this knowledge, the instructor takes the next step: identifying the process for planning and preparing the lecture. The method by which the lecture is delivered and the resource accessories used are integral for the success of instruction.

When instructors are assigned to teach a large group, they should accept the task with enthusiasm because it provides an additional dimension of learning experience relevant to professional self-development, as well as an opportunity to impart knowledge to students.

Glossary

case study An analysis of a real-life patient situation as a way of illustrating information.

debate Structured controversy.

lecture A teaching session in which the instructor is the principal teacher.

pitch of lecture delivery The lecture language is commensurate to the students' level of learning.

References

1. Nasmith, L., & Steinert, Y. (2001). Evaluation of a workshop to promote interactive lecturing. *Teaching and Learning in Medicine, 13,* 43–48.
2. Cox, K., & Ewan, C. (Eds.) (1988). *The medical teacher* (2nd ed.). Edinburgh, UK: Churchill Livingstone.
3. Laidlow, J. M., & Hesketh, E. A. (1995). Developing the teaching instinct. *Medical Teacher, 24,* 364–367.
4. Newble, D., & Cannon, R. (1995). *A handbook for teachers in universities and colleges* (3rd ed.). London, UK: Kogan Page. 378.
5. Gage, N., & Berliner, D. (Eds.) (1991). *Educational psychology* (5th ed.). New York, NY: Houghton Mifflin.
6. Saroyan, A., & Snell, L. (1997). Variations in lecturing styles. *Higher Education, 33,* 85–110.
7. Rowles, C. J., & Brigham, C. (1998). Strategies to promote critical thinking and active learning. In D. M. Billings, & J. A. Halstead (Eds.) (1998). *Teaching in nursing: A guide for faculty*. Philadelphia, PA: W. B. Saunders.
8. Cooper, L., Lawson, M., & Orrell, J. (1997). *Raising issues about teaching: Views of academic staff at Flinders University*. Adelaide, Australia: Flinders Press.
9. Brookfield, S. D. (2006). *The skillful teacher: On technique, trust, and responsiveness in the classroom* (2nd ed.). San Francisco, CA: Jossey-Bass.
10. Pike, R. W. (1995). *High-impact presentations*. West Des Moines, IA: American Media.
11. Zwirn, E. E. (1998). Media, multimedia, and computer-mediated learning. In D. M. Billings, & J. A. Halstead (Eds.) (1998). *Teaching in nursing: A guide for faculty*. Philadelphia, PA: W. B. Saunders.
12. Henschke, J. A. (1975, February). How to use the lecture as a learning/teaching technique with adults. *Baptist Leader.*
13. McKeachie, W. J., Pintrich, P. R., Lin, Y., Smith, D. A. F., & Sharma, R. A. (1994). From teaching and learning in the college classroom: A review of the literature. In K. A. Feldman, & M. B. Paulsen (Eds.) (1994). *Teaching and learning in the college classroom.* Needham, MA: Ginn Press. 75–114.
14. Seeler , D. C., Turnwald, G. H., & Bull, K. S. (1994). From teaching to learning. Part III: Lectures and approaches to active learning. *Journal of Veterinary Medical Education, 21.*
15. McCurry, M. K., & Hunter, S. (2011). Evaluating the effectiveness of personal response system technology on millennial student learning. *Journal of Nursing Education, 50*(8), 471–475.

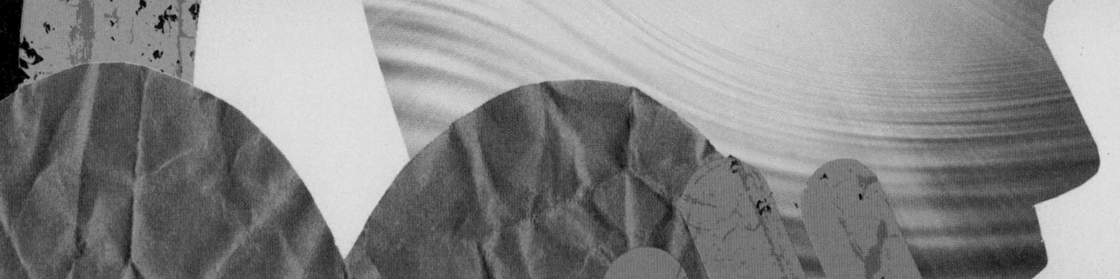

16

Using Technology to Enhance Classroom Learning

Any sufficiently advanced technology is indistinguishable from magic. — ARTHUR C. CLARKE

People interact with their environment through the five senses. The more the senses are stimulated, the stronger is the interaction. Likewise, the more senses are stimulated at one time, the more intense is the interaction. Because learning is a process by which a change in behavior is brought about through experience, one could conclude that the more senses are stimulated during the learning experience, the better the educational experience will be. One of the most common means of stimulating the senses while teaching is to use audio and visual aids, more commonly known simply as "AV." The acronym AV has come to include almost any tools or techniques used to supplement learning, other than a straight lecture presentation. The instructional technology in the AV "toolbox" continues to expand, offering both challenges and opportunities to instructors.

This chapter outlines basic principles of instructional technology. It is not designed to make the educator a technological whiz or graphic designer, but regular practice and student feedback can help growth as an educator who effectively uses instructional technologies when they are appropriate to enhance learning.

CHAPTER GOAL: This chapter familiarizes the educator with effective use of various common instructional technologies.

Teaching Tip >> *When it comes to using instructional technology and creating AV materials, the instructor should know his or her personal limitations. The primary purpose of a class is for learners to master the objectives of the lesson, so do not become distracted by instructional technology or by the creative urge to produce an AV masterpiece. If you are unfamiliar or uncomfortable with teaching technologies, take advantage of learning opportunities that might be available from your school's professional development department or within your local community. You can also find many tutorials online for the instructional technologies discussed in this chapter.*

What is Instructional Technology?

Instructional technology is the software and hardware used to create and transmit audiovisual materials. For example, an electronic slide presentation is created and delivered with a software program, like PowerPoint® or Keynote®, and delivered using a desktop, **tablet** device or laptop personal computer, and a **digital projector**. Educators have an increasing array of instructional technology available to them. As well, student's expectations of how instructional technology is used in the classroom has changed and will continue to evolve.

Many of the instructional technology mainstays of EMS educators 10 to 15 years ago such as 35 mm slide projectors, overhead projectors, VCRs, and blackboards are increasingly being relegated to a storage room. Likewise, some of the instructional technology discussed in this chapter will be out-of-date and irrelevant long before other timeless topics in this textbook.

Instructional technology, just like medicine, is dynamic. Instructors should keep an open mind about adoption and use of new instructional technologies. Giving up the old and familiar to learn new software and hardware technologies is one way to continue to develop as an educator.

Turn on The Tech: Pedagogical Perspective on The Tech-Savvy Student

by Z. Heather Yazdanipour

In the 1960s, two psychology professors at Stanford University, Patrick Suppes and Richard Atkinson, experimented with computers to teach math and reading to elementary students in Paolo Alto, CA. Then in 1970 Bernard Luskin, a UCLA professor, advanced computer-assisted instruction and began to connect media and psychology into what is now the field of media psychology. He has been deemed a media visionary and the father of Computer Supported Collaborative Learning (CSCL). Since those early applications, we have made strides in the E-Learning movement. Today we find ourselves in the next generation of CSCL, E-Learning 2.0.[a,b]

E-Learning 2.0 accepts that knowledge is socially constructed; that learning takes place through conversation and is grounded in collaboration during real-life scenarios. It utilizes the Vygotsky approach of learning via the Zone of Proximal Development.[c,d] Basically, this concept defines the distance between what the student knows independently and what the student has the potential to know through guidance or teamwork with more capable peers. In order for E-Learning 2.0 to be successful, it requires an active and involved educator to provide the student the tools needed for development.

Let us take a look at some tools and strategies of E-Learning 2.0 a little closer.

- *Asynchronous versus Synchronous*: Decide which aspect fits best for each situation.
  - Asynchronous: Participants engage in the exchange of ideas or information without the dependency of others being involved at the same time. It gives students the ability to work at their own pace, in a low-stress environment.
    - E-mail, blogs, wikis, discussion boards, podcasting
  - Synchronous: Involves the exchange of ideas and information with one or more participants during the same period of time.
    - Skype™, Facetime®, chat rooms, virtual classrooms, webinars
- *Blogging*: A quality tool that is no longer limited to the individual doing the journaling.
  - Journal format encourages students to keep record of their thinking over time, facilitates critical feedback by letting readers add comments. Students can provide a personal space online, pose questions, publish works in progress, and link to and comment on other Web sources.
- *Podcasting*: Student-produced is the way to go when it comes to education-based podcasting.
  - Provides a way of publishing educational content to learners. Apple® has been quick to recognize the learning potential of student podcasting. Their podcasting section of iTunes® even has a category dedicated to education.
- *Media Sharing*: Most popular platform in E-Learning because they are user-friendly and highly accessible via mobile devices such as cell phones, personal digital assistants (PDAs), computers, and home gaming consoles.
  - Sites like Flickr® and YouTube™ allow for publishing of pictures and videos of a topic, then allows for annotation and discussion. With Flickr, students can post digital photographs and fellow students can then view the picture and post critical feedback by adding "Hot-Spot" annotations to the image. With YouTube, students can produce a short video on a chosen subject, where it can then be viewed and commented on by classmates and the wider YouTube community.
- *Social Networks*: Although this is a sore spot with some educators (Facebook and Myspace), social networking has become an integral component in implementing E-Learning 2.0.
  - In its simplest form, a social network is a map of specific connections, such as common interests or studies, between the actual individuals or organizations being studied. The commonalities to which an individual is thus connected are the social contacts. It is through these contacts that learning is adopted.
  - It is believed that one of the best ways to learn something is to teach it to others, and social networks truly encompass this mindset. They have been used to foster online communities around extremely diverse subjects like national certification testing.

Although most might think that social networks are not secure, there are many "smart" networks available that allow controlled access to be placed around each individual item posted. There are software companies currently producing social networks especially designed for education,

continues

continued

built from the ground up to support learning. With these software developments, each user receives a personal weblog, file repository (which is podcast compatible), an online profile, and an RSS (really simple syndication) reader (used to publish frequently updated works). In addition, all users' contents can be tagged with keywords, so they can connect with other users with similar interests and create their own personal learning network.

In this age of computer-savvy students, when we educators find ourselves uncomfortable with advancing technology, we should not stand idly by and watch our students, nor should we hinder their progress. Let us not limit E-Learning to just be defined as "electronic"; rather, interpret the "E" in E-Learning as engaging, exciting, energetic, excellent, and emotional. Learning can be and is all of those things and more!

The utilization of technology to connect students rather than separate them is a must. A constructivist teacher creates a context for learning in which students can become engaged in interesting activities, guides them as they approach problems, encourages group efforts, and supports them with encouragement and advice when tackling challenges rooted in real-life situations. This facilitates cognitive growth and learning for both student and teacher.

[a] Harasim, L., Hiltz, S., Teles, L., & Turoff, M. (1995). Learning networks: A field guide to teaching and learning online. Cambridge, MA: MIT Press.
[b] Stahl, G., Koschmann, T., & Suthers, D. (2006). Computer-supported collaborative learning: An historical perspective.
[c] Vygotsky, L. S. (1978). Mind in society: Development of higher psychological processes. Cambridge, MA: Harvard University Press.
[d] Chaiklin, S. (2003). The zone of proximal development in Vygotsky's analysis of learning and instruction. In A. Kozulin, B. Gindis, V. Ageyev, & S. Miller (Eds.), *Vygotky's educational theory and practice in cultural context*. Cambridge, MA: Cambridge University Press.

What is Audiovisual?

Audiovisual (AV) materials are created and distributed using instructional technology. AV is educational instruction provided by means of supplementary teaching aids, such as presentation slides, audio and video recordings, **screencasts**, simulators, and models, to stimulate at least the senses of sight and hearing.[1] AV is also commonly referred to as "multi-media."

The primary use of AV is to enhance students' understanding of the material by supporting and complementing what the educator is saying, explaining, or discussing, thus stimulating the senses and adding to the educator's credibility.[2] AV also facilitates student learning by adding variety to break up the standard lecture; this helps to capture, retain, or regain students' attention.

The most important thing for the educator to remember when planning and using instructional technologies is that the AV material and equipment should supplement—not replace—the learning experience. Occasionally, a presentation may be made up extensively of a high-tech multi-media, which may create the "wow factor!" However, after the "wow factor" wears off, the basic material presented may also fade. To repeat, instructional technologies should supplement and improve the educational process. An instructor should make sure that use of instructional technology does not steal the show by evaluating how the presentation would be received if he or she could not use the instructional technology portion.

Using Audiovisual Materials

Here are a few basic guidelines for evaluating, planning, and using AV materials. Generally speaking, AV should summarize information, illustrate, reinforce, and draw attention to the main points. AV should not consist simply of projected copies of the printed text, and it should not be merely read to students. Moreover, handouts made from presentation slides should not be used as handouts.[3] Instead, create handouts that reinforce key points from the presentation, direct students to additional resources, ask questions to facilitate group discussion, and help students prepare to apply what they have learned to hands-on experiences.

Regardless of the medium, educators should follow these guidelines for effective use of instructional technology:

- It must support achievement of a learning objective.
- It must provide a neutral or positive learning experience for the student.
- It must fit within the allotted time.
- It must be visible, audible, or otherwise accessible to all students.
- It must be cost-effective.
- It must be used legally. That is, there should be no copyright violations; model permissions should be obtained when needed and there is no violation of patient privacy when patient-related materials,

such as ECGs are used (see Chapter 10: Legal Issues for the Educator).

It is important for the educator who is using a complete teaching package (i.e., lesson plans, textbook, AV, handouts, etc.) to review not only the didactic material itself, but also the AV designed for the material. The educator should consider the following when evaluating an educational teaching package, such as those provided by textbook publishers:

- Does the instructor know how to use the AV media provided?
- Is necessary instructional technology available at the teaching site?
- Can the instructor present the lesson as planned without using the instructional technology provided or in a different format?
- Will the course sponsor or administrator allow the instructor to change, alter, or customize the AV material by adding additional presentation slides, skipping sections not relevant to their students, or inserting their own images? Or, must he or she use the AV material "as is"?
- Can the instructor alter the AV material to suit the needs of his or her students or local requirements?
- Is the AV material of good quality? Does it follow basic AV guidelines? (Commercial preparation does not ensure quality.)
- Is the AV material consistent across lessons and units? This consistency is important if a course is to be taught in modules or by multiple instructors.

Teaching Tip >> *The quality of AV material should be judged by its effectiveness to help the instructor meet educational objectives. Students in the same classroom can have widely differing opinions about the quality of AV based on their previous knowledge of the topic. The instructor's overall ability to teach the material will also shape student's opinions of quality. When developing AV material or judging the quality of AV materials packaged with a text book, remember that quality is in large part determined by the vision for the final product and the time and money available to attain that vision.*

The educator should keep in mind a few basic rules for the use of AV materials and technology:

- Know how to use the instructional technology hardware and software.
- Know what to do if a piece of equipment fails during a class; find out where spare parts, such as bulbs, are located and learn how to change them.
- Arrive early enough to ensure that AV materials and instructional technology are in the classroom and ready to use. Do not forget to bring an extension cord or power strip just in case.
- Find out whether the classroom is arranged for the correct use of the instructional technology. Ascertain whether all students will be able to see and hear the AV materials.
- If using a piece of instructional technology later in the class, such as a model or a manikin, cover or hide the equipment so that it is not a distraction for students.
- Make sure whiteboards are clean and clear of writing from previous lessons.
- Have an alternative plan. All technology has the potential to fail, so have a backup plan in the event the material or equipment cannot be used as planned.
- Plan the lesson accordingly, so as not to waste time setting up or operating equipment.

Teaching Tip >> *If the educational program does not have its own instructional technology hardware, like digital projectors, the instructor should reserve it from the institution well in advance. If support is provided from a central service, the needed equipment must be reserved in sufficient time to ensure its availability. Also, just because a piece of instructional technology hardware is "always in the classroom or store room" does not mean it will automatically be there when needed. This is especially true at locations that share resources or for off-site courses. The Saturday that an EMS instructor plans to use the department's digital projector for Advanced Life Support class may be the same Saturday that the Fire instructor plans to use the projector for an extrication class.*

Hardware

AV materials are delivered with instructional technology hardware. Much of the hardware currently available delivers images, video, and audio either separately or together. A digital projector can display static images or animations within presentation slides, full-motion video with or without audio, and

CASE IN POINT

One of the most common problems encountered by educators is connecting their computer to the digital projector commonly expressed as "this is working on my screen but I can't project this image, video, or animation on the big screen." Now what should the instructor do? The teaching plan has suddenly been altered. The instructor might be lucky enough to have an AV assistant quickly available to troubleshoot, but what can the instructor do to salvage his or her presentation? Here are a few suggestions:

- Cancel the class, but this is rarely a viable option and creates inconvenience for both students and instructors. Instructors should prepare to present with or without audiovisual aids.
- Check the connections between your computer and the digital projector. Is a separate audio input required?
- Know how to toggle the screen displays. How to do this varies depending on your computer and operating system.
- The projector resolution may not match the media output resolution. Projecting a video clip may simply not be possible.
- Test the capability of the projector to display the AV material before students arrive. If it is not going to work, simply use the presentation software's ability to "hide" the slide and the students will never know they have missed something.
- Switch to another means of presentation.
- Skip the projected slides altogether and have the students refer to handout material related to the slides.
- Use a whiteboard to present key points, formulas, basic graphics, and so forth. Remember that scores of students were successfully taught this way for years before computers and projectors entered the classroom.
- If an instructor was planning to project a video clip or a video, he or she could have the students break into small groups and write a descriptive script of what should be in such a video. This will force them to think of key points and procedures that would have been emphasized in the video.
- Teach another lesson that does not require the digital projector, or change the class to a skills practice and review session.

If sound is an essential element to the presentation, be sure to have external speakers available. Do not rely on the sound from laptop speakers to project throughout a classroom.

Another common instructional technology failure is not having a power source within easy reach of the digital projector and the instructor's computer. Anticipate this problem and, when you can, travel with a power strip and extension cord. It is also helpful to have presentation remote control that allows you to advance presentation slides at a distance from your computer. Remember that instructional technology is the educator's helper—not the educator's replacement! The instructor must be creative and must think simply to find a solution.

output audio through a built-in speaker or to an amplified audio system.

With the availability of personal computers and digital projectors, the selection of instructional technology hardware is less of a concern for today's EMS instructor than the preparation or selection of AV materials and the actual operation of the instructional technology. Over time, most hardware products have "plug and play" capability, meaning the computer recognizes that it is connected to a digital projector and that you will want to display presentation slides with the digital projector.

Audio

Audio AV materials can be delivered to individuals and groups using a variety of devices, including a videocassette recorder (VCR), DVD player, desktop or laptop personal computer, smartphone, or MP3 electronic audio player. Audio output capability is built into low- and high-fidelity patient simulators.

It is important that the volume be loud enough so that everyone can easily hear. If the device cannot produce enough volume, it must be connected to an amplifier and a sound system. Most DVD players, simulator manikins, **smartphones, MP3 players,** and computers have an "audio output" or headphone jack. An audio output cable is connected from this to the amplifier audio input so that volume can be boosted and distributed throughout the classroom **(Figure 16.1)**.

When an instructor uses any form of instructional technology, he or she should consider moving students so they can hear and see properly. If an instructor has an audio device that is not loud enough to be heard throughout the classroom, students should

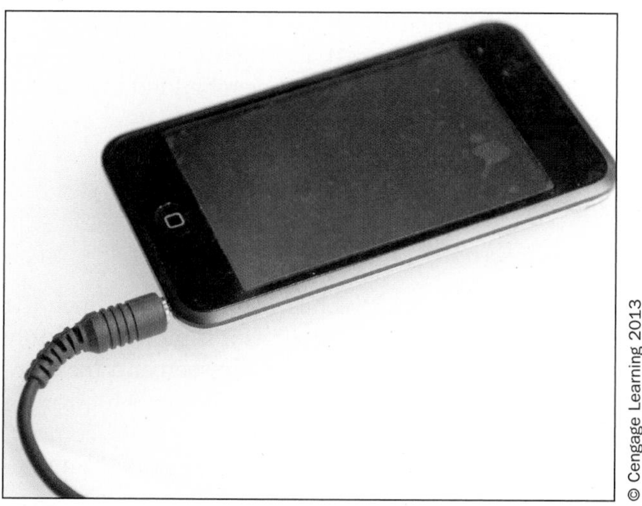

Figure 16.1

Audio devices can be independently connected to the classroom's AV system.

move closer so they can hear. Likewise, handheld audio devices could be passed around the group, or students could individually or in small groups go to audio-listening stations. For example, a breath sound simulator could be a station in the class lab.

Repetition may be necessary for a short audio clip to be effective. A sound recording, such as breath sounds, must be played multiple times to ensure that students not only hear the sound, but understand it. The same applies to video clips. If the class is conducted in a large room such as an auditorium, it may be necessary for the instructor to play the sound multiple times at various locations around the auditorium.

> **Teaching Tip** >> *You can archive audio files, such as breath sounds and heart tones, on the class website, learning management system, or intranet, for students to listen to and review on their own. Similarly you may be able to link students to online archives of breath sounds or have them search, find, and share breath-sound repositories with their classmates.*

Microphones

An important first step for the instructor who is planning a presentation to a large group or in a large presentation space is to determine the number and type of microphones needed. Microphones come in a variety of configurations. Those commonly found in the classroom include a wireless microphone (lectern). This provides clear sound, involves low maintenance, and frees the educator's hands. A wireless hand microphone is sometimes found in areas in which running wires to the podium location would be difficult. This type of microphone allows the educator to move around freely, but it ties up his or her hands. Thus, many educators prefer the wireless lavaliere or lapel microphone. This wireless microphone allows the educator to move within the audience, and to keep his or her hands free to demonstrate skills.

> **Teaching Tip** >> *The instructor must be sure to turn off a wireless microphone after the class session. No one wants to broadcast throughout the classroom private conversations or sounds associated with a trip to the restroom.*

An instructor teaching online or participating in an online Web or video conference also needs a microphone. Many laptop computers include a built-in microphone, but using the built-in microphone can lead to an audio echo or transmitting extraneous ambient noise like the fan inside the laptop computer. Instead of relying on a built-in microphone, purchase a headset and microphone that plugs into one of the laptop's USB ports. An in-line control for muting your microphone and adjusting the audio volume are useful features.

> **Teaching Tip** >> *Learn to place a microphone properly. Place a lavaliere microphone above your nipple line but not so high that it moves when your neck and head move. Also make sure to clip a lavaliere to a stable piece of clothing rather than a necktie that is likely to move as you move. Avoid adjusting your coat or shirt as you speak, as the movement of the clothing will be transmitted by the microphone.*

If more than one audio device is used, an **audio mixer** must be set up. The mixer allows multiple devices to be connected to a single amplifier and set of speakers, thus causing the sound to be "mixed" to a comfortable level. The AV staff usually sets up the mixer and sound amplifier in a classroom, with the educator merely turning the entire system on or off.

> **Teaching Tip** >> *Because of the costs and desirability of microphones and related equipment, most institutions secure these devices in a locked area. The educator should plan to obtain a key or lock combination in advance.*

Cassette Tape Player

If your educational program still relies on cassette tapes for delivering audio AV materials, such as lung and heart sounds, consider alternative media formats, or inquire about the possibility of digitizing audio recordings that are still relevant and effective. Converting audio recordings to .mp3, .wav, or another audio-file format provides more flexibility for storing and delivering audio files to students, as well as incorporating audio recordings into presentation slides.

Digital Voice Recorder

A digital voice recorder is a small, handheld device used to record and play back audio. Do not be surprised if a student, especially an auditory learner, asks if he or she can record the lecture, and then places a digital voice recorder or smartphone with audio-recording capability on the lectern. Instructors may also find a digital voice recorder useful for creating a podcast of their lectures, recording student team performance in the simulation lab, or answering student questions and then posting the audio file on the class website.

Audio Recordings

Audio recordings of dispatch calls, case reviews, and patient assessments can be valuable tools. Audio can easily be recorded on a variety of hardware devices and edited with low cost or free software programs. Smartphones, commonly used by instructors and students, usually have a simple method for recording and playing back audio files. Learn how to transfer these audio files for use in other instructional technologies and incorporation in AV materials. Audio files can be played back over and over again, enhancing the learning process. An audio file can be cued up to ensure that key points are not missed. Students who are auditory learners versus visual learners will find audio files a useful way to prepare for exams. For instance, when a student is learning about different heart sounds, what better way than to hear them? A word of caution when playing audio files to a large group: play short clips measured in seconds or a couple of minutes at most. Instead of playing one long file, pause or break up the file to engage the class with discussion about what they have heard, or what actions they would take next with the information available.

MP3 Players

MP3 players are widely available as stand-alone devices or are built into other devices, like an iPhone or Blackberry. Use available instructional technology to create and distribute .mp3 files to students. One common use is to record and distribute lectures as a podcast. Sound files can also be embedded in a digital presentation.

Visual Aids

Chalkboard (Blackboard)

This less "hi-tech" tool has been a staple since the late 1800s. The chalkboard, or as it is more commonly known, the "blackboard," is easily seen and inexpensive, but it is not usually portable. It serves to provide a large writing surface for listing key points, comparing and contrasting information, and highlighting important points.[4]

Whiteboard (Dry-Erase Board)

The whiteboard is a newer version of the chalkboard, and it has been an integral part of education for years. The whiteboard, as well as the chalkboard, allows the educator to convey spontaneous thoughts, to clarify spelling, and to illustrate ideas.[5]

Whiteboards are most effective when material is written on the board before students arrive, or for quick drawings or explanations designed to enhance classroom discussion. The material once written can be saved for only short periods and cannot be retrieved once the board has been erased. When using this medium, the instructor is required to turn away from the audience—another downside. Educators may prefer to have the information prewritten on the board, or they may investigate another medium altogether.

Teaching Tip >> *A presentation board should always be erased entirely. Erasing a small spot in the middle of some old material to write something new does not take the learner into consideration. When finished with a lesson, the instructor should always erase the whiteboard entirely. Leaving marker ink on the board for a long time makes it more difficult to remove later. It is also good form to leave a clean board for the next instructor. Whiteboards should be cleaned regularly with a special cleaner that protects the surface and makes erasure easier.*

Whiteboards come in all sizes. A large whiteboard fixed to the classroom wall is most common. Some instructors also like to have a small whiteboard that they can easily carry and use when the class is engaged in small group activities, like patient assessment scenarios, or, away from their primary classroom and desks, like practicing splinting and immobilizations skills. A portable whiteboard, sometimes as small as 12″ × 12″, gives the instructor a surface to quickly illustrate important concepts or write key points without returning to the classroom.

Interactive Whiteboard

This modern version of the whiteboard and blackboard provides a multipage, multiuser drawing application. The instructor can display presentation slides, websites, and videos as well as draw designs or charts on the interactive whiteboard. The content, drawings and images, can be saved on a computer for future use. [6]

Some **interactive whiteboards** include touch and gesture technology. Students, just using their fingers, can click and drag objects, write on the board, and interact with the content on the board. If the classroom has an interactive whiteboard, make sure to request training to understand its use and maximize its features to help achieve lesson objectives.

Teaching Tip >> *Give students opportunities to photograph the whiteboard or presentation slides with their smartphones. Many students may find it quicker and more effective to have a digital photo rather than attempt to transpose what was on the board or screen to their notebooks.*

Flip Chart/Posterboard

The flip chart is a low-tech, inexpensive, and easily transportable visual aid. Flip charts can be personalized for a particular situation and prepared in advance. They are great for small meetings, allow for spontaneous thoughts, and provide a way to retain information. Flip charts can help facilitate student–educator communication and can reinforce important points. Using flip-chart paper that has a self-adhesive backing allows the instructor to easily hang the pages on the wall for quick review of key points. This tool offers a valuable alternative to the chalkboard or dry-erase board.[6]

Teaching Tip >> *The instructor must be sure to get approval before taping flip-chart pages onto walls or other surfaces. Also, tape that does not damage the finish should be used. IMPORTANT: An instructor should not write on paper that is placed against a wall or other surface. The marker ink may bleed through.*

Models and Manikins

Not often thought of as instructional technology, static displays and interactive devices such as manikins are an important adjunct to EMS education. The instructor who uses models and manikins should follow some simple guidelines:

- A device or adjunct to be used for teaching must be prepared in advance. This ensures that the device is complete and working well and minimizes loss of class time for preparation.
- The device must be placed in the classroom in such a way that it is not distracting to the students before they are ready to use it. This is especially relevant for new or complicated devices that students may not have seen before. Students should be concentrating on the lesson—not trying to figure out or study a device they have not seen before. Something as simple as throwing a sheet over a manikin or anatomic model before use is effective.
- The instructor must be sure that the model or manikin is correct and is similar to the actual object or patient under discussion. For example, an adult manikin should not be used for demonstration of pediatric interventions.
- The model should be large enough that all students can see all parts of its operation.
- The model should enhance the educational message—not distract from it.
- After the model or manikin has been used, it should be moved aside so it does not become a distraction to students.

Instructors typically think of a model as a fixed object in the classroom to explore anatomical relationships or functions. With a bit of exploration, or even as a student assignment, instructors can access thousands of videos and interactive activities online that show anatomical relationships and physiological functions. Often times these videos can be linked to or even embedded in a class website or intranet.

Teaching Tip >> *When a device that has multiple parts or that requires assembly and preparation is part of the procedure to be presented to the class, the use of a checklist will ensure that the device is ready for use in the classroom.*

Models may be anatomic in nature **(Figure 16.2)**, such as torso sets, individual organs, and cut-away views, or they may be enlarged versions of devices used in the field, such as syringes or laryngoscopes.

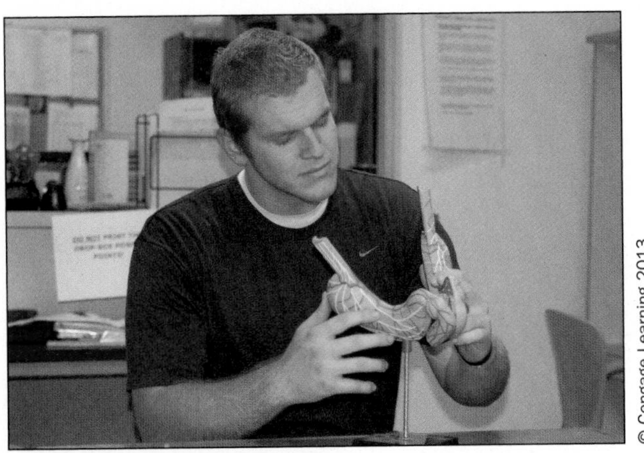

Figure 16.2
Models can be a useful instruction adjuct for helping students to see as well as feel.

Models can also be actual equipment used in demonstrations. To be effective, a model should be easy to set up, easy to use, and easy to maintain.

Human manikins, either whole body forms or anatomic sections, are a useful tool in the classroom. Because many EMS skills cannot be demonstrated or practiced on a live "patient," manikins provide a high degree of fidelity to the real thing. They also allow the instructor to alter responses from the manikin in accordance with student interventions.

Many interactive manikins are available on the market. Prices range from $200 for a simple unit to $50,000 or higher for the more complex ones. The instructor might consider that the simpler the design of a manikin is, the easier it will be to care for and maintain. A manikin should be suited to the skills the student has been trained to acquire, and it should be durably constructed **(Figure 16.3)**.

Teaching Tip >> *Classified ad websites and online auction sites are useful destinations for purchasing gently used models and manikins that may have been retired by other EMS and allied health educational programs. When purchasing used equipment online, make sure to look at pictures of the equipment to judge its condition, ask the seller about the functionality of the equipment, and if available, the seller's reliability ratings. It is probably best to purchase directly from another educator rather than a reseller who knows little about the equipment and the needs of an EMS instruction program. As always, remember: buyer beware, and be cautious about allocating your entire instructional technology budget to a deal that is too good to be true.*

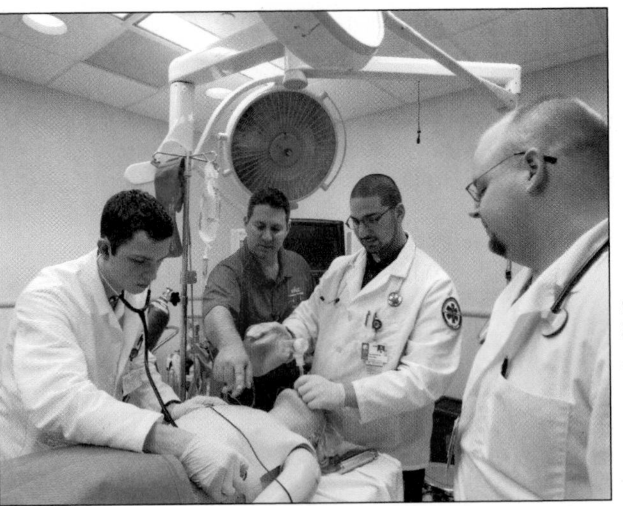

Figure 16.3
Simulation manikins can assist students in "putting it all together" and developing critical-thinking skills.

Projectors

Several types of projectors are in use in today's classroom. Each has its own special place and use.

Overhead Projectors For most educators the overhead projector has been replaced by a fixed or portable digital projector. It is unlikely that transparencies created for the overhead projector are still accurate or relevant to today's EMT or paramedic student. Because of its limited ability to display only transparencies, an overhead projector is not as versatile as a digital projector. The overhead projector is an effective tool to project X-ray films. Many instructors have transitioned to newer technology such as the digital projector.

35 mm Slide Projectors The slide projector, much like an overhead projector, was a staple of EMS education in the past. Educators and clinicians are much more likely to capture new images with a digital camera than a film camera. Publishers have converted their slide collections into digital formats for inclusion in AV materials. If not already done, consider converting an existing slide collection to digital images.

Teaching Tip >> *Many publishers offer presentation slide sets to accompany their texts. These slides may become rapidly outdated. One solution to this dilemma is to pull outdated slides and replace them with slides that have been prepared with the use of presentation software.*

CASE IN POINT

An instructor is teaching an EMT continuing-education class at a local rescue squad. Resources are limited, and he has access only to a commercially prepared presentation slide set that was created to match the third edition of the course textbook. Unfortunately, he is using the current edition, which is the fifth edition. He knows from using the "old" presentation slides that numerous changes have been made to the information, and inconsistencies can be seen between the slides and the current text. What are his options?

- Do not use the presentation slides at all. This will mean that he has to just lecture, ask the publisher for new presentation slides, or prepare his own AV materials.
- Prepare his own AV materials. Creating presentation slides is time consuming, and can be difficult if he lacks experience and comfort with presentation software.
- Edit the presentation slides, and use only those that are still appropriate. Treatments and protocols change, but not so drastically that all of the presentation slides will be useless. Use the "Hide Slide" setting to prevent displaying unnecessary slides to students.
- Look for alternative AV materials from such sources as the state EMS office or on the Web at the NAEMSE *Trading Post*. Contact other instructors to see if they have material that can be borrowed or copied.
- He should not, however, use the old presentation slide set "as is." The outdated material will only confuse students, and if he does not point it out and discuss it, this will reduce his credibility. He should refrain from making excuses for not having current AV materials.

Digital Projectors Both liquid crystal display (LCD) and digital light processing (DLP) projectors are suitable for the classroom. Both project computer presentation software and graphic images through a laptop or desktop computer. Select a digital projector based on your instructional needs. The type of projector you select and the features bundled with the projector will depend on many factors such as:

- Will the **digital projector** be permanently mounted in a classroom, travel between classrooms within the same building on an AV cart, or be packed in a carrying case to be taken to classrooms in other buildings and even other communities?
- How large is the presentation space? An auditorium will require a different digital projector than a classroom for 20 people.
- What is the budget for purchasing a digital projector? Prices of projectors can vary considerably from a few hundred dollars to thousands of dollars. Make sure to factor in lifetime costs such as new bulbs.

When purchasing a digital projector, it is important to understand the difference between brightness and resolution. A projector with more lumens, or brightness, will be able to project a clearer picture in a room with more ambient light than a projector with low brightness. Resolution is the amount of detail the projector can capture and project **(Figure 16.4)**.

A

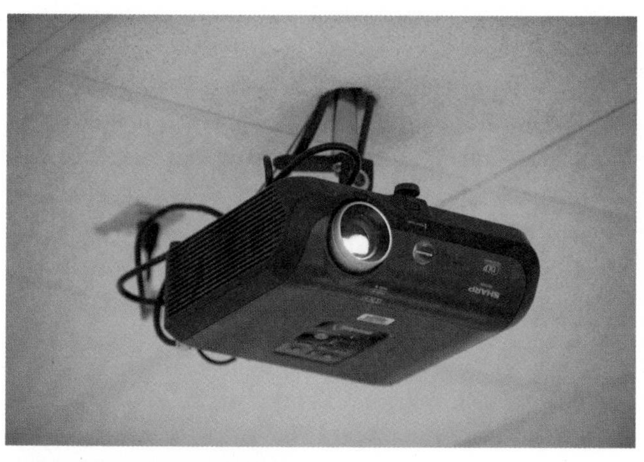

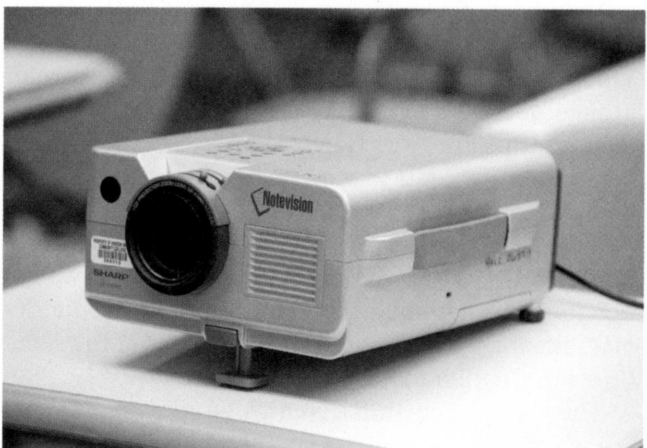

B

Figure 16.4

Digital projectors can be ceiling mounted (A), or portable (B).

Teaching Tip >> *Most digital projectors are compatible with current computer operating systems, including Windows and Macintosh. However, one should always test for compatibility and make sure to have the proper connecting cables. Additionally, digital projectors generate a large amount of heat. Laptop computers must not be placed on top of the projector housing; this might block airflow. The instructor should be sure to follow the manufacturer's recommendation for a cool-down period before turning off the projector.*

Projector Screens

Choosing the right projector screen for a presentation is as important as choosing the right projector. When deciding which screen to use, first determine the size of the room. This will help in deciding appropriate screen size, as will capacity, dimensions, and ceiling height of the room.[6] Once appropriate screen size has been determined, other considerations such as type, format, and material can be addressed. However, a technical discussion of these parameters is beyond the scope of this chapter and is best left to the AV professional.

Teaching Tip >> *In determining the screen size to use, divide the distance from the screen to the last row of the audience by 8, and use the resulting number as the height of the screen. For example, if the distance between the screen and the last row is 120 feet, 120 divided by 8 equals 15; therefore, the screen should be at least 15 feet high.*

Video Equipment

Video equipment can be divided into two broad groups: sources and display devices. A piece of equipment that produces a video signal is the source, and the equipment used to view the signal is the display device.[6]

In the past, the source, such as a 16 mm film projector or a VCR, was the limiting factor. The VCR was at one time the classroom standard as a multimedia device, allowing the student to see and hear at the same time information that is in full motion.

The digital versatile disk (DVD) player replaced the videotape. A DVD does not stretch over time, as a VHS tape does, so the picture remains clear even after the disk has been played many times. DVDs can also be played in computers with a DVD drive. As a large amount of material can be stored on a DVD, publishers can provide multiple scenarios and situations for a lesson. Many textbooks bundle an interactive DVD that the student can use on a personal computer.

There are more devices than ever that can be the video source. A DVD can be played in any device with a DVD player, but with the proliferation of Web-based videos, any device with an Internet connection can be both the video source and the display device. When selecting videos, EMS instructors should consider the availability of online instructional videos that will play back on desktop and laptop computers, tablet devices, and smartphones.

Another matter for consideration for videos is the delivery method. A 25-inch television is the smallest television that should be considered for use in the classroom. Televisions of smaller size would not be seen by students and do not show details clearly enough. A digital projector can also be used to show videos, thus providing a much larger image than is possible on a television. A digital projector may be cheaper than a large flatscreen television, and the size of the image is easily adjustable to the size of the classroom. With the proliferation of tablet computers and smartphones, students are watching more and more Web-based videos on small screens. Instead of playing a video on a large screen, you may choose to just link students to a Web video from the class website or intranet.

Finally, for any video, DVD or Web-based, it is imperative that the educator review the video before the class. You may want to watch the video with students to point out any potential problems. Remember that it is not necessary to show an entire video; select pertinent parts relevant to the learning objectives and show only those segments that do not contain offensive materials.

Embedding Audio and Video

An alternative to using video tapes and DVDs is to capture or create your own video clips. Students can be engaged in small group projects to create videos of assessment and treatment skills. Videos can be embedded into PowerPoint slides, uploaded to a class YouTube channel, or embedded in blog posts.

Cameras

The instructor's camera, whether a digital single lens reflex (SLR), point-and-shoot digital, or camera bundled in your smartphone or tablet device, can capture images to insert into classroom presentations, e-learning programs, or to upload to a class photo-sharing site. Most cameras are able to capture still images and video, and many devices are bundled with software for editing images and video.

A digital camera has a sensor that converts light into electrical charges.[7] The resolution of a camera (detail captured) is measured in pixels. The more pixels the camera has, the greater the details that can be captured. Some advantages of a digital camera include: pictures can be viewed immediately on the camera's LCD screen; pictures can be downloaded to a computer for printing, e-mailing, or posting on the Internet; and unwanted pictures can be easily deleted. Furthermore, digital cameras interface easily with printers to produce hard copy images that can be used for review or evaluation.

If the educator will be demonstrating a skill, he or she should consider using a camera that is hooked to a digital projector or television and can be displayed to the class. This is often easier than the "let's gather 'round the table'" approach used in many classrooms. In larger classes, some students will not be able to see the demonstration; in others, students will see it upside-down and backward. A document camera is a digital visual presenter that connects directly to a video or data projector. It allows real-time big screen and monitor viewing of print documents, 3D objects, photos, or slides. A document camera is essentially a digital overhead projector that can be used in the same way as a traditional overhead projector, which is great for a skills demonstration.[8] However, if the digital camera has a video out, the instructor can save the cost of a document camera by mounting the camera on a tripod, hooking the video-out cable to a television or digital projector, and showing the video. When using either the document camera or a digital camera, the educator can also focus the camera on a book or a sheet of paper and can project it to a television or onto a screen using a digital projector.

Teaching Tip >> *The instructor can ask a student to play the part of a reporter and to capture the images live and up-close with narration.*

Computer-Based Equipment

Although computer-based presentation techniques have been available for many years, the technologic enhancements associated with these methods to deliver education are growing rapidly. These new teaching tools, when used appropriately within a carefully developed lesson plan, can enhance students' learning by increasing their sensory involvement in the learning process.

Computer Presentations

The current presentation standard for the educator is the computer. It can provide a powerful and interesting way to present material. Computer presentations are an adjunct to learning.[4] The most common computer presentation is the slide show, which replaced overhead transparencies and 35 mm slides.[4] Computer presentations are usually shown on a large computer screen or television, or they may be projected onto a screen.[5] **(Figure 16.5)**.

A

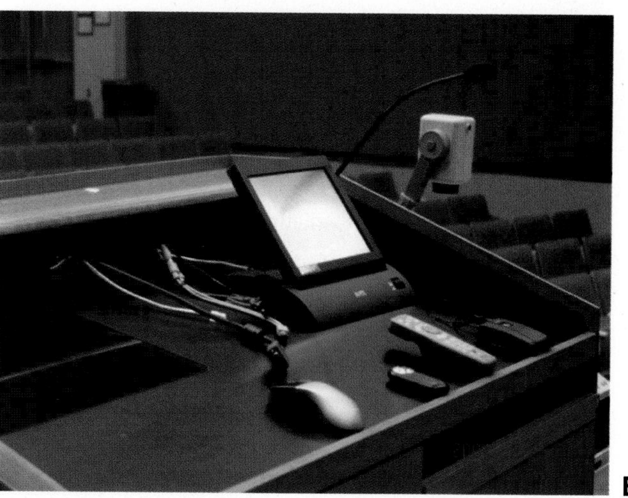

B

Figure 16.5

Presentation software can be delivered through a laptop and portable projector (A), or through a high-end built-in AV system (B).

Presentation software allows the educator to create a presentation with a professional look. He or she can easily include color, graphics, animation, sound, and video. Modifications or revisions can be made easily. The downside involves the cost of the computer and software and the technical problems that can plague the educator. Although this is a highly recommended format, it is always best to have another medium as a backup.

Teaching Tip >> *Knowledge and passion for a subject can usually communicate more effectively than a colorful, jazzed-up presentation of slides.*

Most publishers offer presentation slides as part of their online resource libraries. Slides can be purchased from a textbook vendor or downloaded from a website (such as the NAEMSE *Trading Post,* available at http://www.NAEMSE.org), or the educator can make his or her own slides. Each option has its advantages and disadvantages. When presentation slides are purchased from a vendor, they are usually generic and cover the basic points of a lesson. Frequently, material must be added to a lesson so it follows local practice. An Internet search on a particular topic usually yields a number of possibilities of free downloads. However, one must be careful to verify the information contained in the slides and to check that material has not been taken from copyrighted sources without permission.

Many educators develop their own presentation slides using templates to produce visually appealing slides. Medical graphics are also available as packages from vendors or via the Internet. However, the educator is cautioned to understand the legal restrictions involved in downloading and copying graphics and other files that contain copyrighted material.

Powerpoint® Presentation Tips

- Minimize words using key words only.
- Use no more than seven words per line and no more than seven lines per slide.
- Font size should be 22 points or larger.
- Use numerals instead of text when possible.
- Abbreviate freely.
- Use simple templates without background clutter.
- Consider using graphs instead of tables.
- Use art only when it helps to say something.
- Never use bad art, even if it is pertinent.
- Use animation only when it helps to make a point; otherwise, it is a distraction.
- Use sound only to support points, not to distract the audience.
- Use high-contrast colors—dark background colors with light text or light background with dark text.
- Use hyperlinks to navigate from one slide to another within the presentation (e.g., to move from slide 11 directly to slide 30) or to link to videos stored locally or on the Internet.

Teaching Tip >> *Although many available programs claim to convert presentations from other formats, some features or formatting may be lost in the conversion process.*

Teaching Tip >>

- *While in presentation mode in PowerPoint, you can type the number of the slide and press the enter key and thus jump from slide to slide in the presentation. For example, 1+5+"ENTER" will take you to slide 15.*
- *If you do a presentation and add charts, graphs, or pictures, number all of your slides in the lower bottom corner, then hide the charts, graphs, or pictures that you do not need for every audience. By doing that you may choose to show with selected groups. Make a note of the number and title of each hidden slide, and print the notes for reference at the podium. When you want to show a hidden slide, look at the notes, type in the number of the slide, and press the "enter" key to go to that slide. To continue from where you left off, type in the number of your previous or next slide.*

Internet

A high-speed connection to the Internet that is available in the classroom provides many opportunities for the educator and for students. The instructor can go to websites to show students information, or he or she can demonstrate the availability of additional information on a topic. Presentations can be used directly, without the need for downloading, especially when graphic- or animation-intensive, large files are used. In addition, sites from the major EMS publishers provide up-to-date information on emerging and important EMS-related issues, news, products, and resources. Many EMS websites, blogs, and podcasts offer outstanding educational programs, articles, and resources that can be used to compliment the materials you are presenting in the classroom.

In addition to being a resource, the Internet can be used as a tool for course administration. A class website or course in a learning management system can be established that contains course information, as well as the computer presentations used in class. The instructor can post additional materials, readings, practice exams, scenarios, and so forth, to the website to assist students in mastering course material.

Multipoint Communication (Telecommunications)

Three forms of telecommunication have become increasingly popular over recent years: teleconferencing, video conferencing, and Web conferencing. Teleconferencing uses telephones to link persons from around the world. The most common technique is conference calling.[4] Video conferencing uses satellites or cables, along with teleconferencing, which allows for greater interaction between students and instructors. The fastest-growing type of multipoint communication is Web conferencing. This enables two individuals or groups to communicate via the Internet through voice, video, data, or a combination of the three. One such program, Skype, allows an instructor from across the world to instruct a class using videoconferencing. Using this technology, a doctor, nurse, paramedic, or other-subject-matter expert can interact with a class in real time. Web conferencing is inexpensive, easy to implement, and both students and instructor can participate from the office, home, or classroom.[6]

Accessory Devices

Presentation Remote Control

Radio frequency or infrared presentation remote controls are available; these allow the instructor to move beyond the range of a typical hardwired mouse and to advance the presentation slides remotely. This option is useful when the instructor wants to move around the classroom, or when the computer must be set up away from the presenter.

> **Teaching Tip** >> *An instructor who is using a radio frequency remote device must make sure that it does not interfere with similar devices that may be in use in adjacent classrooms.*

Laser Pointer

A common piece of audiovisual accessory equipment is the **laser pointer**. This relatively inexpensive, small piece of equipment allows the instructor to visually highlight key points during a presentation, without blocking students' view of the material.[6] Some projector remote controls include a laser pointer, which allows the educator to hold only one device while teaching. Because the pointer uses a laser beam, the educator should use caution to avoid projecting the beam directly at any person, especially into the eyes. As with any instructional technology, overuse of the pointer can become more of a distraction than an aid to learning.

> **Teaching Tip** >> *If the educator is nervous or does not have a steady hand, he or she should use a circular motion when highlighting a word or phrase with the laser pointer. This minimizes the impression of shakiness.*

Audience Response Systems

Audience response systems (also called "classroom feedback," "personal response systems," or "clickers") allow the instructor to query students on various topics during a presentation without students seeing how the other students have responded and immediately give feedback.

One type of audience response system is a wireless key pad. Using software bundled with the key pads, the instructor integrates poll or quiz questions into a presentation. When the poll displays, the instructor can open voting. Results can be displayed as votes are cast or after polling has closed.

Polling the audience is a common feature of Web-conferencing systems. There are also online audience response systems that allow students to cast their vote by text message.

Audience response systems are commonly used as games to review information previously covered, but they can also be used during a presentation to assess the group's previous knowledge of the topic, retention of information as it is being taught, or to guide the instructor on how much depth to teach about the subject. They may also be used to gauge student thoughts related to tough questions about ethical issues. When each student responds anonymously, honest feedback is more likely **(Figure 16.6)**.

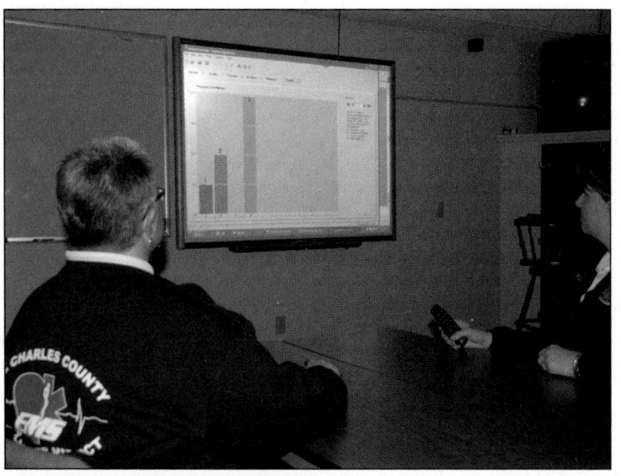

Courtesy of St. Charles County Ambulance District

Figure 16.6

Audience response systems engage learners and provide instant feedback.

Emerging Technology

Any discussion of emerging technology will likely be obsolete by the time you read this chapter. In 2009, tablet computers entered education, seemingly from out of nowhere. When Apple introduced the iPad® it immediately began to change the way we use computers and how we interact in the classroom. With an iPad in hand, the instructor can walk the classroom while presenting, surf the Web, send messages, and play multimedia files all wirelessly **(Figure 16.7)**.

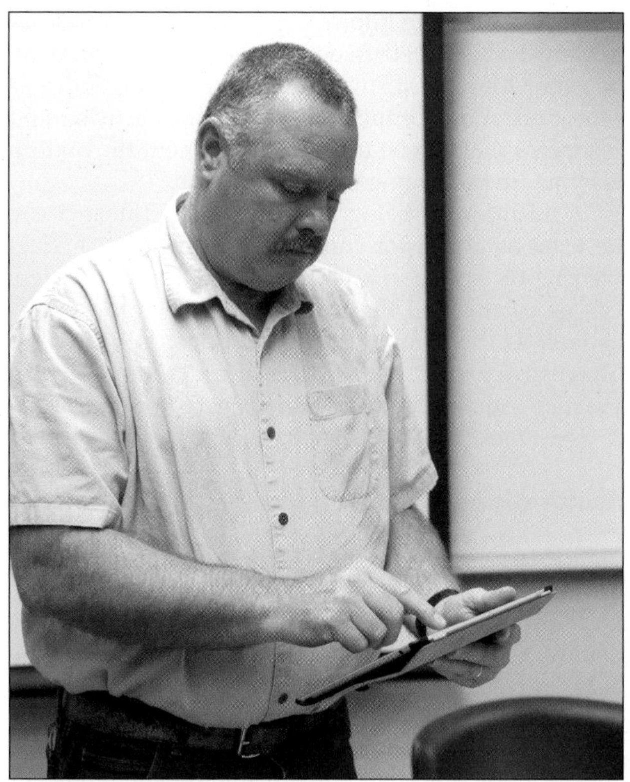

Figure 16.7

Instructors can control multimedia presentations from tablet devices.

There are now many other tablets running on several different operating systems. Some or all your students are probably reading their textbooks on tablets or e-readers, like the Amazon Kindle, or using e-reader apps installed on their smartphones or personal computers.

Smartphones and tablets have created a whole new category of software: the app. There are many apps already available for EMS students and instructors. There are apps to learn and practice 12-lead ECG interpretation, prepare for the National Registry exam, review drug dosages and calculations, look up reference information, and explore human anatomy.

Educational programs, built on immersive single- and multi-player gaming, are a potential emerging technology. Today's high fidelity simulators are actual objects we can physically touch and manipulate. In the future, EMS students may play patient assessment simulation games, provide treatments, and interact with instructors, all while immersed in a virtual environment.

By its very definition, emerging technology will be a regular visitor to the EMS classroom. Emerging technology for patient care monitoring, treatment, and documentation will challenge the instructor to both learn the technology and develop curricula to prepare students to use that technology in the workplace. Keeping an open mind and having a willingness to learn new things, while staying focused on learning objectives, will allow the instructor to cope with the pace of emerging technology and integrate it as appropriate into the EMS classroom.

Summary

The educator's mission is to change students' behavior in a positive way through exposure to meaningful learning experiences. These learning experiences involve stimulation of students' senses to enhance the intake and retention of knowledge, skills, and attitudes needed for mastery of the course objectives.

Instructional technology allows the educator to stimulate more senses in multiple ways to maximize the learning experience. However, the educator must constantly keep in mind that, although instructional technology is a useful tool for presenting educational material, it must not overshadow the educational message itself. Proper use of instructional technology requires planning, preparation, and practice on the part of the instructor.

Glossary

audience response systems Electronic devices to query a group of students during a presentation and share aggregate feedback. Also called "classroom feedback," "personal response systems," or "clickers."

audio Sound.

audio mixer A device that blends sounds from multiple devices that are connected to a single amplifier and set of speakers.

audio visual (AV) Tools or techniques other than lecture used to supplement learning.

instructional technology The software and hardware used to create and transmit audiovisual materials.

interactive whiteboard Electronic whiteboard that provides a multipage drawing application.

laser pointer Handheld device to visually highlight key points during a presentation.

MP3 players Digital device that stores and plays back sounds and videos.

podcast A digital audio recording that can be downloaded from a computer.

tablet computers A compact, handheld, wireless computer device.

smartphones A mobile telephone with capability to perform other computing and imaging functions such as retrieve e-mail and take photographs.

digital The manner in which information is stored in electronic devices such as computers.

screencasts An audio and video screen recording.

digital projector A device that displays and projects computer images onto a screen.

References

1. Audiovisual education. Encyclopedia.com [Internet]. Available at: http://www.encyclopedia.com/printable.asp?url=/ssi/a1/audiovis.html
2. The Virtual Presentation Assistant—University of Kansas. Available at: www.ukans.edu/cwis/units/coms2/vpa/vpa7.htm
3. Guidelines for using AV. Available at: www.2myprofessor.com/Common/guidlines_for_using_audiovisual.htm
4. Parvensky, C. A. (1995). *Teaching EMS: An educator's guide to improved EMS instruction.* St. Louis, MO: Mosby. 121, 125, 131, 145, 148.
5. AV benefits. Available at: http://www.3.uakron.edu/schlcomm/Turner/avbenfts.htm.
6. Polivka, E. G. (Ed.) (2002). *Professional meeting management.* Chicago, IL: Education Foundation of the Professional Convention Management Association. 199, 226–228, 364.
7. HowStuffWorks: how digital cameras work. Available at: www.howstuffworks.com/digital-camera.htm/printable
8. Presentation available at: http:/www.elmousa.com/presentation/menu/htm

Additional Resources

Atkinson, C. (2011). *Beyond bullet points: Using Microsoft® PowerPoint® to create presentations that inform, motivate, and inspire,* (3rd ed.). Redmond, WA: Microsoft Press. ISBN: 978-0-7356-2735-2

DeSilets, L. D., & Dickerson, P. (2009). Graphic design principles for audiovisual presentations. *Journal of Continuing Education in Nursing, 40*(1), 12–13.

University of Minnesota, Center for Teaching and Learning (2011). Active learning with powerpoint. http://www1.umn.edu/ohr/teachlearn/tutorials/powerpoint/index.html

17

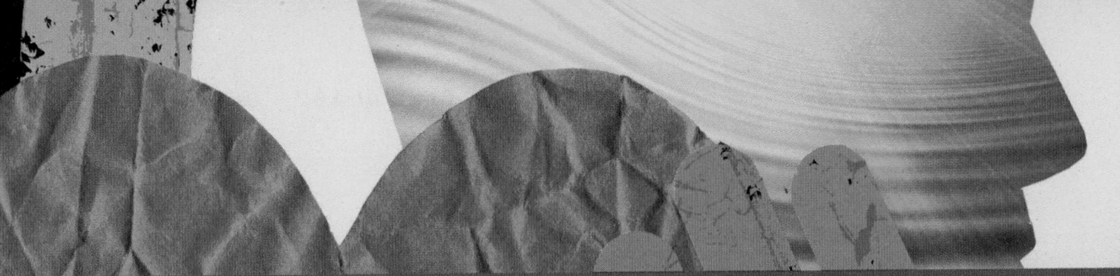

Tools for Distance Learning

Tell me and I will forget, Show me and I might remember, Involve me and I will understand. — CHINESE PROVERB

CHAPTER GOAL: This chapter offers insight into the realm of distance education; it describes different model combinations and provides tools to help instructors focus on teaching and learning within the classroom that has no walls.

Internet-based distributed learning has rapidly expanded across the health professions as an accepted and valuable educational delivery system. By removing the constraints associated with time and distance, the technology provides opportunities for EMS practitioners to access courses and to build on their education and professional development. The term "distributed learning" refers to computer-mediated instruction which uses various information technologies to deliver educational material to students. In contrast, **distance education** is a broad term that describes enrollment in educational courses external to the standard classroom.

Distance education is not a new concept. It offers access to students who otherwise might not enroll into educational programs. For people who have lived and worked in rural or remote locations, distance education via print materials delivered by the postal service has been the mainstay of available education in past decades. Times have now changed! The information and technology revolution has broken barriers and removed obstacles that previously restricted those who wanted to further their education with formal course work. Geographic distances, scheduling conflicts, shift-work rosters, work schedules, and family commitments are no longer a hindrance to those who wish to pursue their education.

Technology has mobilized the way humans communicate and has revolutionized the way they work and learn. With personal computers (PCs) in more than 80 percent of U.S. homes, the PC has become accessible, commonplace, transportable, and affordable to the domestic market. In the United States, three in four households has a PC.[1] Technology advancements, along with rapid expansion of the Internet, and technological applications have brought about a proliferation of opportunities for learning at a distance.

Distance Education in Perspective

Distance education (DE) is a system of education whereby students and teachers are separated by time and distance, so students are not necessarily in the actual classroom at a scheduled time. DE has several name tags which aim to capture the "classroom without walls" philosophy: "distance learning," "distributed learning," "open university," "open and distance learning," "e-learning," "correspondence school," "flexible delivery," "external study," and "virtual education" are some. Although many of the names are interchangeable, a significant difference must be noted here: *distance education* is the term we use when we talk about the *process* of delivering education, and *distance learning* is the desired *outcome* of that educational process.

As a delivery system, DE has been around since the beginning of written language! In the late 1800s, the University of Chicago in the United States offered education via postal service; in Australia, the School of the Air was established in 1944 in an effort to reach children and families in the Outback via two-way pedal radio link; and in 1969, the Open University of the United Kingdom began offering programs that used print and multimedia resources. Distance education was a popular option in the '70s and '80s as it provided an educational opportunity to those who lived too far away from the institutions. During these decades course material and assignments were posted by mail and telephone contact was available if required. Technology has played a significant role in the development of all modes of educational material.

Today, courses have been developed—and will continue to be developed— with the assistance of a wide range of technologies, often in combination, brought together to meet the requirements of the subject. Standard domestic computers have inbuilt applications that facilitate a range of functions. For example, interactive DVDs, audio and video functions, telephone access, and computer conferencing all provide excellent means of bringing life to learning. Lectures may incorporate auditory descriptions, color, video, and animation to deploy a rich learning environment either on their own or in combination with print-based courses. The technology is available for instructors and students to take advantage of fantastic communication tools—both synchronous (at a scheduled time) and asynchronous (at a nonscheduled time). Although students who are enrolled in a course may be geographically scattered across the suburbs, the state, the nation, or throughout the world, communication technology enables distance learners to meet with the instructor and discuss educational concepts through the computer **(Figure 17.1)**.

Advances in telecommunications-based technology have leveraged DE programs to use methods that only a decade ago were thought to be futuristic. Satellite, microwave, fiberoptic, and wireless (WiFi) communications, coupled with video- and audioconferencing and computer conference tools, are part and parcel of the technology interface. From early and rapid expansion into the market place, the online distance-learning market is now growing annually by 10 percent,[2] with more and more students choosing to enroll and study online.[3] The number of students taking at least one online class tripled in the past decade.[4]

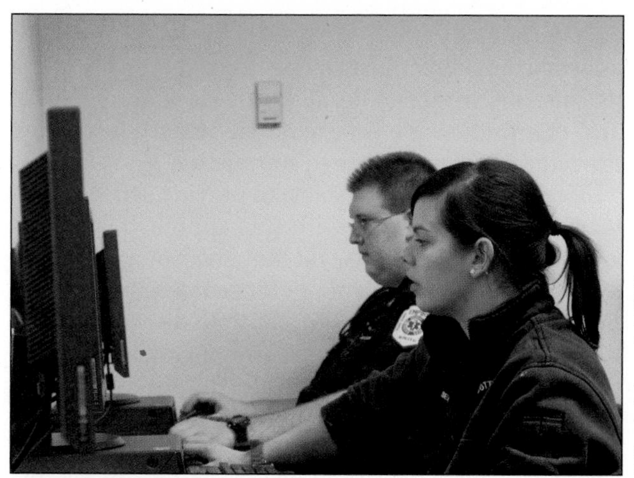

Figure 17.1

Geographic barriers to education are eliminated by distance-education program delivery.

The Internet has become the most common method of information delivery, and across the globe, educational institutions are offering a wide range of programs with most courses coming from the disciplines of education, business, and humanities—which include the health sciences.[5] Within the health care spectrum, online programs for allied health sciences, paramedical science, nursing, health education, and health management are common. Websites that offer or describe such programs include the following:

- Medscape at http://www.medscape.com
- Nursing Continuing-Education Directory at http://www.nurseceu.com
- CMEWeb at http://www.cmeweb.com

Many other sites can be found through online searches and in journal, newspaper, and magazine advertisements.

Online teaching and learning have demonstrated proven performance with student achievement in the university sector.[6] A multitude of studies has been conducted over the past decade to find out about the effectiveness of online learning as compared with traditional face-to-face student classroom learning. These studies have also measured student perceptions and satisfaction with level of knowledge and with various delivery modes. Sufficient documentation has shown that no differences in exam scores have been seen between distance learners and students who have pursued their learning in the traditional classroom. In fact, emerging research indicates that the grades of distance learners are 5 percent higher than those of students who undertake face-to-face classroom learning.[7–9] These findings are supported by scientific studies.[10]

Learning at a Distance

As has been discussed in Chapter 4: Learning Styles, it is well known that learning is highly individualized and that people learn in a multitude of different ways. It is also well known that instructors must employ various teaching methods and techniques to ensure that students understand what they are learning. Similarly, online teaching and learning have specific features that differ from teaching and learning in the traditional classroom and that require due attention.

Online Learning: Student-Centered Learning

The traditional classroom tends be teacher centered; that is, the teacher controls what is to be learned, when it is to be learned, and how it is to be learned. One of the significant differences between learning in the traditional classroom and online learning is the change of focus between learner and instructor—online learning is student centered. The student becomes the controller of his or her own learning. Within DE, some general basic themes underpin all student-centered learning.

The Role of the Instructor Changes

The instructor becomes a guide or facilitator; the instructor guides students through their studies. The focus is on the student's development, interests, and needs.

Students Take Responsibility for Their Own Learning

Students must be self-regulated to meet the demands of learning in isolation, if they are to adhere to task time lines. Although many distance learners are very good independent students, others need a tremendous amount of encouragement to get their work completed on time.

Learning Is Enhanced through Discussion

Technology enhances learning as it provides students with opportunities to discuss lecture content, to talk, share, and collaborate with other students about the course material and related information.

The Instructor Manages Student Learning

The learning process is a shared process; the instructor and the students within the group share information and findings. Learning is ongoing, and students take an active part in the process.

Students Construct Knowledge through Critical Thinking and Problem Solving

This encourages independence and cooperation and promotes understanding and thinking for oneself.

Teaching and Assessment Are Entwined Together

In the classroom setting, teaching is often focused on preparing students for the final test. Online teaching focuses on the learning process.

Collaborative Learning

Learning online promotes, and is ideal for, collaborative learning—that is, an instructional method in which two or three students work together toward a common goal. Although this method is a common practice in the face-to-face classroom with small groups who work together, the virtual classroom uses e-mail, **discussion boards**, **wikis**, and **chat rooms** to foster collaborative learning online. Students can become responsible for each other's learning, and they may nurture mutual success. The collaborative approach to learning is a stimulus for the active exchange of ideas, which, in turn, promotes critical thinking. Online collaborative learning often includes students who have not met each other face-to-face; they have not socialized together nor developed social networks together; thus initially, the personality factor can be absent and the collaborative exercise is bias-free. Collaborative teaching and learning through the written form can, at times, be challenging as contributions to the chat or discussion boards can be void of the individual's true personality and are read and interpreted as written. While some online discussion boards contain a sense of formality, many instructors and course designers include a forum for casual discussions between students. It is within this area that student's raw creativeness can explode into an extremely rich learning environment and social networks develop.

Asynchronous and Synchronous Learning

Any student enrolled in a Web-based course will find that most time spent on course work is done **asynchronously**, that is, independently, and without assistance or direct instruction from the teacher. The website or lecture materials provide a study guide and comprehensive instructional steps that outline the requirements for course completion.

Technology is now available to provide **synchronous teaching and learning**; with this approach, students are in different locations, yet may meet at a prescheduled time to participate in a videoconference, or they may log on to a website for real-time discussion with the instructor. Synchronous learning can be achieved through computer conferencing, during which students and instructor are stationed at their computers. With headsets and microphones, they are able to talk to one another, share documents, and use the whiteboard function to brainstorm ideas or to draw up a model. More commonly, message boards and chat rooms are used for synchronous discussion.

Internet-based DL through the computer is causing a reduced need for other modes of conferencing technology, such as telephone conferencing and videoconferencing.

Characteristics of the Distance Learner

Although it is not possible to regard distance learners as a group with same likenesses, many students share demographic and situational similarities from which a profile of the learner can be typified. Their characteristics are varied; however, their commonalties include the following:

- *Age*: As cited by Thompson, Holmberg reports that the DE learner is usually older than the typical undergraduate student.[11] The 25- to 35-year-old age group tends to dominate, and the 35- to 40-year-old age group is a close contender.
- *Sex*: More female than male students are enrolled in external programs; 60 percent to 70 percent are women.[11]
- *Geographical distance*: As cited by Thompson, Gibson and Graff report that most distance learners reside between 100 and 200 miles (150–350 km) from campus.[11] However, because of the proliferation of online educational programs, students who commute a round trip of less than 30 minutes are enrolling into online courses as a preferred alternative.[5,11–13]
- *Life roles:* As cited by Thompson, Fjortoft reports that more than three-quarters of students who were undertaking a DE postbaccalaureate program worked more than 40 hours per week, and most were married.[11] Other studies by Eastmond claim that up to 90 percent of students who undertake external studies are employed on a full-time basis.[11]
- *Motivation and autonomy:* O'Shaughnessy states that intrinsic motivation and desire for career advancement are significant characteristics of distance learners.[14] Most DE students are self-regulatory, that is, they set aside regular time for study, establish schedules to meet their learning tasks, and do not need regular reminders to get their work completed by the due date. They are autonomous learners.

Therefore, it can be anticipated that the distance learner will most likely have an existing vocation and may be looking to expand vocational interests or gain qualifications that will facilitate movement into a different career path.

Distance Education Within EMS

There is a vast range of courses for undergraduates, graduates, and postgraduates conducted throughout universities and vocational colleges that prepare their graduates to practice within the allied health spectrum. For example, nursing, midwifery, physiotherapy, occupational health, dietetics, and paramedic programs are just some. Nationally and internationally, many universities and community colleges have developed policies that incorporate all courses they offer to have an online presence.[15, 16] Training allied health care practitioners is a major budgetary item for governments to support in its endeavors to provide health care to its citizens, and online access to training health care practitioners is one strategy to address this issue.

In broad terms, many educational institutions have embraced online delivery of education as a strategy to (a) reach more students, (b) utilize available technology, and (c) support the national economy. In terms of distance, time, and work schedules, the cost of training EMS practitioners is high. When one considers the theoretical perspective of education, the sheer volume of large numbers of students, repeat lectures, and classroom or lecture theatre space, DE provides a valuable alternative. DE provides access to education especially for those who have family commitments, who need to work to support themselves, and those who reside a significant distance away from the institution or in rural areas.

While DE is instrumental at delivering theoretical content online, courses that are offered totally online may not meet the psychomotor needs of students;

CASE IN POINT

Flinders University, Adelaide, Australia, has an online presence for every course topic across the university. Students who are enrolled within all health science courses are able to access a variety of theoretical courses entirely online; other courses that have clinical skills mastery require attendance at face-to-face workshops which are programmed throughout the semester.

therefore, provisions within the course structure must incorporate face-to-face clinical skill workshops for psychomotor skill practice and clinical experience.

Structuring Distance Education for EMS

The structure of DE courses within EMS requires unique conceptualization in accordance with the specific profession of the EMS field. Technology can be incorporated in many ways into models for DE programs. Although the choices are numerous, it is very clear that Internet-based instruction has become the leading DE delivery mechanism. Many factors must be identified and figured out before a course can be set up in terms of course content and the mechanism for delivery. A very important early step is to gather together a group of experienced people, content experts and information technologists, to explore suitable possibilities for a particular educational organization. Many universities offer consultancy and mentoring assistance for smaller and independent education providers. This can include training in use of the technology, curriculum design, and online instruction for faculty members. With or without this training, instructors should design distance education to include commonly agreed upon elements of quality online education **(Table 17-1)**.

Determining Course Topics for Distance Delivery

DE is structured to meet the learning objectives of the specific program as determined by the course curriculum. With due attention to curriculum design, theoretical courses within a program can be readily translated into an online course. There is scope for many clinical components to be conveyed through distance modules. For example, topics that relate to the sciences of anatomy, physiology, and pathophysiology, as well as instruction on significant illnesses such as respiratory illnesses of croup, asthma, or pneumonia, lend themselves well to online delivery.

To determine the structure of the online course will require input from the educational institution's faculty members, industry representatives, instructional designers, and technicians. A conceptual map of the course is drawn and this map will reflect the following:

- Course content
- Learning outcomes
- Description of the knowledge and the clinical skills required
- Application of the skills in the workplace
- Elements that describe the performance criteria

Deciding the Structure of the Course

Deciding how the course is to be structured can be challenging. Different topics must be treated differently. The requirements of the curriculum will influence the course design. For example, it might be decided that students will learn the theoretical information online, then gather together for practical skill workshops to develop competence in psychomotor skill performance. Bringing students together for in-class work acknowledges the importance of the social nature of learning.

Decisions must be made about the use of synchronous and asynchronous communications. Will the course be primarily asynchronous, with some scheduled synchronous computer meetings?

Mode of Delivery

The choice of delivery mechanisms relies heavily on available resources, administrative support, comfort level with the technology, and level of available technical support. Each of these considerations is important, no matter what mechanisms are involved. Although Internet-based distribution is exciting, like other forms of educational delivery, it can be done well or poorly. A quality Internet-based program requires that many significant aspects are considered, including the following:

- Are technicians available to set up and maintain the technological aspects of the program?
- Do instructors have appropriate instructional expertise?
- Is enough administrative support available for the ongoing needs of the course?

When the Internet is the chosen mode of delivery, a number of technical and administrative decisions must be made. Some questions that arise include these:

- Will the course be located in the public domain?
- Will the course be housed within a learning management system (LMS)?
- If so, which LMS should be used?

Table 17.1 Rubric to Quality Online Education

	Information about the Course	**Course Statements Details for Successful Course Completion**	**Syllabus**		
Resources to Support Student Learning	The course objectives, assessment details and participation; Technical requirements and technical support	Prerequisites and credit value; Contact details instructor, academic department; Recommended resources; Due dates and instructions for completing assignments; Grading forms and grading scale; The institutions policies; Career support and counseling	Detailed description of the course, the learning objectives and learning outcomes		
	Content Organization and Navigation	**Content Organization**	**Course Content**		
Online Course Organization	Online course content is organized in a logical format which is consistent throughout course documents	Programmed for student time on task; Synchronous or asynchronous activities are scheduled	Delivered in a systematic and logical sequence; Content folders contain relevant learning material		
	Aesthetic Design	**Instructional Delivery**	**Learning Activities are Integrated**	**Activities to Enhance Student Learning**	**Activities for Critical Thinking and Problem-Solving Skills**
Online Course Design & Delivery	The course material looks interesting on the computer screen	Various teaching methods used to encourage student interaction; Student learning is encouraged through use of various technological applications (video, audio, print, discussion, chat); Respect for diverse talents and different ways students learn; Instructor accessible to students	Reading assignments match learning objectives; Activities lead to learning the desired concepts	All forms of media are used to enhance learning opportunities	Problem oriented activities and discussions to promote higher order learning
	Assessment of Student Learning	**Assessment Activities Aligned to Learning Objectives**	**Multiple Assessment Strategies**	**Self-Assessments and Peer Feedback**	**Assessment Feedback**
Assessment of Student Learning	Accepted methods and variety of assignment instruments are used	Assessment items reflect course learning; Evaluation criteria to determine online participation, study groups; Questions fair and reasonable; Scope of assessment activities identified; Authentic and validated assessment of learning	Assignment options to allow for different interests and personal learning styles; Opportunities to demonstrate proficiency in different ways	Student-generated discussion questions and respond to others' discussion	Prompt and substantial instructor feedback

Therefore, it is vital for instructors and administrators to get advice from experienced professionals on these important decisions.

Technology for an Online Course

According to the literature, online courses have become the preferred method of pursuing distance education. Understanding technology that is available, understanding its function, and knowing how to use the system to one's advantage are skills that can be readily mastered. While large institutions of education—universities and community colleges—have implemented online teaching and learning, smaller training providers may still be considering the benefits and advantages. The information that follows is provided for the benefit of smaller educational agencies that are curious about the scope of Internet-based courses.

Learning Management Systems

Learning management systems (LMSs) facilitate the creation of online course work in a World Wide Web–based educational environment. An LMS is a software program that can be used to create entire online courses, or to provide interactive tools that supplement existing courses. Numerous LMSs are on the market; many LMS programs are highly capable, robust, and technical in their components, yet very self-explanatory and easy to use. These include commercial products and open-source (free) LMSs. Organizations are encouraged to find one that best suits their needs. A quality LMS performs three functions:

- *Course structure*: Instructors are able to create course material by uploading lectures, documents, activities, links, and tests onto the website. It is in this structure that the instructional material is contained.
- *Course tools*: These are used to assist the student in participating in the course. Examples of course tools include a message board, a chat room, document sharing, a calendar, password changes, and exams.
- *Course management system*: Administrative features are provided for password authentication, automated grading and test results, student tracking, and generating of statistical data related to the course.

Learning Management System Tools

Functional LMS tools are essential with any Web-based Internet delivery program. A robust LMS will include all aspects of functionality for ease of navigation through the course documentation, information, and delivery. It will have the capabilities to do the things that the instructional faculty want it to do, and it will be simple to use. If an online distance-education program for delivery via the Internet is about to be established, then the list that follows will be helpful to determine the LMS to choose.

Online Course: Functional Tools

A quality LMS will offer the following functions:

- *Course content*. This can be subdivided into the following areas:
  - Topic Information: Description of the course aims and objectives
  - Assessment items: Description of assessment requirements and due dates
  - Statement of assessment: The assessment criteria; how the coursework will be assessed
  - Instruction: Weekly readings, lecture streaming, pod-cast, web-cast
- *Announcements*. These advise students of general announcements that are generated by decisions made during the progress of the course.
- *Assessments*. Documents describe the assessments required for successful completion of the course. The instructional details describe what is to be undertaken, how it is to be presented, and what is expected.
- *Assignments*. This function outlines the theme and content of the coursework to be submitted for appraisal. It provides an outline of the assignment, the inclusions and exclusions, word length, and allocated percentage of the grade. Secondary tabs contained in the Assignment area contain information for students to view that their assignments have been submitted, that the assignment has been graded, and assessment results released.
- *Discussion board*. Online courses require a portal for students to engage with their peers and tutor. The discussion board provides the function where students can upload their responses to tutorial questions, to describe their thoughts and opinions, and to respond to other students' comments.

Within many commercial LMSs, a Wiki tool (a feature that allows students to add and edit content collectively) is available.

- *E-mail.* Many LMSs provide an e-mail function within the program. This is useful as incoming and outgoing e-mail will be relative to the course content thus kept separate from general e-mail.
- *Search.* The Search function is a useful tool that can be used to find documents, programs—or indeed, anything that is stored on the computer! This is particularly useful to users who are not good at filing their documents in the correct place!
- *Who's on line?* This function is useful for students to network with each other, or with the tutor. By clicking on to this capability, course participants can synchronously see who else is attending to their studies, and initiate a chat session with another person. Chat allows instructor and student to communicate in text form in real time. Users must be online at the same time when they communicate. This tool is great for immediate interaction and feedback.
- *Help desk.* For students, or tutors, who are new to distance education, the Help Desk is an area where users can ask questions and receive information about the functions of the LMS.
- *Web links.* In addition to hyperlinks contained within the coursework documents, the Web links provide another area for course developers to upload Web links that are an extension of coursework readings for students to research.
- *Quizzes and tests.* Time-released assessment items are prepared in advance by the instructor and automatically graded within the LMS capabilities.
- *Gradebook.* This feature allows students to monitor their progress throughout the course.

Instructor Management Tools

Keeping track of student access to the course material, their time on task, and record-keeping of their grades is a key function of the instructor's role. Many LMSs will incorporate instructor tools that automatically generate course management functions.

- *Manage course.* This function provides the developer with symbolic depictions that identify the process the link will follow.
- *Assessment manager.* Time-release assessments, grade attempts, and grade allocation are automatically fielded within this function. The instructor is able to create assessment items, choose when they are to be released, make assessment items available to students, and record the student grades.
- *Assignment dropbox.* As students complete their coursework, they are submitted to the dropbox from where the instructors can then view and assign grades.
- *Grading forms.* The developer is able to upload and store grading-criteria forms that will be used during the course.
- *Student tracking.* Many instructors have expressed concern about whether or not students are attending to their studies. This function generates a range of statistical information from which the instructor can make assumptions. For example, the system can generate a Summary of Student Activity, the frequency of Tools that have been used, how often the Course Item is used, as well as group or individual student interaction with the course materials.

While there are a multitude of elements to consider when choosing a LMS, a robust software program purchased from a reputable company will include each of these components.

Instructional Design

Instructional design, the most important part of DE, progresses much in the way that buildings are constructed. An instructional course must be designed in a very specific manner, so that each task is clearly identified with the curriculum, and the exact roles and functions of participants are delineated. Schiffman's model provides a clear pathway that identifies each significant design step that must be addressed at preproduction meetings. First, instructors must conduct a needs assessment, establish program goals and objectives, develop an analysis of specific steps needed to design the program, write objectives, and develop assessment strategies. The next steps involve selecting appropriate media to support the course design, developing instructional materials, and conducting formative assessments. Based on the results of the formative assessment, modifications in program design may need to be made prior to conducting the summative program evaluation.[17]

Conceptual Map for Instruction

Instructional design incorporates the need to draw up a conceptual map of the course instruction.

The conceptual map needs to include a series of annotations and links that provide an overview of how the instruction will be constructed and presented. The conceptual map helps developers think through each element and make decisions about how the content will be presented online. Learning outcomes taken from the syllabus guide the development of the conceptual map, and each of the learning outcomes must be addressed by the instruction. Developers determine the mechanism by which learning outcomes are to be distributed. The conceptual map is influenced by the type of media selected for delivery of the instructional material and by the resources available to produce the material.

Methods for Assessing Learning Online

Learning is assessed according to the processes of the educational institution, and content is determined by the curriculum. LMSs have a range of options for built-in tests and quizzes that can be used for formative and summative exams; and many LMSs provide options for time-release assessments. The assessment items can be produced well ahead of time, uploaded, and programmed for release at a determined time. Additionally, assignments can be locked at a specified time when criteria determine a completion or lapse time. Assignments are usually contained within a secured site. Some examples of test types include multiple-choice, ordering, true or false, and short answer questions. When cleverly constructed, each of these types of testing methods is capable of testing knowledge and comprehension of course work.

Many instructors raise concerns about supervision and exam conduct when the student is required to take the exam from a remote location. Institutions must develop policies to state how this can best be done. Several mechanisms can be put into place to ensure that the right student is taking the right test.

- *Exam passcodes*: An LMS can provide specific exam passcodes that authenticate that the right person is taking the exam.
- *Timed exams*: The exam is scheduled to occur within a specified 24- or 48-hour period. The time is determined at the commencement of the course, so that students are able to schedule the event. Additionally, timed exams are usually of a duration that does not permit the student to look up texts or references.
- *Proctored exams*: The student is required to take the exam at a predetermined location such as the local library. Instructions are provided, and arrangements are made with an overseer before the day of the event. Photo identification may be required.
- *Range of assessment formats*: Course work assessments can be divided into several sections, each of which accounts for a percentage of the overall grade. Online tests, essays, collaborative work, projects, and online discussions can be incorporated into the student's overall assessment.

Online: Assessment of the Domains of Learning

Chapter 4: Learning Styles details the characteristics of how students learn, and there is a wealth of research from the general-education profession that describes learning styles and assessment of each domain of learning: cognitive, psychomotor, and affective. Over the past decade there has been anecdotal argument between health educators about how the different domains of learning can be assessed adequately and comprehensively. There is no argument that online learning is well constructed for assessing the cognitive domain of learning; however, there is continued caution with assessment of the psychomotor and affective domains of leaning.

Assessment of the Cognitive Domain of Learning

The cognitive domain is concerned with the learner's knowledge and information-processing attributes. It involves various mental processes relevant to knowledge. Online assessments can readily be created, implemented, and graded automatically—all without the involvement of the instructor! The assessment items are usually multiple-choice questions, and the assessment of knowledge is solely reliant on the student marking the correct response.

Assessment of the Psychomotor Domain

Clinical educators argue that it is difficult to assess online the psychomotor domain of learning. In response to this, program construction design has students undertake the didactic parts of the course online and then attend clinical workshops to learn the motor application of the skill. Clinical instructors are free to concentrate on the psychomotor aspects of

CASE IN POINT

Volunteer Ambulance Officer, Tammie, lives in the town of Elliston, a farming and fishing community on Eyre Peninsula, South Australia, that has a population of 300 people. It is 170 km from the closest regional city of Pt. Lincoln. Tammie and a small core of other Volunteer EMS personnel provide emergency patient care, on call, to their district.

Following completion of initial mandatory coursework, Tammie enrolled into the Certificate IV in Health Care (Ambulance). She is required to participate in clinical callouts alongside local, certified ambulance volunteers. Throughout her course, Tammie carries out specific learning tasks as determined in the course curriculum and associated with Clinical Development Packages. Study resources include textbooks, worksheets, video, DVDs, and online resources, which are provided by the Education Unit of S.A. Ambulance Service. Tammie's training is supported by regional trainers who conduct regular training sessions at her ambulance station.

In order to complete psychomotor skills and demonstrate clinical competency, Tammie joins a core of other students to undertake regular training via weekend workshops—usually scheduled for six consecutive weeks—at the central town of Wudinna, 160 km away.

skills demonstration without being tied to the background knowledge.

Assessment of the Affective Domain

Similar to assessment of the psychomotor domain, there has been debate over the ability to assess online the affective domain of learning. The affective domain is concerned with the way we do things: behaviors, emotions, feelings, qualities. In response to this, many educational organizations have modified the way they assess the affective domain to accommodate online courses. Examples are: short- or long-answer responses to questions that elicit caring behaviors, having students complete open-ended statements, and having students write an interview transcript that incorporates affective behaviors. While this strategy requires instructors to spend time grading the papers, students are able to respond to coursework that assesses the affective domain of learning.

Faculty Administration Matters

Although an educational organization's student registrar is responsible for general student administration, some administrative matters must be dealt with at the local level. Some examples follow here:

- *Student enrollments must be entered into the LMS.* Student-related policies should mirror the protocol approach used for face-to-face courses. It is prudent for administrators to check the organization's handbook to ensure this has been addressed. If the DE course is about to be set up, the handbook may have to be amended to reflect the change in delivery mode.
- *Student participation.* When an online program expects student participatory activities, instructors may be concerned about what constitutes a reasonable level of student participation or non-participation in the course. Before course commencement, a decision must be made and clearly communicated to students about how the course instructors will grade student participation. A participation policy may need to be developed and a corresponding entry added to the student handbook.
- *Grading collaborative work.* Students enrolled in the course must know how collaborative work will be graded. Without a clear statement on this, disputes can arise between students and faculty. A statement within the course instructions that defines how collaborative work will be graded significantly reduces the potential for problems.

Instructor Skills for Online Teaching and Learning

Many enthusiastic instructors wish to develop their courses into DE format and are unsure how to go about it. If DE is already established at the instructor's educational facility, then the local staff-development department usually offers workshops to provide the skills that instructors need to get started. An LMS will provide a comprehensive guide to assist the instructor in learning the technology, and the Help function within the LMS assists instructors during its use. When purchasing an LMS, the program director should make sure that the vendor includes training as part of the contract. Learning the technology to upload electronic files is not difficult; the challenge lies in learning the pedagogical framework and the different teaching methods available.

The instructor's experiences from classroom teaching provide a range of teaching skills that are readily adaptable to online teaching. Successful online teaching strategies include the following:

- *Posing real-life scenarios*: Students are able to relate learning to clinical practice. Real-life scenarios provide sound foundations from which participants can explore a range of "what ifs" on the discussion board.
- *Asking students for their opinion*: Students bring varied life experiences to the classroom; many will have encountered issues of social and health matters. Students learn from each other.
- *Acknowledging good progress*: Feedback given to students through personal e-mail or the discussion board provides encouragement and allows students to gauge their progress.
- *Maintaining student self-esteem*: Sometimes, the spoken word and the written word are in conflict when nonverbal cues are absent; instructors are encouraged to proofread e-mails sent to students to ensure that students' self-esteem is sustained.
- *Engaging students*: Although students may be many miles away, online tasks and activities that require them to reflect on their learning create an environment that is meaningful to them.
- *Creating and maintaining a learning environment*: This is the tenet of teaching principles.

Teaching Tip >> *Instructors must consider the way students process information; the learning environment that an instructor creates directly affects student learning. Instructors should do the following:*

- *Provide opportunities for students to share ideas.*
- *Provide opportunities for students to feel supported and be challenged.*
- *Empower students toward learning on their own by making course objectives clearly defined and accessible.*
- *Establish relationships with students—relationships are essential if students are to be successful.*
- *Design teaching to reflect high expectations for the success of all students.*

Because online learning does not provide the benefit of classroom visual cues, many instructors may be anxious to know if students are learning through the DE process. Over the past decade, research has generated an influential amount of information about the scope of DE. One study wanted to find out whether two different distance-learning techniques were as effective as classroom teaching for training students at a rural location.[18] This study explored a range of technologies, including two-way audio and computers, and it employed synchronous teaching techniques. Study investigators concluded that "No difference was found" between the two types of study, and they promoted distance-learning techniques as an effective way to provide educational opportunities to rural students. Research from general education and allied health disciplines confirms that learning does occur through DE courses.

Issues of Student Learning

Before a student embarks on an online program, several significant concerns must be considered. Basic computer skills are essential; students who are entering universities or community colleges will have developed computer literacy as part of the schooling, yet mature-aged students might not be as competent as their younger peers. Although keyboard speed may present some limitations, skills for site navigation and basic software applications are required. Many local libraries or community centers offer short courses that teach computer basics. Importantly, potential students require access to a computer with current software and programs to access course material.

Potential students may find it helpful to be informed about course expectations and about how undertaking an online course can affect the home environment. Information packages that contain helpful hints about how to create a home study center and how to plan and attend to learning provide useful information for supporting and optimizing student learning.

Instructors may need to advise students that online learning requires self-regulated discipline because it is easy to defer course tasks in favor of personal commitments. To overcome this, it is recommended that students schedule specific times during the week to be dedicated to course activities and learning so that the benefits associated with accessing the online course can be balanced with personal endeavors **(Figure 17.2)**.

Traditional classroom instruction is usually instructor centered, that is, the instructor is the center

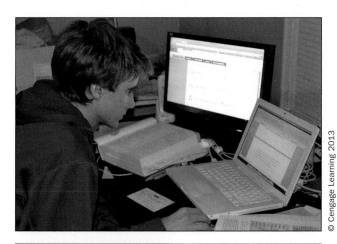

Figure 17.2

Students enrolled in distance-learning courses are able to structure their class time around work time.

of attention, activities revolve around the demands and expectation of the instructor, and students are required to follow the instructor's lead. Online learning offers a different mode; the student is the center of attention, and the student is expected to lead topic activities and learning.

Many students are concerned about and question the equivalence of online learning and face-to-face learning. Although this is a valid query, evidence confirms that the learning that results is equivalent.[19,20] Instructors can help to alleviate student concerns by creating an active, vibrant online community that encourages participation.

Challenges for Distance Education for EMS

With all new initiatives, EMS instructors will face differing personal challenges as they learn to master the skills to deliver online instruction. Some might find the challenges easier than others. Younger instructors might have the advantage of developing their computer and literacy skills from their school days, whereas older instructors might feel threatened to learn a new paradigm of instructional delivery. Alongside of the personal challenges, there also exist external challenges that are drawn from the educational institution, its guiding policies, and its staff-support resources.

Personal instructor challenges:

- *The new online instructor as learner.* The instructor who needs to become a learner to master the change from face-to-face has significant benefits. Progressing through the new learning cycle will give a sense of what the students might experience. Instructors begin to understand their own learning strategies, and, in turn, this will have a flow-on effect into the classroom. While learning a new form of instructional delivery will be a challenge, the outcomes have a positive result.
- *The individual instructor's challenge of reconceptualizing face-to-face to distance education pedagogy.* Seasoned instructors might face the trepidation of moving from highly interactive face-to-face teaching into an online medium, and might need support and mentorship as they learn to master the technology, adapt to accommodate new resources into their teaching practice, and adjust their instructional style to develop and maintain a sense of student community and active participation within the course.

Institutional challenges:

- *The challenge associated with inclusion of field instructors.* The nature of EMS demands strong psychomotor skills which cannot be readily demonstrated through online classes. To support this, field instructors must be encouraged to participate in DE programs so that education and industry cohesiveness can be maintained. This results in the best outcomes for students and for the patients in their care. Arrangements need to be put into place for the field instructors to update their skills, thereby maintaining a strong liaison between educational faculty and field instructors.
- *The challenge of access and equity.* Vocational and higher-education institutions have policies that include access and equity. DE complements these policies by making education available to people who are unable to attend the classroom.

Political and professional challenges:

- *The challenge for EMS educators to provide optimal education programs to return competent paramedics to adequately serve their communities.* Many government leaders from different countries state that their health care system is in crisis and solutions to aid this crisis are constantly being reviewed. There has been an annual increase of 5 percent for emergency ambulance work. [21] In Australia, specific initiatives have been undertaken to reduce the pressure in hospital emergency departments, for example, the Extended Care Paramedic program commenced in New South Wales in 2007, and in South Australia in 2008. Intensive care paramedics undertake further training to provide medical and surgical procedures as a strategic attempt to reduce emergency department overcrowding.

Continuing Education for EMS Providers

While DE is a viable option for a range of courses for undergraduate educational programs within the health sciences, it is also a practicable choice for ongoing- or continuing-education programs and professional development programs, as the students have already developed fundamental skills within their professional practice.

Within most EMS systems, continuing education is a mandatory requirement. Practitioners have a responsibility to keep up-to-date with current and contemporary practices, to incorporate new policies into their practice, and to keep abreast of evidence that impacts care.

Accreditation and regulation boards of professional bodies usually oversee and administer continuing-education programs. Each state and country have different criteria that individual EMS practitioners must meet to retain currency of licensure. EMS accrediting bodies have the expectation that educational programs will reflect contemporary methods by addressing issues of policy, quality of educational program content, access and equity.[22]

The Continuing Education Coordinating Board for Emergency Medical Services (CECBEMS) is the body that accredits continuing-education courses within the United States, including those offered via DL formats. This organization can be found at http://www.cecbems.org; the website provides contact details and information about the process required for newly created continuing-education DL programs to gain accreditation approval.

Summary

Technology has paved the way for change in the delivery of education. A large percentage of students are enrolling in DE options, and DE programs appeal to many EMS professionals for various reasons. DE is a proven method of delivering education, with most educational institutions in the Western world and beyond taking advantage of the technological tools available to take education to those who have previously been unable to access such programs. The convenience and flexibility provided by courses that are free of the constraints of place and time are highly beneficial for learners.

Glossary

asynchronous learning Independent learning without the need to be on line at the same time.

chat rooms A synchronous electronic communication system that resembles actual real-time conversations. Log-on is required to access; all members of the group can view the content.

discussion board A tool to use to communicate with a predetermined group; it is similar to e-mail but is stored and accessed through a Learning Management System.

distance education A system of education whereby students and teachers are separated by time and distance.

learning management system (LMS) Computer software that facilitates the creation of online course work in a World Wide Web–based educational environment.

synchronous teaching and learning Students are in different locations, but meet online at a prescheduled time to participate in real-time discussion with the instructor.

wiki A content-management system where each member of a group can collaborate to develop, design, edit, compile, and produce coursework.

References

1. The Nielsen Company. (2008). Home Technology Report Retrieved 4/6/2012, from http://www.marketingcharts.com/interactive/home-internet-access-in-us-still-room-for-growth-8280/nielsen-internet-access-household
2. O'Leonard, K. (2009). *The corporate learning factbook 2009: Statistics, benchmarks and analysis of the U.S. corporate-training market*. Oakland, CA: Bersin & Associates.

3. Gallagher, S. (2003). The future of online learning: Key trends and issues. The Distance Education and Training Council (DETC) 77th Annual Conference Summary.
4. Chronicle of Higher Education (2011, November 6). Online Learning Trends.
5. Ashby, C. M. (2002). Distance education: Growth in distance education programs and implications for federal education policy. U.S. General Accounting Office Report. GAO-02-1125T.
6. Redding, T. R. (2001). Comparative analysis of online learning versus classroom learning. *Journal of Interactive Instruction Development, 13,* 3–12.
7. Smeaton, A., & Keogh, G. (1999). An analysis of the use of virtual delivery of undergraduate lectures. *Computers and Education, 32,* 83–94.
8. Wade, W. (1999). Assessment in distance learning. *The Journal, 27,* 94–100.
9. Sener, J., & Stover, M. (2000). Intergrating ALN into an independent study distance education program: NVCC case studies. *Journal of Asynchronous Learning Networks*. 4.
10. Fallah, M. H., & Ubell, R. (2000). Blind scores in a graduate test: Conventional compared with Web-based outcomes. *Journal Asynchronous Learning Network*. 4. Available at: http://www.sloan-c.org/publications/magazine/v2n2fallah.asp
11. Thompson, M. M. (1998). Distance learners in higher education. In C. C. Gibson, (Ed.) (1998). *Distance learners in higher education: Institutional responses for quality outcomes*. Madison, WI: Atwood Publishing.
12. Halsne, A. M., & Gatta, L. A. (2002). Online versus traditionally delivered instruction: A descriptive study of learner characteristics in a community-college setting. *Online Journal of Distance Learning Administration*. 5.
13. Smith, S. L. (2001). Student services: The key to distance education programs. National Association of Student Personnel Administrators. Available at: http://www.naspa.org/netresults/
14. O'Shaughnessy, M. M. (n.d.). Designing for the distance learner: The diploma in social integration and enterprise for community development workers. Centre for Cooperative Studies, University College, Cork. Available at: http://www.ucc.ie/acad/foodecon/c_dp3?b.html. Accessed August 1, 2003.
15. McDonnell, A., & Edwards, D. (2000). From the classroom by cyberland: 21st century education for paramedics. *Australasian Journal of Emergency Care, 7,* 231–234.
16. Lord, W. (2003). The development of a degree qualification for paramedics at Charles Sturt University. *Journal for Prehospital Primary Health Care.*
17. Schiffman, S. S. (1995). Instructional systems design: Five views of the field. In G. J. Angin, (Ed.) (1995). *Instructional technology: Past, present and future,* (2nd ed.). Englewood, CO: Libraries Unlimited.
18. Hobbs., G. D., Moshinskie, J. F., Roden, S. K., & Jarvis, J. L. (1998). Education and practice. A comparison of classroom and distance-learning techniques for rural EMT-I instruction. *Prehospital Emergency Care, 2,* 190–191.
19. Boston, R. L. (1992). Remote delivery of instruction via the PC and modem: What have we learned? *American Journal of Distance Education, 6,* 345–357.
20. Simonson, M., Smaldino, S., Albright, M., & Zvacek, S. (2011). *Teaching and learning at a distance: Foundations of distance education,* (5th ed.). Boston, MA: Pearson Education.
21. Ambulance Service of NSW (n.d.). Better meeting the emergency needs of the NSW community: Ambulance Service of NSW extended care paramedic program. E-Library, Australian Resource for health care innovations. http://www.archi.net.au/e-library/workforce/staffing/ecp
22. Council for Higher Education Accreditation (2002). Accreditation and assuring quality in distance education. CHEA Monograph Series, No. 1.

Additional Resources

Allen, I. E., & Seaman, J. (2010). Class differences: Online education in the United States. The Sloan Consortium

http://sloanconsortium.org/publications/survey/pdf/class_differences.pdf

Institute for Higher Education Policy (1999). A review of contemporary research on the effectiveness of distance learning in higher education.

http://www.ihep.org/assets/files/publications/s-z/WhatDifference.pdf

Pang, L. (2003). Global best practices for successful online learning. *International Journal of Learning*, Vol. 10. Electronic (PDF File; 356.550KB), ISSN: 1447–9540, LC03-0179-2003.

United States Distance Learning Association http://www.usdla.org/

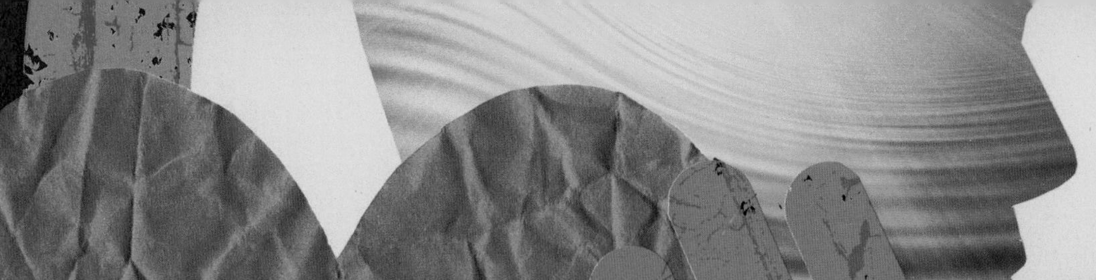

18 Tools for Simulation

A simulation is like a kiss, interesting to read about but much more interesting to participate in. And those that do, tend to repeat the experience. — Coote

Simulation in EMS education can play an essential role in helping students transfer and translate classroom theory into real-world practical application within the relative safety of controlled environments. Implementation of simulation in EMS education should be considered on a continuum—from the very isolated and simple to the large and complex.[1]

In recent years, advances in simulator technology has made the term "simulation" synonymous with the use of **high-fidelity** resuscitation **manikins**. Simulation can, in fact, and should be done using both low and high technology techniques. Any simulation situation is a type of experiential learning designed to mimic, as closely as possible, the real context. The principles of developing effective simulation **scenarios** are similar for low- and high-fidelity simulation. A well-designed simulation evokes emotion and allows students to demonstrate skills, knowledge, and affective behaviors at high levels in a safe environment.

As with any technology, EMS instructors should strive to use simulation resources appropriately. During initial psychomotor skills learning, students should practice specific skills on simpler manikins, task-trainers, or plastic body parts. As the learner progresses and the simulations integrate more simultaneous skills, the manikins also may need to be more complex. While there are numerous advantages to the use of simulation in EMS education, the major benefits include the following:

- Allowing students the freedom to fail
- Allowing students the opportunity to experience high-acuity, low-frequency situations and skills
- Allowing educators to standardize the learning environment
- Allowing students to practice teamwork and communication skills[2]

CHAPTER GOAL: The goal of this chapter is to discuss simulation techniques and technology that uses simulation.

Preparation

When designing any simulated event, careful consideration of the elements needed for effective student learning is essential. Simulator manufacturers often have packaged software that consists of scenarios for simulation sessions. While many of these scenarios are created for nursing and the in-hospital environment, new products created specifically for EMS are emerging. Simulations may be preprogrammed—where the simulator transitions from state to state according to the program, or "on-the-fly"—where the person controlling the simulator manipulates the simulator in response to student decisions and interventions.

In many ways a simulation is a combination of health care, education, and theater. In order for a simulation to succeed, the objectives or goals must align with the skills and the scenarios. An essential component is the **debriefing** session. The debriefing has been compared to an after-action report for a major incident. Components of a simulation session include the following:

- Objectives
- Tasks
- Conditions
- Scenario
- Timeframe
- Participants

- Equipment and setup
- End points and grading rubrics (if evaluation is the goal)
- Debriefing topics or questions

Objectives

To adequately prepare for a simulation session, an instructor should first lay out clear learning objectives, tasks to be completed, and conditions under which the simulation will take place. The scenario should be realistic in content and expectations. A simulation may be very basic and limited in scope or very complex. Factors to consider are student knowledge and experience, equipment and resources available, and the desired outcomes or learning objectives. It is sometimes desirable to adapt real cases, taking care to adjust the level of decision making and "branching" (the number of different directions a simulation may take) and the consequences of the interventions performed. The objectives the learner must demonstrate should help guide the end point and grading or evaluation (if that is the purpose of the simulation). Designating an expected "time-in-simulation" is helpful so that simulations are realistic and manageable for both the student and the instructor. This also will help ensure adequate time is allotted for a thorough debriefing.

Often the terms "simulation" and "scenario" are used interchangeably. Both have a wide range of interpretations. This chapter will use the terms interchangeably. In order to realize the greatest benefit from a simulation session, EMS educators must be thoughtful and deliberate when planning the purpose and scope of any scenario or simulated event. The resources (human and material) needed to effectively conduct the simulation must match the size, depth, and complexity needed to achieve the stated educational objectives. The scope of the simulation may be limited to the resources available within the organization or consortium of organizations planning the simulation.

One helpful tool to begin planning and organizing the simulation is to make lists of the tasks for the students to demonstrate, the conditions under which they should be able to perform these tasks, and the minimum standards to measure successful achievement of the desired competencies, outcomes, or objectives.[3] Some educators have found it helpful to create a **template** or worksheet that allows them to plan and implement a scenario in a uniform and consistent manner.

Tasks

The first step in creating a simulation is to develop a basic list of the overall goals and objectives for the scenario. It is helpful to identify the overall pedagogical goal of the simulation—is it for teaching and instruction or a means of assessing student learning or performance? If the latter, is it formative or summative assessment? Setting objectives for the simulation session is similar to the objectives' development process previously discussed in this text. Objectives can focus on one or more of the three domains of learning (cognitive, psychomotor, and affective) and should be clear, specific, and measurable. An objective such as "The student will perform the five steps involved in bandaging a laceration with active bleeding" is more clear and measurable than "The student will care for the trauma patient." Tasks and objectives may range from simple skill acquisition to complex integration of cognitive, psychomotor, and affective behaviors. Clear and realistic task goals help guide the development of a plan for the simulation.[4]

Educators should also consider the stage of learning that the students are in at the time of the simulation.[5,6] During the initial stages of learning, a simulation should be simple and isolate specific new tasks. At this point in the student's learning, a simulation may consist simply of introducing oneself to a patient or obtaining an accurate set of vital signs. What separates simulation from a simple task exercise is the performance of these tasks in an immersive, realistic setting. During later stages of learning, students should be expected to combine and integrate multiple concepts and tasks, and operate under more realistic conditions. At this point, students may be required to assess and treat a patient with multiple, complex medical issues that require critical thinking, effective communication, and competent procedural care. Summative simulation sessions should be complex and focus on determining whether or not the student is performing at an acceptable level as an entry-level EMS provider. The simulated patient's history, behavior, and acuity should realistically reflect the kind of patients the student will care for in clinical practice.[7]

Since there are limits to the realism and skills that can be performed in the simulated environment, the EMS instructor should, in the early stages of simulation, introduce the students to the rules and limitations of the simulation. Information regarding what a student may verbalize and what skills can be performed on the simulator is critical to delivering a realistic simulation. It may not be enough in a realistic simulation that the student is allowed to verbalize that he or she is wearing gloves. There is a benefit to having the student locate and apply gloves while in the simulated environment.

Students also need to be made aware of what the simulator can or cannot do. Some simulators have pupils that react to light or medications, while others do not. While some simulators will have a blood pressure that can be auscultated, it may not sound exactly like the blood pressure of an actual patient.

Instructors must be aware of the dangers of negative transference and identify any skill or procedure that deviates significantly from the way it is performed on a real patient.

Conditions

Key to achieving the desired outcomes and objectives in a simulation session is the realism of the environment and the ability for the students to "suspend their disbelief" as they move and interact in the simulated environment. Creating an immersive learning environment is essential for allowing the students to practice skills and situations that they will encounter in the clinical environment. Many educational programs conduct simulations in a skill lab or classroom environment. While a stand-alone simulation center is desirable, it is not required for EMS educators to conduct realistic simulation sessions. The key is a realistic recreation of the experience that captures the sights, the sounds, the tactile sensations, and even the smells of the actual environment being simulated **(Figure 18.1)**. The presence of actors or "confederates" to provide a social and environmental context within which the students can operate will add to the realism and allow the students to process multiple sensory inputs while they are practicing critical thinking and complex-factor decision making.

Low light, loud noise, realistic odors, seasonal temperature, tactile sensations, and inclement weather are all factors within the EMS environment. Varying the conditions of simulation can add extra challenges as well a greater degree of realism. While there is a risk of overwhelming the new student with the complex sensory inputs, in the final stages of learning the educator should make every attempt to create intricate, complex, and critical simulations that are as realistic as possible. These should be in sufficient depth and variety as to really test the ability of the provider while still providing the layer of safety that cannot be achieved during a real emergency.

The setting of the simulation is an important factor in creating the illusion of realism. While many simulation centers are built to look like hospitals or in-patient clinical settings, the EMS educator should strive to create simulated environments that mimic the prehospital environment **(Figure 18.2)**. The back of an ambulance is one of the most common simulated environments. Allowing students to practice skills in the relatively confined spaces of an ambulance exposes them to the challenges of this environment. A simulated environment that recreates the motion and the sounds of a moving ambulance adds further realism to the scenarios. Simulations may also take place in a simulated home environment. With a minimum of relatively inexpensive props and furniture, EMS educators can turn a classroom into a home or an apartment. Staging simulations in public spaces

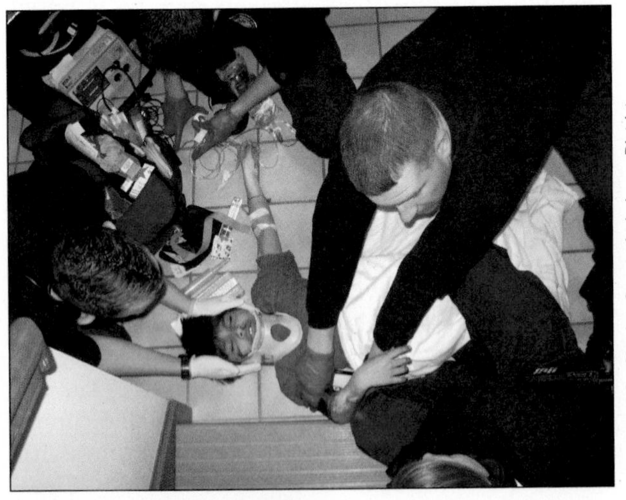

Courtesy of St. Charles County Ambulance District

Figure 18.1

It is important, when possible, to conduct simulations in an environment similar to the conditions that students will face while on the job.

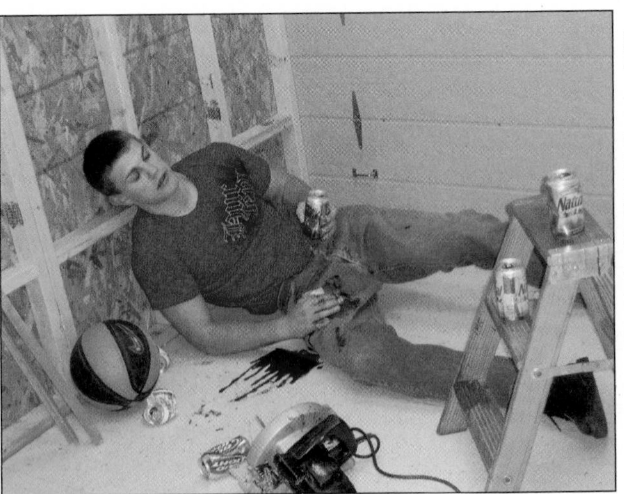

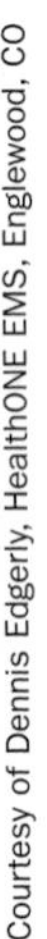

Courtesy of Dennis Edgerly, HealthONE EMS, Englewood, CO

Figure 18.2

Some creative ways to make your classroom into a simulation lab might include simple props.

allows students the experience of caring for patients and interacting in another type of environment they may be exposed to in clinical practice. In order to avoid confusion and misunderstanding on the part if the general public, it is essential that the proper people and organizations be notified when a simulation is taking place outdoors or in a public space. Designating a safety officer (a role that will be discussed in greater detail later) ensures that the public does not mistake a simulated emergency for the real thing.

Simulations can be staged in parking lots, on the grounds of colleges or hospitals, in firehouse or ambulance living quarters, and in other public spaces. This is possible with a programmed patient or, with the evolution of simulator technology, it has become possible to run a high-fidelity simulator with a laptop that communicates wirelessly with the simulator. Several simulator manufacturers for EMS education now offer wireless simulators that are developed with the intent of operations in austere environments. While caution must be taken when exposing these simulators to extreme temperatures or any type of precipitation, the advantage of these "untethered" simulators is that they can be cared for and transported just as if they were real patients, moving from the prehospital to the hospital environment without disrupting the continuity or realism of the simulation.

An alternative to the dedicated indoor simulation lab is the mobile simulation lab. Similar to a stand-alone lab, these mobile classrooms often have a mock emergency department room, or the back of an ambulance inside a large truck. These mobile Sim-labs are often supported by grant dollars and include staff to operate the specialized equipment in them. They have the added benefit of being portable, so educators can take simulation technology to areas that might not have access to such expensive equipment and resources.

While sometimes introducing more distractions, outdoor events generally provide a greater degree of difficulty—uneven terrain, weather. When conducting an outdoor simulation, consideration for the well-being of the participants is paramount. Appropriate attire, equipment, and backup plans in case the educational experience needs to be relocated are essential. Some degree of discomfort is expected, but remember Maslow's hierarchy of needs discussed in Chapter 3: Principles of Adult Learning. If a student is so uncomfortable that he or she cannot concentrate on the lesson, much of the learning may be lost.

Safety should be an overarching concern of educators when planning and conducting simulation sessions. Safety of the participants during simulation training is both psychological and physical. The student must feel comfortable enough to attempt to perform skills and receive feedback without risk of humiliation.[8] This means the educator must develop a high trust level with students. Realism and learning are enhanced by the perception, not necessarily the reality, of risk. Educators must balance that perception of risk with a need for a safe learning environment. If the student perceives that the patient care or the crew safety may suffer if a mistake is made, they will be more motivated and engaged in their learning.

Physical safety is of paramount importance. Every effort should be made to safeguard against the potential injury of a simulated patient or the crew caring for them. Simple precautions, such as the use of inert medications or specialized extrication manikins, are good practices. As simulations become more realistic, it becomes more challenging to keep the risk of injury low. After all, EMS is an inherently dangerous profession and many of the procedures and devices in EMS practice carry a high risk of injury. The educator should consider and mitigate the risks of more dangerous practices in education. It is essential, however, that EMS students practice under realistic conditions. For example, lifting a stretcher poses risk of a back injury, but graduating EMS providers who cannot perform lifts safely while still caring for patients may be of greater risk to patients and the EMS team.

All simulation sessions should include a technical and safety briefing as a part of the presimulation session. Students should be familiar with the equipment and explicitly told what tasks they are expected to perform versus verbalize. Whenever possible, a safety officer should be designated to monitor the simulation and alert participants to potential dangers **(Figure 18.3)**. Students should also be given clear direction on the lifting and moving of simulated patients and the geographical and temporal boundaries of the simulation

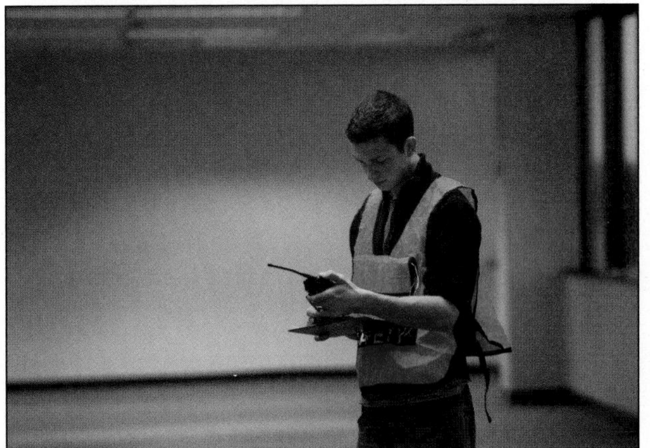

Figure 18.3

Every effort should be made to safeguard against the potential injury to simulated patient or the crew caring for them.

session. All radio traffic should include the words "this is a drill" or similar language to avoid misunderstanding of monitored radio traffic. Finally, as mentioned earlier, it is imperative that whenever a simulation session is being conducted in a public space, proper permissions have been secured and adequate notice has been given to the proper people and agencies.

Scenario

The scenario is the narrative or the story that lays the foundation for the events that will occur within the simulation. The scenario is a combination of "who, what, where, and when" that allows the learners to establish a context within which they will perform. Often the initial scenario is presented to the students in narrative form. Subsequent information, also called "injects," may be supplied by the facilitator or confederates within the simulation that allow the scenario to progress and provide information that otherwise may not be available to the students (the progression of time, X-ray or lab results).

The Scenario Template

Templates are standardized forms that can provide a framework for scenarios. These help standardize the scenario format and make it easier to quickly find key information during the simulation. While there are templates available from the major simulation companies, educators will eventually develop a system for planning, delivering, and refining simulation scenarios that work best for their students and organization. At a minimum, templates should include elements such as the following:

- Goals and objectives, tasks, conditions, and standards
- Expected time in simulation
- Dispatch information
- Patient/scenario summary
- Pertinent patient information (i.e., demographics, medical history, etc.)
- Pertinent assessment, history, and exam findings
- Setting or environment
- Required equipment or supplies
- Identified roles, if extra personnel are involved

If summative evaluation is the purpose of the simulation, the scenario template may include elements needed for evaluation, including critical interventions that are expected from the candidate.

Essential to any simulation is the narrative or story line that drives the simulation. Educators must resist the temptation to create a narrative that is too ambitious or tries to do too much in the time allotted. The story line should align with the goals and learning objectives as stated in the simulation flowchart or template. The story line is a combination of dispatch information, patient information, setting, and expected interventions. The story line (sometimes called the "narrative") is a key component to any simulation, especially a high-fidelity simulation. Story lines can be modeled after actual events to make them more realistic; however, care must be taken to not create a simulation too specific or unusual. With an established story line, anticipated "branching" or consequences should also be considered. *Branching* refers to the potential choices that the student may make, and making a preplan for the consequences of those choices. They are the "if-then" statements in a scenario that allow the person running the simulation the flexibility of responding to the actions of the students as they occur. Branching can add a level of complexity to any scenario, depending on the objectives and story line. To help the evaluator, flow-charts, matrices, or other diagrams that offer a visual map of the scenario can be created to help guide the correct pathway for decisions. Finally, the simulation narrative must be realistic and believable. While it is tempting to make a simulation epic in scale and proportion, the educator must have a clear understanding of the physical, material, financial, and human capital limitations that exist within his or her organization.

While there are many commercially developed simulation scenarios available for the EMS educator, there is a great value in customizing a simulation to meet the needs of the students as they exist for a specific cohort or group. The creation of a good simulation scenario is a combination of lesson plan, short story, and evaluation tool. As a result, the creation of a customized scenario can be very time consuming. EMS educators should consider incorporating a mixture of commercially available and custom-made simulation scenarios into their curriculum.

As mentioned before, the simulation scenario can range from the very simple to the very complex, depending on many factors, including the goals and outcomes, the abilities of the students, and the resources available.

Standardized Patients

Often forgotten as EMS educators integrate simulation technology into their teaching is the invaluable role that role players or **standardized patients** play in the simulated environment. Live patients are ideal for scenarios in which the students need to interact with their patients. In some ways the standardized patient is the ultimate simulator. Educators should integrate the use of these actors into all aspects of the learning experience. However, just as preparation and organization are key in the use of simulations, they are also essential when using human patients in the simulated environment. Actors should be carefully selected, thoroughly trained, and adequately briefed on their roles and responsibilities. A script or a series of "if-then" prompts should be provided to the actors so that they may respond in a uniform and consistent manner when interacting with the students in the simulated environment.

The simulated scenario dictates the types of standardized patients that are appropriate. Elderly patients, patients with pre-existing medical conditions (irregular heartbeat, mastectomy, amputee), and patients representing different ethnic and racial backgrounds provide the students with the ability to interact in a realistic manner with patients who are representative of the diversity of the population as a whole. Former students can greatly enhance the perceived reality, based on their own experiences of managing similar patients or having gone through the simulated scenario before. When attempting a larger scale simulation, such as a mass-casualty incident, reaching out to community groups is a great way to secure patients. The use of children as standardized patients can have a great benefit in that it exposes the students to the pediatric population. When considering the use of children, EMS educators should consider the relevant legal and safety aspects, as these differ from region to region.

Simulation is about creating events that are plausible and realistic in order to give the student the feeling of actually managing an actual event. One of the advantages of using standardized patients is that it allows the learner to experience and the educator to evaluate the affective domain. The real-time interaction and the ability for the student to form a relationship and have meaningful exchanges with the patient are some of the greatest benefits of the standardized patient in the simulated EMS environment. Standardized patient feedback to the student is another advantage. Balancing that, however, is the limitation on the ability to perform certain skills and assessments on the standardized patient. The greatest benefit of the high-fidelity simulator is and will probably always be the ability to perform high-acuity, low-frequency skills in an environment where the errors and mistakes that characterize learning will not have a negative impact on the well-being of the patient.

Recent research has shown that the use of simulation enhances teamwork and may improve patient and provider safety in the field.[9,10,11] The importance of this cannot be overstated. Behavior that is modeled in the classroom will result in changes in the field.[12,13,14] Educators who integrate simulation, balancing high- and low-fidelity simulators with standardized patients, will create in their students a culture of teamwork and collaboration that has been shown to enhance patient safety and reduce errors.

Teaching Tip >> *A culture of safety in the classroom and laboratory can continue with students to their field practice and serve them well.*

Timeframe

The time frame should include the anticipated time that will be spent in simulation and the time that will be needed to conduct a debriefing. If the EMS educator plans running the same simulation multiple times consecutively, he or she must also plan time to reset the scenario. This can be a time-consuming process, as equipment must be disassembled and repackaged and computer programs reset. While there is no rigid rule, a good guideline is to allow twice as much time for debriefing as will be spent in simulation. A 20-minute simulation session should allow for 40 minutes to debrief. If adequate personnel exist, the resetting of the simulation can occur simultaneously with the debriefing session.

Participants

It is essential to identify the target audience for which the simulation is intended. A simulated chest pain patient created for the EMT student will involve different learner outcomes, tasks, and patient progressions than one created for the paramedic student. In addition to the level of the respondent, it is helpful for the EMS educator to know where in their education the students are. There will be different outcomes and expectations for the beginner student as opposed to the student near the end of his or her education.

Equipment and Setup

Simulation includes various amounts and types of equipment; as a result, to ensure familiarity with equipment, facilitators and participants should go through an orientation checklist that identifies the nuances of the scenario. If not completed and familiarized with the nuances, the flow of the scenario can be interrupted or halted, decreasing the value and experience of the simulation.

When conducting simulation, every effort should be made to provide all the patient care equipment required to work through the simulation. The less the student has to imagine or verbalize, the more realistic the scenario. If students going through the simulation are unfamiliar with the patient care equipment, ample time should be allowed for the students to familiarize themselves before they work through the scenario.

"Moulage" (from the French word "to mold") is an important component to increase realism in simulation **(Figure 18.4)**. Both standardized patients and manikins can be moulaged to change appearances or show various types of trauma (bruising, open fractures, burns). Moulaging patients and manikins takes time, but is essential to realism. A moulage kit may include makeup, brushes and sponges, adhesives, mortician's wax or plumber's putty, and latex parts.

Simulation can be hard on manikins and careful attention should be paid to the maintenance—especially on common wear-and-tear items, such as IV arms, surgical airway necks, and intraosseous (IO) limbs. Having students wear gloves keeps the manikins cleaner. Replacement skin and parts are available from manufacturers.

High-tech manikins are controlled by computers and are capable of modeling the wide range of physiological states of adults, infants, and children and replicate complex disease processes and injury patterns. This allows students to experience a broad range of patient presentations and practice a wide range of sophisticated and invasive procedures, such as chest decompression, medication administration, and surgical cricothyrotomy without the risks associated with practicing on human patients.[15,16] These high-fidelity simulators can display realistic assessment findings, including heart and lung sounds, cardiac rhythm disturbances, and other vital sign alterations. They are capable of responding to student interventions in a realistic manner, including airway management and medication administration. From the origins of simulation technology with the earliest CPR and airway manikins to today's high fidelity simulators capable of realistic oxygen/carbon dioxide exchange, simulation in health care has proven to be a rapidly evolving industry with this technology having been proven highly effective in achieving EMS educational goals.[5,17,18]

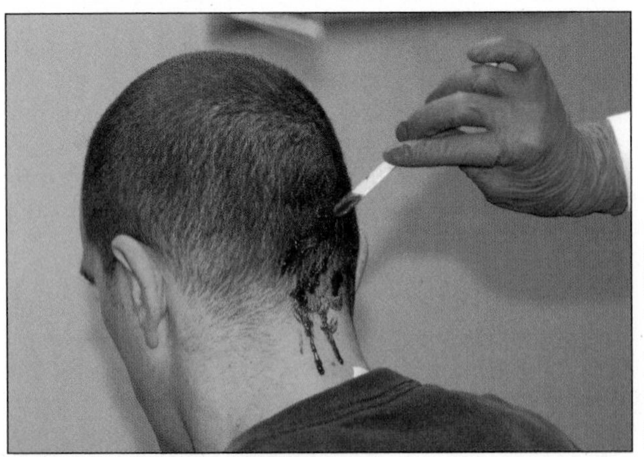

Figure 18.4

Moulage is an important component to increasing realism in simulation.

This sophisticated technology can be very costly.[19] Simulators and task-trainers (isolated body parts that allow students to practice specific psychomotor tasks) can run from four to six figures in cost. Other costs can include parts, maintenance contracts, employee training, and hardware and infrastructure that allow educators to use the simulators in their learning environment. Oftentimes one of the most expensive costs is the investment an institution or organization must make in human capital—investing funds and time for the personnel to maintain, create, and facilitate learning experiences in the simulated environment. Unfortunately, the human resources and time required to preprogram and operate the simulators is often underestimated. It is not uncommon for simulation programs to suffer serious setbacks when the simulation champion leaves the institution, taking with him or her invaluable simulation expertise and knowledge. To make an active simulation lab fully operational, many institutions hire full-time technicians or other personnel.[19,20,21]

Setup of the simulation is crucial to delivering a quality scenario. In order to do so, clear and concise instructions for facilitators, patients, and participants is key to success. Instructions for facilitators need to help guide the facilitator as the simulation evolves and can indicate when intervention by the facilitator is necessary. When using standardized patients, instructions should include limits on what participants and patients can and cannot do. Explicit instructions are needed on how the patient should react to certain questions or lines of treatments, and how they should interact with their environment during the scenario. Instructions for students should be minimal, giving students only enough direction on how to manage the patient(s) and what they are permitted and not permitted to do.

Ground rules for the simulation are another important aspect of the setup phase. These ground rules include a "fiction contract" and expectations. The *fiction contract* is an agreement between the instructor and the student to make the simulation real. The contract can be explicit or implicit, but should be clearly communicated and understood by both the instructor and student.

Expectations of the simulation and consequences of any evaluation also need to be communicated to the students. Students need to understand what is expected of them and how they are to perform during the simulation.[22] During a briefing of the students, the expectations can be reviewed and clarified. It is important to note that briefing the students should be conducted away from the simulation setting and patient(s). This helps to preserve the "realness" of the simulation.

Endpoints and Evaluation

During the simulation, the facilitator assumes the role of the silent observer whenever possible. The facilitator's role is to facilitate the natural progression of the simulation by injecting information and coordinating actions with the technician (in the event that he or she is not also functioning as the technician) to provide a realistic simulation experience that allows the learners to suspend disbelief and immerse themselves in the simulation environment.

Simulation should move toward a specified end point or conclusion. This could be identified as the specified physiological presentation or patient status, or it could be when a certain set of objectives or learner outcomes are (or are not) realized or achieved. Allowing enough time for the student to attempt performance, even if he or she seems to struggle, is important, as valuable learning and confidence building can occur. If the student or team exhibits signs of extreme struggle or frustration, then careful mid-scenario guiding may be appropriate, or ultimately stopping the simulation in favor of a more productive debriefing.

Prompting during a simulation should be kept to a minimum, but may be needed to continue the evolution. The amount of necessary prompts depends on the type of simulation being conducted (formative vs. summative). Limited prompting is an important part of the learning process as it forces the student to apply critical-reasoning and problem-solving skills, which is one of the major goals and benefits of simulation.

It has been shown that safety can be enhanced by using checklists during and after the scenario to ensure key points are discussed.[23] Checklists to score scenario performance have been used by the American Heart Association (AHA) for Advanced Cardiac Life Support protocols since 2003. Using the checklists in simulation-based education showed a 40 percent increase in adherence to AHA protocols after training, and an improvement in performance in simulation and patient care.[24]

Debriefing

The debriefing period can be one of the most beneficial components of the simulation experience, both for the student and the educator.[23] During the debriefing session,students are given the opportunity to examine, reflect on, and discuss the simulation experience. Because simulation challenges the students' perspectives or preconceived ideas on how the situation should have been managed, learning is facilitated. During the debriefing, instructors should promote students' reflections on action and inaction as they are key components of the experiential learning. While the simulation itself may have been rich in content and experience, without a thorough and purposeful debriefing much of the learning may be lost.[24,25]

To enhance the debriefing experience, educators may opt to use recording devices to capture the elements or the entirety of the simulation.[26] The use of video, audio, and vitals-sign-display when recording simulation sessions can provide valuable detailed feedback to students after the simulation. These tools can also help facilitate the self-reflection process. Students at times may not be able to accurately recall all the events of the simulation, or may alter their own perceptions of what actually occurred.

To help students recognize the learning points that arise from the simulation, self-reflection on the events of the simulation should be encouraged of the students who participated. Self-reflection provides students the opportunity to consider their actions and inactions, and how they fit into the overall picture of the simulation.[27] Providing students this opportunity prepares them for events they may encounter in the future when out in the field.

Since simulation is about learning to manage and treat actual cases, applying the lessons learned during the simulation to similar events can facilitate understanding by the students.[28]

Summary

Simulation in EMS education can have a positive impact on the critical decision-making skills, psychomotor skills, and emotions and attitudes of students. Learning occurs when students are faced with a "crisis," which then forces them to alter their frame of understanding and think critically about their actions.[2, 29–34] These feelings should be addressed during the debriefing phase of the simulation.

In the early sixteenth century, manikins (referred to as "phantoms") were used to teach obstetrical skills to physicians in an attempt to reduce the number of women and infants who died during childbirth. Simulation in EMS education today traces its roots to the aviation industry and draws inspiration from disciplines and fields where expertise is required in responding to low-frequency, high-acuity events.

Proper planning, preparation, facilitation, and debriefing are all essential elements of simulation. Each is important to assure that students have a meaningful, safe, learning-simulation experience that promotes key learning objectives. Simulation experiences are another tool to advance student learning within the EMS setting.

Simulation allows EMS educators to standardize the learning experience with a uniform and consistent method of evaluating competency. While students and health professionals in training are required to meet the same criteria for performance and competence, the variable nature of health care and the unique presentation and dynamic of any patient care interaction or situation make it very difficult to measure competence or success based on performance in the clinical environment. Simulation enables educators to gather objective evidence of performance and map the learner's "trajectory"[30] with a great degree of detail and specificity. In a simulated environment, errors can be tracked and the simulation be repeatedly "rewound and restarted"[31] until proficiency is achieved. The ability to standardize the learning experience also enables the educator or institution to evaluate its processes and teaching methodology.[32]

Glossary

debriefing A postevent discussion and evaluation.

high-fidelity manikins Use of sophisticated technology to simulate realistic human physiology such as oxygen/carbon dioxide exchange.

scenarios An outline or plot of a patient situation or projected sequence of patient events.

simulation A type of experiential learning designed to mimic, as closely as possible, the real context.

standardized patient A prepared actor who simulates a patient.

template A standardized form that can provide a framework for scenarios.

References

1. McGaghie, W. C. (2010, January 1). A critical review of simulation-based medical education research: 2003–2009. *Medical Education, 44*(1): 50–63.
2. McLaughlin, M. P. (2010). Medical simulation in the community college health science curriculum: A matrix for future implementation. *Community College Journal of Research and Practice, 34*, 462–276. doi: 10.1080/10668920903235811
3. DeGiusti, M. R., Lira, A. J., & Villareal, G. L. (2008). Simulation framework for teaching in modeling and simulation areas. *European Journal of Engineering Education, 33*(5–6): 587–596.
4. Schneider Sarver, P. A., Senczakowicz, E. A., Murphy Slovensky, B. (2010). Development of simulation scenarios for an adolescent patient with diabetic ketoacidosis. *Journal of Nursing Education, 49*(10): 578–586.
5. King, J. M. (2011, March 1). Teaching advanced cardiac life support protocols: The effectiveness of static versus high-fidelity simulation. *Nurse Educator, 36*(2): 62–65.
6. Wotton, K., Davis, J., Button, D., & Kelton, M. (2010). Third-year undergraduate nursing students' perceptions of high-fidelity simulation. *Journal of Nursing Education, 49*(11): 632–639.
7. Nehring, W. M., & Lashley, F. R. (2010). High-fidelity patient simulation in nursing education. Burlington, MA: Jones and Bartlett Publishers.
8. Blum, C. A., Borglund, S., & Parcells, D. (2010). High-fidelity nursing simulation: Impact on student self-confidence and clinical competence. *International Journal of Nursing Education, 7*(1): Art. 18: 1–14.

9. Kozmenko, V. (2008, January 1). Initial implementation of mixed reality simulation targeting teamwork and patient safety. *Stud Health Technol Inform, 132*: 216–221.

10. Herzer, K. R. (2009, February 1). A practical framework for patient care teams to prospectively identify and mitigate clinical hazards. *The Joint Commission Journal on Quality and Patient Safety, 35*(2): 72–81.

11. American College of Chest Physicians (2008, July). Improving handoff communications in critical care: Utilizing simulation-based training toward process improvement in managing patient risk. *Chest,* Vol. 134, Issue 1.

12. Wayne, D. B., Butter, J., Siddall, V. J., *et al.* (2006). Mastery learning of advanced cardiac life support skills by internal medicine residents using simulation technology and deliberate practice. *Journal General Internal Medicine, 21*:251–256.

13. Batchelder, A. J. (2009, September 1). Simulation as a tool to improve the safety of prehospital anaesthesia: A pilot study. *Anaesthesia, 64*(9): 978–983.

14. Rosenthal, M. E., Adachi, M., Ribaudo, V., *et al.* (2006). Achieving housestaff competence in emergency airway management using scenario-based simulation training. *Chest, 129*: 1453–1458.

15. Chandra, D. B. (2008, December 1). Fiberoptic oral intubation: The effect of model fidelity on training for transfer to patient care. *Anesthesiology, 109*(6): 1007–1013.

16. Cooper, J. B. (2010, January 1). Simulation training and assessment: A more efficient method to develop expertise than apprenticeship. *Anesthesiology, 112*(1): 8–9.

17. Gillett, B. (2008, November 1). Simulation in a disaster drill: Comparison of high-fidelity simulators versus trained actors. *Academic Emergency Medicine, 15*(11): 1144–1151.

18. Fritz, P. Z. (2008, February 1). Review of mannequin-based high-fidelity simulation in emergency medicine. *Emergency Medicine Australasia, 20*(1): 1–9.

19. Weinstock, P. H. (2009, March 1). Simulation at the point of care: Reduced-cost, in situ training via a mobile cart. *PediatrCrit Care Med, 10*(2): 176–181.

20. Tuoriniemi, P. (2008, March 1). Implementing a high-fidelity simulation program in a community college setting. *Nursing Education Perspective, 29*(2): 105–109.

21. Parker, B. C. (2009, April 1). A critical examination of high-fidelity human patient simulation within the context of nursing pedagogy. *Nurse Education Today, 29*(3): 322–329.

22. Simones, J., Wilcox, J., Scott, K., Doeden, D., Copley, D., Doetkott, R., & Kippley, M. (2010). Collaborative simulation project to teach scope of practice. *Journal of Nursing Education, 49*(4), 190–197.

23. Anderson, P. O., Jensen, M. K., Lippert, A., Østergaard, D., & Klausen, T. W. (2010). Development of a formative assessment tool for measurement of performance in multi-professional resuscitation teams. *Resuscitation, 81*: 703–711.

24. Elfrink, V. L., Kirkpatrick, B., Nininger, J., & Schubert, C. (2010). Using learning outcomes to inform teaching practices in human patient simulation. *Nursing Education Perspective. 31*(2): 97–100.

25. Carlson, J., Tomkowiak, J., & Knott, P. (2010). Simulation-based examinations in physician assistant education: A comparison of two standard-setting methods. *Journal of Physician Assistant Education, 21*(2): 7–14.

26. Leonard, B., Shuhaibar, E. L. H., & Chen, R. (2010). Nursing-student perceptions of intraprofessional team education using high-fidelity simulation. *Journal of Nursing Education, 49*(11): 628–631.

27. Birkhoff, S. D., Donner, C. (2010). Enhancing pediatric clinical competency with high-fidelity simulation. *Journal of Continuing Education in Nursing, 41*(9): 418–423.

28. Harder, B. N. (2010). Use of simulation in teaching and learning in health sciences: A systematic review. *Journal of Nursing Education, 49*(1): 23–28.

29. Parker, B., Myrick, F. (2010). Transformative learning as a context for human patient simulation. *Journal of Nursing Education, 49*(6): 326–332.

30. Kneebone, R. (2003). Simulation in surgical training: Educational issues and practical implications. *Medical Education, 37*: 267–277.

31. Dawson, S. (2002). A critical approach to medical simulation. *Bulletin of the American College of Surgeons, 87*(11): 12–18.

32. Hammond, J., Bermann, M., Chen, B., & Kushins, L. (2002). Incorporation of a computerized human patient simulator in critical care training: A preliminary report. *Journal of Trauma, 53*: 1064–1067.

19

Tools for Field and Clinical Learning

Experience develops all our great flute players, but also unfortunately, all our worst players. — PLATO

Clinical education is an essential component of Emergency Medical Services (EMS) education, and the clinical educator may be the most influential teacher an EMS student will ever have. For the purposes of this chapter, the term "clinical educator" refers to all those persons who guide **experiential learning**, including mentors, preceptors, and training officers.

The goals of effective clinical educators are to help transition a student from the theoretical environment of the classroom to the real world of patient care delivery. In addition to being a role model—demonstrating excellent clinical skills and behavior—the clinical educator must be able to recognize and take advantage of opportunities for the student to try a skill, or glean the right lesson from existing circumstances. These are so called "teachable moments" that create long-lasting retention of student learning.

Both employers and patients expect graduates of EMS educational programs to be competent health care providers. Theoretical knowledge and abstract skill performance, although important, are simply not sufficient to prepare someone to work in the hospital or field environment. EMS students, especially paramedic students, must perform as team members and team leaders during real patient care situations if they are to gain a reasonable level of competency and confidence in their abilities.

The previous chapters of this text have focused on more traditional educational models and general instructional methods. These theories and strategies are applicable to all types of instruction, and the clinical educator should take time to become familiar with them.

CHAPTER GOAL: This chapter explores instructional theory and strategy focusing specifically on clinical education, that is, education that is *experiential* and involves the student's observing, participating in, or leading patient care activities in actual hospital or field patient care settings.

Clinical Education

Clinical education in EMS is usually performed under the supervision of an experienced clinician who facilitates learning while still being responsible for patient care. The educator must balance the educational needs for the student while still being an advocate for good patient care.

Clinical or patient care experience for the EMS student most often is acquired in a hospital emergency department (ED) and on an emergency ambulance, although certainly nonemergency clinical areas can provide excellent learning opportunities. For the purposes of this chapter, the term "field clinical" or "field experience" refers to prehospital or outdoor experiences, which may be primarily observation or doing isolated skills as directed by the EMS personnel on the ambulance; "hospital clinical" refers to experiences in a hospital, clinic, or other indoor setting; "field internship" or "preceptorship" is a planned, scheduled educational experience on an advanced life-support unit which includes team-leading skills and the management of prehospital patients and scenes. *Preceptors* are individuals who teach in the hospital or field clinical setting. The Committee on Accreditation of EMS Professions (CoAEMSP) uses this term frequently in their documents and the term will be used in this chapter as well.

The type and scope of clinical experiences vary according to the level of education. Clinical education for entry-level EMS providers, such as Emergency Medical Technician (EMT) or Emergency Medical Responder (EMR) students, is usually limited in scope, objectives, and time. EMT clinical experience often involves observation in a hospital ED or a handful of ride-along shifts on an ambulance. At more advanced levels, such as Advanced EMT (AEMT) or paramedic education, students may perform clinical rotations in a wide variety of hospital departments and health care settings. Specialized units within hospitals, such as operating rooms, cardiac units, cardiac catheterization labs, psychiatric crisis units, burn care units, obstetric departments, and intensive care units are common at this level. Advanced field clinical rotations or internships may also involve experiences with critical care transport teams, law enforcement officers, fire or rescue personnel, other EMS-related service providers, and, on some occasions, air ambulance services. Some programs use innovative and nontraditional settings, such as homeless shelters, skilled nursing and geriatric care facilities, pediatric clinics, immunization outreach programs, and morgues, where students can gain a unique perspective **(Figure 19.1)**.

Experiential Learning

Experiential learning is an educational philosophy that best describes the essence of clinical education. This philosophy is based largely on the original work of John Dewey, with later refinements by the German philosopher Kurt Hahn. At the core of this philosophy of education is the idea that learning begins with an experience. A particular circumstance may require an action on the part of the student, or it may simply be an observation of an action. Once it has been completed or the situation has been resolved, the student reflects on the experience, and with the assistance of a facilitator, draws meaningful lessons from his or her observations, actions, and reflections.

The goal of traditional didactic education in the classroom is for students to demonstrate a practical understanding of the knowledge imparted to them. In class, the student's role may be somewhat passive, although the student is encouraged to be attentive and to participate in class activities. In skills labs, the student is expected to practice and perform step-by-step procedures after they have been properly demonstrated and rehearsed in a linear manner, usually under ideal conditions.[1–4] Less controlled and sometimes frenetic clinical experiences are often left until the final stages of the educational process. Because the quantity and quality of learning during the clinical phase can be unpredictable, clinical education has been sometimes viewed as less valuable than other methods of instruction.[2]

Recently several studies have demonstrated that exposure to patient contacts, especially those that involved advanced life support, increase critical thinking and are directly correlated to successful first time pass rates on the National Registry of EMTs paramedic cognitive (written) exam.[5–9]

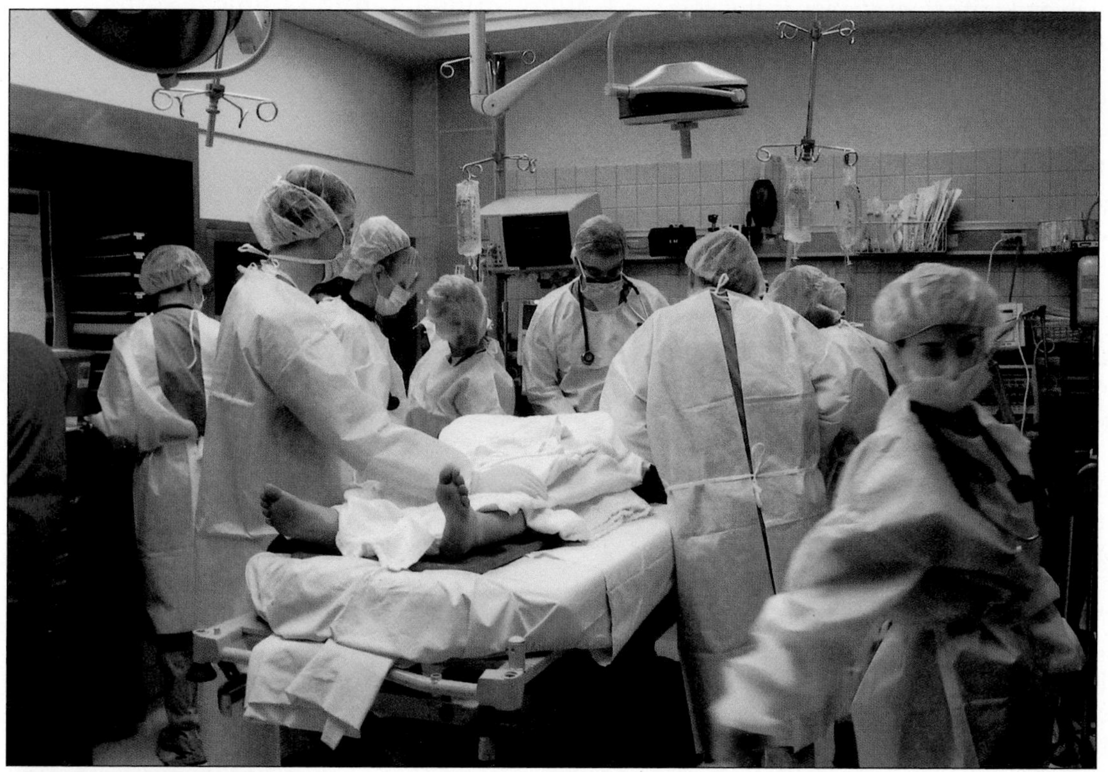

Figure 19.1

Some programs use innovative and nontraditional settings for clinical experience where students can gain a unique perspective.

Participation in clinical education in EMS, however, is also an important step toward the development of confident and competent graduates.[10,11] Unlike the traditional classroom, the "real world" of clinical education requires that students be assertive, take initiative, and eventually direct others to perform tasks.[3] They must be able to assess patients and circumstances, analyze conflicting information, perform technical skills, apply acquired knowledge, and exhibit professional attributes. This requires that the students perform at higher levels of intellectual functioning.[2] Therefore, the importance of an effective clinical-education program for EMS students cannot be overstated.

In clinical education, experience is the catalyst for learning. In the course of treating patients, the student is actively engaging most, if not all, of his or her senses. The student is also immersed in a complex set of thoughts, actions, reactions, and evaluations. Reflecting on these experiences builds a library of knowledge that will help him or her identify similar patterns of disease and injury. This knowledge will aid EMS students to effectively assess and treat future patients.[10]

Experience alone, however, does not necessarily inspire learning. To be educationally sound, experiences should be carefully structured around specific learning goals and should include appropriate orientation, preparation, and critical evaluation.[12] It is the role of the clinical educator to provide background information, to ensure that experiences are put into context, to answer questions, and to direct further learning or review. A proper foundation, combined with timely communication, helps the student to organize learning and makes him or her aware of the fact that learning has just taken place.[3]

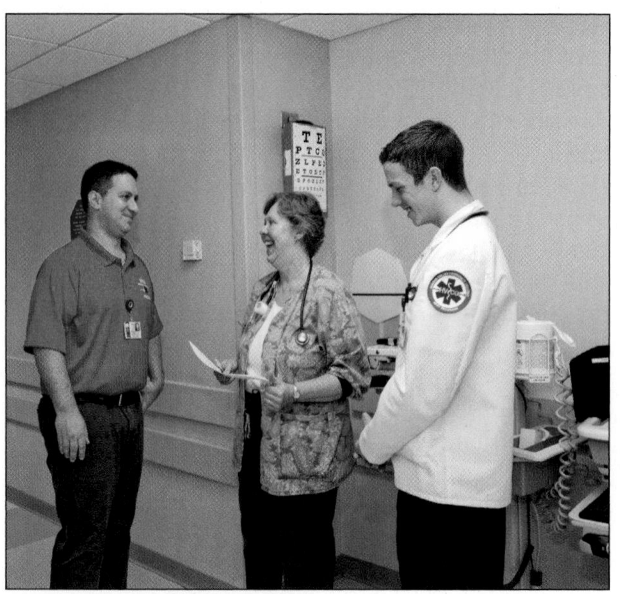

Figure 19.2

Clinical educators must create positive and professional interpersonal relationships with students.

The Effective Clinical Educator

The clinical educator or preceptor, beyond playing a central role during experience-based learning,[13,14] is a role model for students and is seen as an expert in the field.

Above all, clinical educators must create positive and professional interpersonal relationships with students **(Figure 19.2)**. They must lead by example and respect students, display confidence in them, show genuine interest in what they do, and encourage mutual respect. The personal attributes of an educator that promote learning include enthusiasm, patience, friendliness, a sense of humor, flexibility in the clinical setting, and a willingness to honestly admit limitations or mistakes.

Tips for Effective Communication with Students in the Clinical Setting

- Introduce yourself, and use your name.
- Use your students' names.
- Make and maintain eye contact.
- Listen actively, providing verbal and nonverbal cues that you are following the conversation.
- Clarify what is being said by paraphrasing key points and checking to make sure that you understand the communication.
- Do not assume that you understand the student's words or actions until you have heard all of the facts or asked questions that confirm your understanding.
- Watch for context: Most communication is paraverbal (tone, pitch, pace, and power) and nonverbal (behavior, gestures, and actions).
- Do not try to solve problems or give advice; instead, help students explore options to help themselves.
- If you feel that your own feelings are clouding your ability to stay calm and communicate effectively, then take a break and return to the interaction when you are prepared to place students' needs above your own.

Attributes of Effective Clinical Teachers[13,14]

Effective clinical teachers:

1. Create an environment that is conducive to learning with the following:
   - Knowledge of the practice area
   - Clinical competency
   - A desire to teach
2. Are supportive of learners; such support requires the following:
   - Knowledge of the learners
   - Knowledge of the practice area
   - Mutual respect
3. Possess teaching skills that maximize student learning; this requires the following abilities:
   - Diagnose student needs
   - Learn about students as individuals, including their needs, personalities, and capabilities
4. Foster independence so that students learn how to learn;
5. Encourage exploration and questions without penalty;
6. Accept differences among students;
7. Relate how clinical experiences facilitate the development of clinical competency;
8. Practice effective communication and questioning skills;
9. Serve as a role model with excellent clinical skills;
10. Enjoy practice and teaching;
11. Are friendly, approachable, understanding, enthusiastic, and confident about teaching;
12. Are knowledgeable about the subject matter and able to convey that knowledge to students in their practice areas;
13. Exhibit fairness and objectivity in evaluation;
14. Provide frequent feedback and positive reinforcement.

Research shows that student learning is enhanced significantly when clinical educators are skilled at using teaching objectives, able to ask appropriate questions, and willing to provide specific and timely feedback. Additionally, formal preparation and instruction for clinical educators on how to teach in the clinical setting have proved to correlate with better student achievement.[14]

Field Preceptor Job Requirements and Training

For the purposes of this section, the *preceptor* is the clinical educator in the field setting who is working directly with EMS students. Although all levels of EMS students can benefit from clinical and field preceptors, most of the emphasis in EMS clinical education is placed on the AEMT or paramedic-level provider. In fact, the presumption is that if a preceptor can facilitate education for paramedic students, he or she is also qualified to teach EMT students. This may seem logical, but it remains one of the enduring myths of EMS. Providers such as EMRs and EMTs have needs and expectations different from those of advanced-level providers. Paramedic preceptors who usually provide training to entry-level students may not be aware of the needs of providers who practice at the EMR or EMT level. This phenomenon diminishes the advanced provider's oversight value, unless the preceptor is first tutored in the training needs and protocols of EMR or EMT caregivers in the area.

Many EMS programs are measured by the capabilities of their preceptors. Just as with any other educational setting, high standards in both clinical skills and teaching strategies are to be expected. Programs should regularly evaluate performance and develop the skills of preceptors.

Preceptor Job Requirements

A clinical educator for any type of EMS student acts as a role model, and a preceptor's clinical knowledge and patient care skills—including the ability to establish patient rapport—should be carefully screened and evaluated. A preceptor candidate who will be overseeing interns new to advanced life support (ALS) should probably have at least one to two years of concentrated field experience at the level he or she is precepting. Preceptor candidates who will be evaluating interns with previous ALS field experience should probably have at least three to four years of concentrated field experience. It should not be assumed that an expert in ALS or the best-liked employee would make a good clinical educator. The preceptor candidate must be able to deal constructively with adult learners. He or she needs to view interns as active learners with whom the instructor will collaborate to solve problems; they must be seen as students who will require guidance regarding actions of human beings during a crisis, and who will need help to understand how to apply ALS protocols to specific situations.

The following is a list of qualifications exhibited by strong candidates for preceptor-training programs:

- Significant field experience (measured by numbers of emergency patients seen, as well as time spent at the provider level)
- Demonstrated ability to work with people who are learning (not the same skill as caring for patients)
- Experience with planning educational events
- Supervisory and/or critical-incident stress-management training
- Experience or training in conflict management, negotiations, quality improvement, and similar subjects
- Awareness of current EMS research literature and of the value of clinical and educational research (candidate reads current journals and literature, participates in an EMS journal club, attends regional or national conferences, values continuing education)

If available potential preceptor candidates do not possess any of these qualifications, then a different approach should be used for evaluation. For example, a teaching demonstration in front of a select panel or an appropriate audience might prove to be a useful evaluation tool. The candidate should also be observed while providing patient care and interacting with other responders and the public. Potential preceptors should be evaluated on calls rather than by talking with them about responses. Informal and formal interviews should focus on the candidate's attitudes toward and expectations regarding the role of clinical educator.

Role of the Clinical Educator

Through effective hospital and field clinical instruction, didactic knowledge and practical skills are reinforced by experience, which helps to prepare the student to become a competent entry-level clinician.[10]

In general, the role of the clinical educator or preceptor is to do the following:

- Size up the needs of the student.
- Assist the student in creating a plan to facilitate learning.
- Help the student put theoretical knowledge into practice.
- Extend knowledge and learning by relating experience to general theory.
- Promote skills development.
- Promote professionalism.
- Provide feedback to learners about progress toward goals and objectives in the clinical area.
- Be responsive to the needs and concerns of other clinical staff.
- Evaluate, document, and report student progress and achievement.[2]
- Promptly report concerns to program if significant performance or behavior issues occur.

The clinical educator has a particularly challenging role in EMS education. In addition to regular patient care duties, either in the hospital or in the field, the clinical educator must balance the needs of the student with the needs of the patient, bystanders, family members, support staff, and coworkers **(Figure 19.3)**.

By definition, students are not as skilled or competent as the clinical staff with whom they are working. The clinical educator must be willing to allow a student to attempt procedures and other patient care duties. This requires the ability to recognize any opportunity to do so and to perform a quick analysis of the risks to the patient versus the benefits to the

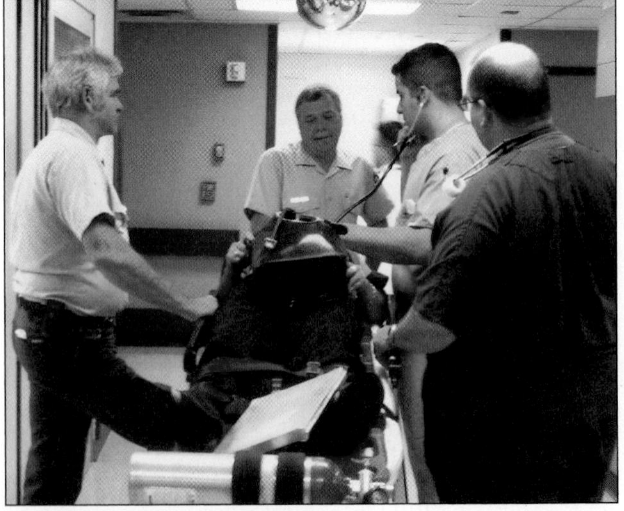

Figure 19.3

The clinical educator must balance the instructional needs of the student with the needs of the patient, bystanders, family members, support staff, and coworkers.

CASE IN POINT

In the early stages of a clinical education, a student's performance may be unpredictable when he or she is attempting new skills. In this stage, the clinical educator should be authoritative and should ask the student to focus on specific objectives before the student encounters them in the next patient. For example, if a student is having difficulty obtaining a patient history, the instructor should try to have the student focus solely on creating a conversation with the next patient. An objective should be introduced for the student to simply introduce himself or herself, then to elicit the patient's name, chief complaint, and history. As the student successfully completes this task with the first patient, the instructor can add additional objectives for the next patient contact, such as obtaining a history from a family member or bystander. Giving feedback and building on small successes increases the student's level of confidence.

student. An effective clinical educator can turn a nonemergent, superficial dog bite into a fascinating description of the importance of infection control, proper wound irrigation and dressing, the mechanism of healing, recognition of rabies or sepsis, and variations in animal and human bites.

More importantly, clinical educators must have enough seniority and trust from coworkers to transfer patient care authority to the student. Eager and well-meaning staff members or EMTs wanting to perform rapid and efficient care can present an unintended barrier to student learning. Experienced clinical educators know to discuss the educational plan with other staff members, whenever possible, before a patient encounter. Students should be identified by a school badge, a distinctive uniform, or a patch reading "EMT Student" or "Paramedic Intern" so as to minimize confusion, particularly when advanced procedures are being performed.

The clinical educator should try to remain in the background as much as possible, seeming to carry on a casual social conversation, or quietly getting a private report from EMTs, family members, and other interested parties for the purpose of creating some space and time for the student to function. At the same time, a seasoned clinical educator should be able to keep an ear and a watchful eye on the student's performance. However, at times, education must be sacrificed in favor of patient care. Then, the role of the clinical educator is to help students reflect on events to find valuable learning points in their observations and in the actions of others.

It is recommended that students make the transition from the role of observer to practitioner, and finally, in the field to team leader.[10] Clinical educators must seek out opportunities for students to function at the level of their current abilities and to develop higher-level abilities. In some cases, students may be able to lead uncomplicated patient encounters, but they may function only as team members in situations that are more complex. The clinical educator must be keenly aware of students' strengths, weaknesses, current capabilities, previous successes, and ongoing challenges.

The clinical educator also plays a key role in reducing high levels of student stress. Evidence suggests that students experience significant stress and anxiety during clinical education.[2,14–16] Performance anxiety can be a serious barrier to achievement when students are unable to concentrate or receive and process information. Although stress and anxiety are common in emergency health care, the clinical educator should be able to recognize when a student's fear is actually preventing learning or inhibiting performance. Once this is recognized, the clinical educator should take steps to create a less-threatening environment, and should focus the student on specific tasks that will serve to build self-confidence.

Steps to help Reduce Student Anxiety[15]

1. Establish a safe relationship.
   - Be empathetic.
   - Deal with mistakes calmly.
   - Emphasize positives.
   - Remember that a trusting relationship takes time to build.
   - Be honest.
2. Build self-esteem.
3. Confront the problem (talk about the anxiety).
4. Draw from the student's past coping mechanisms.
5. If the student appears blocked, give specific direction.
6. Set strict limitations (insist that the student attempt or try to perform).
7. Divide tasks into smaller parts.
8. Set realistic expectations.

CASE IN POINT

A student is embarrassed about removing the shirt of a patient of the opposite sex. Each time this student is supposed to check the patient's breath sounds, he or she hesitates, then moves on to history-gathering questions. This is a case of anxiety masquerading as poor performance. Even though five minutes before the patient contact, the student perfectly described how to obtain breath sounds, the student is paralyzed at the instant of unbuttoning the patient's shirt.

The clinical educator is the best person to help the student get past the overwhelming feelings that are paralyzing him or her. The clinical educator should assist students by first identifying the fear, then rehearsing what he or she will say and do with a mock patient, such as a classmate or a patient that is not threatening. A good strategy is to take "baby steps." The student can be coached to listen to breath sounds through the shirt at first, then coached to raise the back of the shirt only; finally, once the student is more comfortable, he or she can begin removing the shirt altogether while taking steps to preserve the patient's modesty.

Clinical Teaching Strategies

Performance expectations of students at the end of their EMS clinical experiences are high, particularly for paramedic students. In a relatively short amount of time—as little as one to six months—students are expected to observe, practice, and direct field emergency care. Entry-level competency requires that the student master the building blocks of assessment, recognize pathophysiology in actual patients, demonstrate motor skills in adverse circumstances, and exhibit professional behavior in stressful situations. The clinical educator should help students move quickly through the learning process without overwhelming them. The following sections focus on strategies that are specific to clinical teaching and that complement previously discussed teaching techniques.

Do as I Do: Actions Speak Louder than Words

One of the most effective clinical teaching techniques is the consistent modeling of the behavior or skill that is being asked of the student.[2] When the instructor demonstrates the professionalism, technical aptitude, and leadership that are expected, a student learns by observing and emulating behavior. An educator should remember that a student is carefully observing his or her actions before, during, and after patient care activities.

CASE IN POINT

An EMT preceptor is trying to teach professionalism. Upon discovering that the staff lounge in the ambulance base is disastrously dirty with the student sitting idly by, the preceptor begins to clean up. With or without student participation, by emptying the trash and vacuuming, the educator sends a much stronger message than would be sent by verbally expressing disappointment in the situation.

Even if some clinical or operational steps seem redundant and unnecessary to the expert provider, clinical educators should practice all the good habits they would like to see in their students. For example, spending time at the beginning of a shift doing equipment checks and inventory may seem boring and routine to an expert, but it teaches the student that it is important to be thorough and prepared, and to have all equipment in working order. The instructor who arrives on time, well groomed, ready for duty, and wearing a smile teaches the student that he or she takes pride in the work.

When a choice exists between explaining and doing, the clinical educator should choose to *do*. Performing an action or exhibiting a behavior that demonstrates a point will make a more lasting impression on a student than will a simple explanation. The best teaching method is to involve the student in actively demonstrating, practicing, or researching the topic.

Ask Questions

An instructor's effective questioning and answering of questions lead to improved student learning.[17] This reflection on observation and action is an essential element of learning by experience.[18] Clinical educators should encourage an atmosphere where it is safe to ask questions so that no detail is missed; also, the sophistication of the student's inquiries can be a good clue to the instructor about the student's level of progress. Simple questions can be especially important because hospital, EMS operations, protocols, and culture vary dramatically, and it is easy for misunderstanding to occur. Educators can also use questions to help students filter information and focus on the most important issues in patient care.[19]

Questions can be broadly categorized as convergent, where students are asked to analyze or synthesize information, or divergent, where students are asked to extrapolate on a concept. **Convergent questions** seek specific information, whereas **divergent questions** do not have a single right answer.[19]

Research shows that clinical educators have a tendency to pose low-level questions that ask the student to recall memorized facts.[14,19] The clinical educator should be careful not to fall into this common trap.

Examples of Questions Used to Evaluate The Cognitive Domain[13]

KNOWLEDGE (LOWER-LEVEL COGNITION)

Define ______.

List the five principles for ______.

Based on your assignment, what do you recall about ______?

COMPREHENSION

Explain the meaning of ______.

Tell me in your own words what is meant by ______.

Which of the examples demonstrates ______?

APPLICATION

What is a new example of ______?

How could ______ be used to ______?

Show how this information could be graphed ______.

ANALYSIS

What are the implications of ______?

What is the meaning of ______?

What are the key components of ______?

SYNTHESIS OF IDEAS

What are some possible solutions to the problem of ______?

From this information, create your own model of ______.

Suppose you could ______. How would you approach ______?

EVALUATION

Explain the effectiveness of this approach.

Which solution would you choose? ______. Justify your opinion.

What are the consequences of ______?

More effective questioning revolves around asking the student to apply information, think critically, and make decisions. Higher-level questions improve reasoning and eventually lead to improved clinical performance.[19]

The following are some tips on asking effective questions:

- *Slow down.* The slower the question and the longer the wait time for a response, the more time the student has to carefully consider possible answers; thus higher cognitive levels can be expected.
- *Have students compare their actual experience with general theoretical expectations.* This helps bridge the conflict between the classroom (general didactic expectations) and the reality of actual practice. (Examples: Was the patient exhibiting classic signs and symptoms? Is it possible for a patient to have pulmonary edema and bronchospasm at the same time?)
- *Have students provide alternative solutions.* Encouraging students to think creatively about situations will improve their problem-solving abilities. These situations may involve real difficulties that they have encountered or hypothetical scenarios, but they should always be realistic.[1]
- *Have students predict and anticipate changes in patient condition or reaction to treatment.* In addition, have students propose possible plans to address these changes. (Example: What symptoms would you expect of this patient if her condition worsens? Improves? What will you do if there is no improvement after the first medication administration?)
- *Avoid "yes or no" questions.* These types of questions do not provide information about how the student is thinking or arriving at decisions.[20]
- Limit each question to one main thought, and make sure that the question is understandable. Vague questions force students to guess what the preceptor is asking.

Teaching Tip >> *Clinical educators should create an environment that welcomes questions and encourages curiosity. This does not mean that educators must know the answers to all questions. It is best to teach students to "fish for themselves" by showing them where and how to look up reference information. Modeling this continued quest for knowledge encourages lifelong learning that will serve the students well past the day of certification.*

Pairing Students with Preceptors

Unfortunately many EMS services have adopted a policy that "everyone" is a preceptor. Students are often paired with crews based on schedules. This "luck of the draw" method of pairing students can be inconsistent at best, and may result in poor educational experiences as unwilling, untrained, and low-performing clinicians are drafted into a teaching role. EMS clinicians who are interested in teaching need training to become effective preceptors. The common EMS perception that exposing students to a diverse set of clinicians teaches the student many different "styles of care" has not been scientifically tested or proven as a best practice. On the contrary, in early formative stages of learning the student needs consistency, accurate feedback, and gradual skill development. Having too many preceptors may make that consistent feedback very difficult to attain. At least one study has demonstrated that pairing paramedic students with fewer preceptors (the fewer the better) results in a greater number of successful student-team leads.[21]

Care should be given to maintaining impartiality by pairing students with preceptors who can be objective and fair, even if they have had previous working relationships with the student. Cases in which personal relationships between a student and his or her preceptor are already present should be avoided at all cost. A student requesting a specific preceptor should raise instructor concern and further evaluation is necessary.

Pairing a student with the right preceptor can be challenging. Ideally, pairings should be thoughtful, deliberate, and well coordinated. Teaching and learning styles as well as personalities are key components of the pairing. Clinical program coordinators should consider each pairing as an opportunity to develop both the student and the preceptor. Adopting a long-range view of preceptor development in this manner can continuously improve the communication and teaching skills of the preceptor.

Preceptor Training

A combination of innate skills and proper training helps ensure success for preceptor candidates and prepares them for the challenges of teaching adults under stressful circumstances. There is currently no national standard curriculum recommended for EMS preceptors. While various states recommend a minimum number of training hours or topics, no formal EMS research exists on this topic.

The following is a suggested outline of topics that should be included in a preceptor-training program:

- Preceptor roles and responsibilities, program faculty roles and responsibilities
- Legal and ethical issues—confidentiality, harassment, and discrimination
- Principles of adult learning
- Setting goals and objectives
- Effective learning environments
- Teaching methods—communication skills, teaching aids, and questioning techniques
- Purposes of evaluation
- Evaluation criteria and forms, and appropriate use
- Effective feedback methods
- Conflict resolution, mediation, and advocacy for education
- Roles of the team member and team leader
- Effective coaching techniques

The Committee on Accreditation of EMS Professions (CoAEMSP) standards require that paramedic field preceptors receive training. Program coordinators should keep logs of successful training completion and topics covered. This training can best be provided in a partnership between the educational institution and the EMS agency. One acceptable option is to provide some of the training in a distributed format. This can be accomplished with Internet technology, video or self-study packets along with a method to have preceptor questions answered. Clinicians can complete the training at their own pace while at work. This helps cut down on the expense of paying providers to attend training outside their shifts.

Evaluation System

In addition to a preceptor-training module, the field-education program must have a well-defined, written evaluation system for documenting the clinical progress of students. A rating system that removes as much ambiguity as possible from subjective evaluations is valuable. Understanding how one is to be graded can provide a great boost in confidence for the student and can provide a frame of reference for use as he or she moves through the educational process. Having a defendable evaluation tool also makes it easier for students who are seeking a change of preceptor, or who challenge the fairness of their

A Model for Teaching Team Leadership

by Todd M. Cage, M.Ed., NREMT-P

The ability of the paramedic intern to successfully lead a field encounter is in many ways as much of a capstone to the student's academic career as successful completion of certification and licensure exams. Beginning in 1998, the successful completion of *Team Leads* became part of the EMT-Intermediate and EMT-Paramedic curriculum.[a,b] The assessment of ability to lead teams is not unique to EMS, and is seen routinely in the education of medical students and residents.

As each individual is not necessarily born with leadership traits or may not have the life experiences that provide an opportunity to develop leadership skills, these skills should be experienced and practiced in the classroom prior to clinical rotations. A long, academic study in the facets of leadership is not what is needed. The focus of the EMS classroom prepares the student to lead the patient care encounter. The educator has flexibility in how the students will demonstrate leadership, but a foundation is necessary to provide a strong, initial framework from which to work.

DEFINITIONS

Team leader—Someone who leads the call and provides guidance and direction for setting priorities, scene and patient assessment, and management. The team leader may not actually perform all the interventions, but may assign others to do so.[c]

One option for teaching a leadership framework comes from the Agency for Healthcare Research and Quality (AHRQ). The AHRQ is the lead federal agency charged with improving the quality, safety, efficiency, and effectiveness of health care. In 2007 AHRQ released the TEAMSTEPPS® curriculum, which is the first research-based curriculum on crew resource management that is directed at health care settings.[d] Hospitals and other health care organizations across the United States have adopted this curriculum. TEAMSTEPPS® identifies six topics that make team leaders effective: Organize the team; articulate clear goals; make decisions through collective input of members; empower members to speak up and challenge, when appropriate; actively promote and facilitate good teamwork; and be skilled at conflict resolution. In many cases these were based on the expectations that teams had of their leaders.

ORGANIZE THE TEAM

In most situations, team membership is based on the resources assigned to an incident by dispatch protocols and system polices. The purpose of the team leader is to take the incoming resources and choreograph the EMS response.[a,b] Tasks associated with team organization include delegation and role identification.

Delegation: In this phase of leadership, the leader assigns tasks. Often in the health care environment this seems inconsistent, because hospital-based code teams tend to fill necessary roles based on provider type, while fire-based services tend to assign roles based on seat assignments in the apparatus. One way for the EMS provider to think about this task assignment difference is to consider that in many cases, the EMS crew will receive assistance from other agencies. For example, delegation becomes more like integration as first responders move from a basic life-support (BLS) role with CPR and an Automated External Defibrillator (AED) to assisting in an advanced life-support (ALS) code.

Role identification is a sub topic in delegation. The team leader should identify him or herself to the patient and other responders on scene. If the leader is unfamiliar with other personnel on scene, the leader may take the opportunity to identify caregivers and their roles and determine what they have done for the patient so far.

ARTICULATE CLEAR GOALS

In a protocol and algorithm-dominated field, the articulation of clear goals may seem trivial; however, it is the key to a functioning team. The leader will assess the situation, make a plan, and then share the plan so all team members know what is going to happen. The expectation is that everyone is on the same page. In the world of crew resource management (CRM), this is often referred to as the Shared Mental Model.[e] Examples of this would include working with the rescue group at a motor vehicle collision (MVC) to determine how the patient will be accessed and extricated, or advising the team of the plan for splinting a complicated fracture.

MAKE DECISIONS THROUGH COLLECTIVE INPUT OF MEMBERS

Since the landmark *To Err is Human*[f] report, a growing recognition exists in health care that the team leader, whether paramedic, nurse, or physician, is not an island. As a recent change in the health care culture, students should be aware that asking for input from the team is not a sign of weakness. Likewise, it is important for preceptors to understand that, in many cases, the paramedic intern who asks for input about treatment should not be regarded as incompetent. The preceptor should model

continues

continued

team collaboration and ensure the most beneficial treatment plan for the patient is generated.

Also important to note is that since most patients seen by EMS are conscious and alert, they are part of the team as well, which is in many ways the ultimate informed-consent process. As Thom Dick et.al. said in *People Care*,[g] patients have the right to understand that which is being done to them, including the right to consent to or refuse treatment without coercion through intimidation, subterfuge, or outright dishonesty.

EMPOWER MEMBERS TO SPEAK UP AND CHALLENGE, WHEN APPROPRIATE

Since 2000, there has been an increasing realization that errors occur in medicine. Often errors are the result of a sequence of poor decisions and the inability to recognize them early and correct them.[h] One of the primary ways to mitigate this process is to ensure that team members are watching out for each other. The team leader should create a safe environment where team members can feel free to speak up when they see something wrong. This occurs in the surgical theater, where it is accomplished in part by a verbal cue made by the surgeon during the pre-operative brief. Although the precall brief is usually not possible in emergency situations, the team leader should incorporate the verbal cue into the call. A common way to invite the team to participate is to say, "Does anyone have any concerns or does anyone have any suggestions?" The leader should also be aware that his or her body language and verbal responses to feedback and suggestions also serve to communicate how seriously he or she takes the input of others.

ACTIVELY PROMOTE AND FACILITATE GOOD TEAMWORK

A tremendous percentage of the team leader's responsibilities involve communication. A crucial part of team leading is to ensure whether or not the leader's instructions have been understood, and carried out, along with the results. By engaging in monitoring, the leader will ensure that future decisions are not based on faulty assumptions.[h] One practical example of this includes the request for intravenous (IV) epinephrine be administered during a code, but being unaware that IV access had not yet been achieved.

A second tool that should be used to facilitate good teamwork is the briefing. The primary purpose of briefing team members is to ensure that they are focused on the goals and have a shared mental model; this also has the benefit of creating space for inquiry, concerns, and suggestions.[h] To accomplish this, the team leader should check in with different parts of the team and allow them the chance to share their findings. Another method for briefing is called "recapping," where the leader starts at the beginning and covers everything that has been done to date. In many ways this resembles handoff communication that normally occurs at the transfer of care. During cardiac arrest management, recapping can easily be done during the two-minute phase in between interventions, when the primary concern is effective compressions and ventilations and no other interventions are being performed.

SKILLED AT CONFLICT RESOLUTION

Training for conflict resolution in health care is often centered on issues that occur with patients and family members. Additionally, conflict may arise between team members for a variety of reasons. Listening is the primary tool at the leader's disposal in conflict resolution. Although no one methodology will solve every conflict,[h] offer the following guidelines:

- Tackle the problem, not your counterpart.
- The patient needs to be the primary focus.
- Clarify where there may be areas of agreement.
- Acknowledge feelings.
- Treat everyone with respect.

CONCLUSION

In practice, these six leadership activities are not a hierarchy; rather, they are used as often as needed during an episode of care for the betterment of the patient. The common thread in the TEAMSTEPPS® of team organization, articulating clear goals, decision making, team member empowerment, teamwork promotion, and conflict resolution is communication. Consider that these skills can be taught to all levels of EMS providers. Ideally, students should learn these skills early in their EMS education so they can practice them throughout their time in class and clinical. A little bit of practice with some feedback will dramatically increase a student's confidence in leading teams.

[a] U.S. Department of Transportation: National Highway Traffic Safety Administration. *1998 emergency medical technician-intermediate: National standard curriculum.*
[b] U.S. Department of Transportation: National Highway Traffic Safety Administration. *1998 emergency medical technician-paramedic: National standard curriculum.*
[c] U.S. Department of Transportation: National Highway Traffic Safety Administration (2009). *National Emergency Medical Services education standards.*
[d] Agency for Healthcare Research and Quality (2007). *TeamSTEPPS® instructor guide.* Retrieved August 25, 2011, from http://www.ahrq.gov/teamsteppstools/ instructor/index.html.
[e] M. W. Leonard, personal communication, October 27, 2005.
[f] Institute of Medicine (2000). *To err is human. Building a safer health care system.* Washington, DC.: National Academy Press.
[g] Dick, T., Berry, S., Forster, J., & Smith, M. (2005). *People care: Career-friendly practices for professional caregivers.* Van Nuys, CA: Cygnus Business Media.
[h] St. Pierre, M., Hofinger, G., & Buerschaper, C. (2008). *Crisis management in acute care settings: Human factors and team psychology in a high stakes environment.* New York, NY: Springer Berlin Heidelberg.

Cultivating Preceptors: Developing a Culture of Preceptorship

by Dean Vokey, B.Ed., EMT-P

INTRODUCTION

Paramedic education has placed an emphasis on experiential, competency-based learning during the field internship. This emphasis provides students the opportunity to apply classroom theory and skill lab sessions in the real-world classroom of the back of an ambulance under the watchful eye of a preceptor. Key to the success of this learning affirmation is the importance of the preceptor's role. Preceptors are tasked not only with the responsibility for patient care but also the role of clinical teachers, motivators, professional role models, and evaluators of student performance. With this in mind, it should be no surprise that there is a supply-and-demand problem with preceptors. This is due in part to paramedic programs steadily increasing their numbers of accepted students while the availability of preceptors is decreasing, causing paramedics to feel the effects of increased workloads and added responsibilities. To maintain the value of field internships and overall high standards of paramedic education, educators need to consider potential shortfalls in the preceptorship model and develop strategies that emphasize the development and sustainability of preceptorship programs focusing on establishing a culture of preceptorship.

The six R's of Developing a Culture of Preceptorship identify the key areas that focus on recognizing professional responsibilities, finding the right people for the job, providing them with essential skills, avoiding their burnout, providing ongoing support, and recognizing their contribution.

The six R's of establishing a culture of preceptorship:

- Responsibility
- Recruitment
- Readiness
- Retention
- Reassurance
- Recognition

RESPONSIBILITY

As with other health professionals, there is a professional responsibility to participate in clinical education of new practitioners. For paramedics, this provides an opportunity to "give back" to the profession. Experienced paramedics have so much to offer students, not just in terms of skill performance but sharing their experiences and clinical judgment. Educational programs should place heavy emphasis on this aspect of professional responsibility when discussing the roles and responsibilities of the paramedic, and throughout the course.

RECRUITMENT

The next step in establishing a culture of preceptorship is to increase the numbers of preceptors. Right now the most significant challenge facing the preceptorship model is preceptor availability and fatigue. Educational programs are often competing with other programs for preceptors; often this constant stream of students leads to burnout of preceptors. To avoid preceptor fatigue and to increase the numbers of available preceptors, programs should consider developing a Preceptor Recruitment Strategy in response to these challenges. The strategy would focus on attracting new preceptors who exemplify excellence in clinical and professional competency, along with an interest in clinical teaching. This strategy would also set standards for preceptor qualifications: establish minimum years of service and certification level; develop a role description that defines expectations; get the word out that preceptors are needed by posting notices in stations and hospitals and holding information sessions; and develop a selection process, where potential preceptors could be interviewed.

What educators are looking for in a preceptor:

- Willingness
- Experience
- Above-average skills
- Knowledgeable
- Excellent communicator
- Professional deportment
- Responsible
- Caring and empathetic
- Patience
- Commitment

READINESS

Once you go out and recruit the right people for the job, the next step is to prepare them for their new

continues

continued

responsibilities. The goal here is to provide new preceptors with skills and knowledge to ensure they are confident and competent to precept students with a focus on roles and responsibilities, facilitating clinical learning and student evaluation. Most programs provide some sort of preceptor preparation, usually in the form of a workshop. These workshops provide an excellent opportunity for faculty to meet the preceptors and discuss preceptorship issues. The disadvantage of workshops is that it is often a challenge to fill classrooms due to scheduling or getting people to give up a day off to attend unpaid training. Perhaps one solution to increasing participation would be to put preceptor training online, just as many medical schools have done.

Some topics covered in preceptor workshops are the following:

- Roles and responsibilities
- Principles of adult learning
- Motivating students
- Providing feedback
- Conflict resolution
- Evaluating student performance
- Practicum policies and procedures

RETENTION

Now that you have invested in a recruitment and training program and have established a highly trained and committed pool of preceptors, the biggest challenge is to keep them. To achieve this, programs must provide opportunities to keep preceptors involved and interested in the program, such as serving as adjunct faculty, guest lecturers, or participating on advisory committees. Programs must also be aware of the dangers of student overload and its effects on preceptors. If preceptors are constantly bombarded with students, they will steadily get tired of precepting. Some ways to avoid preceptor fatigue include rotating preceptors or limiting numbers of students going to a site. Consider expanding your preceptor pool by establishing new sites and having a recruitment drive.

REASSURANCE

One of the most common complaints from preceptors is that they feel that, other than the occasional site visit or telephone conversation when a problem arises, they do not get the level of support they expect from program faculty. Remaining in constant contact and providing ongoing support is critical to keeping preceptors. Some ways to achieve this include: increasing frequency of site visits; starting a preceptor newsletter or website; establishing a faculty-preceptor committee; and developing a mentoring system where experienced preceptors can provide support to new preceptors.

RECOGNITION

Most preceptors go above and beyond expectations when precepting students. While some preceptors are paid, most volunteer, receiving nothing more than a thank you. Whether they are paid or not, preceptors make a significant contribution to the development of their students, so it is important for programs to recognize their efforts and commitment. Programs would be wise to consider implementing Preceptor Recognition Programs to acknowledge the great work that preceptors do. A small token or gesture goes a long way in letting preceptors know that they are valued.

Preceptor recognition ideas:

- Thank you letters
- Preceptor time as continuing-education credit
- Preceptor awards
- Prize draws
- Free CME courses
- Gift certificates
- Teaching opportunities
- Invitation to graduation
- Preceptor recognition pins, patches, or other uniform insignias
- Trinkets

CONCLUSION

The field internship is an essential component in the development of competent, "job ready" prehospital providers. The key ingredient to the success of this component is the availability of effective preceptors who are committed to clinical teaching. Paramedic programs need to be aware that, as the need for preceptors increases, so too does the demand placed on existing preceptor pools, and preceptor interest may drop due to the added demands. To avoid this scenario and to ensure sustainability of the preceptorship model, programs need to cultivate preceptors and look at ways to emphasize professional responsibility to new preceptors, attract new preceptors, train them, provide ongoing support, keep them interested, and recognize their contribution to paramedic education.

evaluation (see Chapter 22: Other Evaluation Tools, for additional information).

Preceptors benefit from receiving program reference materials, such as a job description that includes reasonable expectations, limits on the numbers of interns (depending on the system, usually one to three per year with a break in between), and communication with the supervisor and school representative to whom they will report.

Feedback and continuing education for the preceptor are highly desirable and should be based on the actual experiences of the preceptor, so as to fine-tune his or her skills and provide information on which the preceptor can base improvements. If possible, the preceptor program and other clinical-education opportunities should be integrated into the provider organization's career ladder. A well-defined training, educational, and feedback system will improve the retention rate of quality clinical educators and will increase the educator's level of job satisfaction.

Tracking and Documentation

Both students and clinical educators must document learning activities thoroughly. Because so many variables are at play and so much information is managed simultaneously, a searchable computer database is one of the best ways of managing all the data being collected. Although these data have to be backed up and safeguarded, it is usually easier to do this than it is to store hard copy forms (paper and pen) in a secure location for a specified time. Although paper forms may be necessary to confirm attendance and document preceptor evaluations, they are not so helpful in analyzing student clinical experiences. Using the power of the Internet to share and manage schedules has become much less cumbersome, but may require expert advice to prevent data loss and to preserve patient and student privacy. Computerized clinical scheduling and skill tracking enable students and faculty to readily assess student progress. These systems provide reporting information to assure students have met program and accreditation requirements.

All records, whether hard copy or electronic, must be maintained in a manner consistent with the privacy practices of every public agency, corporation, and/or educational institution involved. At a minimum, the student should complete a summary of the complaints and field impressions of the patients he or she has encountered, skills that have been both observed and performed both successfully and unsuccessfully, standard patient care reports, and attempts at team leadership. Doing so is vitally important to the field-education process as it actively reinforces learning and teaches the student the importance of keeping detailed records in future practice.

Clinical educators should confirm the accuracy of the student's documentation and should provide a written review of learning activities and performance. The process of reviewing the student's documentation allows the educator to identify patterns in student performance both good and bad, and to record the successful completion of learning objectives.

When possible, students and educators should go beyond the minimum data-tracking and patient-documentation requirements. Students can benefit greatly from a more detailed log of their activity and performance. By tracking detailed information over time, students can also identify patterns in their performance, or lack thereof. A review of the student's experiences will help the educator to anticipate needed learning opportunities or the need for more aggressive coaching.

Additional written work that is helpful in maximizing reflection and learning from experience includes the following activities for the student:

- Keeping a journal of learning activities, emotions, and specific milestones or accomplishments
- Creating a running log of prescription medications encountered (This log can include the

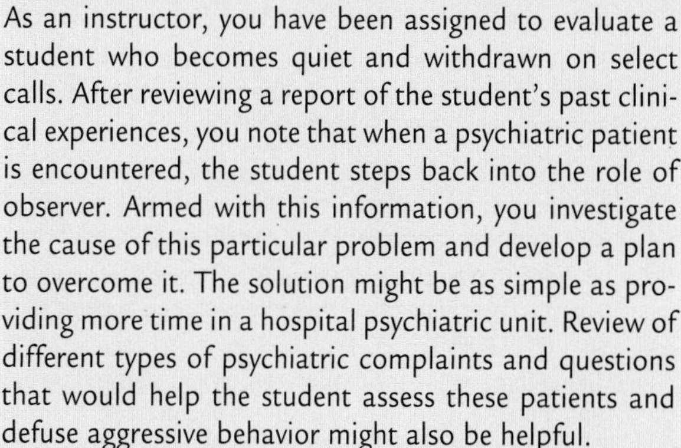

CASE IN POINT

As an instructor, you have been assigned to evaluate a student who becomes quiet and withdrawn on select calls. After reviewing a report of the student's past clinical experiences, you note that when a psychiatric patient is encountered, the student steps back into the role of observer. Armed with this information, you investigate the cause of this particular problem and develop a plan to overcome it. The solution might be as simple as providing more time in a hospital psychiatric unit. Review of different types of psychiatric complaints and questions that would help the student assess these patients and defuse aggressive behavior might also be helpful.

You might discover that this student is shy and afraid, or has a family history of mental illness, which makes the student uncomfortable about talking with this patient. Working with the student one-on-one to discover this and to arrange for the student's personalized help with a counselor could be a life-changing strategy that will help the student grow as a caregiver and as a person.

indications for use, typical dosages and side effects, and a brief description of the diseases the medications are used to treat.)

- Documenting sources of references used to obtain additional information about a patient's disease, injury, or behavior
- Writing patient care reports in prose with the appropriate use of abbreviations (In some locations, patient care reports require only the completion of check boxes and short words. Students who must synthesize and compose full sentences on a relatively blank section of paper with the use of, for instance, the Subjective Objective Assessment Plan [SOAP] method, will be intellectually stimulated.)
- After critical events, answering, in writing, a few questions regarding the nature of the experience (This exercise can spark critical thinking and pattern recognition.)

Preparation and Debriefing

Coming to a clinical experience properly prepared is as important for the educator as it is for the student. If the clinical educator is using a facility with a predictable pattern of patient complaints, volume, or population, much work can take place to maximize learning opportunities when students are present. Careful planning of goals, objectives, and specific activities can focus students, create a very productive learning environment, and make the experience more valuable. For example, a cardiac care unit with a predictable flow of patients with myocardial infarction or angiography is the ideal site for a student to practice cardiac assessments.

Preclinical and postclinical conferences have been found to be useful in the clinical setting.[22,23] In the preclinical conference, the educator can guide students

Guidelines for Clinical Educators

Before the Clinical Session Begins

- Bring references:
  - Drug handbook
  - Medical dictionary
  - Pocket preferences
  - Current SOPs
  - Point-of-care resources
- Set goals for the day.
  - Review and address students' past weakness.
  - List current successes that should continue.
  - If possible, visit the site or department, and determine patient census, patient and staff willingness to work with students, and potential learning opportunities.
- Come prepared with activities that can complement patient experiences or serve as guided tutorials when patient census or call volume is low. Examples of this include the following:
  - Bringing real electrocardiogram (ECG) strips that you have collected over time to practice interpretation and verbalize treatment plans
  - Going through the medication cart or ambulance drug box and randomly selecting medications and quizzing the student on indications, contraindications, dosage, route, mechanism of action, and antidotes or reversal agents
  - Role-playing past patient encounters and having students ask interview questions and verbalize assessment impressions and treatment plans
  - Practicing map reading by listening to other ambulance calls or selecting addresses out of a phone book
  - Performing an ambulance inventory and having students attempt to verbalize three uses for each piece of equipment

During the Clinical Session

- Do not be afraid to look up reference information and ask questions of experts in the presence of students.
- Look for windows of opportunity (sometimes referred to as "teachable moments") to give students a chance to practice skills and direct the team.
- Smartphones are used to store extensive reference material, such as drug reference materials, diagnostic aids, standard operating procedures, and other useful point-of-care material.

After the Clinical Session

- Start by discussing positive aspects of students' performances.
- Make the transition to areas that could be improved.
- Discuss whether the patient presented with typical signs and symptoms; ask about what could have been done sooner.
- Where possible, and without violating privacy, follow up on patient outcomes.
- Discuss some of the emotions noted in the patient and staff members, along with strategies to address those behaviors.
- Ask students to describe alternate methods for assessing and treating patients who were just encountered.

through a goal-setting process that focuses student efforts for the day and sets the stage for later analysis of the experience. Focusing students' activities into concrete steps and assignments also helps to reduce anxiety, wasted time, and misdirection.[15] In the post-clinical debriefing, students analyze their experiences, clarify relationships between theory and practice, and reflect on their actions and feelings, patients' conditions, and the learning process.

Measuring Student Progress and Competency in the Clinical Environment

Currently, little research in EMS education definitively proves the value of clinical learning or explains the best way to track and measure it; however, it seems that something magical occurs when students get hands-on clinical experience. The transition from classroom theory to practical, lifesaving skills can quickly transform students into functional EMS practitioners. Field experience is the setting in which some students and teachers discover that they may not be well suited for a career in EMS, and look for an alternate pathway or an exit strategy. The educator's ability to manage and predict the quantity and quality of clinical experiences needed by the student directly correlates with the success of the clinical-training program. But how does an educator manage and predict what will be needed? Once goals are created, how do educators track student achievement in the field?

The logistics of scheduling, creating documentation, evaluating progress, and keeping records during EMS clinical education can be overwhelming. Scheduling alone can become a logistical challenge depending on how many accommodations are made for clinical sites, preceptors, other classes, and student work commitments. More importantly, tracking the development of student learning and performance in a very unpredictable setting can be very time consuming and too expensive to do with any accuracy or depth. Some programs have a single individual deal with clinical schedules and other clinical logistics and have the class instructor(s) deal with student performance issues. This assists in having one single person consistently control where students are and how they are assigned, especially if more than one class is in clinical at one time. Terminal objectives, such as graduating competent entry-level EMS practitioners, are often not easily measured, and patient census or run volume can vary greatly. Indeed, tracking student progress during clinical rotations is a challenging but essential task for the EMS educator. The educator must create a plan for student learning that is based on realistic expectations, focuses on developing competency, and includes measurable terminal goals and objectives. Students and preceptors should focus on the development of assessment, decision making, and team leadership skills. Progress throughout the internship must be tracked and accomplishments rewarded in the areas of emphasis.

The Challenges

Measuring progress during EMS clinical experiences can often take the form of the easiest, most objective measurement available—time on task, also described as "seat-time" in more traditional educational settings. Hour-based clinical experiences from past EMS curricula were much simpler to schedule and track. Once the student completed a predetermined number of hours, the student's clinical experience was deemed completed, regardless of performance or ability. However, simply completing hour requirements does not necessarily translate to competency in EMS-provider graduates.

Newer educational standards now recommend that students perform multiple successful assessments and demonstrate team leadership skills during patient contacts. Often, as is the case with the paramedic didactic curriculum, the student is required to perform more than a dozen assessments and treatments for a particular complaint before he or she is considered competent. Because patients often present with multiple complaints at the same time and must be simultaneously treated for several differential diagnoses, documentation of student learning may be very complex.

Performance-rating criteria must be straightforward and easy to use because inter-rater reliability can also present a challenge. Many programs find that it can be logistically impossible to keep one student working with the same preceptor over time. As the student moves from preceptor to preceptor, coaching and evaluations may become inconsistent. Likewise, what constitutes a required team leader or a patient contact at the ALS level may vary greatly from one clinical-education site to another. In one evaluation system, the student is successful as a team leader if no prompts are required by the paramedic preceptor(s). For a sample paramedic internship evaluation tool, see Appendix A.

The Solutions

When tracking student progress during clinical training, educators should focus on the following areas:

- Confirming that the student attended the clinical, arrived on time, dressed in appropriate attire, and prepared to work (assess professionalism)
- Keeping accurate counts of the quantity of experiences the student has accumulated and has yet to finish, measured both in time and in number of patient encounters
- Identifying the nature of the illness or injury of patients with whom the student is coming in contact
- Identifying skills that the student has observed and performed during patient encounters
- Documenting instructor evaluation of the student and coaching the student on issues to address
- Continually assessing the student's progress toward completion of the goals stated in the clinical learning plan

Evaluation and Feedback

Educators must provide support and feedback throughout a student's clinical experience because this is a vital part of formative evaluation.[24] Students must have the opportunity to safely attempt, fail, regroup, and try again under the conscientious oversight of their instructor. Constructive criticism should lead to changes in style and habits and to experimentation by the student, all of which should be encouraged. Resultant positive achievements should be highlighted, no matter how minimal or small the progress might be. Educators may feel personally challenged and even frustrated when students are not progressing quickly or steadily. Discussions with peers and frequent breaks can alleviate some of the impatience and self-blame that an educator may feel.

Feedback can be given in many formats. One successful feedback tool that educators find helpful is called SMART. SMART provides educators with the following five guidelines for formatting feedback:[25]

S	*Specific*	Focus on behavior and performance. Give examples.
M	*Meaningful*	Focus on important issues and events. Avoid trivial events.
A	*Appropriate*	Provide balanced and fair review, keeping in mind that students respond best to positive feedback. Choose the right moment to praise improvement. The student must be receptive, and the educator has to stay professional.
R	*Reality based*	Give concrete examples that are based on actual behavior and performance.
T	*Time*	The closer to the event that feedback is given, the more helpful it is.

See Chapter 22: Other Evaluation Tools for more information on evaluation of field and clinical experiences.

Summary

Clinical education is effective when it meets predetermined objectives and provides opportunities for students to become competent and confident clinicians. The effective clinical educator uses actual patient care as the catalyst for learning and tracks students' experiences to plan a rounded clinical education. Many traditional teaching methods can be used in the clinical-education environment. For example, the clinical educator should consistently model the behaviors and skills expected of the student. He or she should ask meaningful questions that enhance student learning and promote critical thinking. The clinical educator must prepare for the clinical student just as in the traditional classroom environment. He or she must also evaluate a student's clinical performance. However, a clinical educator must plan for the unique challenges of educating a student in a busy patient care environment and must work hard to take advantage of a student's teachable moments. Being an effective clinical educator can be vastly rewarding and can make a difference in a student's readiness for a real work experience.

Glossary

convergent questions Seek specific information.

divergent questions Do not have a single right answer.

experiential learning Occurs when students acquire knowledge and skills in a relevant setting.

References

1. Carpenito, L., & Duespohl, T. A. (1985). *A guide for effective clinical instruction,* (2nd ed.). Rockville, MD: Aspen Systems Corporation.
2. Stengelhofen, J. (1996). *Teaching students in clinical settings.* London: Chapman & Hall.
3. Hunt, J. (1981). Dewey's philosophical method and its influence on his philosophy of education. Journal *of experiential education, 4,* 29–34.
4. Shuttenberg, E. M., & Poppenhagen, B. W. (1980). Current theory and research in experiential learning for adults. In *Journal of Experiential Education, 3,* 27–31.
5. Lawler, R., & Chambers, K. (2010, September). Right dose? An examination of a prescription to enhance critical thinking in paramedic students. Oral and Poster Abstract; presentation at the National Association of EMS Educators Symposium, Winner of best research. *Prehospital Emergency Care.*
6. Ricketts, K., Gurliacci, R., & Houston, S. (2010, September). The effect of clinical and field experience on critical-thinking performance for emergency medical technician students taking the EMT readiness exam. Oral and Poster Abstract; presentation at the National Association of EMS Educators Symposium. *Prehospital Emergency Care.*
7. Bercher, D., Wilfong, D., Workman, D., *et al.* (2009, August). Predictors of paramedic program success on the National Registry written examination. Poster Abstract; presentation at the National Association of EMS Educators Symposium.
8. Briguglio, L., Soucheray, C., *et al.* (2009, August). Paramedic student internship experience, critical thinking, and NREMTCE success—phase two: Are paramedic students who perform well on critical-thinking test questions more likely to pass the NREMT cognitive examination? Oral and poster abstract; presentation at the National Association of EMS Educators Symposium, Winner of best research 2009.
9. Salzman, J., Dillingham, J., Kobersteen, J., *et al.* (2006, August). The effects of paramedic student internship experience on performance on the National Registry of Emergency Medical Technicians exam. Oral and poster abstract; presentation at the National Association of EMS Educators Symposium, Winner of best research 2006. *Prehospital Emergency Care.* (2008 Apr–Jun) *12*(2): 212–216.
10. National Highway Traffic Safety Administration. EMT-Paramedic National Standard Curriculum. Washington, DC: NHTSA.
11. Cherry, R. A. (1998). *EMT teaching: A common sense approach.* Upper Saddle River, NJ: Prentice Hall: 32.
12. Davis, B. G. (2001). *Tools for teaching.* San Francisco, CA: Jossey-Bass: 167.
13. Billings, D. M., & Halstead, J. A. (1998). *Teaching in nursing: A guide for faculty.* Philadelphia, PA: W. B. Saunders: 286.
14. Oermann, M. H. (1996). *Research on teaching in the clinical setting.* In *Review of research in nursing education.* New York, NY: National League for Nursing.
15. Meisenhelder, J. (1987). Anxiety: A block to clinical teaching. *Nurse Educator, 12,* 27–30.
16. Kleehammer, K., Hart, L. A., & Keck, J. F. (1990). Nursing students' perception of anxiety-producing situations in the clinical setting. *Journal of Nursing Education, 29,* 183–187.
17. Reese, A. C. (1998). Implications of results from cognitive science research for medical education. *Medical Education Online, 3.* Available at: http://www.med-ed-online.org/f0000010.htm
18. Kolb, D., *et al.* (1971). *Organizatonal psychology: An experiential approach.* Upper Saddle River, NJ: Prentice-Hall.
19. Wink, D. M. (1993, Sept/Oct). Using questioning as a teaching strategy. *Nurse Education, 18*(5).
20. Parvensky, C. A. (1995). *Teaching EMS: An educator's guide to improved EMS instruction.* St. Louis, MO: Mosby Lifeline.
21. Page, D. I., Larmon, B., & Howey, T. (2007, August). A chance to lead: Does having fewer paramedic preceptors result in more student leadership? Oral and poster abstract; presentation at the National Association of EMS Educators Symposium.
22. Worlf, Z. R., O'Driscoll, R. W. (1979). How useful is the preclinical conference? *Nursing Outlook, 27,* 455–457.
23. Matheney, R. V. (1969). Pre- and post-conferences for students. *American Journal of Nursing, 69,* 286–289.
24. Joplin, L. (1997). *On defining experiential education: The theory of experiential education,* (2nd ed.). Boulder, CO: Association for Experiential Education.
25. State of Georgia ASH. Quarry products and State of Georgia Emergency Medical Services Paramedic Clinical Preceptor Program.

Additional Resources

Boney, J., & Baker, J. (1997). Strategies for teaching clinical decision making. *Nurse Education Today, 17,* 16–21.

Bourn, S., & Smith M. (1995). Reliability of EMS instructors as evaluators of practical skills stations. Prehospital Care Research Forum. *Journal of Emergency Medical Services, 20,* 113.

Criss, E. (1998, March). EMS research: Obstacles of the past, opportunities in the present, models for the future. Prehospital Care Research Forum. Supplement to the *Journal of Emergency Medical Services.*

Dowd, S. B. (1994). Clock hours or competencies? *Radiology Technology, 65,* 325–326.

Duke, M. (1996). Clinical evaluation—Difficulties experienced by sessional clinical teachers of nursing: A qualitative study. *Journal of Advanced Nursing, 23,* 408–414.

Grubs, K. (1997, March 14). Eureka: Motor skills mastery. Paper presented at: EMS Today Conference.

Konrad, C., Schupfer, G., Wietlisbach, M., Gerber, H. (1998). Learning manual skills in anesthesiology: Is there a recommended number of cases for anesthetic procedures? *Anesthesia and Analgesia, 86,* 635–639.

Kowlowitz, V., Curtis, P., & Sloane, P. (1990). The procedural skills of medical students: Expectations and experiences. *Academic Medicine, 65,* 656–658.

Margolis, G., & Stoy, W. (1997, September 9). Curricula update: How will it impact those who teach it? Keynote presentation at: Meeting of the National Association of EMS Educators, Second Annual Symposium; Atlanta, GA.

Margolis, G., & Stoy, W. (1998, March). The length of paramedic-education programs in the United States. Prehospital Care Research Forum. Supplement to the *Journal of Emergency Medical Services.*

McGuire, C., & Babbott, D. (1997). Simulation technique in the measurement of problem-solving skills. *Journal of Educational Measurement,* 4.

Sloboda, J. A., Davidson, J. W., Howe, M. J. A., & Moore, D. G. (1996). The role of practice in the development of performing musicians. *British Journal of Psychology, 87,* 287–309.

Snyder, W., & Smit, S. (1998). Evaluating the evaluators: Inter-rater reliability on EMT-licensing examinations. *Prehospital Emergency Care, 2,* 37–46.

U.S. Congress. Emergency Medical Services System Act of 1973 (P.L. 93–154).

U.S. Department of Transportation. National EMS Education Standards (2009)

Wilson, M. E. (1991, July). Assessing intravenous cannulation and tracheal intubation training. *Anesthesia, 46,* 578–579.

PART V

Student Evaluation

In previous chapters, the Emergency Medical Services (EMS) educator has been portrayed as a coach who works closely with students to bring out their best performance and help them achieve learning success. However, the instructor must play another key role—that of evaluator. Just as a coach assesses players at the end of the preseason, the EMS instructor must carefully evaluate whether the student is prepared to play in the "big league" of managing real-world patients in real-world environments.

This vital aspect of the teaching process is often overlooked or "thrown together" at the last minute. Evaluation is a challenging task that requires collaboration and sharing. Without a solid evaluation system that addresses students in all domains, instructors will fail at their goal to graduate EMS providers who are competent in their knowledge, skills, and behaviors/attitudes. This part of the text is designed to jump-start instructors by describing general principles of evaluation, written and other types of evaluation tools, and implementation of the remediation process.

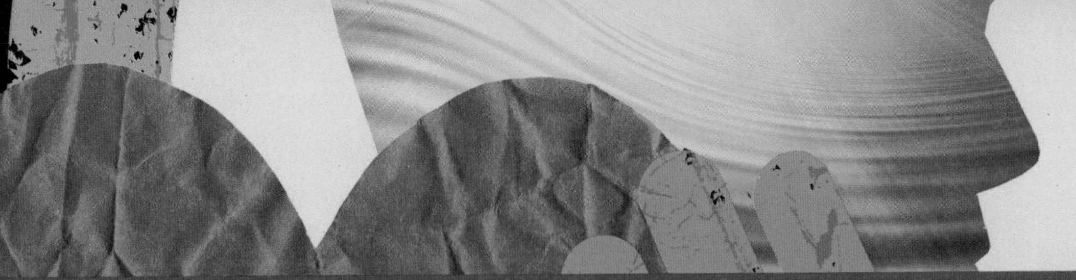

20 Principles of Evaluation of Student Performance

Good people are good because they've come to wisdom through failure. We get very little wisdom from success, you know. — William Sarayan

Evaluating student performance is a task that is often seen as especially daunting. Creating appropriate tools for use in evaluating student performance requires knowledge of the core concepts of purpose, reliability, and validity.

CHAPTER GOAL: This chapter introduces the concepts of purpose, reliability, and validity and applies them to the development of an evaluation strategy.

Evaluation

Student evaluation is an important component of student learning. Although the most common use of student evaluation is to assign a grade, it has other important purposes for students and instructors. And even though the types of student evaluation are numerous, in all cases the process of student assessment should be carefully considered and planned.

Definition

The act of teaching involves facilitating student acquisition of new knowledge, skills, and attitudes. We refer to the process of assessing whether the student has successfully acquired these new capabilities as *evaluation* (although some sources may refer to this process by other terms, such as "assessment"). The program administrator and instructors evaluate many aspects of the educational process during program evaluation. This chapter focuses on the principles involved in evaluating the student's mastery of knowledge, skills, and behaviors.

Multiple Messages of Evaluation

The results of any evaluation contain information that enables the instructor to make judgments. To make appropriate judgments on the basis of an evaluation, the instructor must understand several core concepts. First and foremost, the instructor must be aware that all evaluations combine assessments of the student's acquisition of knowledge and the effectiveness of teaching. Thus, two messages are contained within each evaluation: how well the student is performing, and how well the instructor is enabling learning. The effective instructor carefully considers each evaluation to look for both messages. Barbara Davis writes in her book *Tools for Teaching,*

> . . . tests are powerful educational tools that serve at least four functions. First, tests help you evaluate students and assess whether they are learning what you are expecting them to learn. Second, well-designed tests serve to motivate and help students structure their academic efforts. Third, tests can help you understand how successfully you are presenting the material. Finally, tests can reinforce learning by providing students with indicators of what topics or skills they have not yet mastered.[1]

Importance of Different Tools

The effective instructor does not rely solely on any single evaluation tool. Instructors evaluate student knowledge through formal methods such as written examinations, research projects, practical examinations, and observational reports. Instructors also use informal methods, such as questions delivered in class and homework assignments. Typically, formal evaluations are used to formulate a "grade" for each student, while informal evaluations may not be part of the grading system. Informal evaluation systems are particularly valuable for providing immediate feedback regarding instructional effectiveness. On the other hand, informal evaluations lack the rigor necessary to justify decisions regarding student competency or pass/fail status. Although formal systems provide sound judgment regarding the student's mastery of objectives, formal systems may not be useful in providing feedback for modifying the teaching strategy unless the feedback is provided in a timely manner. The combination of these different formal and informal evaluation systems provides a complete view of student performance.

Teaching Tip >> *The effective instructor uses more than one evaluation tool to evaluate students.*

Importance of a System for Constructing Evaluation Tools

Properly constructing appropriate evaluation tools from scratch can be a challenging task that is generally beyond the scope of a novice instructor. Constructing evaluation tools often requires systems and processes. Even a seasoned instructor may be unable to complete the task alone. When courses are taught and coordinated by individual instructors, an informal network of instructors can accomplish the same tasks as institutional systems that design evaluation tools. Individual instructors can and should work together for the improvement of each instructor's evaluation strategies and tools. Although the processes described in this section for design of evaluation strategy, creation of evaluation tools, and analysis of the effectiveness of these tools may be beyond the capability of a single instructor, they can be effectively implemented by networks of instructors who are working for the common good. Professional associations such as the National Association of EMS Educators (NAEMSE) can encourage these networks. Individual instructors have the responsibility for actively participating in these networks, whether they are formed within a single institution, in collaboration with multiple institutions, or in a cooperative effort between independent instructors.

Evaluation of student performance is a core competency for all those who have a role in instruction. For instance, while preceptors in the clinical environment are unlikely to develop written tests, they definitely conduct observational reports and make assessments of candidates' knowledge. Similarly, all instructors use techniques such as informal questioning to evaluate student understanding. Instructors in all settings, from the classroom, lab, or clinical site, should understand the core concepts of evaluation. They must appreciate the implications of these concepts for their particular setting. Although specific tools may vary, the core concepts of student evaluation are applicable to all instructor roles.

Purposes of Evaluation

The first step in designing an evaluation tool is to decide on the purpose of the assessment. Appropriate design of evaluation instruments begins with consideration of the judgment that will be made from that evaluation. Significant differences can be found when evaluation instruments and tools used to provide feedback to the student are compared with assessments used to determine whether the student is prepared to graduate from an educational program. Differences in design follow from differences in intended purpose.

Formative versus Summative Evaluation

Formative evaluation is the ongoing evaluation of student performance throughout a course. Formative evaluation is important for instructors to gain insight early in the course, while the instructor can adapt teaching methods. Examples of formative evaluation tools include oral questions asked in class, having students write out questions for the instructor's consideration during a break, frequent short quizzes, practical drills, and homework assignments. The intent of these strategies is to provide feedback to students and instructors regarding progress made toward achieving the course objectives. By using formative evaluation, the instructor can modify course structure, adapt presentation strategies, or provide

CASE IN POINT

An instructor in an EMT program is teaching the airway and ventilation portion in a course. During the early phases of the section, she wishes to gain an understanding of how well students are absorbing the information and skills. She decides to give a daily quiz and intends to use the information to adapt her teaching strategy for the next class period. Quiz results will provide feedback to students and to the instructor, so that she can modify her teaching strategy before the time of the unit exam. This is a formative evaluation.

CASE IN POINT

An Emergency Medical Responder (EMR) instructor is approaching the conclusion of the course. Before sending students to sit for certification examinations, he knows he must verify that each student has mastered the knowledge and skills of the curriculum. He administers a final written and skills exam that each student must pass to qualify to take the certification exam. This is a summative evaluation.

remediation during the course. Students use information from formative evaluation to modify study habits and develop an idea of the relative importance of different concepts.

Summative evaluation is the evaluation given to students at the end of a course, or at the end of a unit within a course. Summative evaluation is used to determine whether the terminal goals and objectives of the course or unit were met. Examples of summative evaluation tools include final written examinations, major projects conducted near the end of a unit, final practical examinations, and end-of-course survey instruments. Summative tools provide valuable information on student performance, instructor and preceptor performance, and effectiveness of clinical and field rotations to determine whether course objectives have been met. Unfortunately, feedback from summative evaluations can be used only in future courses.

Most evaluation tools represent a mix of formative and summative evaluation. An example of a mixed tool includes the unit examination. A unit exam is summative in the sense that it is used to assess a student's mastery of a complete block of instructional material. The instructor may require students to pass a unit exam to proceed to the next block of material. There may be little or no time allowed for remediation. The same unit examination may be considered formative in the sense that students will complete several units before they have successfully completed an entire program. Evaluation of each unit gives students feedback on the effectiveness of their strategies for study. Completion of each unit may give the instructor feedback on the integration of different types of material by the students. These formative evaluations occur while the unit exams fulfill the summative role of evaluating student mastery of that particular block of content.

High-Stakes Evaluations

Instructors should consider the stakes of the evaluation before they actually design the instrument **(Figure 20.1)**. A **high-stakes evaluation** is one in which the student's continuation in the program depends on successful completion of (passing) the examination. An example of a high-stakes evaluation is a unit or final exam that the student must pass if he or she is to pass the overall course. High-stakes examinations are usually summative in nature, with little possibility that feedback can be used to modify learning strategies. Students taking high-stakes examinations often experience significant stress. Also, a high-stakes examination typically raises concerns as to how well the examination was designed and if a proper analysis was conducted. With higher stakes come higher standards to defend the examination. In EMS, the highest-stakes evaluation is a certification or licensure examination. Thus, these examinations are subjected to the highest levels of scrutiny.

CASE IN POINT

An EMS instructor is asked by administration to prepare a written examination to be used as part of the screening process for candidates for employment. If a candidate scores poorly on the examination, he or she will not be hired, and no opportunity for retest will be provided. The instructor knows that the exam is a high-stakes evaluation; therefore, it will need careful analysis and construction.

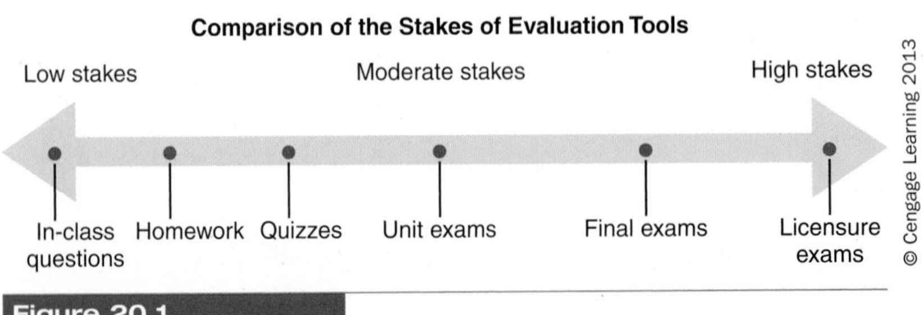

Figure 20.1
Comparison of the stakes of evaluation tools.

Teaching Tip >> *High-stakes examinations must be created and analyzed with rigor so that they can withstand scrutiny.*

Low-Stakes Evaluations

A **low-stakes evaluation** has relatively little effect on whether a student passes a particular course **(Figure 20.1)**. Typically, low-stakes evaluations are used for formative evaluations. Examples include classroom quizzes and homework assignments. Although each individual evaluation may carry relatively low stakes, a number of these evaluations may collectively have a significant impact on the final grade. Low-stakes examinations are typically subjected to little scrutiny. If the instructor is using evaluation instruments of questionable quality, the safest strategy is to reduce the stakes associated with those instruments while their quality is tested and improved as necessary. However, instructors should not consider low-stakes evaluations unimportant. Low-stakes formative evaluations serve the critical purpose of preparing students for higher-stakes evaluations. If an instructor uses only poorly constructed items for low-stakes formative evaluations, students will not be prepared for high-stakes evaluations that use properly constructed items. The instructor should exercise care when selecting items for low-stakes formative evaluations, so that these evaluations will adequately prepare students for final summative evaluations.

CASE IN POINT

An instructor at a community college is using daily quizzes for formative evaluation. All quizzes in the course together count for 10 percent of the final grade. This is an example of low-stakes evaluation. The instructor uses these low-stakes evaluations to pilot test items for future use. If an item is shown to be reliable and valid, then the item is used for unit examinations. This allows for items to be assessed in low-stakes uses, and assures the use of proven items for high-stakes examinations.

Basis for Evaluation

The basis for the evaluation relates to consideration of purpose. A curriculum-based assessment is built on the objectives of the educational program. Performance agreement is the matching of the terminal goals for the course with lesson objectives, presentation of material, and evaluation tools used. In a well-designed and well-conducted course, the evaluation tools match the presented material, which is derived from the lesson objectives. In this way, the evaluation helps students to attain terminal course goals. Mismatch between goals, objectives, presentation, and evaluation leads to difficulties. One symptom of lack of performance agreement is general complaints from students about the examinations. When a performance agreement exists, the examination is a natural and readily accepted component of the learning process.

Evaluations designed to verify the competency of the EMS provider, such as examinations administered by the National Registry of Emergency Medical Technicians (NREMT), are designed in a slightly different manner from those based on a prepared curriculum. Competency evaluations result from a practice analysis. The practice analysis is a formal assessment of specific competencies that are needed for acceptable entry into the role of a provider. The distinction between an evaluation designed to verify competency, based on a practice analysis, and a curriculum-based evaluation is especially important for those instructors who serve as training officers for an EMS organization. These instructors are occasionally called upon to design an evaluation strategy that accurately verifies or reverifies the competency of EMS providers. The specific competencies needed within that particular EMS organization may or may not accurately match course objectives, particularly if the initial training was conducted by a different organization. In a perfect world, there would be agreement between curriculum objectives and practice analysis; however, perfect agreement rarely exists. For example, a delay is typically noted between the implementation of new treatment modalities and the inclusion of new treatment modalities in initial-training programs for EMS providers. Another example involves competencies specific to a particular area of practice. These are critical to the success of the provider, yet are unlikely to be included in a general EMS initial-training program. This makes it essential that the instructor be prepared and willing to modify education standards or standard curricula to meet local needs.

These concepts form the basis of decisions regarding the purpose of an evaluation tool. It is frequently helpful to begin with the question of what will be done with the results. This allows the distinction between formative and summative evaluations. Formative evaluations, used to modify teaching and learning strategies, are associated with lower stakes. Summative evaluations, used to assess students mastery of the blocks of material, are associated with higher stakes. High-stakes summative evaluations require more careful construction than do low-stakes formative evaluations. Summative evaluations may be based on course objectives and used to determine whether students have learned the material covered in the course. Summative evaluations used to verify the competency of students as field providers should be based on formal practice analysis in the expected area of application.

Reliability of an Evaluation Process

For an examination to be an appropriate assessment tool, it must measure consistently. This property is referred to as **reliability**. In other words, an exam with high reliability would produce a consistent result if repeated. If a person weighs in at 150 pounds, a highly reliable scale would produce the same result when the same person is weighed again. Similarly, a reliable exam produces similar results if it is retaken by the same student later. A reliable exam would also produce similar results in different students who have mastered the material to the same degree. Another example can be drawn from target shooting, in that reliability measures the grouping of shots on the target. A tight grouping is said to have high reliability. When an instructor gives an exam, he or she is aiming to measure the degree to which the student has mastered the material (aiming at the same point on the target). The reliability of the exam is dependent on the variation in results caused by extraneous factors not related to the student's mastery of course information **(Figure 20.2)**.

One area of reliability that is particularly troublesome for EMS instructors is **inter-rater reliability**. This is the consistency in scores that different people assign while grading a particular exam. Concern for inter-rater reliability is especially high when the instructor is considering the use of practical examinations and other exams that consist of some degree of subjective evaluation, such as tests containing essay questions. Instructors must exercise special care to ensure consistency between evaluators when these types of exams are used. Inter-rater reliability is assessed through comparison of scores from different evaluators who are scoring the same examination. Several techniques can be employed to ensure inter-rater reliability. Clearly worded behavioral anchors can enhance consistency among items that are scored according to a rating scale. (A *behavioral anchor* is a description of observable behaviors that is linked to specific ratings in an evaluation.) Inter-rater reliability can generally be improved by the use of a greater number of evaluators, although without behavioral anchors, these improvements may be obscured by measurement error. One technique is to have a panel of evaluators grade the same student performance. Another would be to have the student performance repeated for multiple evaluators. Some instructors average scores among evaluators; others eliminate outlying (highest and lowest) scores.

CASE IN POINT

A program director is concerned with inter-rater reliability among part-time EMT lab instructors. The director reviews the skills evaluation forms used to evaluate student performance to ensure that clear criteria and behavioral descriptions are provided for each skill rating. The director uses a spreadsheet to compare the scores of each instructor. The scores for each instructor are consistent, thus demonstrating inter-rater reliability.

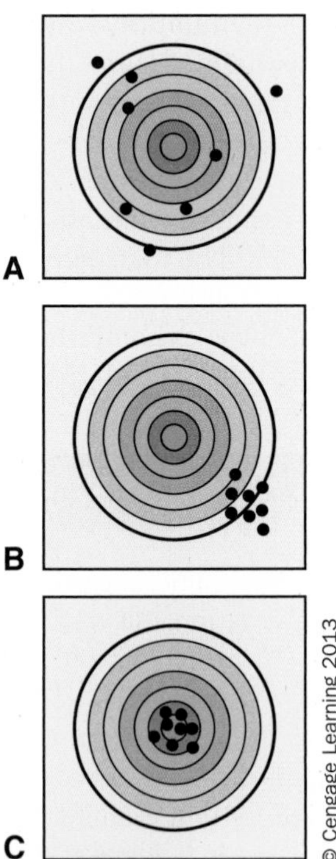

Figure 20.2

(A) An example using the target-shooting analogy of a low-reliability exam. The examination results are not consistent; therefore, comparison with the objectives (the target) is meaningless. (B) An example of an examination with high reliability and low validity. Although preferable to a low-reliability examination, this exam is consistently measuring the wrong stuff. (C) An example of an examination with high reliability and high validity. This tool is measuring knowledge consistently and appropriately.

Testing Exam Reliability

In the ideal world, the instructor could test reliability by administering the same exam to the same students at a later time. Exams that produce consistent results are said to exhibit stability over time. This test of reliability is called "test-retest reliability." Although stability over time is important, this approach to testing reliability has a number of drawbacks. Test-retest is expensive and time consuming. If the time interval between tests is short, students will remember some questions and their responses. If the time interval is longer, students will have learned more in the intervening time, in a sense representing a different group of students.

A different and probably better method of testing the reliability of an examination is to assess the same content using different forms of the test, then comparing the results. Exams that demonstrate consistent results according to this method have demonstrated form equivalence, or "alternate form reliability." A drawback to this method of testing reliability is that there will invariably be some remaining differences in content or difficulty between forms of the exam, making apples-to-apples comparison difficult.

For example, after a new unit exam has been developed for a specific topic such as pediatrics, the instructor can compare the new examination scores with the scores of quizzes that were previously administered. The quizzes contained different items from those in the examination. If scores on the examination roughly match scores on the quizzes, alternate form reliability is demonstrated.

A different method of assessing reliability is to look for internal consistency among examination items. If a survey containing multiple questions is administered, respondents who agree with the statement, "I am comfortable dealing with pediatric patients," should also agree with the statement, "I am comfortable taking care of kids." Examinations can be assessed according to the same principle.

The **split-half method** of testing internal consistency consists of dividing the exam into halves (commonly odd and even questions), then comparing the percentages of correct answers between the two groups of items. The response pattern should be consistent. Of course, the instructor must exercise care to ensure that the two groups of items are comparable in terms of content and difficulty. One drawback of the split-half method is that results of the analysis will change according to how the data are grouped. To correct this weakness, more complex methods of assessing internal consistency, such as **Cronbach's Alpha** and the **Kuder-Richardson** formulas (KR20 and KR21), can be used. These statistical measures assess internal consistency by comparing results for a particular item with all possible combinations of similar items. The Cronbach and K-R methods are typically completed with the use of specialized statistical software.

For example, an instructor in a certification course is using an examination of 40 items without access to statistical software. She assesses the reliability of the examination by comparing scores on the even-numbered items with scores on the odd-numbered items. The scores are roughly equivalent. This is an assessment of reliability performed by the split-half method.

Teaching Tip >> *Instructors must exercise special care to ensure consistency between evaluators when practical exams that consist of some degree of subjectivity are used.*

Validity of Evaluation Process

Reliability of the examination tool is critical, but it is not sufficient by itself. An exam must also measure the knowledge or skills that it is intended to evaluate. This property is referred to as **validity**. Students with more knowledge of a particular subject area would score better on a valid exam than would students without the requisite knowledge. To return to the analogy of the scale, consistent performance of the scale is necessary for that scale to be accurate, but consistency is not enough. A scale can deliver results that are consistently 10 pounds too low and not be accurate. Returning to the analogy of target shooting, a tight grouping is necessary for a consistent bull's-eye, and once the shooter can produce reliable groups of shots, the aim is adjusted relative to the target. A tight grouping centered on the bull's-eye would be considered both reliable and valid. Consideration of reliability is the appropriate first step, but direct consideration of validity is also important.

There are many aspects to consider when assessing evaluation validity. The most important is whether the test measures what it is intended to measure so it

CASE IN POINT

An EMT instructor is building a new exam for use in the trauma section of his course. After drafting a number of questions, the instructor contacts a colleague who is also an EMT instructor to review the drafts. Of 40 draft items, the colleague identifies five that do not seem to match the objectives for the trauma section. The remaining items would be said to have face validity.

will be appropriate and useful for the specific purpose of the evaluation.

The simplest aspect of validity is sometimes referred to as **face validity**, or commonsense validity. Although the concept is now considered to be a simplistic assessment of content validity, it may be useful for the EMS instructor. Review of an examination by colleagues, with their agreement that the test items "make sense," establishes face validity. Assessment of face validity is useful in the initial stages of examination analysis.

Content validity refers to the extent to which examination items accurately represent the wider body of knowledge that is being tested. Examination items should collectively form a reasonably representative sample of the body of knowledge. The depth of material covered in the course should be equal to the depth of items on the exam. For instance, testing advanced life-support (ALS) knowledge by including only items related to basic life-support (BLS) procedures would not provide sufficient depth. Also, the breadth of material on the exam should match the breadth covered in that portion of the class. For example, a test with a medical emergencies section that includes only questions related to cardiology would not provide sufficient breadth. The level of thinking required by examination items should match the level of thinking required for actual practice. High-level critical thinking cannot be effectively assessed through recall-level

CASE IN POINT

An Emergency Medical Technician (EMT) instructor is tasked with building a summative evaluation for a unit on oxygen delivery. To ensure appropriate breadth, the instructor constructs an examination blueprint based on the objectives of the unit (more on blueprints in Chapter 21: Using Written Evaluative Tools). To assure appropriate depth, the instructor also includes criteria for each cognitive level of objectives in the blueprint. These efforts help to ensure content validity.

Criterion Validity

"Criterion validity" (sometimes known as "predictive validity") refers to the ability of an examination to predict performance under other conditions. For example, a unit exam is administered, and results match the results of observational reports in the clinical setting. This examination would have high criterion validity for performance in this particular clinical setting. In other words, a high score on the exam predicts high scores on observational reports. The measurement of this can be achieved through use of a statistical procedure called "regression analysis." In the example cited previously, the score on the unit exam would be the predictor variable, and the score on the observational reports would be the criterion variable. The calculated correlation coefficient would describe the strength of the predictive relationship.

items. Examination items must also be technically correct. In other words, the correct answer must be supported by course content, expert opinion, or science. Basic assurance of content validity can be achieved when performance agreement between course objectives and evaluation instruments is ensured. Evaluation and objectives should agree in terms of breadth, depth, and level of thinking required. Mismatch in any of these areas could cause problems with validity.

It is now generally agreed that validity actually is a description of one's interpretation of examination results, rather than a description of characteristics of the test itself. All examination items test something. The important question is: What conclusions can be drawn from the results? To assess validity appropriately, the instructor must have defined the purpose of the evaluation at the start of the evaluation creation process. Without a clear statement of purpose, the assessment of validity becomes needlessly complex. For instance, in constructing a low-stakes, formative evaluation, assurance of face validity is usually sufficient. If the instructor is constructing a curriculum-based evaluation, checking content validity by comparing it with learning objectives is important. Consideration of criterion validity is key when one is constructing examinations designed to verify competency.

Constructing an Evaluation Strategy

The concepts of purpose, reliability, and validity are central to the construction and administration of appropriate evaluation instruments. Explicit discussion of purpose dramatically improves the chance that stated purpose will be achieved. Analysis and improvement of reliability reduce the chance that results may be due to error rather than representing a true measure of knowledge. Careful consideration of validity assures that the evaluation matches the expected outcome, with clear linkage to learning objectives. Performance agreement among learning objectives, course presentation, and evaluation tools is a core concept to which all instructors must adhere if quality instruction is to be achieved. Even though not all instructors will be called upon to construct an evaluation strategy, the major steps required to construct one should be understood to maximize the quality of implementation.

Step One: Decide on a Purpose

The instructor must make a careful and explicit decision about the purpose of an evaluation. The key is to avoid leaving the purpose assumed, which can lead to confusion. Novice instructors sometimes assume that a test is an end in itself. Each test is nothing more (or less) than an assessment of students' knowledge and/or performance. Patient assessment can be considered as an example. Appropriate interpretation of an assessment finding requires that the EMT understand why the assessment is being conducted. If an EMT student is unclear about the purpose of a particular step in patient assessment, it is unlikely that he or she will respond to patient need with the appropriate action. Just as with any research problem, the first step in constructing an evaluation tool is to have a clear question that the evaluation instrument is seeking to answer. Possibilities include the following:

1. Does the student have the needed skills and knowledge to move into the clinical environment?
2. Has the student mastered the objectives of a particular educational unit?
3. Does the student have more knowledge of the subject than when he or she started the course?
4. Which students have the best mastery of the material in comparison with other students?
5. Is the student competent to work independently as a provider?
6. Is the student progressing toward mastery of the material?

The instructor must remember that each evaluation will carry messages regarding students' performance and the quality of instruction. Each of the purposes provided as examples earlier in this discussion will lead to dramatically different evaluation instruments, as well as to different ways of using the results. For example:

- Does the student have the needed skills and knowledge to move into the clinical environment? This purpose leads to a summative tool with high stakes. It includes aspects of competency verification, which results in the need for evaluation tools with high criterion (predictive) validity.
- Has the student mastered the objectives of a particular educational unit? This purpose also implies the use of a summative tool. Comparison with the stated objectives of the program is needed.
- Does the student have more knowledge of the subject than when he or she started the course? This purpose can be accomplished with the use of a pretest and a post-test. Comparison of results before and after course administration will answer this question, without the need for grades or even determination of a passing score.
- Which students have the best mastery of the material in comparison with other students? This purpose leads to the use of a normative grading strategy (see Chapter 21: Using Written Evaluation Tools for explanation of normative grading). To answer this question, the instructor should grade on the curve, comparing each student's performance with that of each of the other students. This purpose leads the instructor away from establishing pass/fail criteria, or even issuing grades. A ranking of student performance is all that is required to meet this purpose.
- Is the student competent to work independently as a provider? This purpose requires that the test be based on a practice analysis instead of on course objectives.
- Is the student progressing toward mastery of the material? This question implies a formative strategy, with greater emphasis on providing feedback to the student than on grades.

The purpose of each evaluation should be clearly communicated to students and to everyone involved in administration of the test. This helps to prevent misinterpretation of the results. Use of a tool designed for formative purposes to draw summative conclusions can lead to dramatic misinterpretation of test results.

Step Two: Specify What will be Done with the Results

After the purpose has been specified, the instructor must consider the meaning of the results. This follows naturally from a clearly stated purpose. To illustrate this, examples from earlier in the chapter are used here (the purpose is italicized):

- Does the student have the needed skills and knowledge to move into the clinical environment? *Achieving a passing score on the examination is necessary before clinical rotations can begin.*
- Has the student mastered the objectives of a particular educational unit? *Achieving a passing score on the exam is necessary if the student is to move on to the next unit.*
- Does the student have more knowledge of the subject than when he or she started the course? *Comparison of knowledge before and after administration of the course is conducted.*
- Which students have the best mastery of the material in comparison with other students? *Example: students with the top three scores on the examination qualify for preferential selection of their shift schedules.*
- Is the student competent to work independently as a provider? *Achieving a passing score on the field evaluation is necessary for the employee to get off probation and work independently.*
- Is the student progressing toward mastery of the material? *Graded quizzes will be returned to the student and collectively will count for 10 percent of the final grade.* (Note: Because some students will regard assignments without grade impact as unimportant, it is sometimes helpful for the instructor to assign small grade impact to formative assignments.)

Decisions regarding what will be done with results account for the potential stakes of an examination. The importance of these decisions determines the care with which the instructor must assure reliability and validity. The higher the stakes, the more diligent the instructor must be in constructing and using the exam.

Step Three: Select Evaluation Tools

Once the purpose and impact have been specified, evaluation tools are selected. In the ideal world, the instructor would simply select from a bank of valid and reliable tools. Unfortunately, this situation rarely exists. Test-item banks and other tools available from publishers can provide valuable starting points, but these will generally need some modification before they should be used. The instructor should consider the objectives to be evaluated and should select tools that match the domain and level of performance specified by the objectives. For example, high-level psychomotor skills should be evaluated by simulation; however, cognitive objectives can be evaluated by a written examination.

Specific techniques for the construction, use, and analysis of different types of evaluation tools are contained in Chapter 21: Using Written Evaluation Tools and Chapter 22: Other Evaluation Tools.

Step Four: Specify How Reliability Will Be Assured

After examination items have been selected, the instructor must next address the monitoring of reliability. The simplest method for assuring reliability is to reduce reliance on any single test and look for agreement among multiple tests. In essence, this is a form of assessing alternate form reliability. This approach to monitoring reliability is relatively easy and is almost always indicated. Assessment of internal reliability generally is indicated only for high-stakes examinations. For examinations that involve subjective evaluation by more than one grader, such as practical examinations, essay questions, and oral examinations, the instructor should have inter-rater reliability monitored.

Step Five: Specify How Validity Will Be Assured

Face validity and content validity should be checked throughout the item selection and editing processes. As examination items are selected, the instructor and at least one other colleague should review the items for face validity. Referencing the examination key to the stated course objectives can demonstrate content validity. Performance agreement and content validity are assured when each item is referenced to a specific course objective or reference.

> **Teaching Tip** >> *A key to validity includes careful item review by one or more colleagues and referencing of each item according to a specific course objective.*

Criterion (predictive) validity requires the piloting of examination items to test the predictive value of each item. To test predictive value, the instructor must have access to good evaluations of actual performance data, as well as to examination item pilot results. Because most EMS instructors do not have ready access to actual performance data, the applicability of predictive testing is limited for most EMS educational programs.

Because examinations or examination items are commonly reused over multiple courses, it is important that their validity be tested periodically. A regular review process of the examination and key is essential for maintaining currency of the content validity. Testing students on outdated treatment modalities is useless.

Case Studies in Construction of Evaluation Strategy

Many examples exist in EMS education to illustrate how to construct an evaluation strategy. These cases identify each step of the strategy.

Case 1: A Preceptor Seeks to Confirm Progress

The instructor is a paramedic preceptor with a local ambulance service. She seeks to confirm that her intern is making progress throughout the internship and is incorporating lessons learned from previous shifts into development of patient assessment skills.

Purpose

The instructor believes she needs to confirm the student's knowledge of patient assessment and the lessons from previous shifts before beginning the next level of instruction. She decides to assess the intern's knowledge at the beginning of each shift to track the intern's development and guide that shift's activities. The instructor decides that the purpose of these evaluations is fundamentally formative, and that the assessments will not be graded.

Impact

The preceptor decides that providing feedback to the intern is the point of this evaluation. She will use this feedback to assess the effectiveness of the intern's work to date. She will provide the feedback to the intern to focus that shift's work and correct any misconceptions. After a short conversation with the program's clinical coordinator, the preceptor decides not to record the results, but to approach this as an informal evaluation.

Select Tools

The preceptor elects to use an oral quiz of three to five questions at the beginning of each shift. At the end of each shift, she creates three to five questions, based on that day's calls, to ask the intern at the beginning of the next shift.

Reliability

Because the preceptor is the only grader, no problems will occur with inter-rater reliability. She talks with the clinical coordinator about reliability, and together, they decide to review the situation if the intern does poorly on two days of oral quizzes, then compare quiz results with the intern's evaluations in class (checking alternate form reliability).

Validity

The preceptor and clinical coordinator agree that if there are questions about a correct answer, the preceptor will check with the coordinator. The clinical coordinator gives the preceptor a copy of the program learning objectives to be used for reference purposes.

Case 2: An Instructor Seeks to Confirm Mastery

The instructor is teaching a Paramedic course held at a community college. He is teaching at a remote satellite location and works with several adjunct lab instructors to teach the classes. He began teaching last year and does not have the tests used by previous instructors. He is preparing to begin the section on airway management and is considering what to use as a unit examination at the end of the section.

Purpose

In the course syllabus, the instructor told the students that there would be an exam for each unit, and that successful completion of the unit exam was necessary if students were to progress to the next unit. The instructor decides that he is aiming for a summative strategy based on the course objectives.

Impact

The instructor has already decided that passing the exam will be required if students are to progress to the next unit. This is a high-stakes examination, which requires increased vigilance. The exam will have a significant grade impact.

Select Tools

The instructor decides to use a combination of a written exam and practical exams for each skill. He bases the examination on the airway management unit objectives. Written exam items are drawn from a publisher's test bank, and practical examination check sheets are taken from the publisher's instructor resource kit. The instructor proceeds to construct the written examination, along with a key that references specific course objectives.

Reliability

The instructor divides the written exam into content sections so that he can use the split-half method to assess internal consistency. He has been using daily quizzes and expects to compare the results of the examination with those of the quizzes. He knows that he must monitor inter-rater reliability for the practical component, so he makes sure that students repeat each practical station so that different lab instructors can check for consistency. This allows him to assess the consistency of evaluation between practical stations. The instructor prepares lab examiners by meeting with them as a group before the time of the exam for a discussion regarding specific descriptions of acceptable, versus unacceptable, performance.

Validity

The instructor uses an examination blueprint (described in Chapter 21: Using Written Evaluative Tools) to ensure that the breadth of the exam is representative of the entire unit. The instructor edits each item, checking for face validity. He asks a colleague to review the exam for validity as well. He knows that this colleague will ask him to return the favor in the future. He then prepares the examination key, noting the objective and textbook reference that correspond to each item. After final preparation, he sends the exam to his medical director for final review.

Case 3: A Training Officer Seeks to Verify Competency

The instructor in this case is the training officer for an ambulance service. The service has just upgraded its monitor/defibrillators to include 12-lead electrocardiographs. The service director asks the training officer to verify the competency of all providers in 12-lead acquisitions before the new devices are implemented.

Purpose

The instructor is verifying competency in the acquisition of 12-lead electrocardiograms (ECGs). He realizes that although materials are available from the manufacturer, some aspects of the skill are probably not well covered by these materials. This is a summative evaluation that should be based on a practice analysis.

Impact

The service director has made it clear that all providers must pass this test before the devices will be implemented. In a conversation with the service director, the training officer confirms that this will have no impact on performance appraisals, but that each provider must pass the test. Remediation and retest will be allowed until all have successfully completed the exam.

Select Tools

The instructor starts by meeting with the medical director, a representative from the manufacturer, and a field paramedic. This group outlines the specific skills and knowledge necessary for acquisition of 12-lead ECG using the new device. The training officer uses this rudimentary practice analysis to decide that a practical examination is needed. The training officer then has the manufacturer's rep demonstrate the skill, while he identifies the steps required to complete the skill. From this, the practical check sheet will be constructed.

Reliability

The training officer decides to conduct each evaluation by himself, thereby minimizing problems with inter-rater reliability. To help assure stability of the test over many uses, he uses the check sheet that he created, with critical criteria identified. He arranges for the medical director to monitor a random selection of the examinations to ensure reliability.

Validity

The training officer forwards the completed check sheet to participants in the practice analysis meeting to check for content validity. He and the medical director decide to review the first 25 real-life applications of 12-lead ECGs to assess the criterion (predictive) validity of the practical examination.

Summary

An understanding of the principles of student performance evaluation assists the instructor in the selection and development of evaluation tools. The effective instructor uses both formal and informal systems to assess student performance. Evaluation results provide information regarding student performance; they also help the instructor to assess the effectiveness of his or her teaching strategy. Formative evaluations provide feedback to the instructor and the student. Results of the formative evaluations lead to changes in instructional and learning strategies. Summative evaluations contain information regarding student mastery of the objectives; they do not allow modification of learning strategies for the current students.

Reliability and validity are characteristics of evaluation tools. Reliability refers to the ability of the exam to produce consistent results. A reliable exam maximizes the true measurement of knowledge and skills and minimizes the impact of measurement error due to irrelevant details. Validity refers to the applicability of the examination and confirms that the exam actually measures what it purports to measure. A valid examination is technically correct; contains content that is an accurate, representative sample of the wider body of knowledge; and, in some cases, can truly predict future performance. Validity and reliability are important characteristics of evaluation tools. The instructor must be prepared to monitor and improve examination reliability and validity.

As the instructor constructs an evaluation strategy and tools to support that strategy, the most important step is to explicitly identify the purpose of the evaluation. An explicit description of purpose is needed to enable the instructor to select or create the appropriate tool, accurately interpret the results of the evaluation, and decide on best actions to take, as indicated by the results. Instructors who assume that everyone involved understands the intended purpose of an examination are likely to encounter problems. Explicit description of purpose is the foundation upon which successful evaluation is built.

Glossary

content validity The extent to which exam items accurately represent the wider body of knowledge being tested.

criterion validity Predictive validity; the ability of an exam to predict performance under other conditions.

Cronbach's alpha A complex statistical method of assessing internal consistency.

face validity Common sense validity; appears to be evaluating what it is intended to evaluate.

formative evaluation The ongoing evaluation of student performance throughout a course.

high-stakes evaluation One in which the student's continuation in the program depends on successful completion of the exam.

inter-rater reliability Consistency in scores that different people assign when grading a particular exam.

Kuder-Richardson A statistical formula to evaluate internal consistency.

low-stakes evaluation Has relatively little effect on whether a student passes a course.

reliability Consistency.

split-half A test of internal consistency that divides the exam into halves (commonly odd and even questions), then compares the percentages of correct answers between the two groups of items.

student evaluation The process of assessing whether a student has successfully acquired knowledge, skills, and attitudes.

summative evaluation Given to students at the end of a course or unit of learning.

validity Measuring the knowledge or skills that is intended to evaluate for a specific purpose; relevance.

Reference

1. Davis, B. G. (2001). *Tools for teaching.* San Francisco, CA: Jossey-Bass.

Additional Resources

Jacobs, L., & Chase, C. (1992). *Developing and using tests effectively: A guide for faculty*. San Francisco, CA: Jossey-Bass.

National Highway Traffic Safety Administration (2002). National Guidelines for Educating EMS Instructors. Available at: http://www.nhtsa.gov/people/injury/ems/Instructor/TableofContents.htm

Rudner, L. (1994). Questions to ask when evaluating tests. *Practical Assessment, Research & Evaluation, 4*. Available at: http://pareonline.net/getvn.asp?v=4&n=2

Rudner, L. (2001, April). Reliability. *ERIC Digest*. Educational Resources Information Center. Available at: http://www.ericdigests.org/2002-2/reliability.htm

Yu, A. (n.d.). Assessment: Reliability and validity. Arizona State University. Available at: http://www.creative-wisdom.com/teaching/assessment/reliability.html

21

Using Written Evaluation Tools

To those of you who received honors, awards, and distinctions, I say well done. And to the "C" students, I say you too may one day become President of the United States. — George W. Bush

Evaluating students' knowledge is a key task for instructors. This is usually done through the use of written assignments and examinations. Each type of written evaluation has its strengths, weaknesses, and implications for use.

CHAPTER GOAL: This chapter presents information on the construction, use, and analysis of written evaluations.

The Written Evaluation

One of the most common, formal evaluations of student performance is the written evaluation. The instructor can determine whether a written examination is the appropriate evaluation instrument by considering the purpose of the evaluation. Written examinations provide insight on student knowledge, but provide little information about a student's ability to perform a skill or consistently demonstrate a given attitude. Thus, written examinations are most useful for evaluating the cognitive domain. Written exams are not useful tools to evaluate psychomotor objectives. They can evaluate only lower levels within the affective domain. Grading, validating, or compiling results of written examinations is typically easier than other types of evaluations. Because of this, written examinations are easily used with large numbers of students in a single class setting or across multiple classes. Written examinations that rely largely on multiple-choice, true/false, and matching items are especially easy to grade; thus are very useful with large classes. Students should also be exposed to testing strategies that mimic certification examinations to assure that they are prepared. As state and national examinations all have a multiple-choice examination component, the instructor should include that testing strategy in the EMS classroom.

Appropriate selection of an evaluation tool always depends on the proposed purpose of the evaluation. Written examinations are best suited to answer questions such as these:

- What does the student know about the subject?
- Which of the cognitive objectives has the student mastered?
- Does the student have the necessary knowledge to progress to more advanced material or complete the course of instruction?
- Have the scheduled materials been presented adequately?

Properly constructed written exams can operate with high levels of reliability. Because each student is being asked the same questions in the same way during the exam, consistent administration of the test is ensured. Most written examinations provide for consistent scoring, although there are challenges to ensuring reliability with some types of short answer and essay questions. Because written examinations by nature are consistent in administration, reliability is almost exclusively related to the quality of the individual items. This eases the processes of checking and monitoring reliability. Of course, poorly constructed items can, and usually do, have low reliability. Monitoring and improving reliability by assessing and editing examination items promote the appropriate function of these easy-to-use tools.

Similarly, high levels of validity and the ability of the exam to measure what it purports to measure can be ensured by the use of carefully designed and written questions. Written exams generally encounter difficulties in this area. It is very easy to write examination items that assess low-level cognitive objectives, such as recall of key facts. Assessing higher-level thinking, such as problem solving or analysis, is more difficult with written examinations. Because of this, a common error for novice instructors is to assume that students have mastered higher-level objectives simply because they scored well on an examination filled with recall items. Efforts to ensure validity should include consideration of (1) the level of difficulty of required thinking (e.g., recall versus synthesis), (2) the breadth of the material covered (assuring the sampling of items is reasonable), and (3) the depth of the knowledge assessed by test items. This process is referred to as ***blueprinting.***

Each type of written examination item has its strengths, weaknesses, and implications for use. Proper use of written examinations requires an understanding of these strengths and weaknesses. Just as the selection of an evaluation strategy is based on an understanding of the purpose of the evaluation, the construction of a written examination requires the instructor to apply knowledge of test-item types to the objectives that the instructor is attempting to evaluate.

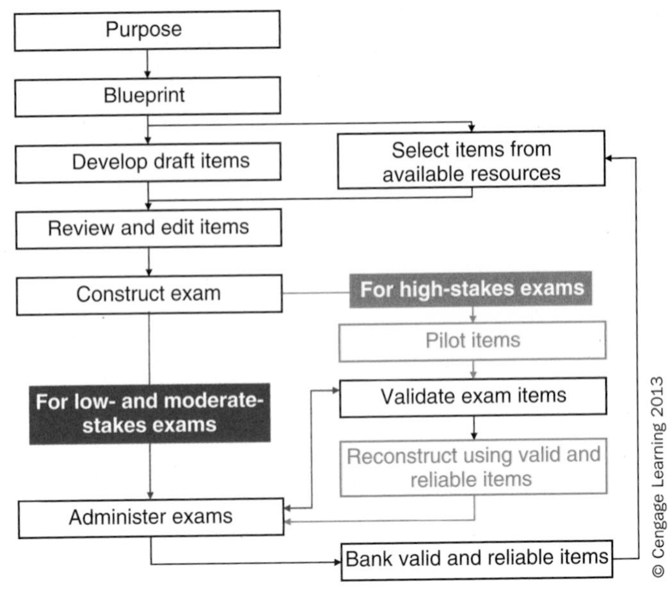

Figure 21.1

Reviewing exam items with other instructors or paramedics and with the program medical director is important for the instructor who wishes to verify the relationship of items to the objectives, to ensure their proper construction, to confirm the correct answer, and to discuss their relevance to practice.

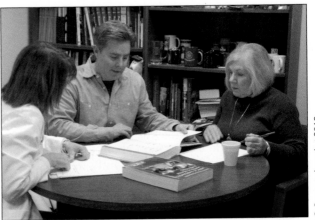

Figure 21.2

It is important that the instructor review exam items with knowledgeable sources (such as other instructors, paramedics, or the medical director) to verify that that they are constructed properly and are relevant to the objectives and the practice.

Construction of a Written Examination

Constructing well-written examination items from scratch can be difficult, but can be learned and refined. Entry-level instructors should focus their efforts on using and building on existing examination items from their educational institutions and other instructors. Textbook publishers and others are sources of exam items; however, many are low-level recall items and will need to be edited by the instructor. Using existing examination items still presents challenges for the instructor. Just because examination items are available does not mean that those items are valid or reliable, especially if they are used for several classes in a row. The instructor still must review and edit examination items.

Construction of a written examination consists of several key steps before the test can be put together. A flowchart of the examination construction process is shown in **Figure 21.1**. The first step is to carefully consider the purpose of the examination. The second step is to blueprint the examination, relating the breadth and depth of the examination to the stated objectives for the course. The third step is to develop or select draft examination items. Draft examination items are then reviewed by other instructors and edited as needed **(Figure 21.2)**. For high-stakes exams, test items should be piloted and validated.

Carefully Consider the Purpose of the Written Examination

The types of written examination items and the content of those items depend on the purpose of the evaluation. Clear differences exist between the breadth of material used for formative exams and that used for summative exams. Elements to consider for purpose include the following:

- Are the subjects cumulative? In other words, is material from previous units to be included? Including some material from previous units is a good method to make sure students keep up with all material.
- What section(s) of the educational standards or course curriculum is being evaluated? To which objectives will the exam be tied?
- Are there limiting factors within the course design that affect evaluation strategy? Examples might include available class time, need for immediate grading and feedback to students, or a large number of students with only one instructor to grade exams.

Blueprint the Examination

Once the purpose has been established, the next step is to blueprint the examination. The blueprinting process is conducted in the following steps:

1. The instructor lists the course objectives to be evaluated by the examination.
2. The instructor assigns a percentage of total questions (or points, if varying numbers of points are to be assigned to each question) written to cover each objective. If necessary, objectives can be grouped together and percentages assigned to each group.
3. The instructor selects exam length. In general, use of more questions increases reliability, but very long tests (with more than approximately 150 multiple-choice items) are much more difficult to develop and administer, and their use does not significantly improve reliability. Fatigue associated with very long examinations can reduce reliability and offset gains from the increased number of items.
4. The instructor multiplies each section's percentage by the total exam length to determine the number of questions needed for each section.

Using the same strategy, the instructor should also construct a blueprint of level of difficulty, based on the level of cognitive material that is being tested (i.e., recall versus synthesis). Instructors may wish to group objectives into categories so that the blueprint does not become overly complex. The instructor should balance the specificity of the blueprint with the complexity. It is rarely useful to specify item selection down to the individual item. If there are several categories in the blueprint with a single item, consolidation of the blueprint is usually indicated.

Generalizing

Instructors are sometimes tempted to assure themselves that students are prepared for examinations by emphasizing the content which is on the test. An example would be the instructor who knocks on the desk when a lecture point is covered on the exam. If students face items that are randomly selected from a large body of knowledge, we can generalize their knowledge of the entire body by their performance on the random sample. The ability to generalize is lost if the students know the sample ahead of time. For instance, if an instructor is trying to evaluate a body of 300 objectives, she might select a random sample of 100 to include on the test. If the students do not know which 100 are on the test, the instructor can be assured that the students are preparing to address all 300. However, if the students know which 100 she chose for the test, the instructor can only be assured that the students prepared for the 100 they knew would be on the test, not the wider body of knowledge. Test preparation should include all objectives in a module, not just those selected for the exam.

Develop or Select Draft Examination Items

From the blueprint, the process moves to the selection or drafting of items for use in the examination. The number of draft items collected should equal at least two times the number of items called for by the blueprint. Having more draft items than called for in each area of the blueprint allows the editing process to select the most promising items to be refined. Some draft items will need extensive editing, and if substantially more draft items are included than needed, items that require considerable rework can be eliminated, if time becomes an issue.

Once an adequate number of draft items has been created or collected, the instructor can begin the review and editing stage. Only those items that have previously been validated can bypass this stage. The instructor should have colleagues and the medical director review the items and assist in the editing process.

Items taken from any commercially available test bank must also be reviewed and edited by the instructor before they are used. When possible, it is preferable for the instructor to employ unbiased editors who have not drafted the selected examination

CASE IN POINT

BLUEPRINTING

An instructor is preparing a written examination to serve as a summative evaluation of the cognitive material for a medical emergencies unit that covers respiratory, cardiovascular, altered level of consciousness (LOC), and abdominal presentations. The instructor prepares a blueprint of the exam.

The first step performed by the instructor is to gather information on the emphasis to be placed on each content area. The instructor begins by consulting the National Registry of EMTs practice analysis, while using three parameters (risk of harm, frequency, and difficulty). He assesses each area for the risk of harm to the patient, assigning the greatest value to the riskiest, a lower value to the next riskiest, and so on. (Results are shown in **Table A**.) He then does the same for frequency and perceived difficulty. He follows by assessing the objectives of the particular course he is evaluating. Counting objectives, the instructor notes that 35 percent of the module objectives are related to cardiovascular, 35 percent to respiratory, 25 percent to altered LOC, and 5 percent to abdominal complaints. Amount of class time spent on each content area is considered next, with the use of percentage allocation. The instructor also asks the medical director and the program coordinator to provide their opinions on the emphasis to be placed in each area, in terms of percentages. Results are averaged, and the totals are slightly adjusted by the instructor so the percentages add up to 100 percent. **Table A** shows the results.

The instructor next considers the level of thinking required for the objectives. He assesses objectives written for the module and determines the percentage of objectives for each content area that is provided for each cognitive level. **Table B** shows the results.

The instructor next combines **Tables A** and **B** to determine the percentage of items that will be needed for each area and each level. This is calculated by multiplying the percentages assigned to each content area (Adjusted Average column from **Table A**) and the percentage of each level shown on **Table B**. The results are shown in **Table C**.

The instructor previously decided that the examination would consist of 100 items of equal weight (each item worth one point). The number of questions required is determined by multiplying the percentage in each column by 100 (the total number of items on the examination). **Table D** shows the number of items needed for each level within each area.

The instructor now knows how many questions of each level and content area are needed for creation of a valid assessment of the student's knowledge of the content for this module of the course. The instructor can now select appropriate items from a test bank and proceed to the editing stage.

TABLE A

	NREMT Practice Analysis			Curriculum Review		Expert Opinion		
Area	**Risk of Harm**	**Frequency**	**Difficulty**	**Number of Objectives**	**Class Time Spent**	**Medical Director**	**Program Director**	**Adjusted Average**
Respiratory	30	40	10	35	30	40	30	30
Cardiovascular	40	20	40	35	30	40	30	34
Altered LOC	20	30	20	25	30	15	25	25
Abdominal	10	10	30	5	10	5	15	11
Total	**100**	**100**	**100**	**100**	**100**	**100**	**100**	**100**

TABLE B

Area	Recall (C1)	Application (C2)	Problem Solving (C3)
Respiratory	25%	30%	45%
Cardiovascular	30%	20%	50%
Altered LOC	20%	40%	40%
Abdominal	20%	30%	50%

(continues)

CASE IN POINT (CONTINUED)

TABLE C

Area	Total	Recall (C1)	Application (C2)	Problem Solving (C3)
Respiratory	30%	7.5%	9%	13.5%
Cardiovascular	34%	10.2%	6.8%	17%
Altered LOC	25%	5%	10%	10%
Abdominal	11%	2.2%	3.3%	5.5%

TABLE D

Area	Recall Items	Application Items	Problem-Solving Items
Respiratory	8	9	13
Cardiovascular	10	7	17
Altered LOC	5	10	10
Abdominal	2	3	6

items or presented the material to students. These editors should consider the following questions for each exam item:

- Are any grammatical or spelling corrections needed?
- Is the item clearly related to a stated course objective? A common mistake is to base items on instructors' presentation materials instead of on the course curriculum. One method to help counter this tendency is to have those providing draft selections also provide an annotated key that references each item to a course objective.
- Has the information/material been presented to the class in a lecture, reading assignment, or other means? Although it is appropriate to ask questions from reading assignments or nonclass content, care should be taken to assure that the content is relevant to core objectives of the course. Some instructors also reference test items to a specific textbook reference to assist with later review and consideration. While this technique is useful to justify a correct answer, it is rarely helpful in justifying why a **distractor** is incorrect. Additionally, higher-level cognitive or problem-solving items are rarely tied to specific reference in the book and may require more clinical judgment than available in the text.
- Is the item constructed appropriately? (See the following sections of this chapter on technical considerations for specific types of items.)
- What is the correct answer that is being sought? If it is a multiple-choice item, is there only one correct (or clearly best) answer?
- Are there any inadvertent hints to the correct answer?
- Is the level of difficulty of the question appropriate?

Teaching Tip >> *Working cooperatively with other educators facilitates item development and editing. This could be as simple as a test-item exchange program between educators. A more complex approach would be for instructors to jointly host an item-writing workshop, inviting participation from a number of educational programs, and allowing all participants to use the results of a day's worth of item writing and editing.*

The Examination Construction Process

After items have been edited, the instructor can construct the examination. Instructors should consider the following guidelines regarding test construction:

- Be consistent in the use of punctuation and abbreviations. For example, periods are used at the end of the distractors if they complete a sentence, but not used if they are incomplete sentences.

Editing Multiple Choice Test Items

Many instructors find editing multiple-choice test items particularly difficult. Collecting a group of instructors to jointly edit draft items can ease the task. This strategy is commonly used by large educational programs and those charged with certification examinations. Invited instructors are instructed to bring a number of draft items as specified by the blueprint. The group then works together to edit the items, projecting the items so that all participants can see the editing process. Sharing editing tasks can improve the questions for a number of reasons:

- The bias and familiarity of the writer does not influence the revisions, as editing is shared between people that did not initially write the item.
- Different options can be rapidly introduced and considered. Having multiple editors approach the task at the same time greatly reduces the cycle time of changes.
- Discussion of types of problems leads to more rapid solution when a number of items are edited together. The editing process speeds up over time.
- Frankly, more heads are better than one. The creativity of solutions builds as more editors are introduced.
- Eliminating local or regional bias or terminology can occur when individuals from a cross section of the country work together on a national exam.
- Ensure that references and resources are transparent. For example, which textbooks or standards are appropriate to the exam?

Of course, there are limits to the benefits based on the number of editors and the time frame. Predetermined criteria for items can be established beforehand to clarify personal preferences and avoid arguments (such as suggested in the following section). While a small group of editors is useful, a large group has difficulty reaching consensus. Fatigue limits creativity; so long editing sessions may be counterproductive. It is usually apparent when an editing team has "hit the wall" and fatigue sets into the group.

- Use a consistent strategy to draw attention to material in the test (underline, bold, italics, or a combination).
- Use capital and lower case formatting consistently for multiple-choice items and for the first word of each option.
- If a separate answer sheet is to be used, ensure that the answer sheet and the test use consistent identification of options (e.g., 1, 2, 3, 4; A, B, C, D; or a, b, c, d).
- Provide clear and complete instructions for the examination—for example, whether the student can write on the test, time limits, whether breaks are allowed, and (specifically for multiple-choice items) whether there is only one correct answer versus whether students should select the *best* answer.
- For short answer questions, students will commonly perceive the amount of space provided for response as a suggestion for length of the answer.
- The exam should be organized in a logical manner, with items from a similar content area grouped together. Some instructors believe that similarly, the examination should begin with the easiest items, moving to harder items. The instructor should note that while these suggestions are intended to improve student satisfaction with the "flow" of the exam, certification examinations are often randomized.
- If several items are related to a single scenario, then those items should follow a logical sequence. Care should be taken to ensure that a single incorrect answer does not jeopardize students' ability to answer the next question correctly. In other words, although a single scenario can be used to set up a number of questions, each question should be capable of standing alone. Additionally, keeping items linked to a single scenario should appear on the same page to avoid confusion.

Pilot use and validation should be conducted before an item is included in a high-stakes examination.[1] Items that demonstrate reliability and validity can then be included in future exams, and items that fail can be returned to the editing process for improvement. A common mistake made by instructors is to pilot examination items using a single source that may not be representative of the intended audience. An example would be asking only other instructors their opinions on items for an entry level examination. Although this may be useful to check content validity, other instructors are clearly not the same population that will be evaluated by the examination items. It is more useful in this situation to pilot the items using a population of other entry-level students.

For low- and moderate-stakes examinations, grading of the exams can be coupled with analysis. Two useful characteristics that can be identified in the analysis are difficulty level and item discrimination. Difficulty level is the percentage of students who answer each item correctly. Item discrimination is the degree to which a correct answer for a particular item is associated with high, overall scores on the exam. Item discrimination is essentially a test of reliability. More on the analysis of written examinations is included later in this chapter.

One critical area for consideration with test items is the level of cognition and difficulty of the items that are used. Certification examinations, such as the National Registry of EMTs, use items that test high-level problem solving. If lower levels such as recall and comprehension are the dominant form of test items within the educational program, then student performance on certification examinations will suffer. In identifying characteristics of educational programs that had high NREMT pass rates, Margolis noted three characteristics directly relating to written testing:

- "Create and administer valid examinations that have been through a review process (such as qualitative analysis)."
- "Incorporate critical thinking and problem solving into all testing."
- "Deploy predictive testing with analysis prior to certification." [2]

Items that test lower levels of cognitive objectives, such as recall, are relatively easy to construct. Therefore, there is a general tendency to choose items that evaluate lower levels of thinking than is intended by the writer. Instructors who are editing and reviewing items should be aware of this tendency and attempt to compensate by consistently assuring that items evaluate problem solving and critical thinking.

Well-constructed and validated examination items are extremely valuable to the instructor and to the evaluation process. This value is effectively destroyed if the security of items is compromised and items are distributed to students in advance of the test. At the very least, this would convert an item that potentially evaluated high-level cognitive thinking into a simple memorization question. As such, validated items should be secured to preserve to the highest degree possible their usefulness.

Examination security can be breached in subtle ways. Letting students know which specific items are to be covered on a written examination is counterproductive in that students may then display false mastery of the material, which is not representative of their true abilities. A written evaluation typically comprises a sample or "biopsy" of the objectives included in the course content. For this reason, if the student knows which specific knowledge areas are contained within the sample from which a broader conclusion is drawn, then the validity of the conclusion is challenged. In this case, the conclusion that the student has mastered the necessary material can extend only to what is directly assessed, and the conclusion that the student has mastered the broader areas from which the sample is drawn cannot be made. Although it is unavoidable that the instructor should have previous knowledge of the test items, care must be exercised to not abnormally focus attention on specific content or items that will be covered in a future examination. An instructor does not *need* to know what specific items are covered on an examination, such as a licensure examination; he or she needs to know only the objectives on which the examination is based. The idea of "teaching to the test" is often considered controversial. Instead of teaching directly to a test, both the teaching and test should be based on a common blueprint. When the examination and course are both derived from a common set of objectives, congruence is assured.

Using Limited Response Items

The instructor may choose several different types of written examination items. Each offers its own advantages and disadvantages. Like other areas of evaluation of student performance, no single tool works for all situations. A combination of different types of examination items provides the strongest validity and reliability.

True/False Items

True/false items offer a complete statement with two possible choices: the statement is entirely true, or it is entirely false. True/false questions can present complex ideas to be evaluated, and they can be easily scored. Additionally, because students can complete them quickly, much more content can be tested in the allotted examination time with true/false questions than with other types of questions. One difficulty is that with only true or false as options, the statement must be either completely true or completely false. For example, if a statement is almost always true, the student is forced to guess whether the person writing the exam was thinking of the 99 percent of the time that the statement is true, or the 1 percent of the time that the statement is false. Another difficulty is that the chance of a random correct answer is 50 percent. In general, true/false questions tend to be very easy or very difficult. The result is that they do not always work well in discriminating between students of varying cognitive abilities. True/false items can be effectively combined with a short answer format by asking students to justify their response. This can be used to assess higher levels of cognition and provide

Examples of True/False Items of Various Cognitive Levels

RECALL ITEM

T/F Positive-pressure ventilation is used for patients with inadequate spontaneous ventilation.

Note that this item is derived from a list of indications. Recall that "inadequate spontaneous ventilation" is a listed indication which enables the student to answer correctly.

APPLICATION ITEM

T/F A patient with cyanosis and a respiratory rate of 10 has adequate spontaneous ventilation.

Note that this item explores whether a situation fits within the category of adequate ventilation. The novelty of the description is important. If a study guide listed this situation as inadequate ventilation, the item would be testing recall. A higher level of cognition is tested by evaluating whether the student can correctly sort novel situations into the appropriate category.

PROBLEM-SOLVING ITEM

T/F The head-tilt chin-lift is the preferred initial method of opening the airway for a child who is unconscious and is not breathing after being struck in the head by a baseball.

Note that this item goes further than categorization. The student is given a novel situation, and asked to evaluate a solution by applying several categories to the situation. First the student must categorize the situation into inadequate ventilation and recognize a need for spinal immobilizaiton. The student must then apply the indications and contraindications of the head-tilt chin-lift to the situation. Again, the novelty of the situation is important to preserve the evaluation of higher levels of cognition. If a study guide said, "being struck in the head is a contraindication of the head-tilt chin-lift," the item would test only recall.

a framework that is slightly more directive than an open short answer.

True/false items should be written in the positive voice, avoiding negatively worded statements such as "is not." It is also important to avoid absolute statements such as "always" or "never." Very few absolute statements are entirely true, and students know this. The practice of taking statements directly out of the text should be avoided, as these are recall items of low difficulty. To help eliminate problems in deciphering handwriting, instructors should have students indicate true or false by circling or otherwise marking among provided selections, rather than having students write "T" or "F."

Examples of How to Edit True/False Items

POOR

T/F Effective splinting always immobilizes the joints above and below the injury.

BETTER

T/F Effective splinting of long bone fractures immobilizes the joints above and below the injury. *(Avoid absolutes.)*

POOR

T/F Oral airways are not used in conscious patients.

BETTER

T/F Oral airways are contraindicated in conscious patients. *(Use positive statements to avoid confusion. Students taking a test will sometimes miss a single word in reading the item and this presents a source for incorrect answers other than lack of knowledge.)*

Matching Items

Matching items typically present two columns of information with the intent that the test taker will select items from one column and match them to items in the second column to form correct statements or direct relationships. This strategy works best with terms and definitions, or with simple concepts and obvious relationships. However, this type of item can be confusing for the student unless very clear instructions are provided.

This item does not work well when one is attempting to assess higher levels of cognitive learning, such as synthesis.

Items to be matched should bear some similarity to each other to avoid making the correct response obvious. In other words, the list of responses should be homogeneous (e.g., do not mix doses with administration routes). With matching items, it is important for the instructor to provide clear instructions such as whether students will use each of the provided possible responses, whether one term can be used once or multiple times, or whether multiple answers are needed to complete a match. Poorly designed matching items are rather simple logic exercises, allowing students to use the process of elimination to greatly improve their chances of selecting the correct answer. The longer and more involved responses should be in the **stem** (the part of the item that is first offered, which may be written as a question or as an incomplete

Examples of How to Edit Matching Items

POOR

1. Cyanosis	a. Used for unconscious patients
2. Nasal cannula	b. Used for airway control in conscious patients
3. Oral airway	c. Delivers low-flow oxygen
4. Bag-valve-mask	d. A sign of poor oxygenation
5. Nasopharyngeal airway	e. Used to assist ventilation

BETTER

1. Provides high-flow supplemental oxygen	a. Bag-valve-mask
2. Provides low-flow supplemental oxygen	b. Venturi mask
3. Provides precise concentrations of oxygen	c. Nonrebreather mask
	d. Nasal cannula

statement), keeping the responses short and simple. During construction, the instructor should take care to avoid giving grammatical cues to the correct answer. Matching sets should not exceed 15 items and should not break across pages. If the instructor is using scannable forms as answer sheets, the number of possible responses may be limited by the form used. This can be a significant limit to the use of matching items.

Multiple-Choice Items

Multiple-choice items are commonly used in national and state certification examinations. Although multiple-choice items are extremely easy to grade and demonstrate high inter-rater reliability (which is why these items are used for certification exams), they are difficult to properly construct. Multiple-choice items consist of three main components: the stem, the distractors, and the key. The stem, as noted previously, is the part of the item that is first offered and can be written as a question or as an incomplete statement. The distractor is an incorrect answer designed to be a plausible alternative to the correct answer. The key is the correct (or best) answer to the stem.

Multiple-choice items can be used to test both low and high levels of cognitive thinking, although constructing multiple-choice items that evaluate high-level thinking is challenging. Multiple-choice items are extremely easy to grade, and they allow for computer scoring of examinations. This makes it possible for a relatively large number of questions to be used, thus increasing the reliability of the evaluation instrument. On the other hand, because valid and reliable multiple-choice items are difficult to construct, the instructor is not able to rapidly develop these items. In other words, constructing the examination items the night before the evaluation is impossible. Because a limited number of responses are allowed with multiple-choice items, these items are unable to evaluate the thinking behind the selection of an answer. One variation on multiple-choice items designed to overcome this limitation is to provide space within which the student can explain a selection, if the student believes that the provided information is not sufficient for a clear choice.

Following are suggested strategies for the proper construction of multiple-choice items:

- Be on the watch for bias cueing (leading students to the correct answer by the way the stem is worded or from grammar choices).
- Negatively worded stems should be avoided. It is easy for students to misread negatively worded stems. Some educators propose that it is okay to use negatively worded stems when the concept tested is an important exception such as when *not* to do something. Medication contraindications are one example of this, such as Nitroglycerin should *not* be administered to a patient with a systolic blood pressure of less than 90 mmHg. Where negative stems are needed, the negative word, such as "not" or "except,"should be underlined or boldfaced so attention is drawn to it.

In general, questions should not build on previous questions. Exceptions to this occur when the sequencing of steps is being evaluated, or when a number of multiple-choice items are related to a single, provided scenario. When a single scenario is used as the basis

Examples of Multiple Choice Items That Test Different Cognitive Levels

RECALL

1. Which of the following parameters is included in the primary patient assessment?
   a. Blood pressure
   b. Level of consciousness
   c. Movement of distal extremities
   d. Bowel sounds

APPLICATION

2. Which of the following assessment findings is most helpful for determining the adequacy of ventilation?
   a. Skin color
   b. Heart rate
   c. Blood pressure
   d. Respiratory rate

PROBLEM SOLVING

3. A patient from a motor vehicle accident presents with decreased level of consciousness, blood pressure of 170/100, heart rate of 60, and a respiratory rate of 10. The skin is pale, cool, and moist. How should you administer oxygen to this patient?
   a. Bag-valve-mask
   b. Nasal cannula
   c. Nonrebreather face mask
   d. Venturi mask

Examples of Bias Cueing

POOR

A patient presents as unresponsive, with no spontaneous respirations, after being hit in the head with a baseball bat. Which of the following would be the most appropriate device to use to secure the airway?

a. Recovery position
b. Oral airway
c. Nasal airway
d. Head-tilt chin-lift

(The term "device" in this example immediately eliminates choices a and d.)

BETTER

A patient presents as unresponsive, with no spontaneous respirations, after being hit in the head with a baseball bat. Which of the following would be the most appropriate means of securing the airway?

a. Recovery position
b. Oral airway
c. Nasal airway
d. Head-tilt chin-lift

(Bias cueing is removed by rewording the stem to remove the clue.)

for several multiple-choice items, the related items should be grouped together, should not break across pages, and may have a box drawn around the scenario and all related questions to ensure that students understand which questions belong to each scenario **(Figure 21.3)**.

- Avoid questions written with a fill-in-the-blank segment in the middle of the stem; these are difficult to read.
- Avoid the use of "all of the above" or "none of the above" as an option. Recognition of one incorrect distractor immediately eliminates "all of the above" as the key. Recognition of more than one distractor as correct immediately indicates "all of the above" as the correct answer. Although "none

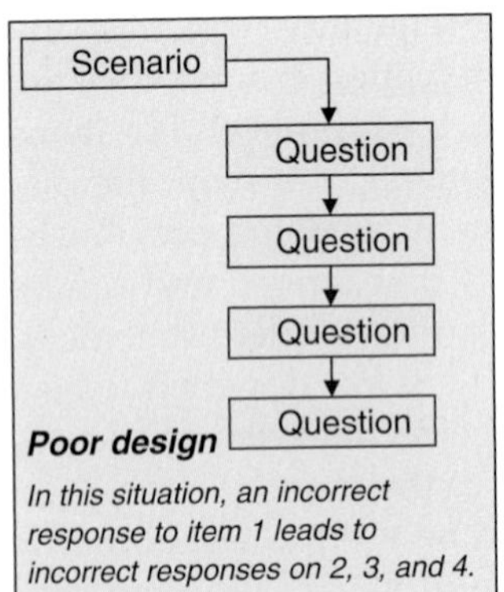
Scenario
Question
Question
Question
Question
Poor design
In this situation, an incorrect response to item 1 leads to incorrect responses on 2, 3, and 4.

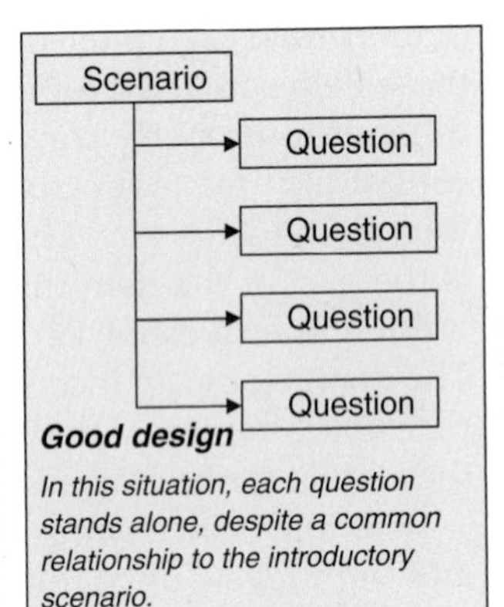
Scenario
Question
Question
Question
Question
Good design
In this situation, each question stands alone, despite a common relationship to the introductory scenario.

Figure 21.3
When a single scenario is used as the basis for several multiple-choice items, related items should be grouped together, should not break across pages, and may have a box drawn around them, along with the scenario, to ensure that students understand which questions relate to each scenario.

Example of Multiple Choice with Fill-in-the-Blank

POOR

You have initiated CPR on a patient in cardiac arrest. As soon as the equipment arrives, connecting ______ would be the next appropriate step.

a. Oxygen

b. Automatic external defibrillator

c. Supraglottic airway

d. Automatic transport ventilator

BETTER

You have initiated CPR on a patient in cardiac arrest. As soon as the equipment arrives, which of the following would be the next appropriate step?

a. Oxygen

b. Automatic external defibrillator

c. Supraglottic airway

d. Automatic transport ventilator

(The blank in the middle of the statement can present unnecessary confusion, and is easily removed by rewording the stem.)

of the above" presents less of a problem, it still presents the student with the ability to use simple logic instead of content knowledge to derive the correct answer. Often, rewriting the stem can prevent the use of "all of the above" and "none of the above" as choices. Additionally, if the instructions for the examination are to select the "best" answer, then use of "none of the above" is inappropriate, as one of the choices will be the best of those provided.

- Avoid the use of "multiple-multiple-choice" items, questions that provide a list of possible components to the answer, with distractors and keys containing different combinations of components. This type of item can be solved with basic knowledge, and these items are actually nothing more than a series of true/false questions. Instructors can easily convert "multiple-multiple-choice" items to a series of true/false items, thus correcting the deficiency.
- Overlapping responses present unnecessary difficulty to students. If the stem asks for a range and a distractor offers a single number, this can be immediately eliminated. Overlap of distractors into the correct range can be very confusing for the student.

Example of Removing "All of the above" as an Answer Choice

POOR

Which of the following would be appropriate care for the patient with a serious chest injury from a motor vehicle accident?

a. High-flow oxygen

b. Spinal motion restriction

c. Rapid transport

d. All of the above.

BETTER

Which of the following would **NOT** be appropriate care for the patient with a serious chest injury from a motor vehicle accident?

a. High-flow oxygen

b. Spinal motion restriction

c. Rapid transport to the nearest trauma center

d. Application of sandbags to the chest

(The easiest way to remove the "all of the above" option is to convert the stem into a negative phrase. In this case, the negative "not" is in boldface and is capitalized to minimize confusion. Also, in the revised example, one of the distractors is lengthened, so the key is not the longest phrase among the choices.) The instructor should recognize that negative stems commonly have reliability problems as mistakes in reading produce measureable rates of error. Although it is easier to change to a negative stem, this may not be the best solution. Creative editing can correct this problem.

BETTER (WITHOUT THE NEGATIVE STEM)

Which of the following would be contraindicated in the patient with a serious chest injury from a motor vehicle accident?

a. High-flow oxygen

b. Spinal motion restriction

c. Rapid transport to the nearest trauma center

d. Application of sandbags to the chest

- Ensure that all distractors are approximately the same length. Common wisdom is that the longest option is usually the correct choice. This is because the writer of the item typically spends the most time with the wording of the correct option (to ensure that it is completely correct) and spends less time with the distractors.

- Ensure that all distractors make grammatical sense. Frequent issues include problems with agreement of plural/singular and a/an. One method of avoiding grammatical cueing is to use complete sentences as the stem.
- Ensure that the correct answer is randomly distributed. A general tendency is for instructors to predominantly use (b) and (c) as the key.

Example of Removing Multiple Multiples

POOR

Which of the following assessment findings is consistent with a patient who is suffering from hypoperfusion due to internal bleeding?

1. Warm and flushed skin
2. Rapid pulse rate
3. Low blood pressure
4. Anxiety

a. 1, 2, and 3

b. 1, 3, and 4

c. 1 and 3

d. 2, 3, and 4

BETTER

Which of the following assessment findings is **NOT** consistent with a patient who is suffering from hypoperfusion due to internal bleeding?

a. Warm and flushed skin

b. Rapid pulse rate

c. Low blood pressure

d. Anxiety

OR, AS ANOTHER OPTION

Questions 12–15 refer to the following statement:

The following assessment findings are consistent with a patient who is suffering from hypoperfusion due to internal bleeding. Circle true or false for each assessment finding.

12. Warm and flushed skin	True	False
13. Rapid pulse rate	True	False
14. Low blood pressure	True	False
15. Anxiety	True	False

Example of Fixing Overlapping Ranges

POOR

Which of the following is a normal respiratory rate for a patient who is 4 years old?

a. 8–16

b. 12–20

c. 15–30

d. 20–40

BETTER

Which of the following is a normal respiratory rate for a patient who is 4 years old?

a. 10–15

b. 16–30

c. 31–50

d. 80–100

(The overlapping ranges present an unnecessary difficulty. The situation is best avoided, even with the addition of a distractor that is far outside the range.)

Example of Ensuring Comparable Length of Answer Choices

POOR

A patient with severe respiratory distress should be transported in which of the following positions?

a. Sitting, if the patient has a normal level of consciousness

b. Supine

c. Prone

d. Recovery position

BETTER

A conscious patient with severe respiratory distress should be transported in which of the following positions?

a. Sitting

b. Supine

c. Prone

d. Recovery position

(Any necessary conditions for the key to be correct are moved to the stem, removing the obvious clue to the correct answer.)

Example of Removing Grammar Cues

POOR

A patient has an injury to the leg with severe pain and bone fragments protruding from the site of injury. This patient has an

a. Closed fracture

b. Open fracture

c. Dislocation

d. Sprain

BETTER

A patient has an injury to the leg with severe pain and bone fragments protruding from the site of injury. This patient has

a. A closed fracture

b. An open fracture

c. A dislocation

d. A sprain

(Grammatical cueing, or grammar cueing, is easily avoided by using a complete sentence as the stem.)

Teaching Tip >> *One method of ensuring random distribution of the correct answer involves the use of a deck of cards. With each item, a card is selected: If the suit is hearts, A is used as the key*

- *If the suit is clubs, B is used.*
- *If the suit is spades, C is used.*
- *If the suit is diamonds, D is used.*

One must be sure to shuffle the deck before cards are chosen.

- Be aware that in constructing a multiple-choice question, instructors tend to distribute the distractors so that two of the three are at the extreme positions, leaving the correct choice among the two middle answers (e.g., if the correct answer is 4, options would typically be 1, 3, 4, and 7). Students are aware of this tendency as well.
- Place responses in a logical order. If the responses are assigned a numeric value, place the lowest numeric response as the first choice, the next highest as the second, and so forth.

Example of the Middle Value

POOR

Which of the following best expresses the range of respiratory rates considered normal for an infant?

a. 12–20

b. 15–30

c. 25–50

d. 50–70

BETTER

Which of the following best expresses the range of respiratory rates considered normal for an infant?

a. 8–12

b. 12–16

c. 18–30

d. 30–60

(Although all cases of the middle value being the correct choice do not need to be changed, the instructor should be aware of the tendency and take care to avoid patterns. Occasional use of an extreme value as the correct choice is appropriate. Although overlapping ranges are seen in this example, the student is being clearly asked to identify which range best describes normal, and the ranges in this case are taken directly from the 2011 AHA PALS provider manual: 12–16 normal for adolescents, 18–30 normal for school age children, and 30–60 normal for infants.)

- Do not create words or abbreviations just to fill a response.
- Do not create humorous or ridiculous options just to fill space. All answers should be plausible to students. The use of humor can create problems with reliability in addition to the fact that it may well be perceived negatively by many students. As humor is culturally and often regionally based, the use of humor is a source of potential bias in the examination.

Using Open Response Items

Open-ended response items can also offer advantages and disadvantages. A combination of different types of examination items provides the strongest validity and reliability.

Challenges of Using the Full Sentence Stem

We have used full sentences as the stem in the examples in this chapter. While this practice easily eliminates grammar and bias cues when compared to blanks and incomplete sentences, use of full sentences as a stem introduces challenges. Full sentences are longer than stems using incomplete sentences. The added length increases the time needed for examinations due to increased reading time. The added length also introduces a source of reliability problems from the unnecessary words. Writing stems as a full sentence is a reasonable practice for novice item writers, but experience with editing should enable more experienced writers to significantly shorten items through the use of incomplete sentences as stems. An example is provided:

A patient presents as unresponsive, with no spontaneous respirations, after being hit in the head with a baseball bat. Which of the following would be the most appropriate means of opening the airway? *(33 words, 167 characters)*

a. Recovery position

b. Oral airway

c. Nasal airway

d. Head-tilt chin-lift

(Editing to shorten the stem would produce a significantly shorter stem that is much easier to read and comprehend. Easy comprehension of key information in the stem is necessary for reliability.)

A patient struck on the head with a baseball bat presents as unresponsive and apneic. You should open the airway by a(n) *(22 words, 96 characters)*

a. Recovery position

b. Oral airway

c. Nasal airway

d. Head-tilt chin-lift

Completion Items

Completion (also known as "fill-in-the-blank") items are statements from which part of the information has been omitted, so students must complete the statement. Enough information must be included for students to glean the intent of the statement without being led to the answer. One issue with open-response items arises when the meaning of the incomplete statement is unclear and several student responses emerge as correct, presenting a problem for the test grader. Items with unclear statements present a challenge for maintaining inter-rater reliability if more than one person is grading the exam. Completion items are not capable of evaluating higher-order thinking such as with problem solving. These items are best used to evaluate recall, especially for key phrases that should be known verbatim or for definitions of key terms.

The provided answer space may present a problem for completion items. If one blank is used for each word of the correct response, the student is presented with a significant clue as to the answer. If only one blank is provided, students frequently assume that the answer consists of one word when multiple words are necessary. Either interpretation lowers reliability of the item.

Tips for writing completion items include the following:

- Omit significant words from the statement, but not so many that it is difficult for the student to determine the intent. For example, "An automated external defibrillator is used to treat ventricular ______." is better than "A ______ is used to treat ______ fibrillation." One method of assuring this is to allow only one blank per completion item.
- Place the blank at the end of the sentence. This shortens the reading time and allows the student to derive the intent of the item before encountering the blank. For example, "______ is used to assess the percentage of hemoglobin that is oxygenated." should be converted to "The percentage of hemoglobin that is oxygenated is assessed by ______."
- As with other item types, avoid taking statements verbatim from textbooks or workbooks. It is particularly tempting to construct completion items by copying a statement from the text and omitting key words. There are two problems with this practice. First, it assures that the item evaluates only recall. Second, statements in texts are heavily dependent on context for the correct interpretation. Without that context, a single sentence frequently becomes ambiguous and difficult to complete the missing words.
- As with multiple choice items, be aware of possible cues from the grammar and sentence construction.
- Ambiguity of grading can be difficult with any open-response item. Because completion items require a very short answer, it is difficult to evaluate the student's thinking behind a particular response. This challenges the reliability of grading. For instance, consider the stem "Pulse oximetry is used to measure ______." While the instructor may intend the answer to be "oxygen saturation,"

reasonable responses may include circulation, shock, distal perfusion, oxygenation, and so on. It is difficult for an instructor to predetermine possible interpretations of an item without piloting the item or using reviewers.

Essay Items

Essay items pose a question or situation for which students are required to provide a relatively long, prose-style answer. Essay items are capable of evaluating higher levels of cognitive thinking, but they also require that the student be capable of expressing this knowledge in coherent, written fashion. Essays can be used to effectively evaluate lower and middle levels within the affective domain. These questions also have the advantage of not being as easily susceptible to student guessing, although students may try to bluff. Because essay items are time consuming for students to complete and for instructors to grade, it is seldom practical to include more than a couple of essay items during a classroom evaluation.

The sole use of essay questions on an examination presents a challenge to validity; this results from obvious problems with the breadth of material. Ensuring reliability during grading is difficult, as many factors other than knowledge can influence the assigned grade. In general, essay questions should be reserved for those objectives that cannot be effectively evaluated with limited-response items.

The instructor should give his or her students advice for and practice with writing essays. This practice can be part of the formative evaluation strategies. The instructor should not give students a choice of questions to answer during examinations. It will be difficult to match the exam blueprint if different students answer different questions. Also, because some questions will be more difficult than others, the test could be unfair. When this choice is presented, each student is actually taking a different examination. Each essay question should be linked to a single objective; the student should avoid attempting to evaluate several objectives with one item.

Tips for writing essay items include the following:

- Avoid using essay items to evaluate recall of facts. Recall items, such as lists and definitions, are better evaluated using items that have less problems with grading reliability such as limited-response items.
- Be clear in the task expected of students. For instance, "Discuss shock." is much less clear than "Describe the various compensation mechanisms for shock."
- In order to evaluate different levels of cognition, one useful strategy is to match the verbs used in the objective to the verbs used in the essay assignment.

Short Answer Items

Between the essay question and the completion item lies the short answer question. Short answer questions are very similar to essay questions, except that essay questions typically require multipage responses, and short answer questions rarely exceed a full page. Depending on the stated objectives, it may also be desirable to avoid requiring the use of full sentences to respond to short answer questions. Allowing students to use bulleted lists or outline forms may provide enough insight for the instructor to effectively evaluate knowledge, while not relying heavily on writing skills. Because they take less time and fewer writing skills for students to complete, more questions can be included. The strengths, weaknesses, and implications for short answer questions are otherwise the same as for essay questions. In most cases, essay questions have little usefulness in the EMS classroom compared with short answer questions.

Writing essay items can be very similar to writing short answer. It is important when writing a short answer question to limit the scope of the question. When limiting the scope, the following may be helpful to convert essay items into short answer:

- Use a subset of clinical conditions; for example, "Describe compensatory mechanisms for *neurogenic* shock."
- Describe the circumstances in more detail; for example, "The patient fell from a height of 20 feet. Describe the implications selecting an appropriate destination for this patient."
- Target the response by providing more detail about the expected response; for example, "Describe the pathophysiology of frostbite, paying particular attention to the role of vasoconstriction."

Teaching Tip >> *Both limited-response items and short-answer items can assess higher levels within the cognitive domain. A simple rule of thumb on which type the instructor should choose is that short answer or essay questions should be used when the time to prepare the examination is short and the time to grade the examination is long. When the time to prepare the examination is long and the time to grade the examination is short, limited response items (such as multiple-choice) are the preferred tool.*

Homework and Research Projects

A variety of homework and research projects can also add to formative and summative student evaluation. Some options are discussed here.

Homework

One tool that is especially valuable as a formative evaluation tool is the routine assignment of homework to be completed by students. Homework should be spread out relatively evenly across the course. Each assignment need not be graded, but many students will interpret the lack of grade impact as lack of importance. Assigning a nominal grade impact to a random selection of homework assignments is recommended to counter this tendency. The instructor should review homework assignments for level of difficulty and should include a mix of easy and difficult items. Encouraging students to collaborate on homework can be a useful practice that helps to build teamwork and peer learning. Frequent assignments, which help to build regular study habits in students, provide the instructor with regular, formative feedback on student progress.

Examples of homework assignments for the Emergency Medical Services (EMS) classroom include assignments from workbooks, completion and definition worksheets, short research projects, targeted discussion in an online forum (discussion board or blog), writing a summary of key points from lecture, and description of care for a supplied scenario. Homework assignments also provide students with examples of what types of problems they will be expected to solve for summative evaluations. To be effective as formative evaluations, homework assignments must be graded and returned to students in a timely manner.

Research Project Assignments

Project assignments based on students' own research are another means of evaluating the ability of students to synthesize information. These assignments are a tool for assessing higher-level cognitive learning. Individual projects allow students to use their own specific learning preferences to complete the assignment. Research projects promote student autonomy, enhance student confidence, and encourage independent learning.

Assignment or choice of topic is an important, yet commonly overlooked, component of the project assignment. Allowing students to choose a topic that appeals to them is appropriate, but the instructor must be an active part of the topic selection and determination of project scope. Students should not waste valuable time on consideration of topics. One way of avoiding this scenario is to prepare a list of potential topics from which students can choose. Controlling the project scope is necessary to ensure that projects assigned to different students are roughly equivalent in terms of difficulty. Many instructors require that students get approval from them on project scope early in the process.

Another option is to prepare guidelines for determination of grades based on the amount of work that students complete. For example, "To get a 'C', the student will complete a written paper of at least 10 pages and a classroom presentation; to get a 'B', the student will also complete at least one optional activity; and to get an 'A', the student will complete at least two additional optional activities. Optional activities include reporting on an interview of a local medical director, creating a project-related website, completing a survey of at least 20 local EMS providers, and creating and demonstrating a working mechanical model related to a particular topic."

A measure of negotiation between the instructor and the student is appropriate in determining scope while still allowing students to express their own talents and learning preferences. It is also helpful for the instructor to reinforce relevance by creating realistic writing scenarios, such as, "Your medical director has asked you to submit a new protocol for the treatment of anaphylaxis. Please submit your protocol, which should include both assessment and treatment sections. Provide at least five sources from peer-reviewed medical journals that support the care you propose."

One problem with project assignments is the tendency of instructors to base the grade on product rather than on process. In most cases, the process used by students to prepare a project is just as important as the product itself. One way that instructors can avoid this trap is by requiring students to submit intermediary steps for consideration and possible impact on grade. An example is to have a "check-in" for the following steps: (1) description of title, purpose, and major points; (2) sources, data, and references; (3) outline; (4) first draft; and (5) final version.

The process of grading project assignments is essentially the same as that used to grade essay items on written exams. Recommendations provided in the "Grading Essays" section can be applied to written components of the project. Criteria for grading projects should be clearly communicated to students as noted in the section on Grading Strategies. The grade may contain components that measure the quality of the product, as well as the effectiveness of the process.

Project assignments are best viewed as a combination of a learning tool and an evaluation tool. As a learning tool, project assignments result in learning that is customized to the individual student's talents and preferences. Project assignments emphasize critical thinking, independent learning, and use of research skills. As an evaluation tool, project assignments permit assessment of high-level cognitive objectives and some affective objectives.

Administering Written Exams

The administration of written exams requires careful attention. An inappropriate environment or ineffective method of administration can significantly impact exam validity.

Environmental Considerations

The classroom setup for a written examination is essentially the same as that used for a lecture format **(Figure 21.4)**. Students should be seated far enough apart to discourage them from looking at each others' papers. Exam proctors should walk the room from time to time so that they are able to see students' faces as well as observe students' space and activity. Appropriate temperature and lighting should be ensured. Special attention should be given to providing a quiet environment.

For examinations that last longer than an hour, the instructor should set clear rules for restroom breaks. It is helpful to have extra copies of the examination and answer sheets, scratch paper, and pencils readily available.

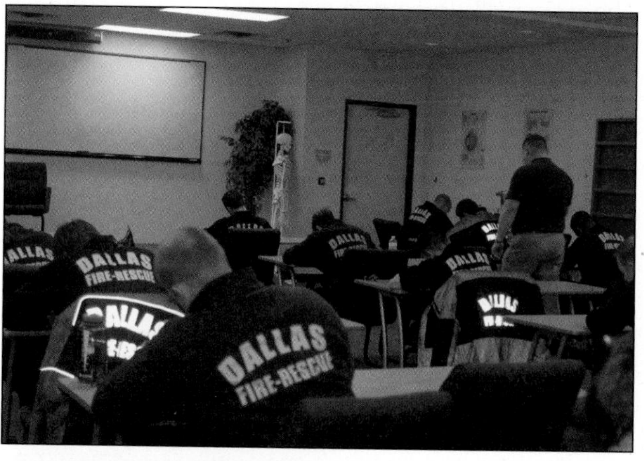

© Cengage Learning 2013

Figure 21.4

Answer sheets and test booklets (face down) can be placed at student seats before the examination. Student notebooks and backpacks should be placed at the back or side of the room.

Proctoring

An instructor should supervise written examinations to discourage cheating and to address problems or process questions as they arise. Lead instructors communicate the importance of examinations by proctoring the examination themselves. Proctors should arrive early and should be prepared to leave late. During the examination, the proctor should monitor the room without hovering over students. The proctor should have a strategy for addressing questions asked by students during the exam. One common strategy is to allow the proctor to answer only questions regarding examination process—not questions related to examination content. Proctors should be cognizant that any communication of content to a student who asks a question gives an advantage to that student over those who did not ask or attempt to fish for clues. The proctor should keep students apprised as to the time by having a clock in the room, writing (and updating) the time on a whiteboard, or periodically announcing the time remaining for the test.

Appropriate proctoring helps to assure the integrity of the examination. Cheating can flourish in an unsupervised environment. The proctor must assure security of testing materials. Looking at other students' answers can be addressed by seating arrangements. Cell phones and other recording devices should be prohibited in the testing environment. Any notes or calculations during the examination should not leave the testing environment. Silence during examinations discourages covert communications. Use of multiple versions of an exam, with differing arrangements of item sequence and distractors, discourages organized efforts by groups of students to each memorize parts of an examination and later reconstruct the examination. Another means to defeat that form of cheating is to revise examinations after each administration. Test development software can make creation of multiple randomized versions easier. Diligent observation by the instructor, combined with clear expectations of integrity, are key to preventing cheating.

Computer-Based Testing

Recent technological developments have enabled more widespread use of computer-based testing in educational settings. Once reserved for high-stakes examinations, these techniques are increasingly available for classroom instructors to incorporate. Computer-based testing as a subset of a wider set of tools is sometimes referred to as "e-Assessment." Testing centers in community colleges and other environments can offer secured, computer-based testing environments, which may be appropriate for high-stakes summative examinations. Other variations exist for use within the classroom. Use of a Learning Management System (LMS), such as Moodle or Blackboard, may include testing modules. This allows for distributed methods of formative assessments and quizzes. Within the classroom, small, remote, voting devices or audience-response systems, sometimes referred to as "I-clickers," can connect to a presentation system. This system can allow an additional layer of interaction within the classroom discussion that can blend a tracked, formative assessment with an informal discussion.

A major advantage of computer-based testing systems is that these systems remove a potential source for error in grading and item analysis. By direct entry into the system, grading and analysis are more efficient. With varying degrees of security, tests can be offered in multiple locations—even in the student's home at a convenient time. Computer systems also allow a greater variety of media to be attached to test items such as pictures, audio, and video. Many different versions of the test can be offered to students, increasing security. Using many different versions of the examination is enabled by the substantial increases in efficiency of grading. Feedback can be offered instantaneously, which is particularly valuable for formative assessments.[3]

These systems typically favor limited-response items. This limits the range of items available to instructors. If large numbers of versions are used, an extensive item bank may be required. Item security may be difficult to maintain, particularly in formative exams linked to an LMS. Cheating may be difficult to monitor if the examination is delivered in a distributed mode, although several varieties of exam security and verification of identity may be used in formal testing centers. The examination process that uses computer-based testing can be subject to a variety of technical difficulties that are not present in paper and pencil versions—such as network outages.

Some self-directed educational programs build computer-based assessment directly into the learning algorithms. Assessments and performance in electronic simulations guide content. These programs, such as the American Heart Association Heartcode ACLS and PALS, combine assessment and learning activities into computer-based simulations. This can effectively combine formative assessment, learning, and summative assessment into a blended set of activities that are seamless to the learner and yet contain sophisticated recorded evaluations of learner abilities.

The National Registry of EMTs, and other certification bodies, use computer testing systems to deliver certification examinations. Although most computer exams use traditional exam theory and are linear, NREMT actually uses a different testing format which is **item-response theory (IRT)**. This exam format provides for a more precise measurement of "xyz" and "abc." More information on IRT is presented later in this chapter. Although IRT is not usually an option to use in EMS classrooms, it seems reasonable that instructors preparing students for NREMT certification would build a degree of computer-based assessment into their programs. The rapid pace of change in technological environments assures that developments in technology-assisted evaluation will outpace the ability of any book to adequately describe current capabilities.

Time Limits

Each student will take a different amount of time to complete the examination. To exert some measure of control over the time spent on the examination, the instructor must set some limits on time. Setting time limits for examinations is a legitimate strategy for (1) preparing students for certifying examinations, and (2) evaluating students' ability to think quickly. The drawback to setting time limits is that students should be able to complete the examination in the time allowed. In estimating the amount of time a student is given to complete an examination, the instructor can give students four times as long as it takes the instructor to complete the test. As an alternative, Barbara Gross Davis, in *Tools for Teaching*,[4] suggests the following timing strategies:

- Allow half a minute per true/false item.
- Allow 1 minute per multiple-choice item.
- Allow 2 minutes per short answer item.
- Allow 10 to 15 minutes per limited essay item.
- Allow 30 minutes per broader essay item.
- Allow 5 to 10 minutes for students to review their work.
- Factor in time to distribute and collect tests.

One strategy to accommodate documented learning disabilities would be to extend the time allowed for an examination.

Analysis of Written Examinations

The analysis and potential revision of written exams are important steps in improving student assessment. The type of evaluation depends upon the examination stakes as well as available resources.

Post-Test Review

A useful strategy after an examination has been administered is to allow class time for students to review the examination as a group with the instructor. This review highlights areas of weakness for individual students, as well as for the class as a whole. Review can also help the instructor to identify areas where the presentation of material did not adequately prepare students for mastery of the stated objectives. It can serve to alleviate concerns about bias when students see what items other students missed. A climate of fairness is promoted when students can discuss questions, answers, or the wording of a question. Although some instructors allow students to retain the examination after classroom discussion, this practice greatly reduces the validity of test items that are reused. Even on low-stakes examinations, students who have access to the previous classes' exams can develop a false sense of security, thinking they are familiar with the content when in fact they are only recognizing items they have seen on previous exams. Teachers may be misled about the students' understanding of material based on answers obtained on previous exams. Additionally, it is neither time nor cost effective to develop new exams for each class, even for low-stakes exams. Conducting a classroom discussion breaches examination security, but the breach is less significant than when students are allowed to retain copies of the examination.

Pilot use and previous validation may not be possible for all examinations, but they should be conducted before an item is included in a high-stakes examination. One possible strategy for pilot use is to present pilot items for formative evaluations, such as quizzes. Another is to have an examination include several (generally not more than 10%) pilot items that do not count toward the exam score; these should be interspersed among regular items. Pilot items that demonstrate reliability and validity can then be included in future examinations. Pilot items that fail validation can be returned to the editing process for revision.

Difficulty Level and Discrimination Index

For low- or moderate-stakes examinations, grading of the examination is coupled with validation of test items. Validation is particularly applicable to limited-response items such as true/false, multiple-choice, and matching questions. Although validation seems difficult, a simplified procedure can be performed by any instructor. The two characteristics of tests that are useful in validation are difficulty level and item discrimination. The difficulty level is the percentage of students who answer each item correctly. The item discrimination index compares the performance of those who scored well on the exam with the performance of those who did not score well on each exam item. Computerized programs will perform the necessary calculations **(Figure 21.5)**, but the same measurements can be easily calculated manually.

Students may find an item difficult for numerous reasons, including that the item may be poorly worded. Adding the discrimination index into the analysis for potential revision of items separates those items that have questionable reliability and validity from those that are appropriately constructed, yet challenging. Items that have extreme difficulty levels (either high or low) will not discriminate as well as those with a difficulty level near 50 percent.

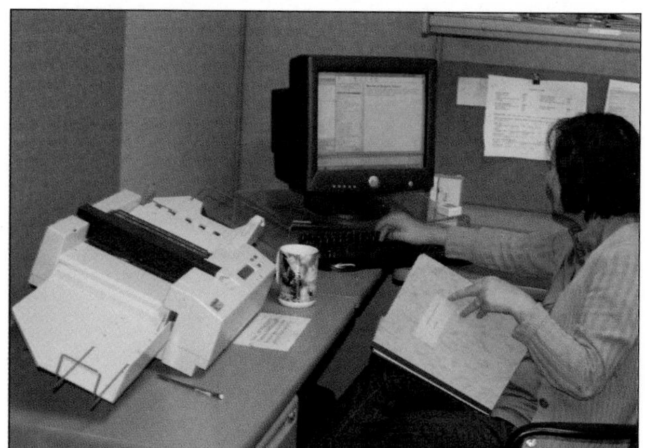

Figure 21.5

Scannable answer sheets and grading software can facilitate quick scoring of multiple-choice exams and provide a means of performing item analysis.

Calculation of Difficulty Index

The following procedure can be used to calculate the difficulty index and the discrimination index for limited response items, such as multiple-choice or true/false questions.

To calculate the item difficulty, the instructor should calculate the percentage of students who had correct responses. The formula for this is ID = (C/T) × 100, where "ID" is the item difficulty, "C" is the number of correct responses, and "T" is the total number of students who took the examination. For example, if 30 students took the exam and 20 answered the item correctly, the difficulty index would be 67 percent. The goal is to use only a few items that more than 90 percent or less than 30 percent of students answer correctly.[4]

As a result, different thresholds are used to indicate the need for revision depending on the difficulty level of the item. When the difficulty level and the discrimination ratio are used, the process shown in **Figure 21.6** can help identify items that need revision.[4]

Negative discrimination indices indicate that students who scored well overall did worse on those particular questions than did students who did not score well overall. Items with a negative discrimination index should be reviewed for validity and revised before they are used again. A common cause of a strongly negative item discrimination index (near to −1.0) is an incorrectly keyed item. Editing of examination items should extend to a check of the answer key as well.

When analyzing items, there are several components of the item that should be considered. Problems with the stem are the most obvious and common to all item types. The stem should be carefully considered to assess for length, ambiguity, and other possible sources for confusion. When evaluating multiple-choice items, consideration should also be extended to examine the distractors. Ideally, incorrect responses should be spread across all possible distractors. The instructor should consider item discrimination and the proportion of each distractor chosen to

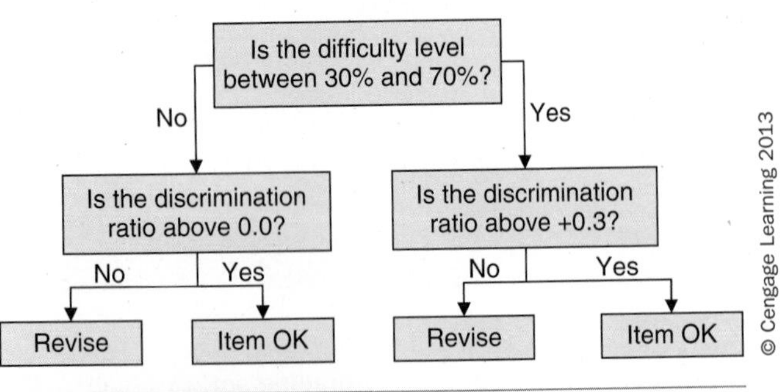

Figure 21.6

The difficulty level and the discrimination ratio can help the instructor identify test items that need revision.

Calculating the Item Discrimination

The purpose of calculating the item discrimination is to compare the response of the high exam performers on each item to the response of the low exam performers. If an item is constructed correctly, the instructor can expect that the high performers get the item correct and the low scorers miss the item. This would be referred to as a "positive discrimination value." The higher the number the better and the more discrimination.If, for some reason, more individuals from the lowest-scoring group than from the highest-scoring group select the correct answer, the result would be a "negative discrimination value." In general, items with a low (or negative) discrimination value would need to be reviewed and probably edited. This negative discrimination would likely indicate that the item was tricky and that high performers read into the item and missed it whereas the low performers got it correct. Other common reasons for negative discrimination include miskeyed items, multiple correct answers, and distractors that are actually lesser known, special case situations. As with calculating item difficulty, calculating item discrimination can be accomplished through the application of simple mathematical skills.

The item discrimination is calculated (in a simplified manner) by completing the following steps:[4]

1. Instructor identifies the exams with the 10 highest scorers and the 10 lowest scorers.
2. For each question, the instructor records the number of students in the top group of 10 who answered correctly. He or she does the same for the bottom group of 10 students.
3. The instructor then computes the discrimination ratio by subtracting the number of students in the bottom group who answered correctly from the number of students in the top group who answered correctly, and dividing by 10 (the number of students in each group). The discrimination ratio will fall between −1.0 and +1.0. The closer the ratio is to +1.0, the more effectively the item distinguishes students who know the material (the top group) from those who do not (the bottom group).

Point Biserial Value

Some test-item analysis programs will report a "point biserial" value for each test item. This statistic is very similar to a discrimination ratio. However, rather than calculating a ratio of high overall performance to low overall performance, the *point biserial* calculates the statistical correlation between an individual item and the overall score on the exam. Calculation of a correlation coefficient is beyond the scope of this text, but the value is returned by several test analysis programs. Like the item discrimination, the higher the point biserial, the better that item differentiates between those with high overall knowledge and those with low knowledge. Also like the item discrimination, this statistic tends to be low when an item is not very difficult. If an instructor has access to point biserial, it can be used in place of the item discrimination to select those items that require further editing.

determine next steps. Distractors that are never selected may not be plausible. If knowledgeable test takers are drawn to a particular distractor (shown by a low or negative discrimination), then that distractor may present a possibly correct answer—usually a special case that only advanced students would recognize. Some testing-analysis software can analyze discrimination for each distractor, greatly easing the task of distractor analysis.

It is important for the instructor to note that the item can have an appropriate difficulty index and discrimination index, but if it does not follow the principles of exam item development and construction, it may not be valid and should not be used.

Grading Strategies

Appropriate grading strategies are as important to validity and reliability as the appropriate exam administration and exam content.

Grading Essays

Grading essays and written assignments can be particularly difficult. Because grading essays is inherently subjective, reliability is difficult to ensure. Some suggested strategies that help to improve reliability in the grading of essays follow:

- Skim all writing assignments quickly before grading them, to gain an overview of the general level of performance and the range of responses.[5]
- Before the writing assignment is given or the test is administered, the instructor should decide on guidelines for full or partial credit. This is referred to as the "analytic method of grading." The instructor assigns a number of points to each designated content area. The instructor decides on partial credit for each area, and totals the points for an easy grade calculation. It may be useful for the instructor to anchor these points to specific words, phrases, or concepts to help ensure reliability.[6]
- Choose examples of student responses to serve as anchors for different levels of performance. The instructor chooses one student response as an example of a good essay, one as an example of middle performance, and one as a poor example. This approach is referred to as the "global method"of grading. It is generally helpful for instructors to also compare responses with those on an "ideal" paper prepared before the assignment.[6]
- Grade essay items question-by-question rather than student-by-student. This allows more meaningful comparison of responses between students. Instructors should shuffle the exams between questions to avoid bias in grading caused by student performance on the previous question.[5]
- Avoid judging assignments on the basis of extraneous factors such as illegible handwriting and the use of pen versus pencil. Judge essays on the intellectual quality of the response. Instructors must remember the purpose of the essay question when they are grading.[4]
- If possible, repeat the grading process a couple of days later. Another option is to use multiple graders. Agreement in grades across independent grading sessions indicates reliability.[6]

CASE IN POINT

An instructor includes an essay item relating to the pathophysiology of shock on a module examination. Five points are assigned to the item. She constructs the following rubric to assist her in grading: (5 points) Clear description of hypovolemic, distributive, cardiogenic, and obstructive shock with at least two examples of conditions that would cause each; (4 points) Clear descriptions but missing clearly relevant clinical conditions for some types; (3 points) Descriptions lack clarity, missing key mechanisms of how perfusion is limited in that type of shock; (2 points) Descriptions or examples only provided for three of the four types; (1 point) Descriptions or examples provided for less than three of the four types.

Norm-Referenced Grading

Normative (or norm-referenced) grading strategies are those that compare student performance with the performance of other students for assignment of a grade. This is commonly referred to as "grading on the curve" The result of this strategy is that a set percentage of students receives an "A," a second group gets a "B," another group receives a "C," and some are given a "D" and an "F." Each student's grade is determined by the group's performance—not by comparison with objectives. This method of grading is commonly attacked because it is based on class performance rather than on comparison of performance with objectives. On the other hand, an advantage of normative grading strategies is that the grading strategy automatically compensates for poorly constructed examinations. If a test is very easy, the curve automatically shifts to require a higher passing score. If a test is very difficult, the passing score shifts lower to compensate. This occurs without additional calculation or analysis by the instructor. A number of variations of normative grading strategies include setting a percentage of students that will receive each grade, assigning grade levels based on natural breaks in the distribution, and assigning grade levels based on a normal statistical distribution. Although purely normative strategies are generally considered inappropriate for summative evaluation in EMS courses, normative strategies are useful for assigning grades to formative evaluations with minimal impact on final grade. Normative strategies are especially useful as an interim grading strategy when piloting evaluation tools are used during formative evaluations.

Criterion-Referenced Grading

Criterion-referenced grading strategies base grade assignment on mastery of course objectives. This approach requires the presence of relatively specific course objectives on which evaluation tools can be based. According to a criterion-referenced strategy, the evaluation is drawn from the blueprint, and setting grades is guided by the degree to which objectives are mastered. One example would be that 90 percent mastery is assigned an "A," 80 percent is assigned a "B," and so forth. This can be based on depth of mastery (90% knowledge of each objective) or breadth of mastery (complete knowledge of 90% of the objectives). A criterion-referenced strategy requires the use of valid and reliable items to ensure fairness in the evaluation process. Because the setting f grades does not automatically adjust for difficulty, tructor must perform additional analysis to set riate passing score.

Setting a Cut Score

In general, the instructor has two strategies from which to choose. In the first, the instructor can build the evaluations, analyze exam items, and set the passing score based on the difficulty of the exam. In the second, the instructor can first set a passing score, then analyze draft items and construct an examination with difficulty appropriate for the preset passing score. In other words, the instructor can either set the passing score to fit the exam or engineer the exam to fit the passing score. Either option is appropriate. It is inappropriate for students to consider a course with an 80 percent passing score "harder" than a course with a 60 percent passing score, without consideration of the relative difficulty of the examinations.

Many educational institutions set the grade levels and passing scores as part of institutional policy. This fits with a common expectation that 90 percent = A, 80 percent = B, 70 percent = C, 60 percent = D, and below 60 percent is failing. Another common expectation is that 70 percent is passing, with grades interspersed. If instructors are teaching with preset passing scores and grading levels, then they must construct examinations of appropriate difficulty to match this preset passing score. The instructor does this by predicting the difficulty level for each item and computing the average difficulty index for all items on the examination. The instructor can then adjust the examination to match the computed difficulty with the preset passing score.

Predicting Item Difficulty

An instructor can use a number of methods to predict item difficulty. The most common is the **Angoff method**. This method is commonly used for high-stakes examinations in educational, certification, and licensure settings. The procedure is to first establish a panel of experts. The panel considers the concept of the "minimally competent candidate," or, in other words, the minimum acceptable level of knowledge. This is not the ideal or average candidate, but the candidate who is barely acceptable. The experts are then asked to estimate the percentage of minimally competent candidates who would answer that item correctly. This is done first with practice items, where the experts' estimates can be compared with actual performance of the item. As the experts rate the items, the consensus that is reached by the experts' estimates forms the Angoff rating. By computing the mean of the Angoff ratings for all items to be included in the exam, the instructor can determine a cut score. Conversion of this predicted cut score into a passing score is a matter of professional judgment for the instructor.

Setting a Cut Score

An instructor who is teaching a paramedic course at a community college is preparing a module examination for trauma. After collecting and editing a number of examination items, the instructor prepares to predict the difficulty by using the Angoff method (see the box Predicting Item Difficulty). The instructor plans to use the information to set an appropriate passing score.

The instructor contacts four preceptors and three lab assistants who will serve as the expert panel. She starts the process by initiating a discussion on the concept of entry-level competency. She describes the concept in this manner: ". . . the idea is to describe the provider who is barely competent. Not a great paramedic, or even a good paramedic, but instead, the paramedic who has just the amount of knowledge to be considered competent." She asks panel members to describe in their own words the depth of knowledge required for entry-level competency related to trauma. The discussion continues for a short time until the instructor believes that the panel has reached consensus on the concept.

Next, the instructor distributes a set of examination items that have been used for past courses and for which the actual difficulty level is known. The instructor projects the item, without the answer indicated, and asks the panel, "What percentage of entry-level providers would get this question correct?" After panel members have given their thoughts, she shares with the group the answer to the item. Panel members are then allowed to reconsider their rating. The instructor then shows the group how the item actually performed (the difficulty level of each item from previous administrations), and the results of each panel member are shown to the group. The panel has a short discussion on the difference between their estimates and the actual performance of the item. This exercise is repeated several times.

After reviewing these practice items, the instructor distributes the ones she will be using for the examination, without an answer key. Each panel member then rates each item as to the percentage of entry-level providers who would answer the item correctly. The answer key is then provided, and panel members are allowed to reconsider their estimate. The instructor collects and averages the results, as **Table E** shows.

The panel of experts has recommended a cut score (minimum passing score) of 70 percent for this examination. The instructor takes this into consideration as she determines the passing score for the examination. She takes into account that during the practice session, the panel consistently predicted rates of correct responses that were slightly higher than the actual values (in other words, during the practice session, the panel slightly underestimated the difficulty of items). She also considers the potential for error and decides to set the cut score for this examination at 60 percent.

(Note: In this case, had the instructor been in an institution that mandated by policy a set passing score, he or she could just as easily use this procedure to predict the item difficulty for each item, then could base item selection on the predicted difficulty to construct an examination of appropriate difficulty for the mandated minimum passing score.)

TABLE E

Item	Judge 1	Judge 2	Judge 3	Judge 4	Judge 5	Judge 6	Judge 7	Average
1	85%	80%	90%	90%	95%	90%	95%	89%
2	75%	65%	70%	85%	80%	70%	80%	75%
3	70%	80%	80%	75%	70%	80%	80%	76%
4	50%	60%	40%	50%	50%	55%	70%	54%
5	50%	45%	40%	50%	50%	50%	55%	49%
6	60%	60%	75%	65%	45%	55%	55%	59%
7	80%	90%	80%	85%	80%	85%	80%	83%
8	90%	85%	85%	90%	75%	80%	85%	84%
9	50%	55%	45%	50%	45%	50%	80%	54%
10	75%	75%	80%	70%	70%	70%	80%	74%
(etc.)								
Total	69%	70%	69%	71%	66%	69%	76%	**70%**

Note: The "total" row is the calculated average for that column.

The Cut Score

The difficulty of the tests an institution uses makes the cut score meaningful. For instance, consider the following two training programs. Program A requires an 80 percent score to pass the final examination. Program B requires 60 percent to pass. Program A uses only examination items with an Angoff rating of at least 90 percent, with an average Angoff rating of 95 percent. Program B uses a range of Angoff scores from 40 percent to 90 percent, with the average Angoff rating of 60 percent. Program B is thus a much more challenging program, despite the lower cut score, because it uses much more difficult examinations.

Item-Respose Theory

Instead of using a set minimum passing score, the National Registry of EMTs determines whether a candidate passes the examination by directly assessing the difficulty of the items answered correctly by the candidate. Traditional examinations give all candidates a set number of items of comparable difficulty and compare performance of candidates by the percentage of items answered correctly. This approach is referred to as a "linear test" and uses classical test theory.

Computer-adaptive testing allows the use of a more precise tool called "item-response theory" (IRT). Using this model, a large test bank is established with items of identified difficulty. (The Angoff method is one way to identify item difficulty.) The computer adjusts the difficulty of items for the candidate based on the candidate's responses. If a hard item is missed, the next question is slightly easier. If an item is answered correctly, the next is slightly harder. And so on. Each question answered correctly is an indication of the candidate's ability. Once enough items are correctly answered to place the candidate's ability with certainty, the test ends. The more items that are answered, the less the error of measurement. The further the candidate's ability from the competency line, the more measurement error is allowable to determine with statistical certainty that the candidate is competent (or not competent). Therefore, candidates who are far above or below the competency line will have relatively few questions. Candidates who are very near the competency line require many more items to accurately determine whether they meet minimum standards of competence.

For this reason, discussions of scores or test length for computer-adaptive examinations that use IRT are not meaningful.

Summary

Properly constructed written evaluations remain the most effective means of easily assessing cognitive objectives. Careful consideration of evaluation purpose ensures that the function of the assessment matches the use of written exam items. Different types of written exam tools have varying abilities to assess diverse types of knowledge. Items such as completion and matching are well suited to testing recall. Essay and short answer items are better for testing synthesis and evaluation. Multiple-choice and true/false items can test different levels of thinking, but construction of items that evaluate higher-order thinking is challenging. Homework can provide valuable formative evaluation. Research projects are another tool that can be used to evaluate higher levels in the cognitive domain. A combination of these different tools provides the instructor with a valid and reliable assessment of a student's mastery of knowledge.

Security of examination materials is important for limited-response tools that prove to be valid and reliable assessments of higher levels within the cognitive domain. Security is not an issue for homework and project assignments, and it is less critical for essay items. Because of the extensive effort needed to properly construct and analyze limited-response items, it is necessary that the security of these items be protected. If security is compromised, items that would otherwise test high-end knowledge become items that test only recall. In addition, compromises of examination security may dramatically change the difficulty level and discrimination index of the compromised items.

Limited-response items are extremely valuable for the EMS instructor. Testing a large number of cognitive objectives with acceptable reliability and validity requires the use of many more limited-response items than essay and short answer items. This also serves to prepare EMS students for licensure examinations, which use limited-response items almost exclusively. Unfortunately, these items become nearly worthless if security is compromised.

Glossary

Angoff method An expert group consensus process to assign item difficulty.

blueprinting Planning the exam to facilitate validity with appropriate level of required thinking, content depth, and breadth.

computer-adaptive testing Allows the use of a more precise tool that is able to adjust the difficulty of items for the candidate based on the candidate's responses.

distractor An incorrect answer designed to be a plausible alternative to the correct answer.

item-response theory The computer adjusts the difficulty of items for each candidate using an algorithm that is based on the candidate's responses.

stem The part of the item that is first offered, which may be written as a question or as an incomplete statement.

References

1. Hertz, N. R., & Chinn, R. N. (2000). *Licensure examinations.* Lexington, KY: Council on Licensure, Enforcement, and Regulation.
2. Margolis, G. S., Romero, G. A., Fernandez, A. R., & Studnek, J. R. (2009). Strategies of high-performing paramedic educational programs. *Prehospital Emergency Care, 13*: 505–511.
3. Cantillon, P. (2010). *ABC of learning and teaching in medicine.* Oxford, UK: John Wiley & Sons.
4. Davis, B. G. (2001). *Tools for teaching.* San Francisco, CA: Jossey-Bass.
5. Jacobs, L., & Chase, C. (1992). *Developing and using tests effectively: A guide for faculty.* San Francisco, CA: Jossey-Bass.
6. Cashin, W. (1987). *Improving essay tests.* IDEA paper, no. 17. Manhattan, KS: Kansas State University Center for Faculty Evaluation and Development.

Additional Resources

Cantillon, P., Irish, W., & Sales, D. (2004, September). Using computers for assessment in medicine. *British Medical Journal, 329*(7466): 606–609.

Case, S. M., & Swanson, D. B. (2001). *Constructing written test questions for the basic and clinical sciences,* (3rd ed.). Philadelphia, PA: National Board of Medical Examiners.

Cashin, W. E. (1987). *Improving essay tests.* IDEA paper, no. 17. Manhattan, KS: Kansas State University Center for Faculty Evaluation and Development.

Clegg, V. L, & Cashin, W. E. (1986). *Improving multiple-choice tests.* IDEA paper, no. 16. Manhattan, KS: Kansas State University Center for Faculty Evaluation and Development.

Frary, R. B. (1995). *More multiple-choice item writing do s and don ts.* Washington, DC: ERIC Clearinghouse on Assessment and Evaluation.

Hertz, N. R., & Chinn, R. N. (2000). *Licensure Eexaminations.* Lexington, KYy: Council on Licensure, Enforcement, and Regulation.; 2000.

Jacobs, L. (2004). *How to write better tests: A handbook for improving test construction skills.* Indiana University Bloomington. Available online at htpp://www.indiana.edu/&tidle;best/write_better_tests.shtml#IV.

Jacobs, L., & Chase, C. (1992). *Developing and using tests effectively: A guide for faculty.* San Francisco, CA: Jossey-Bass.

Johnson, R. R., Squires, J. R., & Whitney, D. (2002). *Setting the standard for passing professional certification examinations.* Tampa, FL: Financial Management Association International.

Margolis, G. S., Romero, G. A., Fernandez, A. R., & Studnek, J. R. (2009, Oct/Dec). Strategies of high-performing paramedic educational programs. *Prehospital Emergency Care,* 13(4): 505–511.

Tucker, S. (2007). *Using remark statistics for test reliability and item analysis.* University of Maryland School of Pharmacy. Available online at http://www.umaryland.edu/cits/testscoring/pdf/umbtestscoring_testanditemanalysis.pdf.

Withers, G. (2005). *Item writing for tests and examinations.* UNESCO International Institute for Educational Planning. Available online at http://www.unesco.org/iiep.

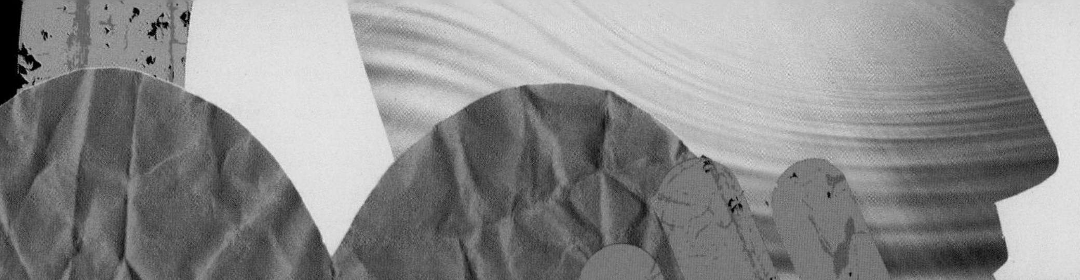

22 Other Evaluation Tools

There are no mistakes, save one: the failure to learn from a mistake. — Robert Fripp

The practice of prehospital emergency medical care requires more than knowledge. Psychomotor skills and appropriate behaviors and attitudes are also essential if Emergency Medical Services (EMS) students are to successfully perform. In addition to written examinations, other evaluations are needed to properly assess student performance.

CHAPTER GOAL: This chapter explores the use of oral examinations, practical examinations, attitudinal assessments, portfolios, and evaluations of student performance in the setting of actual patient care during clinical and field internships.

Evaluation of all Domains of Learning

Bloom's taxonomy describes learning as divided into three domains: cognitive, psychomotor, and affective. Bloom's taxonomy is described in detail in Chapter 8: Goals and Objectives. Most instructors are familiar with the methods used to evaluate the cognitive domain, or knowledge. As discussed in the previous chapter, knowledge is routinely evaluated through written examinations and writing assignments in a variety of educational settings, including the EMS classroom. The psychomotor domain, or practical skills, is better evaluated by observing the student's performance of skills in a controlled environment. Attitudes and behaviors (contained within the affective domain) are dependent on the context. Therefore, evaluation of the affective domain is best done over time and in the applied setting. Attempts to evaluate the psychomotor domain through the use of a written examination seem patently ridiculous to the effective instructor. Selection of the appropriate evaluation tool is guided by the domain of learning that is described by the objective. Written evaluations were discussed in the previous chapter; this chapter describes several other evaluation tools appropriate for the EMS instructor.

The Influence of Learning Styles in Evaluation

Different students exhibit preferences for different learning styles. Learning styles are described in detail in Chapter 4: Learning Styles. Howard Gardner takes this observation further when he asserts that different students actually have different levels of intelligence in various areas, a theory known as **multiple intelligences.**"[1] He describes the areas of intelligence as verbal/linguistic, logical/mathematical, visual/spatial, bodily/kinesthetic, musical/rhythmic, interpersonal/intrapersonal, and naturalistic.[2] It seems appropriate that evaluations can be administered in different ways to allow students to express their mastery of objectives in a manner that is comfortable for them according to their individual styles and talents. An awareness of learning styles and multiple intelligences can help the instructor distinguish between students who have not mastered objectives and those who have difficulty expressing knowledge or skills in a given format. As an example, **Table 22.1** shows how a formative assessment activity using a scenario with a standardized patient who has a cardiac rhythm disturbance can be matched with Gardner's multiple intelligences.

It is recommended that the instructor use various methods of evaluation—not just the ones that play to a student's preferences. Some, and perhaps most, evaluation tools should be standardized and required for all students. However, the instructor must realize that learning preferences and multiple intelligences do have an impact on the evaluation process.

Table 22.1 Elements of Multiple Intelligences Evaluated During a Simulated EMS Cardiac Call

Activity	Intelligence Area Assessed
1. Size-up the situation (look for hazards, determine number of patients, scan the room for patient's general appearance).	Logical-mathematical intelligence Bodily-kinesthetic intelligence
2. Communicate with the patient in a therapeutic manner.	Linguistic intelligence Interpersonal intelligence
3. Obtain the patient's history.	Linguistic intelligence
4. Perform a physical exam and vital sign assessment.	Bodily-kinesthetic intelligence Musical intelligence (breath sounds; heart tones)
5. Place the patient on a cardiac monitor and interpret the electrocardiogram (ECG).	Bodily-kinesthetic intelligence Musical intelligence (listening to the ECG tone to detect rate, regularity) Spatial intelligence (interpreting the ECG morphology)
6. Develop a working diagnosis.	Logical-mathematical intelligence
7. Perform interventions appropriate to the diagnosis (set up the IV line, simulate insertion, secure tubing; calculate the dose; draw up the medication; and administer medication appropriately using safe technique.)	Bodily-kinesthetic intelligence Logical-mathematical intelligence Interpersonal intelligence
8. Perform appropriate reassessment.	Bodily-kinesthetic intelligence
9. Communicate and work collaboratively with other team members.	Linguistic intelligence Interpersonal intelligence
10. Communicate appropriately to the dispatcher and summon additional help if needed.	Linguistic intelligence
11. Move the patient to the ambulance cot in a safe manner; secure the patient; lift the ambulance cot using the appropriate body mechanics.	Bodily-kinesthetic intelligence
12. Reflect on performance during a debriefing with the assistance of faculty and other students.	Linguistic intelligence Interpersonal intelligence Intrapersonal intelligence

For instance, written tests strongly favor those students with preferences and abilities in the verbal and logical areas. Similarly, kinesthetic learners may be favored by the use of practical examinations. Many instructors describe situations in which the student who does poorly on written tests actually performs very well in the field. Allowing some evaluations to vary significantly in form of presentation according to student preference is desirable. This provides the effective instructor with another view of the student's acquisition of new knowledge, skills, and attitudes.[3]

Additionally, the use of various methods of evaluation helps to ensure that all needed competencies are verified. In a review of different methods to evaluate competency in medical evaluation, Gaur and Skochelak noted: "These studies suggest that there is no single standard with which to evaluate medical students and the results of curricular innovations in medicine. None of these tests can be discounted, however, as each may measure a different parameter of competence." Where evaluations agree, we can be sure that the student has mastered a broad range of abilities. Where evaluations disagree, the students' strengths in different skills become evident.[4]

Many of the tools described in this chapter require that multiple instructors be involved in performing evaluations. Effective evaluation of student performance across the domains of learning requires more than a single instructor—it requires a system. This does not mean that instructors who teach courses individually cannot perform meaningful evaluations, but individual class instructors must work together to create tools for evaluation. When the instructor works with the support of others to construct, use, and analyze evaluation instruments within a system, quality evaluation is possible. A recent study of high-performing paramedic-education programs clarified the need for systems of evaluation. Focus groups conducted among programs with several years of high, first-time pass rates on national certification examinations emphasized the need to "provide students with frequent detailed feedback regarding their performance" in "all aspects of the program (classroom, laboratory, clinical, and field) and in all domains (cognitive, psychomotor, and affective)."[5]

Oral Examinations

Oral examinations are evaluations in which the questions and answers are given verbally in an exchange between a student and an instructor or group of instructors. Oral examinations are used to evaluate the cognitive domain and can extend to the affective domain. They may be used to evaluate the speed and confidence of response. The oral exam can evaluate the student's thought process and the thinking behind a particular answer. Oral examinations are similar in purpose to essay questions. Oral exams have the advantage of allowing evaluation by a group of instructors simultaneously. Another advantage is that, different from essay questions, responding to oral questions does not require a high degree of compositional skills; consequently, oral examinations can more closely approximate the expectations of the entry-level EMS professional in the job market.

For an oral exam to be fairly administered, a great deal of concentration is required by the student and the instructors. Any unexpected distractions can affect the test and may have a disparate impact on the student who is being examined when the distraction occurs. The instructor who is conducting an oral examination must exert strong control over the environment to minimize the potential for such distractions. This extends to ensuring that students and examiners minimize the potential for disturbance by having everyone turn off electronic devices. The scheduling of examiners can present difficulties in that they may be expected to evaluate a large number of candidates with little opportunity for breaks. This can lead to uneven evaluation over time. Another potential problem is the identification of trends, leading to unfair emphasis on those who repeat mistakes made by previously examined students. For example, early in the day, the instructor who is testing may consider a mistake somewhat minor. However, as subsequent students repeat a seemingly minor mistake, it may take on greater significance as an error to the examiner, and expectations may change over the day.

Oral exam items should be blueprinted, drafted, and edited in a similar manner as written essay questions. Oral exam items should be scripted and clear instructions given to the examiners to minimize any variation from the script. Without scripting, oral examinations are very difficult to standardize. Examiners must be cognizant of any clues they might inadvertently give to candidates, such as body language, comments, or gestures. By nature, grading of oral examinations is subjective. Ensuring reliability of scoring is also a challenge. One strategy for improving reliability is to use two or more examiners with independent scoring. These scores are later combined into a single composite grade.[6] Clear behavioral anchors are helpful in minimizing subjectivity.

Oral examinations are typically time consuming and labor intensive. Efforts to address the disadvantages of being able to examine only one student at a time are countered by concerns about reliability. Running parallel stations with different examiners, although more efficient, would have a negative impact on exam reliability. Nonetheless, oral examination remains a valuable tool for use in a comprehensive evaluation strategy.

Practical Examinations

Practical skill evaluation is conducted through the use of two major types of examination: the simple skill examination and the situational assessment **(Figure 22.1)**.

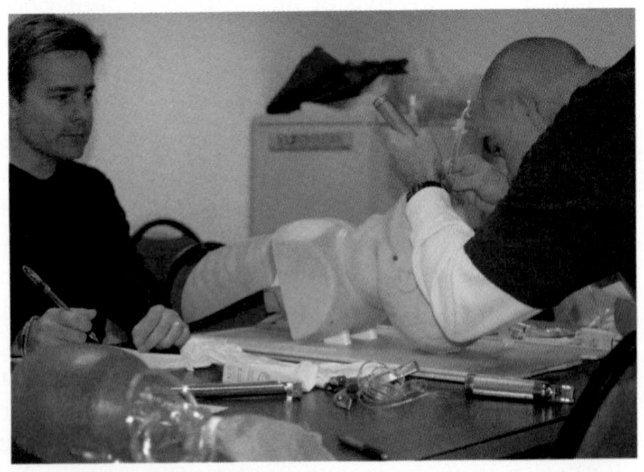

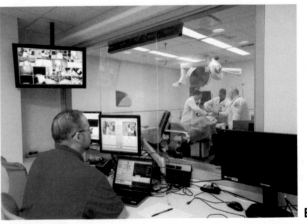

Figure 22.1

Practical-skill evaluation includes the simple isolated skill exam (A) and the situational assessment that evaluates all three domains of learning (B).

The evaluation of a rote mechanical skill is conducted through a simple **task analysis**. This is the easiest skill examination to administer. Simple skill examinations test at middle levels of the psychomotor domain, such as precision, and do not provide significant context for the skills. Situational assessment requires more elaborate simulation and is capable of assessing higher levels within the psychomotor domain, such as articulation, and elements of the cognitive and affective domains. For more information on setting up scenarios or simulations, see Chapter 18: Tools for Simulation.

Skill Evaluation

When a skill evaluation is conducted, the skill is first defined and the expected degree of proficiency is determined. Checklists are available for most skills, such as National Registry Practical Skills Examination sheets and commercially available products **(Figure 22.2)**. If checklists are not available, a performance checklist is developed from a **task analysis**, which provides a comprehensive list of the steps to be performed. Each step should include objective criteria, so that different examiners can agree on the criteria for successful completion of the step. It is usually best for instructors to keep the number of steps on the checklist to a minimum. This reduces errors in evaluation by allowing the examiner to observe the task as it is performed and complete the performance checklist afterward. The checklist should prioritize steps and list them in sequence. Critical steps should be identified, and important aspects should be weighted appropriately. Failure to properly perform any critical step results in failure of the exam. Whenever possible, the examiner should avoid qualifying or writing out the behavior; instead, the examiner should use the checklist to indicate whether a step was performed or not. The checklist should also provide any information that the examiner would need to give to the candidate. The more closely the examiner sticks to the script, the more reliable the evaluation is likely to be with various students and examiners.

To assess performance at the precision level of skill acquisition, context need not be provided and simple skill examinations can be used. Before the skill is tested in context, it is appropriate for the instructor to conduct simple skill evaluations to ensure that the student can perform the skill perfectly in isolation. Testing in context is done through the use of situational assessments. Situational assessments present the student with simulated scenarios; instructors evaluate the responses and judgments of the candidates in these specific situations. Situational assessments are more difficult to develop and deliver than are simple skill examinations. It is important that the situation and responses be simulated as accurately as possible.

The use of a programmed patient (also known as a "standardized patient") is useful in conducting situational assessments. A *programmed patient* is an actor who plays the part of the patient. Programmed patients are provided with descriptions of what responses they should give to candidates when patient assessment is conducted. *Moulage* is the simulation of injuries with the use of makeup and special effects. Additional actors may be used to play the part of family members and bystanders. The environment of the situation should be as realistic as possible. This may require that simulations be conducted in office areas, restrooms, and outdoors rather than in the typical classroom.

A common problem with skill evaluations (both simple skill evaluations and situational assessments) is the tendency for examiners to allow candidates to verbalize elements of the skill. This can occur for a variety of reasons, including lack of appropriate equipment for the candidates to use. When candidates are allowed to verbalize components of a skill evaluation, validity is destroyed by the conversion of what would have been an evaluation of the psychomotor domain into a cognitive evaluation.

Another frequent issue is the consistency of administration of the examination. Unless carefully controlled, each scenario is likely to be presented in slightly different ways, leading to problems with reliability. This is countered by the careful attention of examiners in presenting information consistently. An instructor can ensure reliability by providing a script to examiners and insisting on compliance with the script.

Objective Structured Clinical Examination (OSCE)[7]

One tool that is commonly used in medical education is the Objective Structured Clinical Examination (OSCE). The OSCE is a combination of a situational assessment and a subsequent oral (or written) examination. Students are exposed to a scripted clinical situation. For instance, students could encounter a situation in which a history is provided and they are told to assess the patient. Examiners use a standard checksheet to record which assessments were conducted. Each student is then given an oral or written examination regarding different elements of the scenario. Because the interaction is scripted and later questions standardized, cueing by instructors is minimized. Reliability increases with scripting and the use of objective criteria.

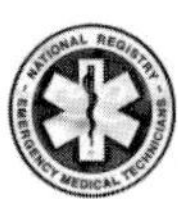

National Registry of Emergency Medical Technicians®
Emergency Medical Technician Psychomotor Examination

BVM VENTILATION OF AN APNEIC ADULT PATIENT

Candidate: ______________________ Examiner: ______________________

Date: ______________________ Signature: ______________________

Actual Time Started: __________

		Possible Points	Points Awarded
Takes or verbalizes appropriate body substance isolationprecautions		1	
Checks responsiveness	***NOTE:** After checking responsiveness and breathing for atleast 5 but no more than 10 seconds, examiner informsthe candidate, "The patient is unresponsive and apneic."*	1	
Checks breathing		1	
Requests additional EMS assistance		1	
Checks pulse for at least 5 but no more than 10 seconds		1	
***NOTE:** The examiner must now inform the candidate, "You palpate a weak carotid pulse at a rate of 60."*			
Opens airway properly		1	
***NOTE:** The examiner must now inform the candidate, "The mouth is full of secretions and vomitus."*			
Prepares rigid suction catheter		1	
Turns on power to suction device or retrievesmanual suction device		1	
Inserts rigid suction catheter without applying suction		1	
Suctions the mouth and oropharynx		1	
***NOTE:** The examiner must now inform the candidate, "The mouth and oropharynx are clear."*			
Opens the airway manually		1	
Inserts oropharyngeal airway		1	
***NOTE:** The examiner must now inform the candidate, "No gag reflex is present and the patient accepts the airway adjunct."*			
Ventilates the patient immediately using a BVM device unattached to oxygen [Award this point if candidate elects to ventilate initially with BVM attached to reservoir and oxygen so long as first ventilation is delivered within 30 seconds.]		1	
***NOTE:** The examiner must now inform the candidate that ventilation is being properly performed without difficulty.*			
Re-checks pulse for at least 5 but no more than 10 seconds		1	
Attaches the BVM assembly [mask, bag, reservoir] to oxygen [15 L/minute]		1	
Ventilates the patient adequately -Proper volume to make chest rise (1 point) -Properrate [10 –12/minute but not to exceed 12/minute] (1 point)		2	
***NOTE:** The examiner must now ask the candidate, "How would you know if you are delivering appropriate volumes with each ventilation?"*			

Actual Time Ended: __________ **TOTAL** 17

Critical Criteria

___ After suctioning the patient, failure to initiate ventilations within 30 seconds or interrupts ventilations for greater than 30 seconds at any time
___ Failure to take or verbalize body substance isolation precautions
___ Failure to suction airway **before** ventilating the patient
___ Suctions the patient for an excessive and prolonged time
___ Failure to check responsiveness and breathing for at least 5 seconds but no more than 10 seconds
___ Failure to check pulse for at least 5 seconds but no more than 10 seconds
___ Failure to voice and ultimately provide high oxygen concentration [at least 85%]
___ Failure to ventilate the patient at a rate of at least 10/minute and no more than 12/minute
___ Failure to provide adequate volumes per breath [maximum 2 errors/minute permissible]
___ Insertion or use of any adjunct in a manner dangerous to the patient
___ Failure to manage the patient as a competent EMT
___ Exhibits unacceptable affect with patient or other personnel
___ Uses or orders a dangerous or inappropriate intervention

You must factually document your rationale for checking any of the above critical items on this form (below or turn sheet over).

Figure 22.2

The National Registry of Emergency Medical Technicians (NREMT) *BVM Ventilation of An Apneic Adult Patient* skill sheet is a good example of a skill checklist.

Inter-Rater Reliability

Inter-rater reliability can be a major problem with practical examinations. A well-constructed performance checklist can help reduce problems by not allowing examiners to qualify observations; instead, they must report and record whether a step was performed according to established criteria. Even with excellent checklists, reliability is a frequent problem when a single examiner observes the student's performance. A panel of examiners can help reduce reliability concerns. Another technique for improving reliability is the requirement of multiple iterations for a set type of skills being evaluated (e.g., successfully managing four of five trauma scenarios, each evaluated by a different examiner).[8] A third technique for improving inter-rater reliability is to use a norming process to assure that evaluators are assessing performance in the same manner. In a norming process, multiple evaluators would grade the same performance and compare evaluations in order to minimize differences. While not adjusting the test, adding video or audio taping of performance can help to assure reliability by introducing a mechanism that allows for later review of performance to assure fair grading.

High-Fidelity Simulations

Extremely realistic situational assessments (also known as "high-fidelity simulations") have the capability of evaluating all three domains of learning in context. As such, these types of assessments are powerful tools for verifying mastery of objectives. These assessments present a rare opportunity for the instructor to evaluate the student's integration of needed knowledge, skills, and attitudes. Many courses use these assessments as a component of summative evaluations.

Affective Evaluations

Evaluation of the affective domain can be challenging for instructors; however, it is an important component of student evaluation. The National EMS Education Standards state that students should be evaluated in all domains, including the affective domain.

Rubrics

A useful tool for affective evaluations is the **rubric**. Rubrics are helpful evaluation tools anytime there are multiple facets to the evaluation as each component part can be broken down. In addition to student affective evaluations, rubrics can facilitate the evaluation of presentations or scenarios. The rubric converts a list of characteristics into a graded set of observable criteria to be completed by the evaluator. Construction of the rubric consists of first identifying the characteristics to be evaluated. For instance, the following characteristics have been drawn from the 2009 National Emergency Medical Services Education Standards:[9] integrity, empathy, self-motivation, appearance/personal hygiene, self-confidence, communications, time management, teamwork/diplomacy, respect, patient advocacy, and careful delivery of service. A rating scale is then selected. A common rating system is 5 = excellent, 4 = above average, 3 = average, 2 = below average, and 1 = unacceptable. A National Academy of Sciences review found: "The weight of evidence suggests that the reliability of ratings drops if there are fewer than three, or more than nine, rating categories. Recent work indicates that there is little to be gained from having more than five response categories. Within that range (three to five), there is no evidence that there is one best number of scale points in terms of scale quality."[10]

Teaching Tip >> *Another common rating system is 0 = unacceptable, 1 = acceptable, and 2 = excellent. Another alternative is to simply indicate that performance meets or does not meet the stated objective.*

Teaching Tip >> *To prevent clustering of scores at the middle value of a rating system, the instructor should use an even number of choices.*

When the rubric is completed, observable behaviors are provided for each level of performance. The 2002 National Guidelines for Educating EMS Instructors[11] provides a rubric for the characteristic of appearance/personal hygiene.

The rubric can be completed by a number of evaluators. By providing relatively detailed descriptions of affective characteristics, different evaluators can conduct assessments with some degree of inter-rater reliability. These tools should be provided to the student at or near the beginning of the course. Rubrics can be used for formative evaluation, and they provide valuable feedback to the student. Concrete examples of unacceptable conduct should be provided to the student. Because affective behaviors are situation-dependent, these examples should provide as much context as possible. When the discussion is framed in terms of observable behaviors rather than vaguely worded attitudes, student resistance to feedback

Sample Rubric[11]

Point Value	Criteria
1	Inappropriate uniform or clothing worn to class or clinical settings. Poor hygiene or grooming.
2	Appropriate clothing or uniform selected most of the time, but the uniform may be unkempt (wrinkled), mildly soiled, or in need of minor repairs; appropriate personal hygiene is common, but occasionally, the individual is unkempt or disheveled.
3	Clothing and uniform are appropriate, neat, clean, and well maintained; good personal hygiene and grooming.
4	Clothing and uniform are above average. Uniform is pressed, and business casual is chosen when uniform is not worn. Grooming and hygiene are good or above average.
5	Uniform is always above average. Nonuniform clothing is business-like. Grooming and hygiene are impeccable. Hair is worn in an appropriate manner for the environment, and student is free of excessive jewelry. Makeup and perfume or cologne usage are discrete and tasteful.

is minimized. The more concrete and objective the feedback, the better it will be received. For instance, challenging a student that "he is sloppy" is likely to produce a defensive reaction from the student that the evaluation is an opinion. On the other hand, noting three dates in which the student reported to a clinical site unshaven with a wrinkled uniform is more likely perceived as a clear standard instead of a personal opinion. In some cases, the instructor may wish to have students fill out rubrics on each other, a technique known as **360-degree evaluation.** This is particularly valuable when group projects are assigned to class members. Group members can provide valuable feedback to each other regarding teamwork skills. Of course, summative evaluations of affective characteristics should also be conducted. The same rubrics can serve as summative tools.

Rubrics can fairly easily be converted to surveys that the student can use for self-assessment. Self-assessment is a useful formative strategy. Affective evaluations should be completed by the primary instructor and can also be completed by secondary and lab instructors who spend appreciable amounts of time with the student. The instructor who uses these affective rubrics in the clinical setting and internship can assess the degree to which a particular behavior is consistently exhibited in the applied-care setting. These assessments provide valuable feedback to the student, and can be significant indicators of future behavior. A 2004 study of medical students found that records of unprofessional conduct in medical school was correlated with future disciplinary action by a state medical board.[12] Evidence of predictive validity such as this makes evaluation of the affective domain a critical part of assuring future professional conduct.

Impact on Grades

Converting rubric scores to grades is relatively easy. The degree of grade impact of affective evaluations is a matter of professional judgment for the instructor to decide. This excerpt is from the 2011 CoAEMSP Interpretations of the CAAHEP Standards and Guidelines: "As important as the cognitive and psychomotor domains, the program must teach, monitor, and evaluate (i.e., grade) the attitudes and behaviors of the students, including interpersonal interactions."

An acceptable affective evaluation should be required for each student to pass the class. Some programs will also use affective evaluations as a part of course grades. The use of rubrics ensures a criterion-referenced strategy. Averaging scores from multiple evaluators can help ensure reliability. Content validity can be assessed through expert review, in a manner similar to written evaluations. Use of rubrics helps the instructor convert a subjective evaluation of the affective domain, with poor reliability, to a more objective and reliable assessment. It is important to note that the student must achieve the minimum expected standard in each domain of competency. Ratings for poor behavior and excellent knowledge should not average into a passing grade, just as a student with excellent behavior and substandard knowledge should not pass.

Surveys

Another tool that is used to evaluate the affective domain is the completion of surveys by students. This tool is especially useful if the course is relatively short, and the purpose of the evaluation is to look for a change in behavior from precourse evaluation to postcourse evaluation. Surveys can be constructed as a series of statements for which students indicate the degree to which they agree with the statement. It is useful to use a Likert-rating scale to indicate varying levels of agreement, for example, 5 = strongly agree, 4 = agree, 3 = neutral, 2 = disagree, and 1 = strongly disagree. By assessing the same objective with a number of different statements, the reliability of each statement can be assessed through a variety

CASE IN POINT

An EMS instructor is tasked with designing a summative affective evaluation for paramedic students. The list of characteristics is drawn from the National Emergency Medical Services Education Standards list of characteristics of professionalism in the clinical behavior/judgment section. She then consults the interpretation of program accreditation standards, and notes that there should be at least one comprehensive affective evaluation of each student, separate from affective components of clinical/field evaluations. Keeping this in mind, she decides to use a three-point rating system, with categories of "unacceptable," "average," and "exemplary." In the interest of including her advisory committee members in the process, she schedules a meeting for the representatives of EMS services and hospitals on the advisory committee to anchor the rating system with observable behaviors.

She begins the meeting by leading a discussion of the list of characteristics to develop consensus on the specific affective objectives to be evaluated. She follows with a discussion of the rating levels. She describes "unacceptable" as needing improvement before a student can successfully complete the program. She describes "average" as the minimum level required for entry-level competency. She describes "exemplary" as performance that makes the student a role model for that affective characteristic.

She begins with the area of integrity. She starts by discussing the "average" category, minimum entry-level competency. She reminds everyone that this is the same level used for standard setting for a written exam. She asks the group what behaviors or examples they can cite for students they believe are in this category. Working on a white board, she consolidates these ideas into a few statements of observable behaviors. The group works to achieve consensus on that list. As the group works, they realize that several had slightly different ideas of how integrity applied to EMS. The list of observable behaviors created a shared, common understanding of how to apply the imprecise concept of integrity to the specific actions of the EMS student.

Working from the discussion of minimum acceptable competency, she leads the group to describe characteristics for the "unacceptable" category. They recognize that most statements would be less than the "average category" in terms of degree or consistency of behavior. For instance, the minimum standard included the statement: "always tells the truth." The group then developed "sometimes doesn't tell the truth" as a less consistent performance in the same area. Some concepts are expressed only in the "unacceptable" category. For example, cheating was described by the group as unacceptable, even though that concept was not expressly listed in the minimum acceptable statements.

She leads the group next on clarifying the behavioral anchors for the "exemplary" category. The group struggles with this for the subject of integrity. They tend to view integrity in terms of acceptable or unacceptable, with little ability for students to excel. After some discussion, they identify a few behaviors that illustrate exemplary conduct. As an example, the group identified courage to directly and appropriately challenge other students' poor behavior as a description of excellent conduct within the area of integrity.

The group then moves on to the next characteristic on the list and repeats the previous steps.

of statistical tests, such as **split-half** or **Cronbach's alpha** (see Chapter 20: Principles of Evaluation of Student Performance, for further explanation of reliability tests). Surveys can also be used to assess the mastery of affective objectives related to the comfort level of the provider, such as "I am comfortable providing care for pediatric patients." Surveys are better than behavior-based rubrics for evaluating objectives that relate to confidence and comfort level because abstract characteristics like confidence are not easily assessed by observation of behavior. Thus, for affective objectives that are easily translated into observable behaviors, the rubric is the preferred tool; student surveys are more accurate for assessing internal characteristics.

Portfolio Projects

Research projects were discussed in the previous chapter. A variation on the traditional research paper is the use of a portfolio project. Portfolios are discussed in greater detail in Chapter 13: Tools for Individual Learning. Grading strategies used for portfolios vary considerably, depending on the specific forms of presentation used. Grading intermediate steps provides important feedback and an opportunity to provide formative evaluation. Basing a portion of the grade on the results of the intermediate assessments is recommended. Guidelines for grading the written components are provided in the previous chapter. Other formats for presentation of information should have separate grading criteria. In grading written work, it is important to look past the handwriting and style to evaluate the content. Similarly, in evaluating other formats, it is important to look past the stylistic elements to evaluate the content of the presentation. It is helpful to use rubrics to assess alternative presentation formats. Instead of trying to create brand new rubrics, the instructor can modify rubrics through commonly available sources such as Rubistar.[13] Building the rubric with the student or group helps to ensure that the grading criteria are well known to the student. The student can then use the rubrics as a self-assessment tool when working through the final stages of the project. If students are working together in a group to complete the project, the instructor should evaluate the interpersonal skills used. This can be done with the use of rubrics constructed for this purpose. The instructor who directly observes the group working together can assess teamwork. A combination of self-assessment and 360-degree evaluation can also be used.

Portfolio projects can be used to evaluate different domains and appeal to different learning preferences. Portfolios take time for the student to develop as components are usually developed over the duration of the course. This allows the project to serve both as a learning tool and as an evaluation tool. These projects can be a challenge for the instructor to grade, and rubrics may have to be created for each of the styles of presentation. Fortunately, generic rubrics are available. Typically, generic rubrics are designed for teachers in elementary and secondary schools; they may require some degree of modification by the EMS instructor.

Paramedic Portfolio Competency Package

In 2009, paramedic-education programs around the United States joined in a coordinated project to document psychomotor competency through a body of evidence. This body of evidence was known as a "portfolio," rather than single skills attempts or a single summative exam. The group was convened by the National Registry of EMTs (NREMT), which was exploring a more effective method to demonstrate consistent skill proficiency than with a single skill exam. The concept in that initial group, and subsequently with additional programs, included: (1) setting a minimum number of practice attempts for students in the laboratory setting; (2) having a preceptor evaluate those same skills in the hospital setting on real patients; and (3) field preceptor evaluation of the skills.

The laboratory component of the package includes 24 formative evaluation instruments that have many details to assist in learning the details of the skill. Peers are used to assist in the development of skill proficiency, allowing for more practice time in lab. Once proficient, as evaluated by an instructor in the discrete skills such as Comprehensive Adult Physical Assessment, Intravenous therapy, or Nasotracheal Intubation Adult, students move into a scenario phase where they begin to demonstrate competency in those same skills integrated within the context of a simulated patient situation. This is where the more complex responsibilities of patient assessment and management, along with the ability to correctly execute the individual skills, are learned. Scenario lab instruments include Team Leader and Team Member and students are evaluated by peers and instructors. The next progression of the portfolio package is demonstration of skills in the clinical setting on real patients and evaluated by a preceptor. The skills include clinical evaluation instruments for skills, such as medication administration, blood glucose, and 12-lead ECG acquisition, and also include an "impression/differential diagnosis" section and a "treatment plan" section to facilitate discussion of these areas and development of judgment. Students must interact with the patients and perform skills.

The final component of the portfolio package is the field internship setting with actual patients, and with preceptor supervision and feedback. Preceptors who are trained in methods of evaluation and the specific internship tool are utilized to guide student practice and evaluate the student in all domains.

Often, student performance declines slightly at the beginning of each new phase of portfolio documentation. The goal of the portfolio package, however, is to document the development of proficiency over time, so variations in performance level are expected. When programs can demonstrate a completed portfolio that documents multiple iterations of each skill and patient-management situation by multiple evaluators including peer and faculty evaluators, over a sustained period of time, a final summative examination may not be necessary for program completion.

The National Registry of EMTs continues to evaluate and support this project and is currently working to identify characteristics and methods of evaluation of team membership and leadership. The skills-proficiency tools are provided to programs without cost and are available at http://www.NAEMSE.org on the *Trading Post*.

Applied Care Evaluation

The primary goal of an EMS educational program is to prepare graduates to function competently as EMS providers. It is impossible for the instructor to fully simulate the environment and conditions of a medical emergency. Therefore, some degree of evaluation in the actual setting in which care is being provided is necessary. Instructors must supervise the experience because they may still be unsure about the competency of the student at this early stage. Evaluating the student in the hospital and field environment is difficult. Among the challenges are maintaining appropriate patient care during the evaluation experience, ensuring reliability of the evaluations, and working with a team of preceptors. Appropriately conducting evaluation in the applied care environment requires well-constructed evaluation instruments that match the clinical experience to the objectives, a team of high-quality preceptors, and a systematic approach by the primary instructor.

Global Rating Scales

The most commonly used tool for evaluating student performance in the clinical setting is a set of global ratings of performance. When this tool is used, a set of characteristics are listed, along with a Likert-type scale for each. In some cases, a short description is provided for each rating.

Global ratings are easy for the preceptor to complete. They can be constructed and completed very quickly. The major difficulty with global-rating scales is that without extensive training and continuous reminders, inter-rater reliability is very difficult to achieve. Many instructors compensate for this lack of reliability by requiring that a large number of ratings be performed by multiple preceptors. Other instructors bolster reliability by providing detailed descriptions for each rating, effectively converting the global-rating tool into a rubric.

Other Evaluation Tools

Neal Whitman, in *A Guide to Clinical Performance Testing*,[14] describes a model for using other tools to evaluate student performance in the clinical setting. Whitman draws distinctions between aspects of evaluated performance that are related to a specific objective in the course and aspects that are not well described by course objectives. This is discussed in terms of whether predescribed specific steps are to be performed (as in patient assessment), or the specifics are not predescribed (as in scene management) as illustrated in the text box above.

Objectives Matrix

	Specifics Preestablished	Specifics Not Preestablished
Objectives	Checklists	Observation logs
Other aspects	Critical incident forms	Anecdotal records

Checklists as Whitman describes them would be very similar to those checklists used in skill evaluations and simulations. Observable aspects would be listed in well-constructed checklists, generally in the order in which they should be performed **(Figure 22.3)**. The preceptor indicates whether the student performed the step or not. Preceptors should be discouraged from making qualitative ratings. In some variations, the checklist includes categories for whether the step was performed correctly, performed incorrectly, or not observed **(Figure 22.4)**. Affective components can be evaluated with rubrics that contain observable behaviors associated with levels of performance, instead of checklists. A sample internship evaluation tool is provided in Appendix A.

Observation logs list the various objectives, and open space is provided beside each in which the preceptor can note how that objective was met during the encounter. For example, an objective might be: "The student keeps the patient's family informed." Preceptors would make notes next to this objective when they observe that objective being performed. Although checklists work well for those skills and qualities that can be standardized for nearly all patient encounters, observation logs should be used when the specifics of skills and qualities are heavily dependent on the situation.

Example of Global Rating

The student uses assistants well:

1	2	3	4	5
Consistently fails to direct assistants		Uses assistants well most of the time		Consistently makes best use of assistants

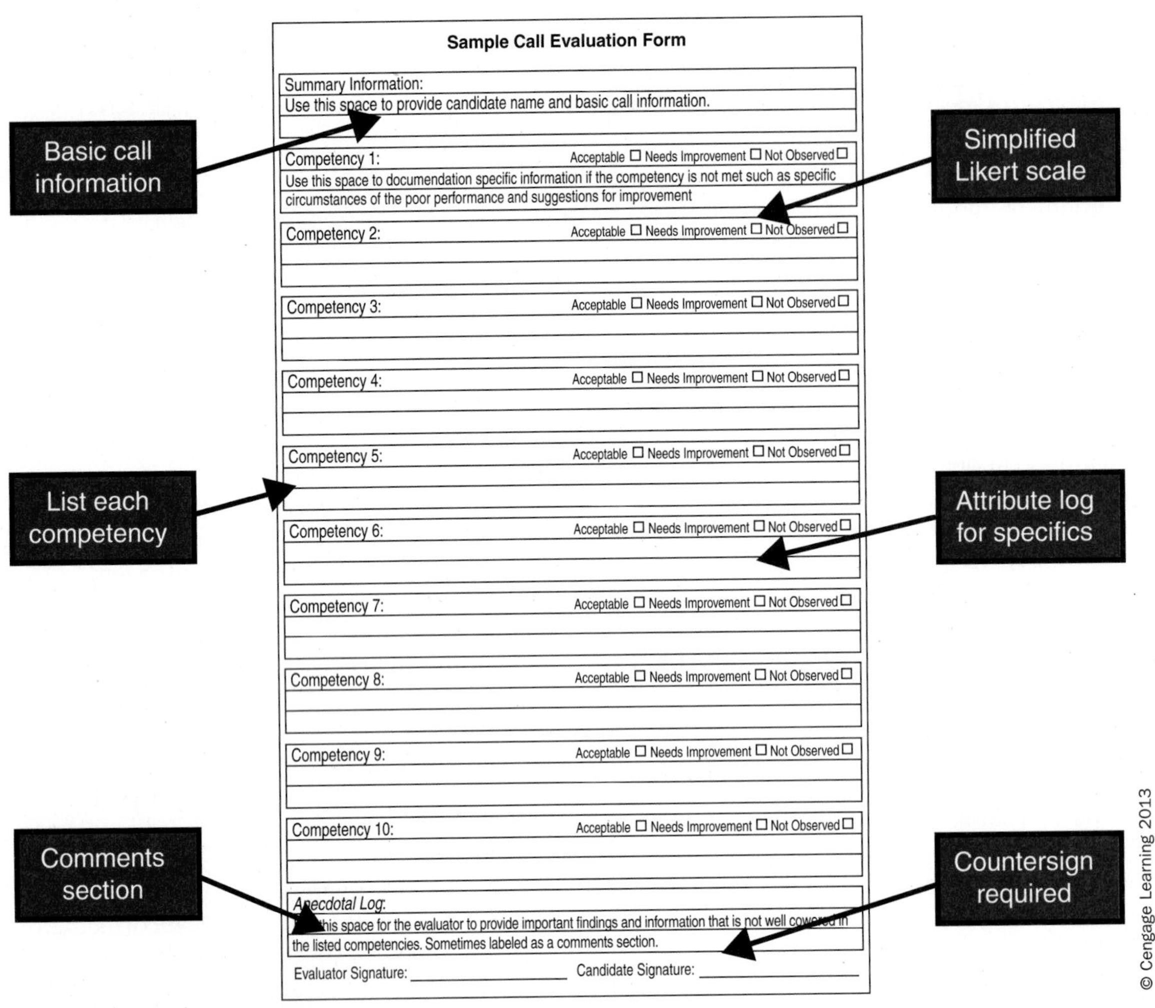

Sample Call Evaluation Form

Summary Information:
Use this space to provide candidate name and basic call information.

Competency 1: Acceptable ☐ Needs Improvement ☐ Not Observed ☐
Use this space to documendation specific information if the competency is not met such as specific circumstances of the poor performance and suggestions for improvement

Competency 2: Acceptable ☐ Needs Improvement ☐ Not Observed ☐

Competency 3: Acceptable ☐ Needs Improvement ☐ Not Observed ☐

Competency 4: Acceptable ☐ Needs Improvement ☐ Not Observed ☐

Competency 5: Acceptable ☐ Needs Improvement ☐ Not Observed ☐

Competency 6: Acceptable ☐ Needs Improvement ☐ Not Observed ☐

Competency 7: Acceptable ☐ Needs Improvement ☐ Not Observed ☐

Competency 8: Acceptable ☐ Needs Improvement ☐ Not Observed ☐

Competency 9: Acceptable ☐ Needs Improvement ☐ Not Observed ☐

Competency 10: Acceptable ☐ Needs Improvement ☐ Not Observed ☐

Anecdotal Log:
This space for the evaluator to provide important findings and information that is not well covered in the listed competencies. Sometimes labeled as a comments section.

Evaluator Signature: ______________ Candidate Signature: ______________

Figure 22.3
Sample call-evaluation form.

Critical incident forms are used to identify a specific aspect of performance, and the preceptor describes the situation when a positive or negative example is observed. As an example, the characteristic might be: "Promotes interagency cooperation." When the preceptor observes the student bringing water to the incident commander on a fire scene, the preceptor would make notes on the critical incident form to describe the positive example.

Anecdotal records are simply a means of describing any other behavior that the preceptor deems relevant. Space for anecdotal comments is often provided on evaluation forms. Anecdotal records are valuable for capturing information that is not well described in advance by the other tools. Use of anecdotal records acknowledges that no evaluation system is perfect, and that all tools will invariably miss some important aspect of performance.

The effective instructor uses a combination of the previously described evaluation tools to form a system for observational reports to be completed by the preceptor of the experience. An effective strategy is to use a pyramid approach to the evaluation system. This consists of a report for each clinical encounter; these reports form the base of the pyramid. These encounter reports could include components of checklists, observation logs, critical incident forms, and anecdotal records. The preceptor would then complete a report for the entire shift (the next tier on the pyramid) and combine information from encounter reports. This has the advantage of giving the student a degree of perspective on how the patient encounters combine to form a general impression for the shift. A number of shifts would be combined into a summative report for the entire rotation, forming the next higher tier on the pyramid. This builds from formative evaluation into a summative tool. An overall summary would be included at the end of the clinical cycle. Each tier builds on information obtained from the lower tier **(Figure 22.5)**.

Sample Summary Evaluation Form

Summary Information:
Use this space to provide candidate name and basic call information.

	Acceptable	Needs Improvement	Not Observed
Competency 1:			
Characteristic 1a	☐	☐	☐
Characteristic 1b	☐	☐	☐
Characteristic 1c	☐	☐	☐
Characteristic 1d	☐	☐	☐
Characteristic 1e	☐	☐	☐
Competency 2:			
Characteristic 2a	☐	☐	☐
Characteristic 2b	☐	☐	☐
Characteristic 2c	☐	☐	☐
Characteristic 2d	☐	☐	☐
Characteristic 2e	☐	☐	☐
Competency 3:			
Characteristic 3a	☐	☐	☐
Characteristic 3b	☐	☐	☐
Characteristic 3c	☐	☐	☐
Characteristic 3d	☐	☐	☐
Characteristic 3e	☐	☐	☐
Competency 4:			
Characteristic 4a	☐	☐	☐
Characteristic 4b	☐	☐	☐
Characteristic 4c	☐	☐	☐
Characteristic 4d	☐	☐	☐
Characteristic 4e	☐	☐	☐
Competency 5:			
Characteristic 5a	☐	☐	☐
Characteristic 5b	☐	☐	☐
Characteristic 5c	☐	☐	☐
Characteristic 5d	☐	☐	☐
Characteristic 5e	☐	☐	☐

Attribute Log

Use this section as a free from space to have evaluator note the specifics associated with any deficiencies. Have the evaluator associate any notes in this section with the specific characteristic by the use of a box as shown.

Anecdotal Log:
Use this space for the evaluator to provide important findings and information that is not well cowered in the listed competencies. Sometimes labeled as a comments section.

Evaluator Signature: ____________ Candidate Signature: ____________

Basic shift information

Simplified Likert scale

List each characteristic

Attribute log for specifics

Comments section

Countersign required

Figure 22.4

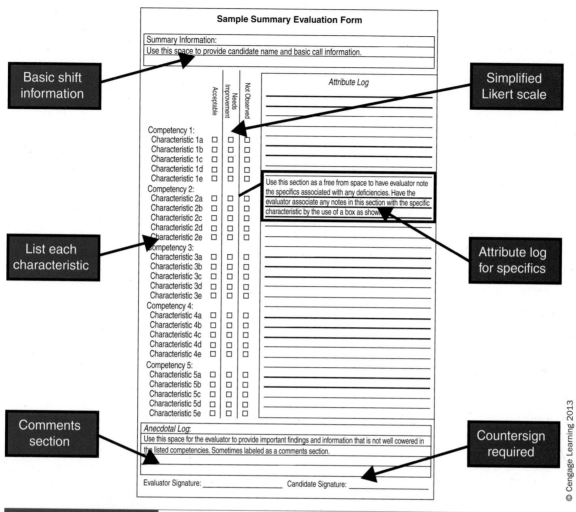

Sample skill-evaluation form.

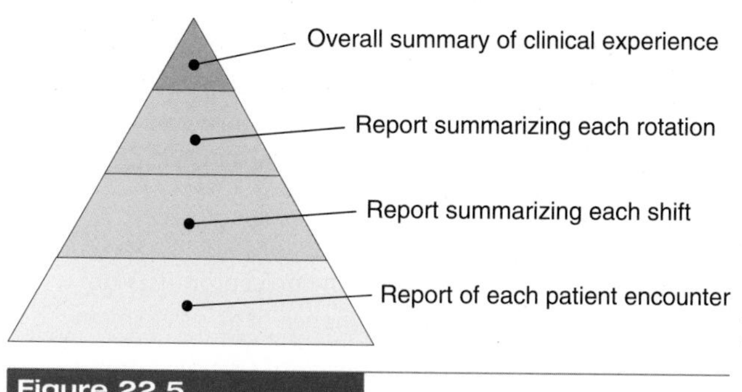

Figure 22.5

Pyramid approach to the evaluation system.

Selection of Experiences

The instructor should provide student experiences in relevant areas. For initial courses of instruction, guidelines for clinical experiences can be drawn from The National EMS Education Standards, accreditation standards or state EMS regulatory agency documents. The instructor should review these guidelines before beginning to instruct a course. Working from these guidelines, the instructor can plan for relevant clinical experiences. Early clinical experiences are typically used to evaluate student performance of skills on actual patients.

The student is usually moved from specialized areas of the hospital (such as labor and delivery) to more relevant areas (such as the emergency department) and then to the field environment. This model illustrates the concept of scaffolding experiences. The instructor should evaluate each clinical area according to two dimensions. The first dimension is one of educational experiences. In other words, what can the student learn in this environment? Educational experiences in the applied care environment should be clearly linked to educational experiences in the classroom and lab to build relevance. The second dimension is one of evaluation potential. In other words, what conclusions can the instructor draw from evaluations of the student performance in the given environment? For example, say a paramedic instructor requires venipuncture experiences with the hospital laboratory team. The student will learn the variation of vein locations and will learn techniques for finding a vein. The student can be evaluated on finding veins, and successfully accessing the vein to draw blood. This may be a necessary precondition before intravenous infusions on patients are allowed. However, the instructor should not draw the conclusion that the paramedic student can initiate intravenous lines after observing performance only of venipuncture in lab settings.

Preceptors

In most cases, the lead instructor is not able to directly observe the performance of all students in the hospital or field setting, so preceptors must be used. A *preceptor* is defined as a teacher who is an identified experienced practitioner who provides transitional role support and learning experiences during the hospital or field setting.

Preceptors should be proficient in the environment in which they perform. However, subject matter expertise is not enough. In fact, many students take lessons from preceptors to heart much more than they do lessons from the classroom instructor **(Figure 22.6)**. This can be effective if the lessons from the preceptor are aligned with those given in the classroom. If the lessons conflict, significant problems can arise. Thus, preceptors must be aware of the basic principles of adult education. They must also be aware of their role, and they must know what is being taught in the classroom. Regular communication between preceptors and instructors is necessary. Preceptors should be trained in the use of the evaluation instruments they will be expected to use.

Some instructors experience difficulty in assuring preceptors that negative impressions are appropriately documented in the hospital or internship phases of education. In some cases, the preceptor is willing to share the experiences informally with the instructor. There can be many reasons for this, ranging from difficulty in using the forms to fear of confrontation. Occasionally, meeting directly with preceptors informally can help the instructor identify mismatch between formal and informal communications. Training on evaluation instruments and assuring preceptors that negative ratings are taken in context can also help. Assuring that lines of reporting results from the preceptor to the educational program are independent of the student is helpful in minimizing the fear of confrontation that some preceptors feel.

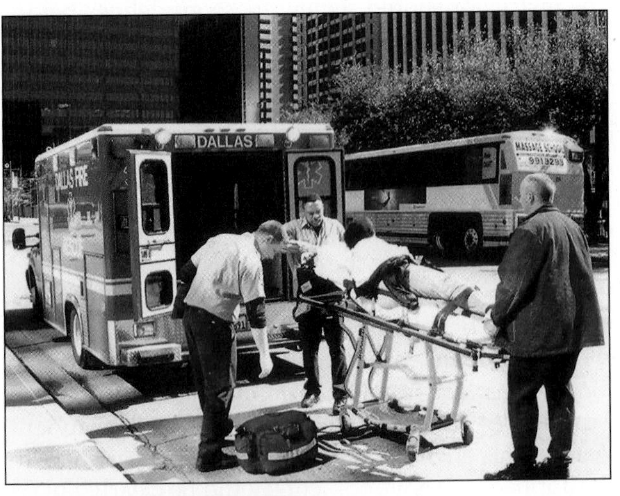

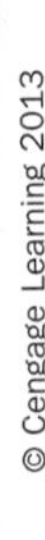

Figure 22.6

Feedback from preceptors is often instrumental in student learning. Feedback should be documented on the student-evaluation tool.

CASE IN POINT

A clinical coordinator is revising the documentation tools used for students in a paramedic program during their field internships. She decides that because different types of forms will be required for different elements, each student will be given a notebook with a set of forms to be completed by the preceptor. Each notebook contains the following, which are designed for up to 15 shifts with a preceptor:

- Forty call evaluations, each including an observation log that lists 10 objectives that can be demonstrated during any call
- Fifteen shift evaluations, each including an observation log that lists 10 objectives; these can act as a tool for the preceptor in summarizing the day's performance
- Twenty performance checklists for patient assessment, to be completed by the preceptor after observing the intern's performance of an assessment
- A knowledge checklist for each of several common protocols used by the service, to be completed by the preceptor after the student applies each protocol to an ambulance run
- Eight rubrics for affective objectives, to be completed by the preceptor on every other day of the internship
- One summary evaluation, along with a global rating for each objective, to be completed by the preceptor at the end of the internship

Integration of Evaluation with Patient Care

A unique challenge to evaluating student performance in the applied care setting is the integration of educational goals, evaluation goals, and provision of excellent clinical care to the patient. It is essential that preceptors be prepared to meet this challenge. In terms of the educational goals of clinical experiences, the applied care setting is extremely effective in allowing students to experience the consequences of poor decisions. These lessons are extremely powerful and are likely to be retained by the student. However valuable these teachable moments may be, the educational value of having to deal with poor decisions must not be allowed to affect the patient. The preceptor must be prepared to intervene if it appears that the patient will suffer from a student's mistake. If the patient will not suffer, though, a valuable opportunity to drive a lesson home may be created.

With regard to the goals of evaluating student performance, preceptor intervention can present difficulties. It is difficult for the preceptor to hold a student accountable for a mistake that was never allowed to occur. Intervention should occur just at the "point of no return," when it is apparent that the student will not realize and correct the mistake. If the preceptor frequently intervenes too early, the student may become hesitant and unwilling to commit to a decision. If the preceptor provides clues to the intervention, such as by asking, "Are you sure you want to do that?" on all critical steps, and not just when a poor decision is in progress, the evaluation has greater validity. Mastering this fine balance is an important skill for preceptors.

Even with extensive clinical and internship opportunities, it is unlikely that the student will be evaluated on all skills in the clinical environment. The instructor must be prepared to extrapolate from the results of evaluations that have been conducted. This extrapolation should be reasonable, based on the types of situations in which the student has demonstrated acceptable performance. For example, it is unlikely that all students will have the opportunity to manage a cardiac arrest in the applied care environment.

The instructor may choose to extrapolate from the student's actual performance in caring for a critically ill patient and from simulations of cardiac arrest, to conclude that the student can adequately manage a cardiac arrest in the field. This is a matter of professional judgment for the instructor, who combines personal opinion with input from the program director and the medical director. It is helpful to have guidelines regarding minimum exposure to different types of patients experiencing different types of emergencies. However, it is not feasible to require every student to see all types of calls. Reasonable extrapolations must be made.

For a sample paramedic field internship evaluation tool see Appendix A.

Teaching Tip >> *State regulations and program accreditation requirements typically have rules regarding minimum exposure for patients chosen from various age groups (e.g., adult and various pediatric age groups), types of complaints and emergencies (e.g., cardiac and respiratory), and procedures (e.g., initiating IV access and drug administration).*

Summary

By combining written evaluations with other evaluation tools, an integrated strategy can be developed for assessing each of the domains of learning. Creating an effective evaluation strategy begins with careful consideration of the purpose of the evaluation. This purpose may be tied to a curriculum, using established objectives to anchor the evaluation tools used. The purpose may likewise be to verify competency with evaluations based on a practice analysis (that can be used to build objectives). It is sometimes helpful for the instructor to divide course objectives among the domains of learning, as the domain will be a significant consideration in the selection of evaluation tools. Based on the objectives, the instructor can decide on which tools will be used to evaluate student performance. Cognitive objectives can be effectively evaluated through the use of written examinations, oral examinations, and research projects. Psychomotor objectives can be assessed with practical examinations, simulations, and evaluations of student care of patients in a supervised clinical experience. Affective objectives can be evaluated through writing assignments, oral examinations, and surveys at lower levels. Higher levels can be assessed through behavioral observations (with rubrics) that occur during class and lab as well as during the clinical and field components of a course. Regardless of which domain area is to be evaluated, students must be given previous knowledge of what objectives will be applied and to what degree they will be expected to perform.

When an integrated approach is used, a number of tools are required for effective assessment of the student. No one single tool will be capable of assessing the depth and breadth of objectives for the typical EMS course. The use of multiple tools also helps to ensure reliability of the evaluation process; consistency of results from different tools can be assessed. The grade assigned to a course should include elements from each of the formal evaluation tools. Each tool can be weighted according to the stated purpose of the evaluation strategy and the course objectives. Each tool will have strengths and weaknesses. By thoughtfully combining tools, the instructor can effectively minimize the weaknesses of each individual tool.

Based on the evaluation strategy chosen, specific tools and items can be selected and edited, and evaluation instruments constructed. The resourceful instructor collects tools and items from commonly available sources, instead of constructing each from scratch.

Effective instructors also carefully edit each item and tool to ensure that the item has content validity for their particular course. Items are then analyzed to confirm reliability and validity. Over time, instructors can collect a powerful toolbox of evaluation instruments.[15,16] Although security is an issue for written examinations, other types of evaluation instruments are better shared with students. For example, students can use performance checklists and rubrics for meaningful self-assessment. Whether the student has prior knowledge of components to be assessed does not matter because knowledge is not being tested—performance evaluation is the object of these instruments.

Another point of view is to look at the evaluation of student performance as a set of progressive steps to be followed by the instructor. The use of formative evaluation is coupled with learning activities. Formative evaluation allows the student and the instructors to modify the learning strategy to ultimately master the course objectives. This mastery of course objectives is assessed through the use of curriculum-based summative evaluation tools. Appropriate instruments are combined after the instructor considers the appropriate domain of the objective drawn from the curriculum. The curriculum and the student together are tested through competency verification, which is a summative evaluation based on a practice analysis.

Evaluation of student performance can be complex. The results of each evaluation convey two intertwined messages that the instructor must decipher. The first of these messages is information regarding the performance of the student. The results of each evaluation can tell the instructor how well the student is performing. The effective instructor realizes, though, that the performance of the student is integrally tied to the performance of the instructor. This is the second message carried by the results. Poor results may reveal that the student is performing poorly, or they may indicate that the instructor has not provided adequate learning opportunities for the student to master the material. Of course, this assumes that the evaluation itself is giving accurate and meaningful results. To decipher these multiple messages requires an understanding of the fundamentals of student evaluation.

Proper selection, construction, and analysis of evaluation instruments help to assure the instructor that evaluation is providing meaningful results. Proper formative evaluation provides feedback to the instructor about whether the learning activities have adequately prepared the student. With these fundamentals, the instructor can decode the results of tools that evaluate student performance.

Glossary

360-degree evaluation Feedback that utilizes many sources of evaluation, including peers.

Cronbach's alpha A statistical method to assess internal consistency.

multiple intelligences The theory that different students have different levels of intelligence in various areas.

rubric An evaluation tool that defines criteria for each degree of expected performance when there are multiple facets to the evaluation.

split-half A test of internal consistency that divides the exam into halves (commonly odd and even questions), then compares the percentages of correct answers between the two groups of items.

task analysis Provides a comprehensive list of the steps to be performed for a skill or process.

References

1. Gardner, H. (1993). *Multiple intelligences: The theory in practice*. New York, NY: Basic Books.

2. Gardner, H. (2006). *Multiple intelligences: New horizons*. New York, NY: Basic Books.

3. Sparks-Langer, G. M., Starko, A. J., Pasch, M., *et al.* (2003). *Teaching as decision making: Successful practices for the secondary teacher,* (2nd ed.). Philadelphia, PA: Prentice Hall.

4. Gaur, L., & Skochelak, S. (2004, May 5). Evaluating competence in medical students. *Journal of the American Medical Association, 291*(17): 21–43.

5. Margolis, G. S., Romero, G. A., Fernandez, A. R., & Studnek, J. R. (2009). Strategies of high-performing paramedic educational programs. *Prehospital Emergency Care 13*(4): 505–511.

6. Jacobs, L. C., & Chase, C. I. (1992). *Developing and using tests effectively: A guide for faculty*. San Francisco, CA: Jossey-Bass.

7. Harden, R. M., Stevenson, M., Downie, W. W., & Wilson, G. M. (1975). Assessment of clinical competence using objective-structured examination. *British Medical Journal, 1*: 447–451.

8. Davis, B. G. (2001). *Tools for teaching*. San Francisco, CA: Jossey-Bass.

9. National Emergency Medical Services Education Standards 2009. National Highway Traffic Safety Administration (NHTSA). Available online at http://ems.gov/pdf/811077a.pdf

10. Milkovich, G. T., & Wigdor, A. K. (Eds.) (1991). Committee on performance appraisal for merit pay. Commission on behavioral and social sciences and education, National Research Council. *Pay for performance: Evaluating performance appraisal and merit pay*. Washington, DC: National Academy Press.

11. National Highway Traffic Safety Administration (2002). National guidelines for educating EMS instructors. Available at: http://www.nhtsa.dot.gov/people/injury/EMS/Instructor/Tableofcontents.htm

12. Papadakis, M. A., Hodgson, C. S., Teherani, A., & Kohatsu, N. D. (2004, March). Unprofessional behavior in medical school is associated with subsequent disciplinary action by a state medical board. *Academic Medicine 79*(3): 244–249.

13. RubiStar (2003). *Create rubrics for your project-based learning activities*. Lawrence, KS: Advanced Learning Technologies Center for Research on Learning at the University of Kansas. Available at: http://rubistar.4teachers.org

14. Whitman, N. (1982). *A guide to clinical performance testing,* IDEA paper No. 7. Manhattan, KS: Kansas State University Center for Faculty Evaluation and Development. URL: http://www.theideacenter.org/sites/default/files/Idea_Paper_07.pdf

15. Accreditation Council of Graduate Medical Education and American Board of Medical Specialties (2002). Toolbox of assessment methods, Version 1.1. Available at: http://www.acgme.org/Outcome/assess/Toolbox.pdf

16. Accreditation Council of Graduate Medical Education and American Board of Medical Specialties (2000). Table of toolbox methods. Available at: http://www.acgme.org/Outcome/assess/ToolTable.pdf

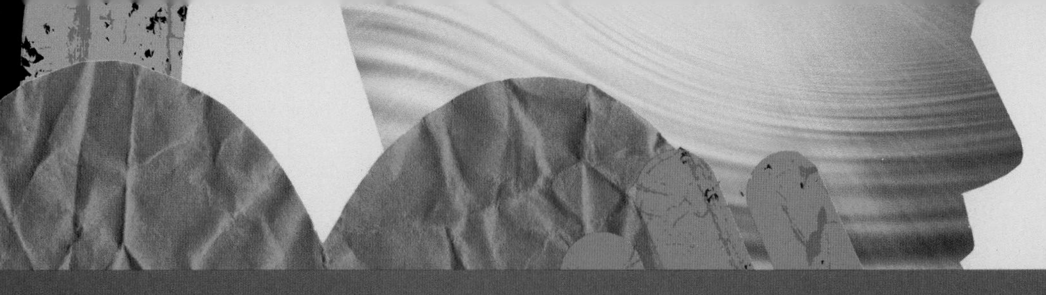

23 Remediation

You won't find a solution by saying there is no problem. —William Rotsler

What should an educator do when a student does not meet the program's performance standards?

Performance standards provide the foundation for all levels of the Department of Transportation National Highway and Traffic Safety Administration National EMS Education Standards (the Standards) with terminology such as "competencies, clinical behaviors and judgements."[1] However, education standards typically do not provide specific learning objectives, explicit guidance on how to measure goals or objectives, nor do they advise how to conduct an effective remediation (retraining and retesting) process. Although this allows for a great deal of flexibility, it may not provide enough structure for the novice instructor.

In addition to the Standards, additional performance standards are found in state, regional, and local regulations for Emergency Medical Services (EMS) education. Because regional guidelines are typically written to allow for flexibility in programs, they also may not contain specific evaluation or remediation processes. An instructor should use these references to provide the foundation on which to build an evaluation system for an educational program.

When a student does not meet the established performance standard, two options are available to the instructor: remediation, or removing the student from the educational process. When an evaluation system is in place for an educational program, a remediation process should also be included as a component of that system.[2] To be most effective, the remediation process must be clearly articulated and understood by all members of the educational team and by students.

CHAPTER GOAL: This chapter will define the purpose and process of student remediation.

Teaching Tip >> *The instructor has the greatest control of the remediation process when policies and procedures are in place before remediation is ever needed.*

Remediation Defined

The term **remediation** is derived from the root word "remedial," which means to correct a deficiency.[3] The suffix "-ation" refers to an act or process. Therefore, the definition of *remediation* is the process of analysis and identification of deficits (or problems) and a plan for retraining or improving performance before retesting is undertaken. The implication for evaluation is that performance standards would be achieved by each student. One must realize there is no guarantee that all students shall achieve the performance standards following a remediation process. Remediation is a critical component of any educational process because it provides solutions for situations in which students do not meet the performance standard. In these cases, the educational program must effectively respond with actions that go beyond the typical educational process (i.e., apply additional effort to help a student achieve competency). Research indicates that many, if not most, students require remediation at some point in their academic careers. It should be noted that up to 90 percent of community college students needed remediation in literacy and mathematical skills.[4] Given this statistic, it is readily evident that any educational process must assure that remediation is included as an essential aspect of the instruction design and development of the instructional offering. If this vitally important aspect of instruction is not included in the process, one would surely expect to see a higher failure rate.

Additional reasons besides the threat of low success rates must drive the need for remediation. The educational process is a partnership between the student and the educational team, and a successful student outcome is a reasonable expectation. In this partnership, it is also reasonable to assume that the educational team will be an advocate for student success. In this environment, a remediation process is an appropriate tool designed to facilitate success.[5]

One aspect of the student-educator partnership that is difficult to design is a system that allows for remediation but does not compromise program integrity or fairness to the other students in the program. On the basis of student performance in a particular course, an instructor may feel one student "deserves" a second chance, and that another does not. Without a defined remediation system in place for guidance, the potential for bias is greater.

When to Remediate

Remediation should follow a student's failure to meet an expected standard during an evaluation process. The remediation may be related to a deficiency in the cognitive, affective, or psychomotor domain. The remediation process should be initiated as soon as the breakdown is identified. Students should not be allowed to continue until remediation and reevaluation have taken place. Because of the schedule of some courses, this may mean that remediation must occur quickly. Frequently, educational systems mistakenly allow the student to proceed in their educational program without establishing the foundation of instruction required to assure success. Programs should create methods to provide counseling or tutorial programs for those students who need additional information or clarification on a specific topic.

Any type of evaluation, whether formal, informal, formative, or summative, can trigger the remediation process (Chapter 20: Principles of Evaluation of Student Performance describes different evaluation types in detail).

The importance of remediation as an integral part of the evaluation process cannot be overemphasized. Student advocacy is a primary role for every EMS educator, just as patient advocacy is a primary role for every EMS provider.[1] In addition to discussing and describing student advocacy as a value, it is important that the instructor provide the necessary tools to accomplish this task.

Although the range of students who may require remediation is not yet fully known, mounting evidence suggests there is a need for it in every educational program.[4] Given this need, educational programs must plan for remediation by establishing deliberate steps and processes. A defined procedure allows classroom educators to focus on *how* to provide remediation for specific students, rather than getting bogged down in determining *whether* they should or can provide remediation. The administrative team for the program should create the remediation policies and procedures. The student handbook, syllabus, policies and procedure manual, and other program documents should contain policies and procedures that clearly outline the process. The remediation policy should also be provided to students during program orientation.

CASE IN POINT

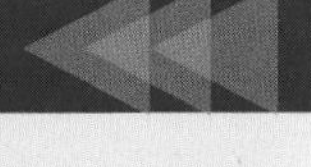

A student has just performed a series of skills associated with IV therapy and drug administration. During the student's demonstration, the instructor noted several times that the student repeated the same mistake; she placed an uncapped needle on the table as she prepared other steps of the process. When the instructor critiqued her performance and provided feedback, the student told the instructor that she knew she made the mistake and will "do better next time." Since the student repeated the mistake several times, the instructor is unsure whether the pupil actually does know the proper procedure, or if she was just being sloppy because it was a simulation and not a real patient encounter. A formal remediation cycle may be used to correct this mistake and then the student can be retested. In this case, the amount of time spent on the actual retraining may be minimal. In the remediation process, the student will be required to demonstrate proper skill performance and to provide evidence that she really does know the procedure.

Steps in the Remediation Process

Once an evaluation reveals the inability of a student to meet an expected standard, the educator should initiate the remediation process. In some cases, the student may recognize this inability to perform independently and will discuss concerns with the instructor; this discussion may result in initiation of the process.

Educators should refrain from using the term "failure." It is an appropriate term for the situation;

however, an educator should seldom use that word when referring to a student. It is essential for educators to speak about outcomes and results in the educational process. Scores are established in the education of students that can determine if students have met the expectation of the program or if remediation is required.

The remediation process includes the following five steps:

1. Conduct an assessment of possible reasons for the student's performance deficit.
2. Determine the cause of the performance deficit (**attribution**).
3. Develop a remediation plan.
4. Implement the plan.
5. Reevaluate.

To ensure fairness in the remediation process and to maintain program integrity, a thorough assessment of the student's performance (be it cognitive, psychomotor, or affective) should take place prior to a remediation plan being developed and implemented.

Information gathered during this step assists the instructor to determine whether remediation is permissible, possible, and appropriate. Information regarding the cause of a student's inabilities (outcomes or results), from the student's perspective as well as from the instructor's, is needed to make this decision.

The second step in the process, during which the root cause for the student's issues are identified, is known as "attribution." Attribution helps identify the level of responsibility shared by the instructional process, educators, and the student. Attribution has a significant impact upon the remediation process.

Assessment Phase of Remediation

The assessment phase of the remediation process may reveal helpful information for the student on any of the following topics:

- Need for study skills enhancements
- Need for evaluation for learning disabilities
- Need for developmental or remedial classes
- Need to obtain additional clinical experience
- Need to work on affective skills such as communication
- Understanding of the sacrifices necessary for the course
  - Contact for helpful resources
  - Schedule adjustments for work and family
  - Access to financial or other support

Teaching Tip >> *If the instructor does not conduct a thorough front-end analysis to identify the problem, he or she may not identify the actual cause for the student's inability to meet expectations, and the remediation plan may not be successful.*

Once the problem has been identified and retraining is determined to be possible and appropriate, a remediation plan is developed. For the plan to be finalized, the student must agree to the terms and conditions, including the consequences of repeated failure. Once the plan is in place, the retraining can begin. The progress of the student during the retraining process should be closely monitored. Once retraining has occurred, Step 5, reevaluation, can occur. **Figure 23.1** illustrates a remediation algorithm.

Step 1: Conduct an Assessment of Possible Reasons for Failure

Prior to each class, a diligent educator reviews the steps of remediation and covers this information with the students as the class starts. Students

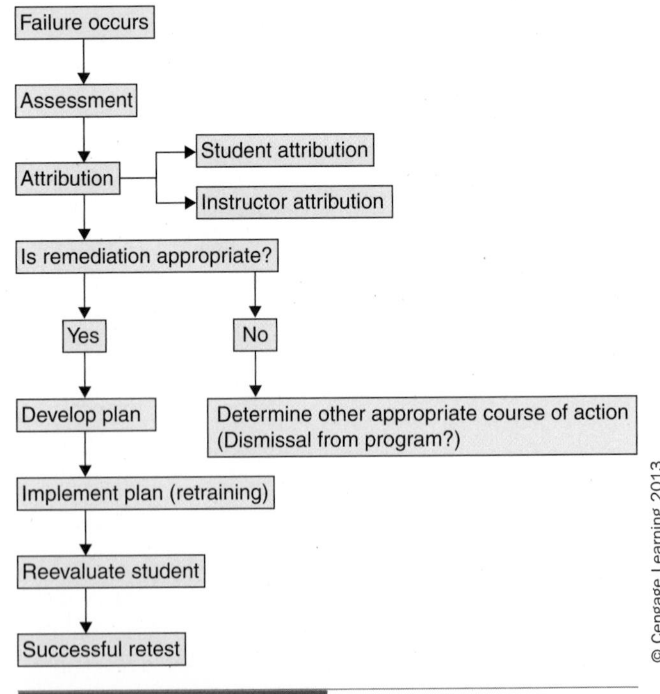

Figure 23.1
Remediation algorithm.

should be provided with, and sign, a copy of the program policies and procedures including those relating to remediation. Faculty and students should know where and how to access them. Once a failure occurs, the instructor should review the remediation policy and procedure early in the process to ensure compliance with established rules of the program.

The following questions are useful in determining if a student is eligible for remediation, and in deciding whether remediation is possible and appropriate:

1. Is there a standard in place that indicates what level of student involvement is required for remediation to be provided?
   - Does the policy identify a score or range of scores required for remediation to occur?
   - Is there an attendance standard?
   - Are other criteria specified (e.g., limits on total number of attempts at remediation and retesting allowed in a program)?
2. Can remediation be accomplished in a timely manner to allow the student to continue in the program?
3. Are appropriate resources available for providing remediation?
4. How committed is the student to the remediation process and to improving his or her performance?

Time constraints are a critical factor to be analyzed. For example, if the course schedule does not permit enough time for remediation to take place, it may not be appropriate to proceed with retraining. If the time frame for retraining is not adequate, a second failure may result during the retesting phase. As the course continues to move forward, the student will be faced with the additional burden of keeping up with new material while attempting to achieve success in the retraining required. Resource considerations are vitally important in the development and implementation of a remediation plan. Many programs have limitations on their equipment and supplies; some share resources among several simultaneous courses. Remediation requires careful scheduling and cooperation. The need to provide resources for remediation for one student can seriously disrupt programs that operate with tight resource constraints, adding additional importance to the need for incorporating remediation considerations into the evaluation process.

The most costly aspect of most remediation events is the cost for faculty and staff to plan and deliver retraining for a student. Some systems pay personnel for the additional time needed to address remediation. A program must be willing and able to address these additional costs for remediation in the design of the program.

The final decision regarding eligibility for remediation usually requires an understanding of the reason for the failure. If it is determined that the decision rests solely with one instructor, bias can enter into the decision-making process. Input from other faculty members or a consistent committee of the educational team can help reduce this bias.

CASE IN POINT

(PART 1 OF 2)

An educator is teaching an Emergency Medical Responder (EMR) course. The course is 48 hours long and adheres to the Standards and to the state EMS agency regulations.

The syllabus states that students are required to successfully pass three testing cycles during specified parts of the program to be eligible to take the state EMR test for certification. Each test consists of two parts: 50 multiple-choice questions and three psychomotor skill tests based on appropriate scenarios. The syllabus further states that students who fail the exam process are allowed to retake that part of the test one time. It also states that failure a second time results in dismissal (removal) from the program. One student just failed the practical examination portion for the first testing cycle. What should happen next?

A process allowing for remediation is included in the evaluation system for this course. The syllabus identifies three testing points that have relatively high stakes: (1) students must successfully complete each examination to be able to continue in the course; (2) in the event a student fails testing, one retesting opportunity is provided before dismissal; and (3) remediation should occur after failure of the first attempt and before a retest is attempted.

Teaching Tip >> *Because of the commitment to student advocacy, when educators are unsure whether a remediation attempt should proceed or are unclear of the standard in place, it is best to allow the student to attempt the remediation process.*

Educational program strategies and educator knowledge and experience are important considerations in the assessment phase, but the student's role in the process is also critical. There is significant anecdotal evidence and action research (nonscientific or pseudoscientific evidence) on student attitudes and their impact on learning. Educational psychologists are placing greater emphasis on attitude. If the real cause of the failure is primarily attributed to the student and the student is unwilling to acknowledge that fact, then successful remediation may not be possible if the student is not willing to correct the behavior.

Step 2: Determine the Cause for Failure (Attribution)

Evidence suggests that attribution may be the single, most important component affecting the remediation process.[6] To develop a meaningful remediation process, the educator must identify the root cause of the student's failure.

Intuitively, we know that incorrect problem identification can lead to implementation of the wrong or an ineffective solution. Therefore, seeking multiple points of input can assist the instructor to identify the correct cause. In addition to reviewing the instructional process and evaluation instruments, the educator should interview the student and consider seeking input from instructors in all settings in which the student has participated, including the classroom, lab, clinical, and field settings. It may also be appropriate to seek input from the medical and program director.

Teaching Tip >> *The instructor must maintain the student's confidentiality during this process. Discussion of the issue of failure should be limited to appropriate members of the educational team.*

The educator should demonstrate active listening and implement clear communication skills when interviewing the student. A seasoned educator realizes that most students are very emotional during this time, and that it is important to maintain professionalism and perspective.

It is common for the educator to assign a different attribution to the failure other than what the student believes to be the cause. For example, a student believes the reason for failure was inadequate time to prepare for the examination, but the instructor believes the root cause is that the student missed a practical skill development section. The impact of conflicting attributions on the solution is significant.

Teaching Tip >> *More often than not, failure of a student, regardless of the cause, affects the instructor as well as the student. Input from members of the educational team outside the situation should be considered to help limit bias and provide objectivity.*

Student Attribution

One way that the educator can identify the student's attribution of the cause for failure is through an interview. The instructor should ask open-ended questions and should approach the interview in a nonjudgmental manner. It may be appropriate for the instructor to emphasize to the student that he or she is working on an educational solution to the problem. The instructor may find it helpful to tell the student that the goal of the remediation process is to determine what strategies will most likely result in the student's passing on the next attempt.

Teaching Tip >> *Some students lack the maturity to accept responsibility for their action or inaction. The instructor should focus energies on developing a solid plan with the intent that the student will eventually accept responsibility in the failure. If the student's action or inactions cannot be rectified, additional actions will be required.*

As the educator conducts the interview, it is important that the student's commitment to improving performance be assessed **(Figure 23.2)**.[6] The instructor may find it necessary to make decisions regarding the student's abilities to succeed on future attempts. If the student does not possess the necessary tools (cognitive, affective, or psychomotor abilities), the resultant remediation plan may need to include strategies for developing these abilities. Inclusion of the program and medical directors in the decision process may be required.

As the instructor works through the process of attribution, it is important to ascertain whether the student ever successfully demonstrated the standard. This may reveal whether the student is capable of attaining the standard. If success was demonstrated previously, then the instructor should determine what has changed. Perhaps the progress of the student was not monitored appropriately, which allowed for uncorrected poor performance. If the instructor does not have evidence of successful attainment of the standards, corrective instruction should be provided to the student.

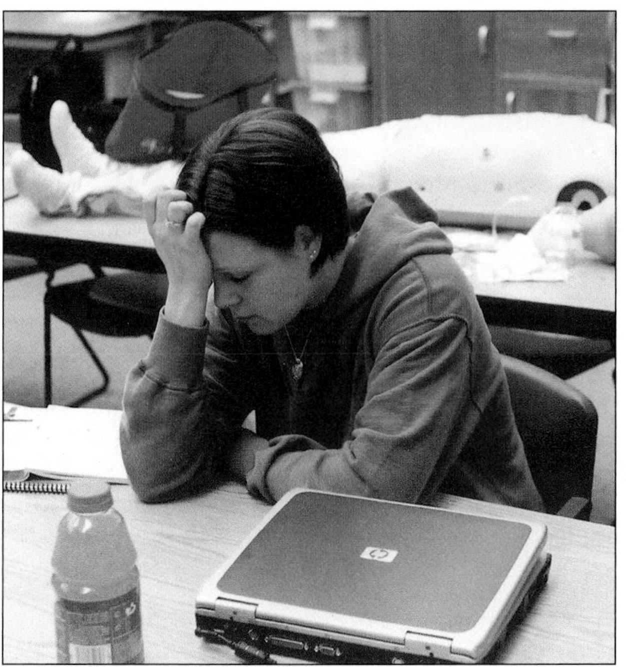

Figure 23.2

Student commitment to improving performance is imperative if the student is to succeed.

Program Attribution

It is important for the instructor to examine what possible role the educational process played in the failure. It must be ensured that the faculty understood and articulated the performance standard clearly to the student. Was the student informed of one standard, yet tested for another? The instructor must ensure that the goals and objectives of the course appropriately match the testing process.

The educator must analyze the evaluation process. Were the correct instruments used to evaluate students? Have these instruments been validated? Are they reliable? The evaluation section explains these processes in detail.

The educator must also analyze the learning plan. Was the plan appropriate and effective? Was adequate time allotted for students to learn the material? Were adequate teaching strategies used to appeal to the student's learning style or preference? Did the learning plan allow for reinforcement of concepts, and did it test for understanding? Were activities designed to facilitate the learning of metacognitive (critical-thinking) processes?[7] Findings from the program attribution may indicate the need for changes and improvements in the course.

Multiple Attributions

Frequently, student failure is caused by multiple attributions. In many cases, the attributions identified by the student and the educational team do not match. The interrelationship between education, performance, environment, and student needs is complex. The instructor should consider the effect that each of these has on student performance.

The next *Case in Point* highlights two program problems: not enough manikins for students, and not enough instructors. One-on-one instruction may

CASE IN POINT

(PART 2 OF 2)

The policies and procedures indicate that remediation is allowed and encouraged for the student who requires additional interactions. During the problem assessment interview, the student is unclear about why he believes he failed, but he says he wishes he had been allowed more time to practice the skill.

As the educator reviews the course syllabus and schedule, he notes that the practical skill development session has many skills listed on the sheet. Because of time constraints, although the instructor demonstrated all the skills, the students did not get appropriate practice time. The instructor also determined that many of the students did not perform very well on the practical exam, even though only one failed to demonstrate proficiency of the required skills. The educator immediately contacts the program coordinator to discuss rearranging the schedule to allow for additional practical skill time and permission to retest the entire class. A private skill session is also arranged for the student who failed to complete the required tasks.

On retest, all students pass.

CASE IN POINT

A program has an inadequate number of manikins for all students to actively participate during class. A shy student feels that the instructor is paying more attention to the other students and withdraws. The instructor is dividing his attention between too many students and does not notice that the student is withdrawing. When the student fails the examination, he blames the instructor for not providing appropriate instruction. The instructor counters that the student is not assertive and seems unwilling to practice skills. Every instructor must consider the impact these multiple attributions have on the development of a successful remediation plan.

result in successful retesting of the student in this case, but unless the program can allocate additional resources, the problem will most likely reoccur.

The teachable moment is a concept employed at all levels of EMS curricula. It describes the opportune time to provide valuable information to people closely affected by traumatic emergency situations. For example, some EMS agencies often visit households within weeks of a bicycle crash to provide helmet safety information. In other departments, EMS crews or supervisors discuss home safety with older adult patients and their families after an older adult experiences injury related to a fall.

People are often willing to listen to advice and direction provided by professionals during these teachable moments. However, confronting a student while he or she is discussing attribution is usually *not* a teachable moment. Receiving a failing grade on an examination may be devastating to life plans and goals, and the student may be very emotional. It may not be helpful for the instructor to try to convince a student that his or her attribution is incorrect at this time.

Although students can benefit from understanding and accepting personal responsibility for failure, the student attribution interview may not be the best time to approach the subject. Experience and strong interpersonal skills will assist an educator in deciding if and when it is appropriate to confront a student about his or her perception of attribution. It is critical for the instructor to determine whether the remediation plan can account for the student's attribution.

Step 3: Develop a Remediation Plan

Input from both the student and the educational team is used to develop the remediation plan (see sample remediation plan document in **Figure 23.3**). The remediation plan should clearly describe the process and the expected outcomes for the student and instructional team. It should define any work (e.g., reading assignments, homework, or self-study) that is to be completed independently by the student, and should describe the type of assistance that is to be provided by the instructor. A timeline for the remediation should also be included, clearly identifying when the process will begin and end, including an estimated total number of hours that the retraining process should require. The plan should describe the length of time the student and instructor may spend together and should suggest the amount of time the student will consider spending on independent work or study. If appropriate to the plan, the instructor can include the dates and times that progress reports will be issued. The plan should also identify the date and time of retesting, specify what type of retesting will occur, and tell about any observers (e.g., the medical director or other instructor) who will be present during retesting. The expected standard for successful completion should be reinforced, and the consequences of any failure to comply with the terms specified in the remediation plan should be described. The consequences of failure of the retest should also be described.

The instructor should review the finished plan to ensure that it complies with the program remediation policy. The completed document, when signed by the student, instructor, program director, and medical director, is sometimes called a **learning contract**. Copies of the document should be provided to all parties involved, and one should be maintained in the student's permanent record.

> **Teaching Tip** >> *It may be helpful for another member of the educational team to review the plan before it is finalized to ensure that it is reasonable and appropriate.*

If the educational methods are not identified as the cause for the failure, they may then become the basis for the retraining methods used in the remediation plan. For example, the teaching strategy can shift from a group approach to a targeted process for the student's individual learning style and preference. If, on the other hand, the educational method is attributed as the cause of failure, adjustments to the educational methods should be made. An educator cannot continue to do the same thing and expect different results.

Step 4: Implement the Plan

The instructor must monitor the student's progress closely during remediation, ensuring that all involved parties are performing as described in the plan. The instructor should maintain progress reports and regularly provide the student with corrective feedback. The student should be held accountable for his or her actions as outlined in the plan. Careful documentation is critical; in the event of legal challenge, the educational team will be called upon to provide evidence to show how they advocated for the student.

Step 5: Reevaluate

Remediation plans require that both the student and the educator make sacrifices in time and resources, and the stakes are often high. The educator must

Student Name: ______________________ Date: ________________

The above student has failed to attain a passing score on the following evaluation(s):

____.

A remediation plan has been approved for this student with the following conditions:

Describe all expectations and outcomes for each of the following. Include specific work required like reading assignments, independent study, skills development sessions, etc. As appropriate include how many hours will be provided.

Student expectations and deliverables:

1.

2.

3.

Program expectations and deliverables:

1.

2.

3.

List each deliverable and the date required for completion:

Item: ________________________________ Due date/time: ____________________________

Item: ________________________________ Due date/time: ____________________________

Item: ________________________________ Due date/time: ____________________________

A retest will follow the completion of remediation. List each evaluation tool to be utilized and required passing score.

Describe the consequences of noncompletion of the remediation process or failure on the retest.

Signatures:

______________________ ______________

Student Date

______________________ ______________

Instructor Date

______________________ ______________

Program Director Date

______________________ ______________

Medical Director Date

The original document will be placed in the student's permanent record. Copies of this document will be provided for each member signing above.

Figure 23.3

Remediation plan template.

CASE IN POINT

A student fails a cognitive anatomy test on the circulatory system. During the problem assessment, the instructor determines that the student possibly learns best through visual instruction. For the remediation plan, the educator provides the student with some pages from an anatomy coloring book and lends the student a heart model for the weekend. The instructor also provides the student with several Web addresses for sites with cardiac content. The student spends an hour with the instructor answering questions. On retesting during the next class session, the student attains a very high score. The instructor adds more visual elements to all future class presentations.

carefully evaluate the tool that will be used to retest the student to ensure that it is fair and objective. All tools should undergo validity and reliability testing and should be approved by the program director as well as the medical director. The instructor must decide whether the same evaluation tool will be used to retest the student. A psychomotor skill test will most likely use an identical tool, but the scenario used to prompt the student to perform the skill may be different.

Using the same tool for a written exam will likely increase the score without necessarily resulting in an increase in the student's knowledge level. Having seen the exam and identifying what was missed may lead the student to correct only those specific item errors, with no increased knowledge or improved understanding. Consequently, retesting a written exam with a different tool provides a more accurate measure for determining that true remediation has occurred. Educators should seek advice from other members of the educational team if they are not sure about reevaluation decisions.

If retesting involves an instrument with a high level of subjectivity, such as a psychomotor skill test, the instructor should consider using an independent evaluator who has limited knowledge of the student's previous results.

An educator must ensure that the grading of the reevaluation tool complies with the policies for remediation. Depending on how the policy is written, it may be appropriate for the original grade to remain unchanged, with the grade book indicating that a "pass" occurred on retest, or it may be appropriate for the two grades to be averaged. Another process may be appropriate as well; this decision should be based on how the policy is written.

Summary

Remediation is needed when a student does not obtain a passing score or achieve acceptable performance on an evaluation. The remediation process is an integral component of the evaluation system, and it is a reasonable expectation for a program that values student advocacy to have a process in place. Remediation helps maintain partnership within the educational process. Students should be informed of the remediation process well in advance and know what to expect if they need it.

Remediation is necessary for many students. It will not be appropriate in all situations, but it is important that clear guidelines and policies be established before the need arises. With deliberate design, the process can maintain program integrity and provide fair criteria for all students.

Glossary

attribution The root cause(s) of the student's performance deficiency.

learning contract A document mutually agreed to by the student and faculty that defines activities and behaviors that must be met in a specified time frame to achieve specific objectives.

remediation The process to analyze and identify performance deficiencies and develop a plan to improve that performance.

References

1. National Highway Traffic Safety Administration (2009). *National EMS Education Standards.* (DOT HS 811 077A). Washington, DC: Department of Transportation.
2. Boylan, H. R., Bonham, B. S., & Rodriguez, L. M. (2000). What are remedial courses and do they work: Results of national and local studies. *Learning Assistance Review, 5*: 5–14.
3. *Riverside Webster's II Dictionary,* (rev. ed.) (1996). New York, NY: Berkley Books.
4. Spann, M. G. Jr. (2000). Remediation: A must for the 21st century learning society, Policy Paper. Denver, CO: Center for Community College Policy, Education Commission of the States. (Available from ESC Distribution Center, 707 17th St. Suite 2700, Denver, CO 80202–3427.)
5. Colby, A., & Opp, R. (1987). Controversies surrounding developmental education in the community college. *ERIC Digest.*
6. Benner, P. (1982). From novice to expert. *American Journal of Nursing, 82*: 402–407.
7. Adult Education Resource Information Service (1999, September). *Adult learning. ARIS information sheet.* Melbourne, Australia: National Languages and Literacy Institute of Australia.

24

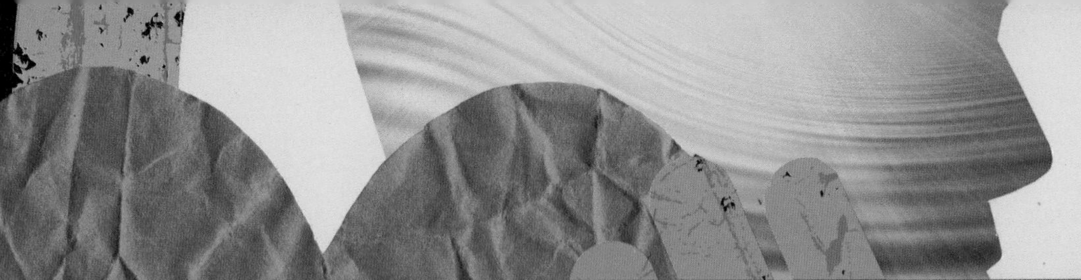

Administrative Issues

It is a mark of an educated mind to be able to entertain a thought without accepting it. — Aristotle

Whether a seasoned veteran or a new education program administrator, conducting a successful class is much like running the hurdles at a track meet. Good preparation and a solid administrative infrastructure will help the program director or coordinator scale the "hurdles" with deftness and finesse. A good academic leader sets the vision, assesses the environment, builds consensus, encourages and mentors the team, communicates effectively with all stakeholders, abates risk, ensures quality, creates and monitors the budget, and plans and evaluates the work. Educators carryout the plan. Lack of effective planning can leave the track littered with the agony of frazzled and discouraged educators, grievances, budget variances that threaten program viability, and students who fail to meet academic goals, or worse, experience harm due to program liability.

Although tending to administrative issues may be the primary responsibility of a course coordinator or program director, every educator has a role in administration of the course, from documenting attendance and enforcing conduct rules, to completing student evaluations. Additionally, every educator should have a basic understanding of, and appreciation for, administrative tasks to maintain order; to protect the institution, program, and faculty from liability; and to ensure fairness and consistency with students. Paying close attention to administrative policies and procedures can also promote the best possible educational experience for students and everyone else involved in the program.

CHAPTER GOAL: This chapter discusses general administrative matters common to most programs and instructors as well as issues with which the program director or course coordinator should be familiar.

Chapter Format

Administrative issues are not just the purview of the program director. Every member of the educational program team—from director to instructor, medical director, and administrative and support staff—need to appreciate the importance and necessity for administrative issues and proper administrative follow-through. This is especially challenging in EMS education because educational programs are defined and regulated by a number of external forces. The first part of this chapter presents an overview of administrative issues germane to all EMS educational programs, regardless of venue or offering institution. The second part of the chapter addresses those issues of importance to the individual course instructor, and the final section describes issues and information important to the program director.

The reader is encouraged to review Chapter 10: Legal Issues for EMS Educators, as a number of issues discussed in this chapter have a basis in laws and regulations presented in the chapter.

It may seem that running an EMS educational program is a confusing and monumental undertaking, especially if the program is a "one-person shop" or "one full-time person shop" supplemented by part-time instructors. The challenge lies in determining how to juggle national, state, local, and institutional issues and still teach. This can indeed be a challenge, and one way to transition into this role is to find a mentor.

Conducting a program with excellent results takes more than transitioning good street providers into the classroom to impart their knowledge to the next generation of EMS personnel. It is a good place to start, but most quickly discover that they do not even know what they do not know and need to come up to speed as fast as possible. *Details make a difference and egos need to be left at the door!* The best place to begin is to find a program demonstrating best-practice models and superior outcomes and seek a mentoring relationship with that instructor or program director. This program need not be in EMS; it could be another health-related field or one suggested by a dean or other academic leader. This can assist in creating an administrative infrastructure that provides a sound foundation upon which an excellent program can be built, sustained, and ever improved.

Administrative Foundation

This section provides an overview and introduction to national, state, and local issues, consensus documents, and regulations that affect EMS education. As with any such broad overview, the reader is cautioned that state and local authority has final jurisdiction; thus, not all of the material presented may be applicable to each specific program.

National-Level Curricular and Administrative Issues

The National Highway Traffic Safety Administration (NHTSA), a division of the U.S. Department of Transportation (DOT), is currently recognized as the lead federal agency for the development of national EMS consensus documents. The Emergency Medical Services for Children (EMSC), a division of the Maternal and Child Health Bureau (MCHB) within the Department of Health Resources and Services Administration (HRSA) partners with NHTSA to support and promote many EMS activities.

The *EMS Agenda for the Future* is a consensus document developed in 1995 and 1996 with funding from NHTSA and EMSC. The purpose of the document was to "predict the future by creating it."[1] It has served as the guiding force to drive change across the country and impacts EMS providers, health care organizations and institutions, governmental agencies, and policy makers.

As a follow up to the *EMS Agenda for the Future*, NHTSA and EMSC convened a task force in January of 1998 to discuss the EMS educational system and the high variability of EMS scopes of practice around the country. Out of that task force, the *EMS Education Agenda for the Future: A Systems Approach* document was developed using the same extensive peer-reviewed process that was so successful for the *EMS Agenda*. The EMS *Education Agenda* sets the vision for increasing the quality, structure, professionalism, and accountability for EMS education, thus advancing EMS education in the same light as medical, nursing, and other health profession programs. It builds on the broad concepts from the 1996 *EMS Agenda* to outline steps to enhance the consistency, quality, and efficacy of EMS education, with the goal of increased competency among program graduates. The document includes an educational system with the following five integrated national EMS core components:

- Core Content
- Scope of Practice Model
- Education Standards
- National certification
- Education program accreditation[2]

The system prescribes a high degree of structure, coordination, and interdependence among the five components (**Figure 24.1**). Both *Agenda* documents are important reading for anyone who is or wishes to become an EMS educator. These documents may be obtained by visiting several websites. Two of the easiest to find important documents or links to them are http://www.naemse.org and http://www.ems.gov.

National EMS Core Content

The National EMS Core Content document was published in 2005 by NHTSA. Led by the National

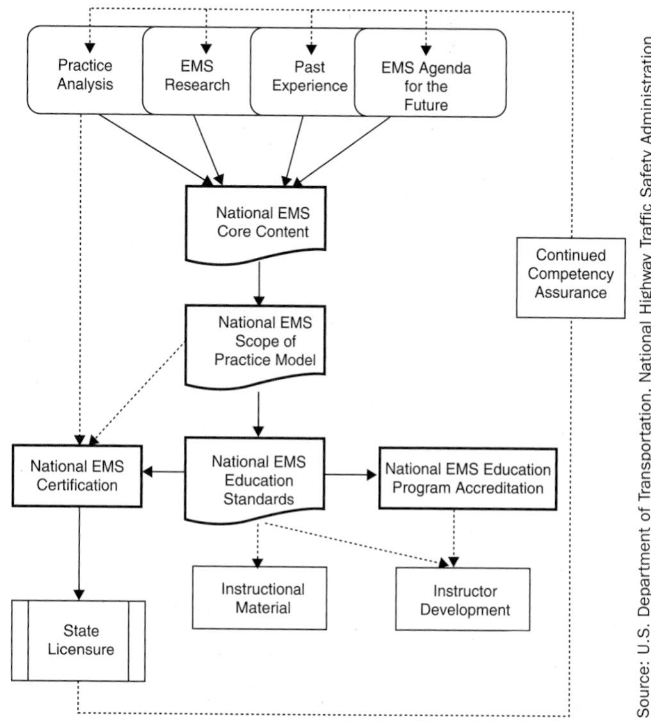

Figure 24.1
EMS Education System Components.

Association of EMS Physicians (NAEMSP) and the American College of Emergency Physicians (ACEP), the document defines the entire domain of EMS knowledge and skills without assigning the skills into any specific provider level.[3] At the time it was published, 39 different levels of licensure still existed in the United States.

National EMS Scope of Practice Model

The National EMS Scope of Practice (SOP) Model (2007) project was led by the National Association of State EMS Officials (NASEMSO) and the former National Council of State EMS Training Coordinators with other EMS community participants. The document was published by NHTSA and identifies four levels of EMS providers: Emergency Medical Responder (EMR), Emergency Medical Technician (EMT), Advanced EMT (AEMT) and Paramedic.[4] Each provider level designates specific skills and scope of practice that are intended to be a floor for that level nationally. The hope is that the SOP model will be adopted by states to ensure consistency between states and promote reciprocity.

National EMS Education Standards

NHTSA and HRSA (EMSC) contracted with the National Association of EMS Educators to create the National EMS Education Standards ("Standards") (**Figure 24.2**). Approved by NHTSA on January 30, 2009, the document identifies competencies, clinical behaviors and judgments, educational infrastructure, and the depth and breadth of content to include at each level, and serves as a guide for program personnel in making appropriate decisions about what material to cover in class. The document encourages educator creativity and flexibility to tailor courses to local needs and facilitates alternative delivery methods.[5]

Feedback was swift; educators and regulators found that transitioning from a prescribed curriculum to the Education Standards was such a paradigm shift that adoption was going to be difficult-to-impossible without some additional resources. In response, companion documents, called *Instructional Guidelines* (Guidelines), were published for each level of practice. They provide elaboration of the content of the Standards but are quickly becoming outdated as the body of EMS knowledge evolves. The Guidelines are intended for short-term guidance as programs adapt to the new model and are specifically *not* intended to be part of the Standards. A *Gap Analysis Template* was published in July 2009 for states and programs to use in planning the transition. The document identifies the knowledge, skill, and infrastructure differences between old NSC and the new Education Standards.[6]

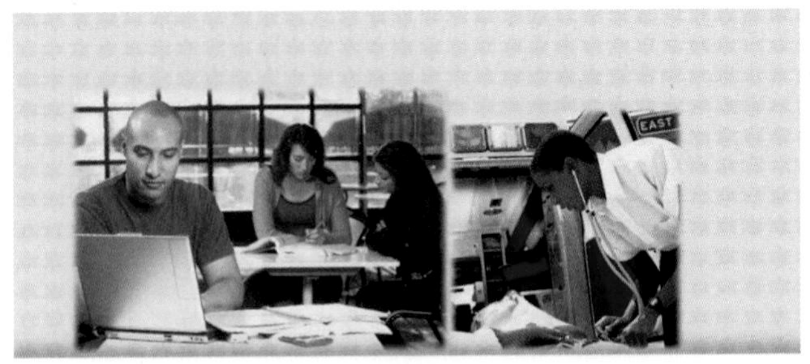

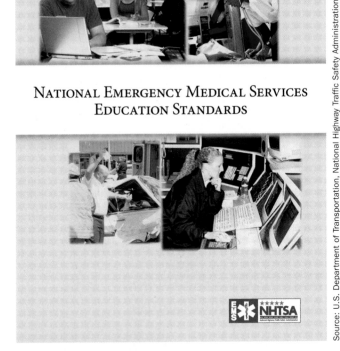

Source: U.S. Department of Transportation, National Highway Traffic Safety Administration

Figure 24.2

National Emergency Medical Services Education Standards.

National EMS Certification/Credentialing

The creation of a single national agency process for EMS credentialing was also proposed in the *EMS Education Agenda.* As currently the only such national organization, the National Registry of EMTs has assumed this role. The Education Agenda proposes that reciprocity from state to state will be easier and more efficient if all states require graduates to utilize the same credentialing agency. The NREMT is currently the only EMS registry agency that is accredited by the National Commission for Certifying Agencies (NCCA), the accreditation body of the National Organization of Competency Assurance (NOCA). NOCA is the recognized authority on accreditation standards for professional certification of organizations and programs. The NREMT also identifies requirements for recertification of registration. In some states, continuing-education (CE) and recertification or relicensure requirements are also managed through the biennial NREMT reregistration process.

National EMS Education Program Accreditation

The last component of the *EMS Education Agenda* is National EMS Education Program Accreditation. In the *Agenda*, the accreditation described is programmatic accreditation that is intended to be tied to national certification. Only paramedic candidates who have graduated from a Commission on Accreditation of Allied Health Educational Programs (CAAHEP) accredited program will be allowed to take the NREMT paramedic exam. Although the concept of national certification married to national accreditation in the Agenda includes all levels of certification, only the paramedic level currently has movement to accomplish this. CAAHEP does not accredit programs that are shorter than one academic year (two semesters).[7]

Although not mentioned in the *EMS Education Agenda*, accreditation also exists for EMS continuing-education programs. The Continuing Education Coordinating Board for Emergency Medical Services (CECBEMS) reviews and accredits applications for EMS-related CE. Applicants must demonstrate sound educational design, physician oversight, relevant references that are current and appropriate in breadth of coverage, and appropriate educational infrastructure.[8] CECBEMS accreditation is particularly useful because it makes it possible for students to earn CE credit at national or regional EMS conferences conducted outside the student's home state, or for students to obtain CE through distance-learning options like the Internet.

State-Level Administrative Issues

The governance of EMS is the responsibility of each state. Each state's laws or statutes and their attendant regulations or administrative rules contain specific directives regarding the education, scope of practice, and credentialing of EMS personnel. The location of each state's lead EMS agency varies, but it is typically found inside the Department of Public Health, the Department of Public Safety, the Office of Emergency Management, or it is established as a separate state agency or division. The state EMS agency is often organized into sections that may include (but not be limited to): licensure and certification; training and education; trauma systems; special populations (e.g., EMSC, elderly); data collection, emergency preparedness and response; ambulance licensing and operation; other strategic trends (stroke, STEMI); communications; information technology; resource funding, allocation and utilization; and medical oversight. Each state should have an EMS Act or other enabling legislation outlining its scope, function, and authority.

The lead agency is usually given the authority to develop, adopt, and periodically update rules and regulations that implement the relevant laws or statutes. Time is generally allowed for input and feedback from stakeholders who have an interest in the proposed changes in rules and regulations. The state legislature, however, is still responsible for ensuring that the intent of the statue is preserved.

Each state has statutes unique to its jurisdiction. Some are more prescriptive than others and some delegate more responsibility to the state EMS agency or a local governmental office. In addition to the state EMS agency, the Department of Education of each state frequently has additional or similar laws that regulate the establishment of educational institutions and the qualifications of instructors, including those who offer EMS educational and training programs.

Each EMS educator must be familiar with the state's rules and regulations regarding education and training where they teach. States may require that EMS instructors or course coordinators have a particular credential in order to teach, as well as appropriate continuing education to continue to teach. A voluntary national EMS instructor-credentialing exam does exist from the National EMS Educator Certification and more information can be found at the website of NEMSEC.org.

States may also require that educational institutions meet specific minimum regulations before beginning operations. The states, in most cases, do not accredit educational programs, although they may use the terms "accredit" or "accreditation." The states typically provide authorization to the program based on content, organization with time specifications, objectives, operation, educators, and/or outcome criteria. Accreditation is, by nature, based on a structured self-appraisal that is overseen by professional peers—not by state regulators or any governmental entity.

In addition, instructors must be able to access the statutes and/or rules if students request the information or ask questions that must be answered within the context of the law or regulations. It is a good idea for instructors to include information as to how students can access these documents within the student orientation materials.

Local Issues

Most local jurisdictions do not have specific regulations related to EMS or emergency services education. However, general local ordinances and regulations such as zoning laws, noise regulations, taxes, and so on, may apply to an educational institution providing EMS education. The other possible source of local administrative issues may relate to EMS educational programs that are designed to serve the needs of a specific response agency such as the local county ambulance district or city fire department. Admissions, class schedule, length of program, location of classes, and so forth may be specified in the training-program contract. It is important that any such contractual relationships clearly define the role of the instructor, the educational institution, and the response agency as related to student performance, discipline, and dismissal. Such issues may have special implications for personnel employed by unionized agencies. However, the educational institution should not compromise its educational standards or quality to meet such requirements.

Institutional Issues

Each educational institution will have its own set of rules, regulations, and procedures for delivery of an educational program. It is imperative that the program director, instructors, medical director, and administrative staff know and follow them. Failure to do so may result in, at the least, confusion and inconvenience, and more seriously, harm to students academically and financially. Program and institutional accreditation is predicated on the adherence to such regulations.

Program Director-Related Administrative Issues

Admission Policies

Admission to an EMS program may be open to anyone with or without minimum eligibility criteria being in place (open vs. limited enrollment). Some programs require minimum reading, writing, and math assessment scores or the student must satisfy other placement criteria that should be specified in the admission requirements. These prerequisites are designed to ensure that students have the necessary reading-comprehension, computational, and written communications skills to be successful in the program prior to enrolling in and paying for the course.

The admissions process may require a prospective applicant to attend an informational meeting and submit the following: an application, verification of meeting the minimum age requirement, official high school transcripts or GED results, college transcripts, proof of a current driver's license, proof of a current EMT license (if applying to paramedic classes), and current CPR for health care provider card. It is important to note that it is not appropriate to ask a potential student's age; only whether or not the individual meets the minimum age requirement.

Some programs have a competitive admission process that gives higher standing for admission to those with general or science-specific academic course credits, EMS or other patient care affiliations and/or experience, military service, or higher assessment scores. Regardless of the setting or type of admission process, it should be fair, nondiscriminatory with objective and defendable criteria, and meet the needs of the local EMS community and training program. Criteria should be clear and published so it is easily accessed by all applicants. Prospective students should be told how to prepare academically and experientially to increase their chances of admission. Policies should be carefully crafted with the assistance of admissions personnel and the approval of deans or comparable administrators who oversee the EMS educational programs. Policies must be closely followed and should be consistent with state and federal laws and regulations. (See Chapter 10: Legal Issues for EMS Educators for additional information on legal requirements related to program admission.)

Course Policies/Handbook

There are many layers of rights, obligations, deliverables, expectations, consents and agreements inherent in a student-program relationship. The name of these documents may vary from institution to institution, but the contents should always include the key issues identified in this section. The more common names for these collections of policies and documents are "student policies" or "student handbook."

Elements that should be included in the handbook/policies for students and faculty are the following:

- Program description; general content to be presented and methods of instruction
- Student outcomes/competencies; general objectives and expected learning outcomes
- Program and course calendar and/or schedule of topics; general activities by course or dates with major assignments or required projects and due dates
- Content topics with corresponding readings; possible references, useful websites, library hours, and so on
- Equipment or materials needed (e.g., stethoscope, penlight)
- Health and immunization requirements

- Attendance, tardiness, and class participation policies; how attendance affects students' grades if applicable
- Special instructions or items that are not self-explanatory (e.g., parameters for an oral report, lab etiquette, or logistics for student participation)
- Student evaluation criteria for all program components including classes, lab sessions, hospital and field clinical, and internship
- Statement of expectations for appropriate professional (affective) behavior at all times during any component of the program, with grading criteria
- Dress code/uniform requirements for class and hospital and field experiences
- Scheduled examination dates
- Grading criteria and explanation of final grade computation
- Statement/policies regarding academic dishonesty
- Course drop dates and payment refund policy
- Policy on missed exams and late assignment submissions
- Student grievance policy
- Class rules (e.g., talking or eating in class)
- Technology rules (e.g., use of electronic devices during class and/or examinations)
- Classroom, lab, clinical, and field safety policies and procedures, including the emergent reporting and evaluation of body substance exposures or injuries
- Instructional support services available
- Inclement weather policy
- Standard precautions and body substance isolation methods and the proper use of personal protective equipment (PPE)
- Functional job description and disability accommodations policy
- Equal opportunity statement
- Roles and responsibilities of the program medical director in student evaluation and sign-off for Registry or state testing

It is imperative that each student sign a statement that provides written proof that he or she has been given access to those policies/handbook, understand their meaning, and agree to follow them. Without this written verification, students could challenge sanctions for noncompliance with policy provisions claiming that they were never informed, and be successful in their appeals. The signed acknowledgement page from each student with a copy of the specific handbook/policies should be kept on file for every cohort of students. Instructors should also read every word of the student handbook/policies and follow the policies to the letter. The documents(s) should be reviewed before the beginning of each new program and adjustments made as needed. Every class seems to have someone who artfully uncovers an unsuspected loophole and challenges program conventions, governance, or operations because the policies were unclear, ambiguous, or silent on a particular topic. Thus, experience becomes a painful catalyst for closing up and cementing over those gaps.

Colleges or universities will already have general policies in place that have been vetted by the institution's attorneys. Instructors must align any program-specific policies with the college's documents. If a student handbook must be created for the first time, a good strategy is to seek out examples from respected high-performing programs or from published examples in peer-reviewed literature. Veteran instructors often have an established network of colleagues who are usually more than willing to share resources if asked. Gain permission prior to using or adapting their verbiage and cite sources in the document. The student handbook/policies is a contract between the program/institution and the student. Consequently, these documents should be thoughtfully prepared, realistic, and changed as little as possible during the program.

Disability Accommodations

EMS educational programs should not discriminate against otherwise qualified individuals with a disability. However, students are expected to demonstrate the physical capacity to perform all the essential functions of the profession during the course with or without reasonable accommodation. Some include information on access and disability services in the syllabus; others place it in the student policies/handbook. Wherever noted, it is important that the program specifies the essential functions of the program so the prospective students can self-identify their ability to successfully complete the program. A functional job analysis for the EMT and Paramedic was conducted in 1992 by Ohio State University as part of the EMT-B NSC revision and is available on various websites.

After admission to the program, students should be instructed, if applicable, to make written requests for accommodations for documented disabilities to the course coordinator or program director. Programs may not discriminate for admission based on a disability covered by Americans with Disability Act of 1973. (See Chapter 10: Legal Issues for EMS Educators.) Given that processing such requests may take a few weeks, the request should be submitted before the course begins or as early in the course as possible, and must be accompanied by documentation from a professional confirming and describing the disability with recommended accommodations. An individual representing the teaching institution with expertise in disability issues may be needed to ascertain if the individual making the disability diagnosis and recommending the accommodation is qualified to do so. The program will need to review whether the accommodations are reasonable for the program to make based on resources. Students should know that, although all students with a disability may not be able to successfully complete the course, the law was enacted to provide access to job training. Accommodations made during the course do not guarantee an accommodation for the National Registry of EMT or many state exams. Students should request specific accommodations to the NREMT and/or the State EMS office according to their criteria.

Religious and Cultural Accommodations

With the ever-increasing diversity of our population as well as the desire of foreign students to enroll in training programs, it is not uncommon to have a student from a different culture, ethnicity, or non-Judean-Christian religion. Students may request special accommodations due to religious beliefs, practices, and cultural norms. How the instructor responds to these requests is often guided by institutional policy. However, the policy may not take into account such activities as outside-of-class clinical and field experience and personnel requirements.

One of the more common issues encountered involves student participation in clinicals. Religious observance of the Sabbath may limit or prevent a student from scheduling a clinical or field internship on Saturday. Likewise, students may want to schedule around Sunday worship. Traditionally, institutional calendars observed only major Christian holidays such as Christmas, Good Friday, and Easter. However, more and more institutions, school systems, and governments are recognizing the Jewish high holy days as well, and possibly other ethnic religious holidays. Even if an institution does not observe these days, students may request an excused absence for their personal observance. Most institutional policies on religious holidays either allow individual students to be absent on these days or encourage instructors to allow makeup assignments. Regardless of the policy, the student is still responsible for any material or work missed. And it goes without saying that instructors should not schedule major class activities such as tests, cadaver labs, and so forth on such days.

Muslim students are required to pray five times per day at prescribed times. There are restrictions on where the prayers can occur, such as in an area where blood is present. Thus a student in a clinical setting may not be able to meet this obligation or will need to be allowed to find a suitable area. Students may also bring their prayer rug or mat with them to class or clinical and field sites.

A concern that may arise with some students is the religious requirement to maintain a beard. Services utilized for field internships may have requirements related to using self-contained breathing apparatus (SCBA) that preclude the wearer having a beard. This issue has been addressed in a number of legal challenges, and most services have a policy to address or accommodate this religious practice.

Dress codes also need to take into consideration religious and cultural requirements and norms. This is most often seen in relation to headscarves and the covering requirements for women. This may also be a concern for students in lab sessions where certain areas of the body are exposed to practice procedures or skills, especially in a coeducational class. Again, the instructor should try to provide reasonable accommodations.

Equal Opportunity Statement

Programs that receive federal dollars are required to have an Equal Opportunity Statement that declares the program's commitment to nondiscriminatory practices. Statutory references that support the statement may also be listed. For example:

> To the extent provided by applicable law, no person shall be excluded from participation in, denied the benefits of, or be subject to discrimination under any program or activity sponsored or conducted by The University of ____________ or any of its component institutions, on the basis of race, color, national origin, religion, sex, age, veteran status, or disability.
>
> It is the policy of The University of ____________ to strive to maintain an educational and work environment free from impermissible discrimination. In addition to compliance with all applicable federal and state laws and regulations, no person is to be the subject of discrimination on the basis of sexual orientation.

Grievance and Appeals Process

All students have the right to lodge complaints and to receive due process for the resolution of grievances that may be lodged against the program, instructors, or other students. Programs should follow institutional policies that address the process steps and protections inherent in a grievance process. A grievance should be resolved at the lowest level possible.

Ensure that all investigative materials and all findings and meeting proceedings are maintained in strictest confidence and are disseminated only to the parties permitted access due to their direct involvement in the situation. The person bringing the grievance must be afforded full immunity from retaliatory actions stemming from the act of bringing a grievance ("whistleblower protections").

The program should include an appeal process for discipline that prevents a student's academic progression and/or results in suspension or dismissal prior to the terms of the discipline being imposed, unless the nature of the allegation is so egregious that an immediate suspension or dismissal is deemed necessary by the program director.[1] As a first step, the student and instructor should discuss the situation and their points of view face to face. Students should be able to present a defense or rebuttal to the allegations against them, or their perceived reasons for unacceptable performance, without fear of reprisals or retaliation. If the faculty member affirms the decision for disciplinary action, the student could be given several options for appeal.

Some EMS programs have a standing student-affairs committee composed of class peers who are empowered to hear an appeal on matters related to discipline in an informal process and to render an opinion. This opinion may or may not be binding on the student or the faculty member depending on the program policy.

If the student remains unhappy with the outcome, he or she should have the option of appealing to an unbiased program administrator or a hearing board that is empowered to review the facts and affirm, modify, or reverse the disciplinary recommendation(s). The involved student and the faculty member recommending disciplinary action should have the right to be heard by a neutral fact-finder in a fair hearing.[9]

Inclement Weather Policy

It is a matter of policy whether an educational program stays open or adjusts their academic schedule during bad or inclement weather (**Figure 24.3**). This may be determined at the program level or it may be imposed by the academic institution with which the EMS program is affiliated.

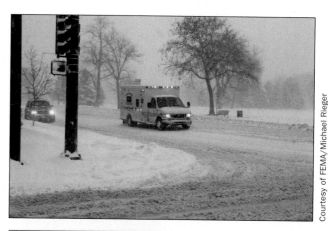

Courtesy of FEMA/Michael Rieger

Figure 24.3

It is a matter of policy whether an educational program stays open or adjusts their academic schedule during bad or inclement weather.

The foundational concern should always be the safety of students and faculty and the policy should clearly state that. The purpose of the policy is to specify conditions under which class schedules may need to be altered or modified based on inclement weather and to allow flexibility to usual and customary attendance policies. The policy should state who is authorized to make the decision to invoke the policy, cancel class, or to resume normal class schedules. The following considerations should be contemplated as the policy is developed or reviewed.

- What are the implications if a class is cancelled in terms of student objective achievement (is it the day of a major exam?); revenue stream to the educational institution; salaries paid to employees of EMS agencies who are detailed to class as their duty assignment, and so forth, and how should these be addressed?
- What elements need to be included in the policy, such as a flexible approach authorizing a late start or an abbreviated class schedule for the session, authorizing students to arrive late without penalty, up to canceling the class?
- What is to be included in the notice?
- How will the program communicate to students and faculty that the schedule is altered or a class has been cancelled? One of the greatest challenges is the method by which these changes are effectively conveyed to all students and faculty with enough advance notice for them to take appropriate action. Variations in commute times and distances and methods of transportation will cause inclement weather to pose different challenges to different folks. Communication options may include:

local radio or television station community-service announcements; phone tree activation; website, e-mail, text message or pager notices; or a voice-mail message on the program's main phone line. Also specify in the policy how long the policy will remain activated or classes remain cancelled, depending on the significance of the weather disruption.

Program Evaluation

A major administrative responsibility is program-evaluation oversight and management of necessary changes. Periodic evaluation of achievement of program goals is essential to maintain and continuously improve program quality. The 2009 Education Standards Educational Infrastructure section describes needed evaluation of program instructional effectiveness and evaluation of program organizational and administrative effectiveness (p. 60). Additionally, the CoAEMSP requires that accredited paramedic programs annually assess their resources and program outcomes.

The process of EMS program evaluation can be very extensive, involving a number of different evaluative dimensions and perspectives. However, for the purposes of this book, a simple approach designed to help the individual instructor evaluate an EMS training program will be presented. It is important to recognize that program evaluation is just part of a larger scheme of assessment that includes instructor evaluation, course evaluation, and student outcomes.

Evaluation of a program at any level can be divided into two major approaches (just like the evaluation of student progress): formative and summative evaluations. Formative evaluation involves an ongoing evaluation designed to assess program effectiveness while the program is in progress. Formative evaluations could include student cognitive or psychomotor examinations, how students are doing on course work, as well as having students evaluate the instructor's teaching methods and the clarity of information delivered. Maybe the first lab session could be followed up by an informal discussion on how it worked, if students had an adequate amount of time in their specific groups, and if they had an adequate amount of time with the instructor to become comfortable with the skill. Formative program evaluation can result in "in-flight corrections" so that the program director and instructors can adjust the program to better meet student needs, or review specific material again since students were not completely successful on their quizzes. Ideally, formative evaluations will provide feedback to the instructional staff and the institutional administrative staff on all aspects of the program, including instructional effectiveness, the classroom/skills lab environment, hospital experiences, and student performance. The formative evaluation can serve as verification that the stated goals and objectives are being attained, or as identification that they are not being met, so corrections can be made.

A summative program evaluation is a retrospective review of the program after it has been completed. This would potentially include an evaluation of instructors and their teaching and availability and attentiveness to student needs, an evaluation of lab and clinical experiences to identify availability of resources and how the experiences prepared the students for the next step in the program. Additionally, obtaining information from others than the students is very helpful. For example, hospital personnel can identify how the experience worked for them and if communication was adequate between school and hospital and if students were appropriately prepared for the experiences. Field experiences should be evaluated from the student perspective as well as the field preceptor perspective, so that any problems or suggestions can be identified and corrected or improved. Ideally, formative and summative evaluations should complement each other and provide a total evaluative picture of the program.

Another set of terms often associated with course and program evaluation is "outputs" and "outcomes." Outputs are the statistical results of the program or course; they include measures such as number of students completing the course, student contact hours, tuition generated, and so forth. Outcomes are often nebulous and difficult to measure directly. An outcome is designed to measure the impact of a course or program on a group or area. For instance, if a service conducts a training course on geriatric mental emergencies for its paramedics, the outcome that one would expect to see would be an improvement in the quality of care provided to geriatric patients with mental conditions and, ultimately, a decrease in negative outcomes as a result of these conditions. Although outcomes are important, they are often not used or required for evaluation of an individual course because they are difficult to quantify and effects take time to occur. However, program outcomes should be measured using a metric that may include such measures as employee and employer surveys.

Paramount to performing any type of evaluation is deciding on the measures to be used in the evaluation. These should be decided during the program development process and not as an afterthought once the program has begun. Possible measures or sources of measurement include the following:

- *Course objectives.* This is the "gold standard" for evaluation because this measures whether or not the participant met each of the objective requirements for the course. Evaluation forms should be sent to the graduates of the training program between 6 and 12 months after completing the program to give feedback about the training program they completed and how well they were prepared for field practice.

- *Student completion rates.* The number of students successfully completing the course provides some indication as to the effectiveness of the course, provided a uniform standard for determining successful completion is applied.
- *Comparison with other courses.* This will work only if the courses are identical, such as with a comparison of two EMT courses that are conducted according to the same national standard.
- *Certification/licensure rates.* If a course prepares the student for some level of certification or licensure, attainment of that certification level is a good measure of course success.
- *Job placement and continued employment.* Are students who have completed a course able to obtain jobs and function effectively in those jobs? Evaluation forms should be sent to the graduates of the training program between 6 and 12 months after completing the program to give feedback about how prepared the graduate felt about obtaining and functioning in an EMS job.
- *Standardized testing.* Standardized tests or other evaluations given to students at the end of a course that compares them according to an established norm can be used. These standardized tests need to be validated examinations that are appropriate for the level of students in the educational program.
- *Student and graduate satisfaction evaluations.* How did students feel about the course and what was its value to them? Such surveys can be given at the conclusion of the course and followed up some time later, perhaps after the provider has been employed in the field for a specified time.
- *Employer satisfaction evaluations.* These measure employers' assessments of graduates' knowledge, skills, and professional behaviors. They are typically conducted about six months after the graduate student has been on the job.

Just as programs are evaluated, individual courses should be evaluated as well. The conscientious instructor will want to make sure that the course he or she is teaching is accomplishing its objectives while it is ongoing. If a problem is noted, it can be corrected to ensure a positive learning experience. Gagne and Briggs, in their book *Principles of Instructional Design*, list the following as examples of data that can be collected during a formative evaluation.[10]

From the observer:

- In what respects are (are not) the materials and media employed in the manner intended by the designer?
- In what respects does (does not) the teacher carry out the procedures and make the decisions intended?
- In what respect do (do not) the students follow the general procedures specified?

From the teacher:

- What practical difficulties are encountered in conducting the lessons?
- How would you estimate the degree of interest or absorption of students in the lesson?
- What difficulties were encountered in carrying out the intended teaching procedures?

From the student:

- How likely are you to choose to do the things you learned in this lesson?
- How likely are you to recommend this lesson to a friend?
- What are the results of a test of performance based on the lesson's objectives?

How the instructor goes about obtaining these data will depend on a number of factors, including course length, course type, number of students, and available time. Some possible approaches to evaluation include the following:

- Giving course evaluation questionnaire to students periodically
- Taking time out from class to discuss with students how the course is going
- Using standardized measures such as giving the same test to all sections of a course, or comparing results of previous course measures with those of the current course
- Using an outside observer of a course lesson as a resource
- Having a "neutral third party" visit with students alone and discuss the course(s)
- Asking students to list the pros and cons of the course anonymously

Regardless of the input received by the instructor through either a formative or a summative evaluation, the important thing is that the instructor must be prepared to render some judgment as to the course's worth. Boyle lists the following as program characteristics that should be considered when one is making a judgment about an educational course or program: quality, suitability, effectiveness, efficiency, and importance.[11] By using a combination of formative and summative evaluations, the instructor will be better able to evaluate a program in the many dimensions required to provide an effective learning experience.

Budgeting and Financial Planning

Part of the planning process must include creating a budget. A budget is a financial plan for coordinating resources and expenditures over a selected period of time. Hospitals, EMS agencies, and educational institutions prepare many types of budgets such as capital, cash flow, and operating. The capital budget plans for the acquisition of major assets with a dollar value over a predetermined threshold and with an anticipated life cycle of three to five years or more. The cash flow budget is typically a month-by-month plan for revenues received and expenses paid. A program director is most directly concerned with the operating budget.

An operating budget identifies the expected resources and expenditures of an entity for a given future period, usually one year. It provides a basis for evaluating the financial performance of the program while helping to control costs and communicating short-range plans and financial requirements within the organization and externally to the community.

Prerequisites for the development of an operating budget are the following:

- Include a statement of the purpose or mission of the program.
- List the specific objectives the program is expected to accomplish during the budget year.
- Identify who is responsible for submitting specific sections of the budget.
- Describe the current operations in terms of revenues, expenses, and services accomplished.

This requires an intact reporting system that highlights program activities and the attendant financial information.

Steps in Developing an Operating Budget

An orderly, systematic approach to developing a budget will assist in assuring that resources are available to meet program needs. The budget must account for all expenses and income.

1. Justify Work Units Consumed, Programs Conducted, Outputs Produced, and So On

Does the program need to continue what it does, the way that it is currently done? Is there any opportunity for economies of scale or increased efficiency? Since salaries typically consume over 60 percent of an educational program's operating budget, *efficiency is often gauged in terms of staff productivity.*

Productivity is defined as the amount of output (service) per unit of input (hours of work), or in assigned and taught student-contact hours or semester hours. Consider how many educators or educator hours (full-time equivalents [FTEs]) are budgeted per class hour or per number of students. If valuable educator time is consumed in low-skill or clerical tasks, consider if an investment in technology or the addition of support staff actually pays for itself in improved efficiency. Additionally, the institutional and program mission for research and institutional and professional service may be components of academic institutions, and time should be included for those activities when possible.

Programs use different metrics to measure productivity. Each program should create a measuring stick that works for the program and use it as a benchmark. If the program runs low on educator-to-student or staff-productivity ratios and outcomes are poor, additional faculty may be needed. If the program runs high on educator-to-student ratios and outcomes are poor, the educators may be inefficient or ineffective and money may be wasted. An evaluation of the current plan is called for and perhaps a new direction is needed.

Budgeting is an art and people are not widgets. Productivity measures can be heavily influenced by staff maturity in terms of experience and advancement on the learning curve and must be considered in budgeting FTE time. It is expected that new educators will take longer to prepare and process class materials and function as effective learning coaches than those who have been in their positions for several years. Mentoring takes time, but it is worth the investment. Consider the impact on program costs if new educators were left on their own to conduct a program by trial and error.

Seasoned educators being asked to do things in a new way, such as online teaching or to use new technology, may also experience a temporary erosion in productivity that requires additional faculty hours during the transition.

Determining a target productivity ratio can be aided by conducting time and motion studies where staff are actually observed and timed while doing various tasks. The findings are plotted and distilled into a reasonable and expected norm.

What is the effectiveness of the program? Again, metrics may vary. Some will use pass/fail rates on credentialing exams; others may look at student retention or satisfaction rates or performance assessments from preceptors, managers, and/or students. Perhaps the best measure would be the quality of patient care performed by graduates after they transition from class to the workforce. Adding additional dollars to a program is not guaranteed to improve effectiveness. Conduct a complete root-cause analysis of the performance gaps before determining that a budget adjustment is the answer to your problem.

2. Prioritize Program Outputs

What would be the impact to the program, organization, EMS service providers, community, or patients if any item in the budget was denied or cut? What are the core services or line items that must be preserved and protected at all cost? Can the program manage without that extra box of 4X4s, but not a working bag-valve-mask? Although this is a somewhat simplistic analogy, educators must find cost savings when absolutely necessary. Reasoned justifications should be included in the analysis.

3. Forecast Service Demand

In the case of an educational program, the budget must consider student enrollment projections and whether they are increasing or decreasing. If possible, the program should look at trends for student volumes for the past five years. Service providers can assist in assessing the need for more employees and whether they will need more, less, or the same number of EMTs and/or paramedics in the next year. Consider if the current workforce is soon to retire within the next three to five years. Also consider if there are any other environmental factors that impact planning such as an economic downturn, or availability of EMS jobs; consider whether a competing program closed or expanded, or whether a fire-science program at your college made EMS education a mandatory part of their curriculum. Another impact is how national education standards have changed that will require longer and more expanded classes than in the past.

4. Project Revenues

Consider all possible revenue streams. These might include tuition, student fees, grants, donations from philanthropy, or subsidies (depending on your affiliation). As tempting as it sounds, the program cannot just raise tuition fees to meet inflated cost projections. Anyone affiliated with a college is locked into a tuition cost per credit hour cap that cannot be changed mid year just because more capital is needed. Thus, if a program is to operate within its means, the program must maximize revenue and minimize costs or there will not be a program.

5. Estimate Personnel and Other Expenses

An essential component of zero-based budgeting is to project all costs to the program as accurately as possible. It is not wise to rely on historical trends and just add 5 percent each year.

Program managers must consider whether a cost is responsive or driven by changes in service volume or the number of students. Those that fluctuate by volume are considered "variable." Those that remain constant, uninfluenced by volume, are called "fixed." For example, at least a portion of the primary instructor's salary cost is typically fixed. The time spent in the administrative work of planning and organizing a class should vary little whether there are 10, 20, or 30 students. Thus, it is preferable to fill all class openings to maximize revenues for programs that have heavy fixed costs.

On the other hand, the total costs associated with lab instructors are strongly driven by volume or number of students. If one assumes a consistent ratio of five or six students per lab instructor in class labs, far more instructors would be needed for a class of 40 than for a class of 20. These expenses would vary based on the number of labs scheduled for the class, the amount of supplies needed per student, and so on.

Another consideration for personnel is the amount of educator time and resources needed to plan for program revisions. Actual outputs can be measured in relative value units (RVUs). For example, if an RVU is defined as 60 minutes of an employee's time, all work units taking 60 minutes would be one RVU. Consider all the tasks that must be completed by staff members based on current and projected student and class volumes and assign a time value to them. Compare their anticipated work units against the number of hours they are authorized to work. The process is laborious when done the first time, but it is necessary.

One full-time equivalent (employee) (FTE) is usually budgeted in the range of 2,080 work hours per year. This does not take into consideration nonproductive hours consumed when using vacation, sick, bereavement, jury duty, education, leave of absence, military deployment, meeting, continuing-education, orientation, or holiday time. Those items will need to be factored in as a general productive to nonproductive time ratio depending on the nature of the benefit package and budgeting model. For employees, also factor in FICA expenses and other benefit costs such as insurance coverage and matching funds for pension plans.

Other salary outlays may include money for a medical director, lab instructors, guest faculty, or independent contractors who may be hired by the program for particular deliverables.

The program manager must evaluate assets in terms of capital and noncapital supplies and equipment and determine what is in stock and what is needed to conduct a quality class based on student and program projections

A general ledger chart of accounts is created to project costs. Beside salaries, suggested line items may include but are not limited to the following:

- Professional fees: guest faculty, consultants
- Telephone; pagers
- Equipment repairs
- Other repair; maintenance services
- Supplies: instructional
- Supplies: noninstructional
- Books and publications
- Travel
- Equipment rental
- Marketing
- Licenses; permits
- Dues
- Employee continuing education and development
- Accreditation fees
- Criminal background checks and drug screening and costs related to physical examinations and immunizations/titers if borne by the program and passed through to the students
- Clinical and field internship scheduling and skills tracking software/license
- Depending on the nature and location of the program, professional liability coverage for educators and students

Accounts may be added or adjusted based on specific program configuration and needs.

Look at all class activities. What disposable or consumable supplies or equipment will be needed for each class or lab based on the number of students? What is the cost of each item? How many will each student use or need? Multiply these variables by the number of students to get the projected cost figures for each item. EMS programs are lab intensive. Instructors need to create authentic simulations and scenarios that require the use of real equipment in good working order. These instructional costs can be large and must be planned for to conduct a quality program.

Points to consider:

- *Try to never pay full or list price.* Make it a practice to work closely with vendor reps to negotiate discounted pricing or locked-in pricing for several years in return for a commitment to use their product for a specified period of time or to guarantee a minimum order number during that time.
- *Compare cost, quality, and features.* One of the advantages of our competitive market economy is the option of selecting from a large variety of texts, tools, supplies, and equipment. Price points can vary widely for products of equal quality; continuing to buy from the same place may not be effective. Although it may take some time to investigate various options for purchases, it will pay off in the long run.
- *Seek out economies of scale.* Program personnel should attempt to negotiate a better cost per item by purchasing products in bulk that will be clearly used during the year. Consider creating a buying group locally to become eligible for preferring pricing.
- *Institute tight inventory controls.* The cost of waste and creative procurement (theft) from supplies can be significant and methods to minimize or eliminate these problems are worthwhile.

An alternative method of budgeting variable costs is to drill them down to the cost per student and then estimate budget projections based on the number of anticipated students. Medical-surgical and pharmacy supplies are good examples of variable costs that change based on the size of the class or number of labs conducted. This figure can be used when negotiating the need for a tuition or fee increase.

Lastly, consider indirect costs that may be related to overhead if a prorated fee for classroom/office space, housekeeping, maintenance, utilities, insurance, and so on is paid.

6. Adjust the Figures to Reach a Balanced Budget

Adjust the figures as necessary to reach a balanced budget (revenues equal or hopefully exceed expenses) unless an unfavorable variance (negative profitability margin) is acceptable.

If there is a disparity between resources available and resources needed, attempt to realign the budget as necessary. Adding FTEs is very difficult for most programs in a difficult economic climate. However, reducing them should not be the knee-jerk response when asked to cut the budget. People (educators) are the program's most valuable asset. Program personnel need data and information before submitting a pie-in-the-sky budget. Budgets must be based on facts, not emotional pleas.

Introduction to Accreditation

According to *The New Oxford American Dictionary*, *accreditation* is to "give authority or sanction to [someone or something] when recognized standards have been met." In the context of education, *accreditation* is defined as a *voluntary* standard conferred by a *nongovernmental* organization with the purposes of quality, accountability, and improvement.

Accreditation is either institutional or programmatic (also called "specialized" or "professional"). In order to be an accreditation agency, the accreditor must be recognized or approved by either the U.S. Department of Education or the Council for Higher Education Accreditation (CHEA).

Institutional accreditation evaluates the entire institution without judging specific programs within the institution. Examples are: the Southern Association of Colleges and Schools (SACS) or Middle States Colleges and Schools (MSCS), The Higher Learning Commission of the North Central Association of Colleges and Secondary Schools (NCA) as well as other types of recognized institutional accreditors.

Programmatic accreditation, which may also be called "specialized accreditation," pertains to a specific educational program, typically one that prepares students to practice for a particular occupation. These types of accrediting bodies apply standards for curriculum and profession-related specifics and may be associated with a professional organization. The only nationally recognized accreditation currently available for EMS education is provided through the Commission on Accreditation of Allied Health Education Programs (CAAHEP). CAAHEP has a committee for EMS called the Committee on Accreditation of Emergency Medical Services Professions (CoAEMSP). It is one of 17 Committees on Accreditation affiliated with CAAHEP. Before January 1, 2000, this committee was called the Joint Review Committee for the EMT-Paramedic (JRCEMT-P). Other educational programs accredited by CAAHEP include those for medical assistants, diagnostic medical sonographers, and other clinically related occupations. The only CAAHEP accreditation for EMS is at the paramedic level. CAAHEP does not currently accredit educational programs that are shorter than one academic year (2 semesters) and consequently it is unlikely that Advanced EMT, EMT, and EMR programs would become eligible to be accredited in the CAAHEP system.

The primary purpose of educational program accreditation is the protection afforded to students when the program is evaluated according to specific standards and benchmarks. In addition, accreditation provides a measure of protection for the program and the institution, for the health care community, and for society at large, particularly the patients. Accreditation promotes the professionalism of EMS as practitioners achieve the high standards it requires. Potential students can identify programs and institutions that are accredited—a fact that likely provides them with a measure of assurance that their tuition will not be wasted. Although peer review does not guarantee quality, it is a reasonable indication that the educational program infrastructure meets or exceeds commonly accepted practices. Institutions of higher learning usually accept transfer credits from accredited programs.

Beginning the accreditation process, paramedic programs submit a self-study report, first as an initial self-study and then every five years thereafter as a continuing evaluation. This report is a program self-evaluation based on specific standards for accreditation that follow a format of systematic evaluation. After the self-study document is submitted and reviewed, a site visit is conducted by peers who visit the program and talk to instructors, students, graduates, advisory committee members, employers of graduates, clinical and field preceptors, and other educational stakeholders. After the site visit, the program is sent a findings letter based on the site visit report and is asked to make adjustments as needed. All information is used to make an accreditation action recommendation by the CoAEMSP board to CAAHEP. Additionally, achievement of the program objectives with outcome measures is revisited annually and continued attempts to improve the program are documented.

Despite program variations, there are some educational program elements that are generally required by overseeing authorities such as state EMS officers. Some examples include the following:

- Educational programs typically must use, at a minimum, curricula or follow educational standards approved by the state's lead agency. This may include specialty curricula not available nationwide and/or content that covers expanded scopes of practice adopted by that state that varies from the National Scope of Practice Model and National EMS Education Standards.
- If clinical or field experience is to be obtained, clinical instruction plans and written agreements may need to be obtained in advance.

- Classroom, laboratory, and practice resources, as well as access to a library with appropriate reference materials, must be adequate for student needs. Opportunities for the student to accomplish skill competencies in the field environment must be ensured if required by the program curriculum or National EMS Education Standards.
- The educational program must have or make provisions for students to obtain liability insurance if a clinical component is required.
- The program must have a physician medical director who possesses the background and experience to competently provide medical oversight for EMS educational programs.
  - The National Association of EMS Physicians publishes excellent resource documents for novice EMS Medical Directors. Examples include: Clinical Aspects of Prehospital Medicine, Vol. 1, and Medical Oversight of EMS, Vol. 2 (Pak ISBN: 978-0-7575-6140-5); Evaluating and Improving Quality in EMS, Vol. 3 (ISBN: 978-0-7575-6073-6), and Special Operations Medical Support, Vol. 4 (ISBN: 978-0-7575-6079-8).
- All educational program personnel, including the program director or coordinator and primary or lead instructor, must be properly credentialed in terms of certification or licensure and academic preparation. CAAHEP-accredited paramedic program directors must have a minimum of a bachelor's degree.
- Preceptors or field-training officers who supervise students in the hospital or field environments should be qualified, appropriately trained, and their performance monitored and measured. CAAHEP-accredited programs must provide specific training to preceptors.
- An advisory committee should establish and monitor program goals and should include various stakeholders, including graduates and employers of graduates, receiving hospital personnel, clinical preceptors and others.
- Individual student records must be maintained including application, certifications currently held, transcripts of hours and performance, and documentation of clinical and field experiences.
- The student selection process must be clearly outlined and followed.
- The educational program must supply information to each student at the beginning of each program, including the following:
  - Course objectives
  - Student handbook
  - Required hours or competencies
  - Minimum acceptable scores on testing or performance measures
  - Attendance requirements
  - Disciplinary policy
  - Grievance procedures
  - Practices that safeguard the health and well-being of the student
  - Fees; payment options

Medical Director's Role in an EMS Program

The medical director, (**Figure 24.4**), is an essential component of an EMS educational program and can be a potent force for positive change in the classroom or in the clinical and field settings. Physician oversight is commonly required by the state EMS agency and is identified in the 2009 Education Standards Educational Infrastructure as a necessary component at all levels of EMS education. Additionally, active participation of the medical director is required for the national accreditation of paramedic programs (CoAEMSP) standards. As a practicing physician, the medical director can be a powerful advocate and therefore instrumental in moving a program toward its organizational development goals. He or she can

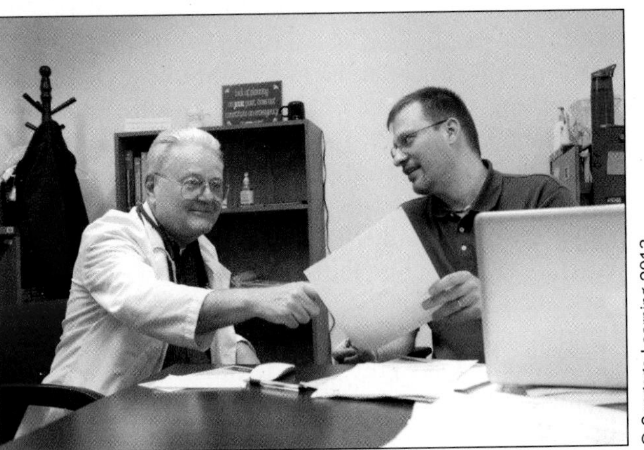

Figure 24.4
The Medical Director is an essential component of the EMS educational program, and should approve the medical accuracy of the course content and all examinations.

Starting a New Program

Creating an educational infrastructure depends on the type of program to be conducted. An essential first step in creating an administrative infrastructure is to engage in a strategic-planning process with the goal of writing a clear and compelling plan that identifies tactics and strategies to implement over the short-, intermediate-, and long-range planning horizons. If done well, this document serves as a blueprint for success, gives the program clear direction, helps it adapt to environmental threats and challenges, and secures needed resources.

Questions to ask and answer:

- Why does the program exist?
- What are the core values of the program?
- What ethical or philosophical constructs will be embraced?
- Where is the program going or growing in the next year, three years, and five years?

Foundational to setting future goals is a clear, concise, and easily articulated statement of the program's "mission" or "purpose." In one or two sentences, distill the essence of why the program exists. Most organizations write very comprehensive, sometimes flowery, and wordy mission statements that almost no one can recall or recite. In stark contrast, one of the most profound health care organization mission statements is simply phrased "Patients first." Another uses "Everything matters" over their logo. Everyone, at every level, can remember that and it leaves no doubt in anyone's mind what the organization stands for.

Next, create a vision of where the program should be in the next five years. Consider how the program should be viewed in the broader educational arena, what linkages or accreditations will be accomplished, what services will be provided, and what are the desired levels of excellence or outcomes to be achieved?

Third, the core values should be identified to drive educational planning and decisions. Consider the beliefs and world views that are embraced by the organization and program. The next step is to view the program from a perspective that emphasizes the impact of external factors, like a change in national education standards and/or scopes of practice or a tight economy. Consciously position the program to be self-directing and driving innovation, rather than being reactionary and a victim of change.

An important part of this process is to conduct a "SWOT analysis" of the program's internal strengths and weaknesses juxtaposed against opportunities and threats in the external environment. The SWOT analysis identifies the following components.

S	Strengths	Analyze program strengths.
W	Weaknesses	Identify program weaknesses.
O	Opportunities	Determine opportunities for growth or improvement.
T	Threats	Consider potential present or future threats to the program.

Internal strengths and weaknesses should be evaluated based on: financial return on investment and budget variances; quantity and quality of education based on defined outcome measures; performance assessment of leaders, educators, preceptors, and providers; physical facilities; and technological resources. It may be helpful to group external considerations into categories such as: professional or practice; economic and financial; legal or regulatory; political; competitive or collaborative.

Armed with this information, develop practical goals, objectives, tactics, or tasks to address the key issues. Segregate the goals into functional units sometimes called "key result areas" (KRA). An example of a broad subheading or KRA would include program administration. Tactics in this area may address issues related to the following:

- Medical oversight
- Program leadership
- Collaboration and communication with local EMS educational programs, hospitals, EMS agencies, and other stakeholders
- Community partnership agreements
- Program accreditation
- Curriculum development
- Policies and procedures
- Asset management in terms of human and economic resources

While strategic plans are visionary by nature, they must also be practical. It is very frustrating and counterproductive to create a plan that has no chance of being successfully implemented. If a large gulf exists between "what is" and "what should be," identify and prioritize steps to improve the program based on available resources. This permits reasoned decisions in an economically challenging environment.

Create an implementation plan that details and sequences the steps, assign the persons accountable for completing each task, and specify due dates, keeping in mind that these are dynamic, rather than static documents.

(*continues*)

Starting a New Program (*continued*)

If this is a new class start-up or you need to justify new resources, craft a business plan. The six major sections of a business plan are as follows:

- An executive summary: One to two page abbreviated summary of the plan
- A business problem to be addressed: Environmental assessment driving the requested change
- The available options to address a problem or an opportunity. (Use the SWOT analysis technique, then define the option, an analysis of the benefits and risks, feasibility, direct and indirect costs, issues and assumptions for each option. Options may be rated based on criteria such as improved efficiency, enhanced quality, staff cost, lost productivity, cost of remodeling and equipment, process-change feasibility, and marketing requirements.)
- The preferred option: summary of rationale for preferred option
- Implementation and evaluation: Required activities, timelines, responsible individuals, milestones of progress, and measures of success
- Appendix: Feasibility studies, research or surveys, quotes from vendors; worksheets with cost detail; other supporting documentation[12]

also be responsible for securing the financial and community support necessary to be successful. Too often, the medical director is not used to his or her full advantage and programs struggle to meet students' needs without the assistance of this important ally.

The medical director should do the following:

- Review and critique educational content and verify medical accuracy.
- Review major examinations for *medical* accuracy, validity, and relevance.
- Provide oversight for medical instruction, supervision, and evaluation of students.
- Monitor progress of students and the program.
- Cooperate and collaborate with the program director.
- Assume responsibility for the medical quality of the program and for delegated responsibilities.
- Attest to entry-level competencies of students before graduation.
- Understand EMS and EMS education and have knowledge of the local medical community.
- Serve as an active advisory board member and facilitate interaction between the educational institution, the instructional staff, and community stakeholders.

For all these duties and others that may arise during the course of the medical director's tenure, he or she should likely be provided some degree of monetary compensation. Payment for serving as an EMS educational program medical director should be commensurate with the time and complexity committed toward meeting the program's goals and objectives.

Instructor-Related Administrative Issues

The role of the individual course instructor goes beyond that of being a well prepared, knowledgeable, and effective classroom or lab instructor. The instructor also has a responsibility to know and understand, follow, and enforce rules, regulations, and policies in the classroom. Often the instructor is on the "front line" of such issues. This section presents some common administrative issues that the typical EMS educator may encounter.

Instructor Contract or Agreement

In most academic institutions, it is important that all instructors have a formal contract. This not only protects the individual instructor, but the institution as well. The program director or even a part-time course instructor may find it necessary to ask a friend or colleague to fill-in or teach a specific part of a course. It is important that such arrangements be formalized, especially if there is compensation involved.

The instructor contract is usually a formal document developed and approved by the hiring institution. At a minimum, it should include the following:

- Specific course(s) or responsibility of the instructor
- Date, time, location of the course(s)
- Compensation
- Specific requirements such as filing syllabus, reporting grades, and so on

- Access to facilities and location for meeting with students
- Contact person for assistance with administrative support
- Information on how the instructor will be evaluated

The instructor contract, as stated above, protects the instructor. It also protects the students and the hiring institution; therefore, it is important that contracts be completed and on file for all instructors each semester or program period, even if the same instructors are used each time.

Institutions may require programs to have on file specific criteria for hiring instructors. These should include academic preparation, experience, and teaching experience/preparation. Likewise, nondiscrimination and EEOC requirements should be provided.

Course Syllabus

A syllabus usually describes the body of instruction to be conducted. The form and title of this document may vary based on local requirements. The format may be set as a standard by the educational institution with which the EMS program is affiliated, or it may be created at the instructor's discretion based on the nature and complexity of the class. It may be as short as a couple of pages, or it may be much longer depending on the level of detail presented. Many elements in the syllabus may be drilled down into greater detail in another document such as the student handbook or course policies, if not included in the syllabus.

Whatever the form, the syllabus is an important resource for students and faculty. Educators should design a clear, complete, and current document that answers students' questions and prevents misunderstanding, complaints, and other problems. A well-written syllabus can determine the outcome of a dispute between the instructor and a student. Careful writing is essential to develop a syllabus that stands the test of an institutional or legal challenge. Each student should receive his or her own copy of the syllabus and/or student handbook at the first class meeting and have any questions clarified. Instructors should review key points in the syllabus and student handbook and make sure all students are familiar with issues that affect them. Copies of these documents may also be available through electronic media and the Internet. Many programs and institutions of higher learning develop websites that archive these documents for quick access.

A syllabus may contain the following basic information:

- Course title and description, course number
- Instructor's name, contact information (an e-mail and telephone number for students to use), office location, and hours
- Any prerequisites
- Course dates, times, location(s), (semester), year
- Program goal to graduate entry-level practitioners who are competent in their knowledge (cognitive domain), psychomotor skills (psychomotor domain), and professional behaviors (affective domain)
- Required textbooks and/or educational resources plus details on where these can be purchased or consulted

Affective Evaluation Requirements

The Education Infrastructure section of the 2009 Education Standards identifies "student assessment" components that include student evaluation in all domains at all levels. This includes affective evaluation or the evaluation of professional behavior. So, just as a minimum score is required on a final exam in a course, and final skills exams must be passed, the professional behavior must also be satisfactory or the student does not pass. All domains of learning must be evaluated and deemed to be competent for the student to graduate (**Figure 24.5**).

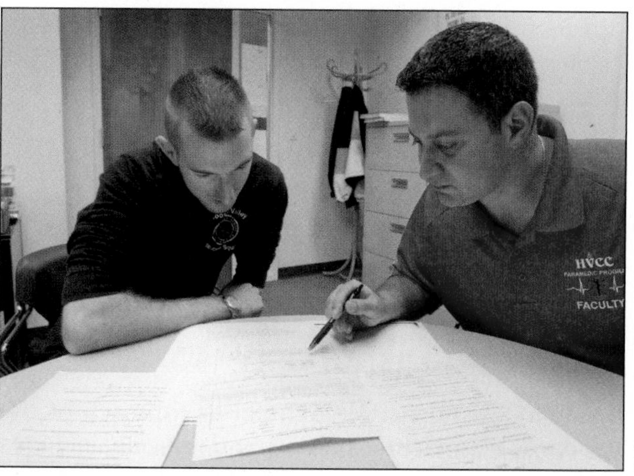

Figure 24.5

Affective evaluation is a key component in determining a student's final evaluation.

The Standards also identify 11 affective/professional behavior characteristics for all levels of EMS providers in the Clinical Behavior/Judgment section on Professionalism (p. 60). These characteristics are the following:

- Integrity
- Empathy
- Self-motivation
- Appearance/personal hygiene
- Self-confidence
- Communications
- Time management
- Teamwork/diplomacy
- Respect
- Patient advocacy
- Careful delivery of service

EMS educators need to demonstrate, teach, and coach students toward achieving competency in these areas first by modeling them in the classroom, lab, and clinical and field settings. Student actions that do not demonstrate appropriate behavior should be promptly identified and discussed with the student and documented. This requirement is an academic requirement of the program and failure of the affective domain evaluation constitutes academic failure of the course. (Various methods of evaluation of the affective domain are discussed in Chapter 22: Other Evaluation Tools.)

Teaching Tip >> *Model accountability: Students and other educators cannot break the habit of denial and lack of accountability unless they replace it with another behavior such as accepting responsibility and being accountable. Primary instructors should model the desired behaviors they expect of students. This starts by having everyone acknowledge the clear goals and objectives they are striving to meet.*

Academic Dishonesty

Academic dishonesty is defined as a breach of the standards of academic integrity and typically includes cheating, plagiarism, collusion, falsifying academic records, and any act designed to give unfair advantage to the student. In many programs, the cost of academic dishonesty can be suspension or permanent expulsion from the institution. Consequences could also include a failing grade along with a disciplinary record that may affect the student's future employment or educational opportunities. A dishonest or incompetent student who becomes a dishonest or incompetent EMS practitioner produces unconscionable consequences.

Academic integrity and honesty are essential values for all EMS providers and health professionals. EMS personnel, especially paramedics, must often independently care for patients who require the most urgent and invasive interventions without benefit of immediate medical consultation or assistance. Their ability to perform accurately and rapidly critically affects patient mortality and morbidity, and educators must ensure that these practitioners possess the knowledge, skills, and behaviors required to perform the job well.

An understanding of how and why students cheat may help instructors deter dishonest behavior. A survey of educators conducted on its website by the National Association of EMS Educators in 2008 revealed that the leading causes of cheating in EMS were failure to study, laziness, a "desire to just get their ticket punched," time pressure, and poor supervision. There seemed to be an undercurrent of belief that personnel and vehicles needed to remain on the street and how the tests and CE hours got accomplished was not as important as the fact that they stay compliant with requirements and regulators by the most expeditious means possible. A study conducted by researchers at the University of British Columbia and published by the American Psychological Association in September 2010, examined the behavior of university students over 10 years and found that many who cheated are not afraid of punishment, are amoral, and have a strong sense of entitlement. They reported that students who cheat ranked high for three personality disorders: psychopathy, Machiavellianism (manipulativeness), and narcissism. Others were simply unprepared.[13]

An evolving area of concern is online education where the opportunities for academic dishonesty abound, including "short cutting" or "beating the system"; for example, spending little or no time with the educational content, going straight to the test and being done in a matter of minutes (because they already had the questions and/or key), or learning how to change an answer once it had been marked incorrect. CECBEMS has created rigorous standards for content and testing standards for CE vendors and educators who want approval for online courses.[14]

In today's culture, many believe that cheating is appropriate to help them get results at all costs and is not morally wrong, as everyone is doing it.[15] In 2010, it was discovered that 28 Haverhill, Massachusetts

Southwestern School of Health Professions, Academic Dishonesty Recommendations—a Guide for Faculty[17]

THE RESPONSIBILITY OF THE FACULTY

Confronting academic dishonesty is the shared responsibility of faculty and students, although faculty members are called upon to play a leadership role. An attitude of intolerance by faculty can play an important role in its prevention. In keeping with a "no tolerance" policy, faculty members should add the following statement to their examination papers to be signed by all students: "I have neither given nor received assistance on this exam (paper, project, presentation, etc.)." Or, faculty may choose to have students handwrite the statement and sign it.

WAYS IN WHICH STUDENTS MAY COMMIT SCHOLASTIC DISHONESTY

During examinations:

- Signaling to another student with coughs, hand signals, or other body language
- Concealing notes on hands, caps, or shoes, or in pockets
- Writing in small note books or "blue books" prior to an examination
- Writing information on boards or desks, or keeping notes on the floor
- Obtaining copies of a test in advance, without permission (e.g., during an earlier exam period offered by the faculty member)
- Passing examination information from an earlier class to a later class that day or week
- Leaving information in the restroom
- Exchanging exams after they have been distributed so that neighbors have identical test forms
- Changing a graded paper and requesting that it be regraded
- Failing to turn in a test and later suggesting that the faculty member has lost it
- Stealing another student's graded test paper and writing one's own name on it
- Recording two answers—one on the test form, one on the answer sheet
- Marking an answer sheet to enable another student to see the answer
- Transmitting answers for an exam to a student in a testing area via a pager
- Encircling two adjacent answers and claiming to have had the correct answer
- Stealing an exam for someone in another section or for placement in a test file
- Storing test information on a cell phone, tablet, or other electronic device

On a paper, lab, or other type of assignment:

- Destroying or removing library materials to gain an academic advantage
- Obtaining reports or assignments from websites
- Fabricating data for lab assignments
- Failing to contribute as an equal partner in group assignments

GENERAL TIPS FOR COMBATING SCHOLASTIC DISHONESTY

1. Incorporate professional ethics content into program curricula and reemphasize on a regular basis.
2. At the beginning of the program, use the institution's standard scholastic dishonesty language from the Guidelines for Students and orient students to the information. Emphasis should be placed on the fact that scholastic dishonesty will not be tolerated. (Example: "Any student who commits an act of scholastic dishonesty is subject to discipline. Scholastic dishonesty includes but is not limited to cheating, plagiarism, collusion, the submission for credit of any work or materials that are attributable in whole or in part to another person, taking an examination for another person, any act designed to give unfair advantage to a student or the attempt to commit such acts.")
3. At the beginning of each course, review scholastic dishonesty guidelines in course syllabi and reiterate the importance of honesty.
4. Make a clear distinction, in front of the class, between group assignments and expectations of sole effort.

TIPS FOR COMBATING SCHOLASTIC DISHONESTY DURING EXAMINATIONS

1. Separate students and/or assign seats. Move a student who appears to be copying from another student to another seat.
2. Distribute different test forms (or rearrange the order of test items) and inform students of that practice, particularly for large classes. Change tests each semester.

(continues)

Southwestern School of Health Professions, Academic Dishonesty Recommendations—a Guide for Faculty[17] (*continued*)

3. Require that proctors remain in the testing room, and occasionally walk around the room throughout the testing period.
4. Enforce silence during the testing period.
5. Do not return exams for students to keep or to write down exam items.
6. Check desks and the surrounding area for unauthorized materials, including textbooks and papers.
7. Issue a blank piece of paper for students to use to cover their answer sheets.
8. Require students to remove caps, hats, and sunglasses during the testing period.
9. Use caution in allowing students to use programmable calculators.
10. Provide clear directions concerning rules to follow for the examination period (e.g., whether the student can go to the restroom, whether the student can access anything from his or her backpack).
11. Collect pagers and cell phones.

TIPS FOR COMBATING SCHOLASTIC DISHONESTY ON PAPERS/ASSIGNMENTS

1. Provide clear directions on each paper/assignment concerning allowable collaboration or absolute independence.
2. Do not use take-home exams.
3. Assign paper subjects or assignments in such a way that the student is unlikely to be able to purchase assignments from a "paper mill" or find a relevant paper on the Internet.
4. Be attentive to higher vocabulary or more journalistic than academic writing style and other clues that may flag a paper as inconsistent with the knowledge and style of the student writing it.
5. Share with your colleagues websites offering papers for students.
6. Have students write the following statement on each independent assignment: "I have neither given nor received aid on this assignment."
7. Search the Internet by topics assigned so as to be familiar with websites on the Internet.

TIPS FOR COMBATING SCHOLASTIC DISHONESTY ON CLINICAL ASSIGNMENTS/EXPERIENCES

1. Thoroughly orient preceptors to student objectives and expectations.
2. Have clinical faculty/preceptors sign off student assignments in clinical settings, including papers or logs.
3. Have faculty present in the clinical area.

EMTs were accused of fraudulently obtaining their recertification by documenting CE hours that were never legitimately earned. Their cases turned out to be the tip of the iceberg. More than 200 EMTs in that state were suspended for allegedly falsifying CE records.[16]

The cases in Massachusetts were followed by other headlines alleging academic dishonesty in EMS programs around the country, giving rise to public uncertainty regarding those they traditionally regarded as their heroes and emergency health care safety net. It is critical that educators understand why cheating or educational fraud occurs and do everything possible to correct the root cause and exact engineering and process controls to abate the risk. The document, Southwestern School of Health Professions Academic Dishonesty Recommendations, a Guide for Faculty, describes ways in which students may cheat and details how instructors can prevent various types of academic dishonesty.

Institutional policies vary as to what an instructor should do when he or she suspects that academic dishonesty is occurring or has occurred. All instructors should be familiar with institutional policies on confronting a student, taking up an exam, documenting the allegation, and recommending consequences and/or disciplinary action. Academic dishonesty is typically considered by institutions as a disciplinary issue rather than an academic issue and students are entitled to full due process. It is paramount that nothing be done to prejudice the student's rights. (See Chapter 10: Legal Issues for EMS Educators for more information.)

General Classroom Management

Managing students in any classroom can be a challenge. Decisions about classroom management require knowledge of students' rights.

Right to Fail

It is important for instructors to recognize that students have a right to fail. What this means is that if a student elects to not meet course requirements as clearly delineated in the syllabus, he or she will receive the appropriate grade. As an example, if a student comes to class and sits in the back and plays games on his or her computer throughout the class, and is not a disruption or distraction to other students, he or she has the right to do so. An instructor may establish classroom behavior requirements such as no talking, no use of ear buds or electronic devices, and so forth in the best interest of the class as a whole. However, the basic principle is that if students' behavior is not illegal, immoral, disruptive, or distracting, they have the right to engage in such actions and accept the consequences. Of course this should not abdicate the instructor's responsibility to attempt to motivate and counsel such students.

Right to Access

Students pay tuition to attend an educational institution and thus have a right to have access to what they have paid for. This may seem straightforward, but it is not uncommon for instructors to inadvertently violate this right. A common example is the "locked door policy" in which an instructor locks the classroom door at the beginning of class preventing any late-arriving students from entering; the idea being that students need to be on time and if they are not, they are denied access. However, the student has paid for the right to attend that class and as long as his or her coming late is not disruptive to the class, he or she has the right to do so. This does not, however, prevent the instructor from having an attendance policy or connecting tardiness to the course grade.

It is important for instructors to understand the rights of students and to realize that they have the right to make choices about their education. Instructors should also be aware of institutional policies and definition as to what constitutes a class distraction and/or disruption and their responsibility to deal with students who cause them. Of course in an emergency service's academy setting, the instructor can set more stringent classroom behavior requirements due to the formal relationship with the students.

Arbitrary and Capricious Grading

Even with the best-written syllabus and clearly defined grading criteria for a course or assignment, a student may take exception to a grade he or she receives, often accusing the instructor of being unfair, or worse, malicious in assigning the grade. Ideally, the student calmly meeting with the instructor can settle such disputes. However, situations may arise where the student and instructor meet an impasse and the student feels compelled to take his or her concern to the next level, usually the program director or department chair. Students have the perception that the director or chair can overturn or change a grade assigned by the instructor, which in many institutions is not the case. The basic principle in play is that the instructor is the sole master of the classroom in academic matters, the idea of academic freedom being the basis. What the program director can do is to serve as a mediator between the student and the instructor. If mediation fails, institutions usually have in place a policy for adjudication of such disputes, especially if the charge is arbitrary or capricious grading on the part of the instructor.

To prevent such disputes, it is important for the instructor to grade all assignments fairly and equally and to follow exactly any grading parameters or criteria listed in the syllabus. The use of a grading rubric which clearly shows the criteria, weight, and value of each component of an assignment or critical facts or concepts in written assignments, will go a long way to prevent allegations of unfair grading, as well as providing the student with a detailed analysis of his or her grade (**Figure 24.6**). A rubric is also useful when multiple sections of a course are offered and taught by different instructors such as in a "shadow program" for students with a varying work schedule.

Electronic Devices

Prohibiting students from using electronic devices in the classroom as learning aids remains controversial. Prohibitions against ringing cell phones and beeping pagers is an established and acceptable practice, but limiting the use of laptops and tablets presents a number of issues. An institution or program may have a policy on such usage, therefore negating this as an issue for the instructor. But for instructors who must make their own policy, it is important to keep in mind the reason for such prohibition. Often instructors limit usage because they do not want students playing games, watching movies, or using social media during class, feeling that it is more important for the student to be paying attention and listening to them. The question then becomes: is this about supporting student success or instructor ego? Remember, students have the right to make decisions about their success or failure in a class.

When making decisions about electronic devices, it is important to understand who the students are and what is "their" normal. Today's students live in a world integrated with electronic devices. Social communication

Student Presentation
Evaluation Form

Presenters: ________________ ________________ ________________

Your comments and suggestions are needed to improve the presenter's ability to speak in front of an audience. Please feel free to give honest feedback about the presentation.

Introduction -established "need to know" -defined objectives -outlined main points	Excellent ____ Good ____ Fair ____ Poor ____ Comments: ________________
Organization of program -flow in logical order	Excellent ____ Good ____ Fair ____ Poor ____ Comments: ________________
Knowledge -knowledge of subject matter -terminology, language, vocabulary	Excellent ____ Good ____ Fair ____ Poor ____ Comments: ________________
Teaching qualities -preparedness -effective use of time -personality, appearance, voice	Excellent ____ Good ____ Fair ____ Poor ____ Comments: ________________
Delivery -composure, eye contact -gestures, enthusiasm	Excellent ____ Good ____ Fair ____ Poor ____ Comments: ________________
Teaching Aids -effective use of teaching aids -equipment in working order	Excellent ____ Good ____ Fair ____ Poor ____ Comments: ________________
Conclusion -main points recapped -objectives accomplished	Excellent ____ Good ____ Fair ____ Poor ____ Comments: ________________
Overall presentation	Excellent ____ Good ____ Fair ____ Poor ____ Comments: ________________

Figure 24.6

Example of a grading rubric for a student presentation.

between individuals is as likely to be by text message as by face-to-face or telephone. Information is immediately available to them via the Internet and Web-enabled smartphones. According to the annual Beloit College Mindset List for 2014, most freshmen do not know how to write in cursive.[18] So given this demographic, is it good educational strategy to deny students the tools that have become an integral part of their daily lives? Perhaps what should be done is to educate students in the proper etiquette of using such devices. Even better would be designing educational activities to integrate the devices into the learning schema.

Instructor Evaluations

The instructor plays a central role in the teaching and learning dynamic. In the case of EMS education, an instructor evaluation is required by accrediting bodies and often by state regulatory agencies. This is especially true for educational programs that result in professional certification or licensure. In institutions of higher education, these evaluations serve a number of purposes, such as forming the basis for contract renewal, pay increase, tenure review, accountability, or union contract requirements.

Most evaluations follow an approved and standardized format and are conducted by a program director, chair, or dean based on personal observation, student evaluations, peer evaluations, and outcome criteria (**Figure 24.7**). They should also include a self-evaluation completed by the instructor.

For a proper instructor evaluation to occur, it is imperative that the purpose of the evaluation be clearly defined and stated and not be subject to instructor retaliation. Instructor evaluations fall into two broad but overlapping categories: evaluations done to evaluate and rate the performance of the instructor and instructor evaluations obtained for the purpose of improving the instructional experience. It may seem that both approaches ultimately accomplish the same objective, that is, to improve the learning experience, and they ultimately do, but for different reasons. Areas of evaluation should include classroom teaching components such as meeting class objectives, clarity of information delivery, class control and interaction, as well as availability to students, student advocacy, student counseling, exam development, lab planning and implementation, and others.

Using student evaluations of the instructor for performance evaluation is a reasonable approach given that the instructor's role is to assist students in meeting course objectives. However, such evaluations must be taken in the context of the course material, the instructional process, and the standards established by the instructor. The question to be constantly asked is whether the student evaluations reflect a true measure of the instructor's performance, or the personal feelings and biases of the students. A "hard" instructor may receive low ratings because of the high standards he or she has established for the class, even though he or she is doing an effective job of teaching. Likewise, the nature, motivation, and ability of the students must be considered in any performance evaluation. Often, instructors teach entry-level EMS courses to personnel who have other interests but are required to complete EMS training as part of the job training. Such students may express their frustration or lack of motivation through the instructor-evaluation process.

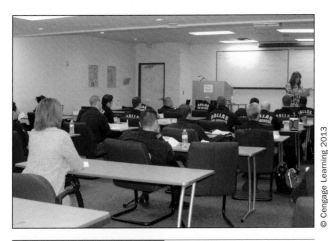

Figure 24.7

Most instructor evaluations follow an approved and standardized format, and are conducted by a program director, chair, or dean.

Regardless of the purpose or nature of the performance evaluation, the institution or agency should have in place support to assist instructional personnel. This applies not only to inadequate or marginal instructors, but to "good" instructors as well. In academic institutions a faculty development center or teaching laboratory can provide help in evaluating an instructor's classroom performance and in providing strategies for improvement. In smaller institutions money should be budgeted for faculty development.

The performance evaluation for one class or based on one observation is merely a snapshot in time of the instructor's performance. Everyone has good and bad days, and some topics and subjects are taught better than others. To provide a more complete picture of an instructor's performance, a more comprehensive tool, such as a teaching portfolio, is needed. The teaching portfolio provides an opportunity for the instructor to present his or her "teaching life" in a complete and organized manner. A teaching portfolio could contain the following items:

- List of all courses taught over a particular time
- Syllabi of past and present courses
- Past evaluations—both performance- and student-based
- Examples of innovative or creative teaching approaches or student-centered strategies developed by the instructor
- A statement of the instructor's teaching philosophy and what he or she expects to accomplish through the teaching
- The instructor's future plans related to instruction and teaching

More information on teaching portfolios can be obtained through the Center for Teaching and Learning (CETaL) at the University of Texas at El Paso (see http://www.utep.edu/cetal/).

When conducting a performance evaluation, the assessor should do the following:

- Use a standardized form that has been institutionally or agency approved.
- Provide a means for the instructor to acknowledge that the evaluation has occurred, most often by

signing the form. This acknowledges that the evaluation has taken place, but not that the instructor necessarily agrees with or accepts the findings of the evaluation.

- Provide a time for consultation with the instructor after the evaluation has been completed to discuss the findings and to identify strengths and weaknesses.
- Provide the instructor with a copy of the evaluation.
- Provide a means by which the instructor can refute evaluation findings in a formal manner. This is especially important when the evaluation has a direct effect on continued employment and promotion.
- Consider videotaping the instructor during the class in which the assessment is done as a means of recording instructor performance and minimizing subjectivity.

Formative Instructor Evaluations

If the instructor evaluation is to be a truly useful tool to drive improvement, consideration should be given to conducting interim evaluations during the course. This allows the instructor to receive feedback while there is still time to make changes to improve performance, and thus better assist students in meeting their objectives. A good time to give such evaluations is at midterm or after major modules in the course. Conducting such evaluations lets students know that the instructor values their input and is willing to make changes in their best interest. It also signals that the instructor is seeking constructive feedback. Depending on the course length, students may be given multiple opportunities to evaluate the instructor. Because such midcourse evaluations are often not "official," the instructor can tailor the evaluation to obtain the most feedback from students.

Summative Instructor Evaluations

This evaluation usually occurs at the end of the course and is often completed by course participants. End-of-course instructor evaluations are often mandated by institutions and accreditation bodies. Feedback to the instructor is provided so that he or she may recognize strengths and areas for improvement or change. Some institutions use a two-part evaluation consisting of a standardized form that may be machine-readable and a second form that contains open-ended questions. The open-ended form is designed exclusively for feedback given directly to the instructor; the machine-readable form is used to rank instructors on an institution-wide basis and may be used as a performance evaluation.

The common practice of gathering course evaluations from participants at the end of the course has positive and negative aspects. Positive aspects include the following:

- Convenience—participants are in class and have scheduled time to complete the evaluation.
- Response rates are high because the participants are in class.
- Students have the entire course perspective on which to base their evaluation.
- Evaluations given after final participant course evaluation and results are anonymous, so students have no fear of retaliation by the instructor.

However, some disadvantages to this approach should be considered, including the following:

- Participants may feel "forced" to complete an evaluation.
- If the evaluation is the last thing to be completed before the student leaves, especially with 1-day seminars, the participant may rush through the evaluation and not give it much thought.
- Any positive feedback given to the instructor about the course is lost because the course has already been completed.
- The participant may be "motivated" or "pumped up" about the course, especially if it will result in a new certification with the expectation of being able to perform at a new level. This may cause the participant to have a positive bias toward the instructor and the course.
- The participant may focus unduly on a recent negative or positive event with the instructor instead of on the whole course experience.

Given the limitations of the traditional end-of-course evaluations, some instructors and institutions wait for a time after the course has been completed to send participants the final instructor evaluation. The main advantage to this approach is that students have had time to reflect on their educational experience and the instructor's ability to facilitate their learning. The downside is that return rates may be poor in that participants can self-select to respond. In addition, responses may be slanted toward those participants who feel strongly, either positively or negatively, about the instructor.

Summary

EMS educational program administration involves many facets. The program director must remain current on many issues, including national standards and curricula, national accreditation, national and state credentialing, and state standards and requirements for course oversight and administration. Local and institutional requirements must also be met so the integrity of the program can be maintained and the institution and its employees protected. Administrators should work towards the goals of increased innovation, decreased duplication, enhanced quality, and better use of resources.[19] Attention to administrative matters is essential for safeguarding the reputation of the program and its faculty and for raising the professional standards of EMS. Beyond the legal and ethical considerations, doing so will enhance the quality of the program, abate risk, and protect the public.

References

1. National Highway Traffic Safety Administration (1996). *Emergency Medical Services agenda for the future.* Washington, DC: U.S. Department of Transportation.
2. National Highway Traffic Safety Administration. (2000). *Emergency Medical Services Education Agenda for the Future: A Systems Approach.* (DOT HS 809 042). Washington, DC: U.S. Department of Health and Human Services.
3. National Highway Traffic Safety Administration. (2005). *National EMS Core Content.* (DOT HS 809 898). Washington, DC: U.S. Department of Transportation.
4. National Highway Traffic Safety Administration (2007). *National EMS scope of practice model.* Washington, DC: U.S. Department of Transportation.
5. National Highway Traffic Safety Administration (2009). *National EMS education standards.* (DOT HS 811 077A). Washington. DC: U.S. Department of Transportation.
6. National Association of EMS Officials. (2009, July 17, 2009). 2009 National EMS Education Standards Gap Analysis Template. *Implementation of the national EMS Education Agenda Web Site.* Retrieved 03/23/2012, from http://www.nasemso.org/EMSEducationImplementationPlanning/Toolkit.asp
7. Commission on Accreditation on Allied Health Educational Programs, Policies and Procedures (2011, September). Website. Retrieved 03/26/1, from http://www.caahep.org/documents/file/PolicyManual.pdf
8. Continuing Education Board for Emergency Medical Services. (2012). Explanation of CECBEMS Approval Process Retrieved 03/23/2012, from http://www.cecbems.org/applications/approvalProcess.aspx
9. Haidinyak, G., & Walker, G. C. (2005). Don't let the grievance process cause grief. *Nurse Educator, 30*(2): 73–75.
10. Gagne, R. M., & Briggs, L. J. (1979). Principles of instructional design, (2nd ed.). Fort Worth, TX: Harcourt, Brace, Jovanovich.
11. Boyle, P. G. (1981). *Planning better programs: The adult education association professional development series.* New York, NY: McGraw-Hill.
12. Berg, J. G. (2010, November 8). Getting down to business with a business plan. *Nursing Spectrum (Illinois),* 26–31.
13. Williams, K. M., Nathanson, C., & Paulhus, D. L. (2010). Identifying and profiling scholastic cheaters: their personality, cognitive ability, and motivation. *Journal of Experimental Psychology: Applied, 16*(3), 293–307.
14. Eastham, J. N., & Zietlow, V. (2008, July 8). *Will cheating kill EMS online education?* http://www.emsworld.com.
15. Callahan, D. (2004). The cheating culture: Why more Americans are doing wrong to get ahead. Orlando, FL: Harcourt.
16. *Lowell Sun* (2011). Former Massachusetts firefighter guilty in EMT fraud. *JEMS.com, June 10.*
17. Reprinted from University of Texas Southwestern Medical Center, Southwestern School of Health Professions.
18. Beloit College. (2014). The Beloit College mindset list for the class of 2014. *The Mindset List* Retrieved 3/23, 2012, from http://www.beloit.edu/mindset/2014/
19. Youngberg, B. J., & Weber, D. R. (1998). Integrating risk management, utilization management, and quality management: Maximizing benefit through integration. Chapter 4. In B. J. Youngberg (Ed.), *The risk manager's desk reference.* Gaithersburg, MD: Aspen Publishers: 27–42.

Additional Resources

Abruzzese, R. S. (1992). Evaluation in nursing staff development. In R. S. Abruzzese (Ed.), *Nursing staff development: Strategies for success.* St. Louis: Mosby-Year Book: 235–248.

Alexander, M. (2006). *Foundations for the practice of EMS education.* Upper Saddle River, NJ: Pearson Prentice Hall: 168–171.

Bastable, S. B., Gramet, P., Jacobs, K., & Sopczyk, D. L. (2011). Health professional as educator: Principles of teaching and learning. Sudbury, MA: Jones & Bartlett.

Bloom, B., Madaus, G., & Hastings, J. T. (1981). Evaluation to improve learning. New York, NY: McGraw-Hill.

Board of Regents of State Colleges v. Roth, 408 U.S. 564 (1972).

Gushee, M. (2009, January 9). Student discipline policies. ERIC Clearinghouse on Educational Management: *ERIC Digest*, No. 12. http://www.ericdigests.org/pre-922/policies.htm.

Nichols, J. O., & Nichols, K. W. (2000). The departmental guide and record book for student outcomes assessment and institutional effectiveness, (3rd ed.). New York, NY: Agathon Press.

Page, J. O. (2004). Discipline with due process. In J. Fitch, (Ed.), *Prehospital care administration* (2nd ed.). San Diego, CA: JEMS Communications/Elsevier: 73–82.

Stepien, W., Gallagher, S. A., & Association for Supervision and Curriculum Development (1997). *Problem-based learning across the curriculum: An ASCD professional inquiry kit.* Alexandria, VA: Association for Supervision and Curriculum Development.

Suver, J. D., Neumann, B. R., & Boles, K. E. (1995). Management accounting for health care organizations, (4th ed.). Santa Monica, CA: Bonus Books.

University of California. (2008, October 20, rev.), 100.00 Policy on student conduct and discipline. http://www.ucop.edu/ucophome/coordrev/ucpolicies/aos/uc100.html.

Vaughan v. State, 456 S.W.2d 879, 833 (1970).

Wiggins, G., & McTighe, J. (2005). Understanding by design (expanded 2nd ed.). Alexandria, VA: Association for Supervision and Curriculum Development.

Williams, K. M., Nathanson, C., & Paulhus, D. L. (2010). Identifying and profiling scholastic cheaters: Their personality, cognitive ability, and motivation. *Journal of Experimental Psychology: Applied, 16*(3).

Zoll Data Systems (2006). Defining KPIs to maximize business performance. KPI White Paper.

APPENDIX A

Field Shift Evaluation Worksheet

FIELD SHIFT EVALUATION WORKSHEET

STUDENT NAME　　DATE　　EDUCATIONAL PROGRAM　　CLINICAL SITE:

Page ___ of ____　　TIME IN:　　OUT:　　PRECEPTOR:　　UNIT or STATION:

DIRECTIONS: Each contact must be rated by the student FIRST, and rated by the preceptor SECOND. Mark student ratings in the row marked "S" and preceptors in row "P". Comment on any discrepancies on back. Preceptors complete shaded sections.

RATINGS*: **NA** = Not Applicable; not needed/expected **0** - Unsuccessful -required excessive or critical prompting; includes rating of "not attempted" when student was expected to try; **1**- Marginal - inconsistent - Not yet competent; **2** - Successful/Competent no prompting.

Patient Age Gender	Impression and/or Differential Diagnoses	LOC, Complaints, Event/Circumstances	Summary of Treatments Rendered successfully by student	Circle Patient Contact Type	Rater	Clinical Objectives: Pt. Interview + HX gathering	Physical Exam	Field Impression Tx Plan	Skill Performance	Communication	Professional Behavior (Affect)	Team Leadership	Preceptor Initials	COMMENTS and IMMEDIATE PLAN FOR IMPROVEMENT FOR NEXT CONTACT
1.				ALS	S									
				BLS	P									
2.				ALS	S									
				BLS	P									
3.				ALS	S									
				BLS	P									
4.				ALS	S									
				BLS	P									
5.				ALS	S									
				BLS	P									
6.				ALS	S									
				BLS	P									
7.				ALS	S									
				BLS	P									

Comment on any unsatisfactory ratings or discrepancies:

Overall plan for improvement for future shifts:

Student reported ❑ on time, ❑ well groomed, ❑ in uniform and prepared to begin their shift. Yes ❑ No ❑	Student knows equipment location and use. Yes ❑ No ❑
Behavior was professional: ❑ Accepts feedback openly ❑ Self Motivated; ❑ Efficient; ❑ Flexible; ❑ Careful; ❑ Confident	Student helps clean-up and restock, unprompted. Yes ❑ No ❑
Student asked relevant questions and participated in learning answers, used "downtime" to its highest potential. Yes ❑ No ❑	Student left site early (did not complete shift). Yes ❑ No ❑

Preceptor would appreciate a ❑ **phone call** or ❑ **email** from the instructor (please provide contact info below). Yes ❑ No ❑

STUDENT SIGNATURE	I agree to the above ratings: Preceptor SIGNATURE

Clinical Objectives:

Pt. Interview HX Gathering: Student completes an appropriate interview and gathers appropriate history. Listens actively, makes eye contact, clarifies complaints, and respectfully addresses patient(s). Demonstrates compassionate and/or firm "bedside" manner depending on the needs of the situation.

Physical Exam: Student completes an appropriate focused physical exam specific to the chief complaint and/or comprehensive head-to-toe physical examination.

Communication: Student communicates effectively with team, provides an adequate verbal report to other health care providers, and completes a thorough written patient narrative.

Field Impression + TX plan: Student formulates an impression and implements an appropriate treatment plan.

Professional Behavior Objectives: The student demonstrates they are

- **Self motivated**: Includes taking initiative to complete assignments, improve/correct problems. Striving for excellence. Incorporating feedback and adjusting behavior/performance.
- **Efficient**: Includes keeping assessment and treatment times to a minimum, releasing other personnel (first responders) when not needed, organizing team to work faster/better.
- **Flexible**: Includes making adjustments to communication style, or directing team members; changing impressions based on findings;
- **Careful**: Includes paying attention to details of skills, documentation, patient comfort, set-up and clean up; Completing tasks thoroughly.
- **Confident**: Includes making decisions, trusting and exercising good personal judgment, being aware of limitations and strengths;
- **Accepts feedback openly**: Includes listening to preceptor and accepts constructive feedback without being defensive (interrupting, giving excuses).

Team Leadership Objective: The student has successfully led the team if he or she has *conducted a comprehensive assessment* (not necessary performed the entire interview or physical exam, but rather been in charge-of the assessment), as well as *formulated and implemented a treatment plan* for the patient. This means that *most* (if not all) of the *decisions* have been made by the student, especially formulating a field impression, directing the treatment, determining patient acuity, disposition and packaging and moving the patient (if applicable). Minimal to no prompting was needed by the preceptor. No action was initiated/performed that endangered the physical or psychological safety of the patient, bystanders, first responders or crew. (Preceptors should not agree to a "successful" rating unless it is truly deserved. As a general rule, more unsuccessful attempts indicate willingness to try and are better than no attempt at all.)

Ratings: **NA** = Not Applicable; not needed/expected – This is a neutral rating. (Example: Student expected to only observe, or the patient did not need intervention) **0** - Unsuccessful -required excessive or critical prompting; includes rating of "not attempted" when student was expected to try; This is an unsatisfactory rating; **1**- Marginal - inconsistent - Not yet competent; This includes partial attempts. **2** - Successful/Competent no prompting; ***NOTE: Ideally, students will progress their role from observation to participation in simple skills, to more complex assessments and team leadership. Students will progress at different rates and case difficulty will vary. Students should be active and ATTEMPT to perform skills, assess/treat patients and lead encounters early-on even if this results in frequent prompting and unsuccessful ratings. Unsuccessful ratings are <u>normal and expected</u> in the early stages of the clinical learning process when student needs prompting. Improvement plans MUST follow any unsuccessful or inconsistent ratings.**

Courtesy of NREMT Paramedic Psychomotor Competency Portfolio

Glossary

360-degree evaluation Feedback that utilizes many sources of evaluation, including peers.

ABCD model A model to write objectives in which the audience, behaviors, conditions, and degree required to achieve the objective are clearly defined.

active behavior The student is actively thinking or doing something to learn.

affective domain Learning in terms of feelings, emotions, attitudes, and values.

affiliation agreements An agreement between the academic or educational institution and a clinical facility.

analysis The cognitive domain level that requires separation of whole concepts into individual, smaller parts to analyze their meaning and understand their importance.

analytic thinking Processing information in a logical, sequential manner.

andragogy The art and science of teaching adults.

Angoff method A way to predict item difficulty.

application The cognitive domain level that relates classroom information to real-life situations.

archetypal pattern recognition Traits, behavior, or symbolic pattern recognition.

articulation The fourth stage of psychomotor skill development is to blend the skill with the cognitive and affective dimensions of a skill or procedure so that the learner understands the "whys" and "whens." The psychomotor domain level that occurs when proficient and competent performance of the skill, with personal style or flair occurs.

"ask, pause, and call" technique A questioning technique where the instructor waits for a longer time—up to 30 seconds—before allowing a student to answer a posed question.

assault Occurs when one person places another person in reasonable fear of immediate harm or physical contact.

asynchronous learning Independent learning without the need to be on line at the same time.

attribution The root cause(s) of the student's performance deficiency.

audience response systems An electronic tallying system whereby the instructor receives feedback from the audience or class to specific, posed questions. Also called "classroom feedback," "personal response systems," or "clickers."

audio Sound.

audio mixer A device that blends sounds from multiple devices that are connected to a single amplifier and set of speakers.

audio visual (AV) Tools or techniques other than lecture used to supplement learning.

auditory learning Learning through sounds.

autonomy Independence.

battery A physical, unlawful touching of another person without consent.

bias Unreasonable judgment.

Bloom's Taxonomy A description of the domains of learning developed by Dr. Benjamin Bloom.

blueprinting Planning the exam to facilitate validity with appropriate level of required thinking, content depth, and breadth.

case study An analysis of a real-life patient situation as a way of illustrating information.

categorization of the value The student organizes his or her own values that have characteristics in common into a relationship or hierarchy that has characteristics common to based on what has been learned in class, through skill demonstrations, and during personal experiences, as well as through the influence of those the student holds in esteem.

characterizing The affective domain level that requires development of one's own value system that governs behavior.

charlatan Persons who claim knowledge or skill that they do not possess.

chat rooms A synchronous electronic communication system that resembles actual real-time conversations. Log-on is required to access; all members of the group can view the content.

classroom feedback systems See definition for audience response systems.

clinical coordinator Schedules and tracks hospital and other clinical training rotations.

cognitive domain Learning that takes place through the process of thinking; it deals with facts and knowledge.

collaborative learning A group learning activity.

command response A requirement of the student.

composure Has to do with how the learner reacts; maintaining a sense of calm under stress.

comprehension The cognitive domain level that focuses on interpretation and understanding meaning.

computer-adaptive testing Allows the use of a more precise tool that is able to adjust the difficulty of items for the candidate based on the candidate's responses.

conceptualization of the value The student identifies the basic concepts of the new value as characteristics that are common to any one value already held.

constitutional protections The U.S. Constitution prohibits any level of government from violating constitutional rights. Congress has enacted a law, 42 U.S.C.A. § 1983, that allows persons to sue a governmental actor who violates their constitutional rights. EMS educational institutions and instructors may be considered governmental actors if they receive government funding or are contracted by the government.

content validity The extent to which exam items accurately represent the wider body of knowledge being tested.

context-based learning (situated cognition) A learning strategy that places the lesson within the actual situation in which it will be used.

convergent questions Seek specific information.

cooperative learning A group learning activity where the students are jointly responsible for learning outcomes.

copyright protection Protection afforded to original works of authorship fixed in any tangible medium of expression.

criterion validity Predictive validity; the ability of an exam to predict performance under other conditions.

critical thinking As described by John Dewey: ". . . the active, persistent, and careful consideration of a belief or supposed form of knowledge in light of the grounds which support it and the further conclusions to which it tends." Higher level cognitive skills, or problem solving skills.

Cronbach's alpha A statistical method to assess internal consistency.

cultural competency Awareness of beliefs and customs of cultures.

culture Amalgamation of customs, experiences, languages, and beliefs common to a defined group.

debate Structured controversy.

debriefing A postevent discussion and evaluation.

defamation The sharing of true but private information that injures the reputation of another, or the intentional or reckless making of a false statement. There are two types of defamation: libel and slander.

digital The manner in which information is stored in electronic devices such as computers.

digital projector A device that displays and projects computer images onto a screen.

discussion board A tool to use to communicate with a predetermined group; it is similar to e-mail but is stored and accessed through a Learning Management System.

distance education A system of education whereby students and teachers are separated by time and distance.

distractor An incorrect answer designed to be a plausible alternative to the correct answer.

divergent questions Do not have a single right answer.

domains of learning Categories of learning that include cognitive, affective and psychomotor.

evaluation The cognitive domain level where mastery of cognitive concepts is achieved to allow judgments and decisions about information.

experiential learning An active learning process that engages all senses; learning by doing; this type of learnig occurs when knowledge and skills are acquired in a relevant setting.

face validity Common sense validity; appears to be evaluating what it is intended to evaluate.

facilitation Assisting a learner in discovering information or abilities for him or herself; to make easier.

FERPA Family Education Rights & Privacy Act of 1974 that prohibits release of a student's personally identifiable information except under certain circumstances.

field coordinator Schedules and tracks field EMS rotations.

formative evaluation The ongoing evaluation of student performance throughout a course.

forming stage Team members encounter one another for the first time, attempt to define the task assigned to them, and start to determine the future course.

fraud Misrepresentation, or the making of a false statement with intent to deceive, that causes actual harm to someone who reasonably relies upon it.

global thinking Processing information by seeing the whole before the parts.

goal A broad statement of instructional intent.

grievance A wrong considered as grounds for a complaint and potential lawsuit.

high-fidelity manikins Use of sophisticated technology to simulate realistic human physiology such as oxygen/carbon dioxide exchange.

high-stakes evaluation One in which the student's continuation in the program depends on successful completion of the exam.

higher order thinking Has to do with Bloom's higher cognitive levels to include analysis, synthesis, and evaluation; critical thinking, problem solving.

HIPAA The Health Insurance Portability and Accountability Act, which protects the medical privacy of patients.

imitation The first phase of psychomotor skill development that occurs as a student repeats and mimics a skill demonstrated by an expert.

independent learning labs (learning resource center) An area with technology and various resources available to students to help them acquire cognitive, affective, and psychomotor skills.

independent thinking Processing information alone.

instructional technology The software and hardware used to create and transmit audiovisual materials.

interactive whiteboard Electronic whiteboard that provides a multipage drawing application.

inter-rater reliability Consistency among evaluators or evaluation methods.

item-response theory The computer adjusts the difficulty of items for each candidate using an algorithm that is based on the candidate's responses.

kinesthetic learning Learning through touch.

knowledge The cognitive domain level that focuses on memorization and recall.

Kolb theory Describes two ways that learners can transform experience into knowledge—reflective observation and active experimentation.

Kuder-Richardson A statistical formula to evaluate internal consistency.

laser pointer Handheld device to visually highlight key points during a presentation.

learning contract A document mutually agreed to by the student and faculty that defines activities and behaviors that must be met in a specified time frame to achieve specific objectives.

learning management system (LMS) Computer software that facilitates the creation of online course work in a World Wide Web–based educational environment.

learning style A preferred method of learning.

lecture A teaching session in which the instructor is the principal teacher.

lecturer Content expert who presents selected didactic material.

low-stakes evaluation Has relatively little effect on whether a student passes a course.

manipulation The second phase of psychomotor skill development that occurs as a student practices a skill and begins to create his or her own method or style of skill manipulation.

Maslow's Hierarchy of Needs A theory that identifies an incremental series of human needs. Individuals must satisfy the lower level needs to achieve the higher levels.

mastery Achieving goals and objectives established for a specific skill or knowledge area.

mentor An experienced person guiding a less experienced person toward a goal.

metacognition simply put, thinking about thinking; literally, "in the midst of knowing"; an awareness and control of one's thinking.

misrepresentation Fraud, or the making of a false statement with intent to deceive, that causes actual harm to someone who reasonably relies upon it.

mnemonics Using patterns to assist in recall.

MP3 players Digital device that stores and plays back sounds and videos.

multiple intelligences The theory that different students have different levels of intelligence in various areas.

naturalization The fifth level of psychomotor skill development where the skill becomes a habit and is performed flawlessly without much conscious effort; the level of psychomotor skill that represents mastery.

negligent referral The inappropriate recommendation of an individual that misrepresents qualifications or character.

norming stage Team establishes and maintains ground rules.

objective A specific, measurable learning outcome.

organizing The affective domain level where the learner integrates new, refined, or different beliefs into their existing value system.

passive behavior The student is not engaged or active but only receives information or ideas.

pedagogical features Features of a book designed to enhance student understanding.

pedagogy The art and science of teaching children.

performance agreement Concordance of goals, objectives, content, and evaluation tools.

performing stage Team develops the ability to work through group problems, and results begin to occur.

philosophy of education A personal statement that reflects the educator's beliefs and attitudes about their approach to education.

pitch of lecture delivery The lecture language is commensurate to the students' level of learning.

podcast A digital audio recording that can be downloaded from a computer.

power Control.

practical lab instructors Persons who teach in laboratory settings.

preceptor Practicing paramedics or health professionals who instruct EMS students in hospital or field clinical setting.

precision The third level of psychomotor skill development where the skill is practiced without mistakes in a controlled environment without distraction or variation.

primary (lead) instructor A person who is qualified to provide leadership or supervision over a series of courses or entire EMS program.

problem-based learning (PBL) An instructional method by which the instructor creates a complex, well-structured problem that a group of students tries to solve.

problem-centered learning Learning placed in the context of a real-life situation. It requires application of knowledge from many subjects.

program coordinator Educator responsible for program logistics.

program director Assumes overall program responsibility.

program medical director The physician responsible for medical oversight of the program and assuring terminal competency through monitoring testing and program evaluation.

psychomotor domain Learning that takes place through the attainment of skills and bodily, or kinesthetic, movements.

qualitative Non-numerical observations that show underlying dimensions or patterns of relationships.

quantitative A measurement or information based on quantity or numbers.

receiving The affective domain level that occurs as the student acquires awareness of the value or importance of learning information and expresses a willingness to learn.

reliability Consistency.

remediation The process to analyze and identify performance deficiencies and develop a plan to improve that performance.

responding The affective domain level where the student actively participates in the learning process and begins to derive satisfaction from it.

risk management The process of preventing, or at least minimizing, harm or loss to a business, organization, or person.

role playing A group process that involves students in a dramatization.

rubric An evaluation tool that defines criteria for each degree of expected performance when there are multiple facets to the evaluation; a measurement tool that establishes a framework for evaluation.

safe classroom An environment in which the student feels little risk of emotional harm while actively participating in learning activities.

satisfaction response A voluntary response that brings on a sense of self-esteem.

scenarios An outline or plot of a patient situation or projected sequence of patient events.

scholarship High standards and/or quality of academic achievement.

screencasts An audio and video screen recording.

self-directed learning Learning without instructor presence.

sensory acuity Ability to perceive fine detail.

simulation A type of experiential learning designed to mimic, as closely as possible, the real context.

smartphones A mobile telephone with capability to perform other computing and imaging functions such as retrieve e-mail and take photographs.

social thinking Processing information effectively while multi-tasking in a group setting.

Socratic method A method of questioning that uses the practice of asking, rather than telling, to arouse curiosity in the subject matter so students will arrive at their own conclusions rather than being told the "right" answer.

spatial awareness Awareness of the location of one's extremities in relation to their body and the environment.

split-half A test of internal consistency that divides the exam into halves (commonly odd and even questions), then compares the percentages of correct answers between the two groups of items.

standardized patient A prepared actor who simulates a patient.

stem The part of the item that is first offered, which may be written as a question or as an incomplete statement.

storming stage Team members jockey for position as they struggle to define the team's leadership.

student-centered instruction/learning Puts the learner at the center of the educational event and incorporates innovative, active teaching strategies such as group work, case studies, role playing, writing assignments, and so on.

student evaluation The process of assessing whether a student has successfully acquired knowledge, skills, and attitudes.

summative evaluation Given to students at the end of a course or unit of learning.

syllogism A type of argument in logic that contains a major and minor premise and a conclusion.

synchronous teaching and learning Students are in different locations, but meet online at a prescheduled time to participate in real-time discussion with the instructor.

synthesis The cognitive domain level that combines pieces of information into new and different whole ideas.

T.H.I.N.K. A model or system; a mnemonic used for a model to teach critical thinking skills which stands for "T" - total recall, "H"- habits, "I" - inquiry, "N" - new ideas and creativity, and "K" - knowing how you think.

tablet computers A compact, handheld, wireless computer device.

tactile stimulation Activation of the sensation of touch, texture, temperature, and other touch sensations.

targeted internship experience A focused area of clinical experience (hospital or field) through which learning is enhanced or remediated.

task analysis Provides a comprehensive list of the steps to be performed for a skill or process.

teacher-centered instruction/learning Instruction that focuses on the teacher and thus, primarily, the lecture format.

template A standardized form that can provide a framework for scenarios.

Theory of Margins A model that examines the relationship between power (ability) and load (demands on learner).

thinking style The method by which an individual prefers to make decisions.

tort A private or civil wrong or injury, other than a breach of contract, for which the law allows a remedy.

transformational learning A learning theory centered around creating change in perception and thought.

validity Measuring the knowledge or skills that is intended to evaluate for a specific purpose; relevance.

valuing The affective domain level in which the student perceives that a behavior has worth or value.

visual learning Learning through imagery.

wait time A concept in questioning techniques that gives time to students to think about questions posed to them and to ponder their response.

whole-part-whole instruction A teaching technique that first provides the big picture, then breaks it into separate parts and steps, then completes the technique with another overview of the big picture.

wiki A content-management system where each member of a group can collaborate to develop, design, edit, compile, and produce coursework.

willing response The student agrees to respond from something inside the student.

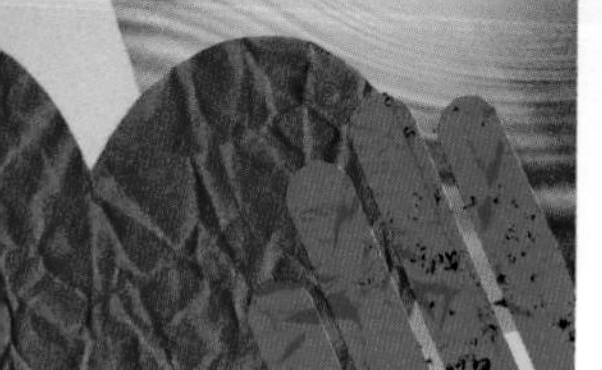

INDEX

Information in figures and tables is indicated by *f* and *t*.

A

B

C

D

E

F

G

H

I

J

K

L

M

N

O

P

Q

R

Z